Breast Cancer: New Horizons in Research and Treatment

Breast Cancer: New Horizons in Research and Treatment

Edited by

Jeffrey S Tobias MD, FRCP, FRCR
Consultant in Clinical Oncology, University College
London and The Middlesex Hospital, London, UK

Joan Houghton BSc
Director, Cancer Research Campaign and University
College London Trials Centre, Royal Free and University
College London Medical School, London, UK

I Craig Henderson MD, FACP, FRCP (Edin)
Adjunct Professor of Medicine, University of California,
San Francisco, California, USA

A member of the Hodder Headline Group
LONDON
Co-published in the United States of America by
Oxford University Press Inc., New York

First published in Great Britain in 2001 by
Arnold, a member of the Hodder Headline Group,
338 Euston Road, London NW1 3BH

http://www.arnoldpublishers.com

Co-published in the United States of America by
Oxford University Press Inc.,
198 Madison Avenue, New York, NY10016
Oxford is a registered trademark of Oxford University Press

© 2001 Arnold

British Library Cataloguing in Publication Data
A catalogue record for this book is available from the British Library

Library of Congress Cataloging-in-Publication Data
A catalog record for this book is available from the Library of Congress

ISBN 0 340 74216 X (hb)

1 2 3 4 5 6 7 8 9 10

Commissioning Editor: Joanna Koster
Project Editor: Sarah de Souza
Production Editor: Rada Radojicic
Production Controller: Fiona Byrne

Typeset in 10/12 Minion by Saxon Graphics Ltd, Derby
Printed and bound in Great Britain by The Bath Press, Bath

What do you think about this book? Or any other Arnold title?
Please send your comments to feedback.arnold@hodder.co.uk

Contents

Contributors

Ingvar Andersson MD, PhD
Chairman of Radiology, Department of Diagnostic Radiology, Malmö University Hospital, Malmö, Sweden

I Basnett HBBS, MSc, EFPHM
Deputy Director of Public Health, Camden and Islington Health Authority, and Honorary Senior Lecturer, London School of Hygiene and Tropical Medicine, London, UK

Michael Baum ChM, FRCS, FRCR
Professor of Surgery, Department of Surgery, Royal Free and University College Medical School, London, UK

John R Benson MA(Oxon), DM FRCS (Eng), FRCS (Ed)
Senior Surgical Registrar and Honorary Lecturer, Chelsea and Westminster Hospital, London and Imperial College School of Medicine, London, UK

Valerie Beral FRCP, F MedSci
Professor of Epidemiology, Imperial Cancer Research Fund and Cancer Epidemiology Unit, The Radcliffe Infirmary, Oxford, UK

Gianni Bonadonna MD, FRCP
Director, Division of Medical Oncology, Instituto Nazionale Tumori, Milan, Italy

Susan A Brooks PhD
Senior Lecturer in Cell Biology, School of Biological and Molecular Sciences, Oxford Brookes University, Headington, Oxford, UK

J Bunker
Visiting Professor, Cancer Research Campaign and University College London Trials Centre, University College London Medical School, London, UK

Alan Coates MD (Melb), FRACP, AStat
Chief Executive Officer, Australian Cancer Society, Sydney, New South Wales, Australia

Jack Cuzick PhD
Head, Department of Mathematics, Statistics and Epidemiology, Imperial Cancer Research Fund, London, UK

Roger Dansey MD
Associate Professor of Medicine, Barbara Ann Karmanos Cancer Institute/Wayne State University, Detroit, Michigan, USA

Tim Davidson ChM MRCP FRCS
Consultant General and Breast Surgeon, University Department of Surgery, Royal Free Hospital, London, UK

David DeFriend MD, FRCS
Consultant Surgeon, Department of General Surgery, Torbay Hospital, Torquay, UK

D Gareth R Evans MD, FRCP
Consultant in Medical Genetics, St Mary's Hospital, Manchester, UK

Giuseppe Giaccone MD, PhD
Deputy Head, Division of Medical Oncology, Academic Hospital Vrije Universiteit, Amsterdam, The Netherlands

Roberto Grilli MD
Head, Unit of Clinical Policy Analysis, Laboratory of Health Services Research, Mario Negri Institute, Milan, Italy

I Craig Henderson MD, FACP, FRCP (Edin)
Adjunct Professor of Medicine, University of California, San Francisco, California, USA

Carol Hermon MSc
Chief Scientific Officer, Imperial Cancer Research Fund Cancer Epidemiology Unit, The Radcliffe Infirmary, Oxford, UK

Joan Houghton BSc
Assistant Director, Cancer Research Campaign and University College London Trials Centre, University College London Medical School, London, UK

Anthony Howell FRCP
Professor in Medical Oncology, Department of Medical Oncology, Christie Hospital NHS Trust, Manchester, UK

Anthony Leathem MB ChB, MD
Senior Lecturer in Surgery, Department of Surgery, University College London, London, UK

Alessandro Liberati MD
Head, Laboratory of Health Services Research, Mario Negri Institute, Milan, Italy

Richard R Love MD
Professor of Medicine and Family Medicine, Madison, Wisconsin, USA

Richard G Margolese MD, FRCS
Director, Department of Oncology, Jewish General Hospital, and Herbert Black Professor of Surgery, McGill University, Montreal, Quebec, Canada

CK Osborne MD
Department of Medical Oncology, Christie Hospital National Health Service Trust, Manchester, UK

William P Peters MD, PhD
President, Director and CEO, Barbara Ann Karmanos Cancer Institute, Detroit, Michigan, USA

Herbert M Pinedo MD, PhD
Head, Division of Medical Oncology, Academic Hospital Vrije Universiteit, Amsterdam, The Netherlands

Michael Pollak MD
Professor, Departments of Medicine and Oncology, McGill University, Montreal, Quebec, Canada

Peter M Ravdin MD, PhD
University of Texas Health Science Center, Department of Medicine/Medical Oncology, San Antonio, Texas, USA

Dianne L Riley
Cancer Research Campaign Clinical Trials Centre, King's College School of Medicine, London, UK

Stefan Rydén MD, PhD
Associate Professor, Consultant in Surgery, Department of Surgery, Angelholm Hospital, Angelholm, Sweden

Christobel Mary Saunders
Senior Lecturer/Honorary Consultant, Department of Surgery, Royal Free and University College Medical School, London, UK

Udo Schumacher
Professor of Anatomy, Universitäts-Krankenhaus-Eppendorf, Anatomisches Institut, Hamburg, Germany

Petr Skrabanek (deceased)
Department of Community Health, University of Dublin Trinity College, Dublin, Ireland

Stephen Sutton BA, MSc, PhD
Senior Scientist and Reader in Social/Health Psychology, Health Behaviour Unit, University College London, London, UK

Kathryn J Thirlaway
Research Psychologist, Cancer Research Campaign Psychosocial Oncology Group, Department of Oncology, University College London Medical School, Bland Sutton Institute, London, UK

Hazel Thornton
'Saionara', Rowhedge, Colchester, Essex, UK

Jeffrey S Tobias MD FRCP FRCR
Consultant in Clinical Oncology, University College London and The Middlesex Hospital, London, UK, and Chairman, CRC New Studies Think Tank for Breast Cancer

Pinuccia Valagussa
Chief, Operations Office, Instituto Nazionale Tumori, Milan, Italy

Cornelis JH Van der Velde MD
Surgeon Department of Surgery, Leiden University Medical Center, Leiden, The Netherlands

Jan Hein van Dierendonck PhD
Cell Biologist, Department of Surgery, Leiden University Medical Center, Leiden, The Netherlands

Henk-Jan van Slooten MD
Leiden University Medical Center, Department of Surgery, Leiden, The Netherlands

Foreword

My Mother died of metastatic breast cancer on my birthday (31 May), 25 years ago, in the year I embarked on my academic career as Senior Lecturer in the Department of Surgery at the University Hospital of Wales. I am writing this forward in the last week before I retire from my Chair of Surgery at University College London on my birthday, 31 May 2000. Seven years ago my Sister, the youngest of five siblings, was diagnosed with breast cancer, and is alive and well to this day. Although I am the last to rely on anecdotes in lieu of evidence, I believe that the extreme contrast in the experience between my mother and sister's case effectively bracket my professional life time's experience of the disease.

My mother Mary (God rest her soul) was the matriarch of a large orthodox Jewish family with extreme academic ambitions in the days before households were equipped with electrical appliances. Throughout the dark days of the second world war and the blitz, she selflessly brought up a family of five children, together with a variable number of waifs and strays displaced by the war or orphanhood. In those days the big 'C' was unmentionable and stigmatised; in fact to this day I am unaware of the cause of death of my maternal grandmother, although I have my suspicions. The first I knew of my mother's impending death was witnessing her climbing upstairs in the house, holding her back and dragging her foot. This image is clearly imprinted in my memory as it was on one of those rare visits to the family household by a young surgeon preoccupied by his professional development and impossible workload, together with his own family of three children under the age of seven. My mother dismissed my enquiries by claiming it was yet another bout of 'sciatica'. Ultimately the skeletal metastases from her breast cancer were diagnosed and her right breast was discovered to be replaced by malignant tissue. How long it had been there, whether she was aware of this or not because of her inherent modesty, will remain a mystery. Although treatment was palliative in intent, the toxic side effects of the chemotherapy at the time, haunt my memory. Worst of all from her point of view, was the complete loss of her beautiful raven locks. Her hair, always piled high in a complex chignon, was a constant source of pride, and her baldness inadequately covered by scarf, was a source of shame. Furthermore, and to my

lasting shame, I failed to challenge my Father's wish that my Mother should be denied knowledge of her diagnosis. Clearly she was no fool and must have known what was going on, because out of the four medical sons she had mothered, it was always me, the 'breast cancer specialist', that she came to for explanations. Inevitably the last few months of her life for me were spoilt by the charade we played – I knew that she knew, she knew that I knew that she knew, and yet never was I allowed to discuss her illness with her in an open fashion. She suffered very badly from the pain of skeletal metastases with the side effects of chemotherapy adding insult to injury, until eventually there came the time for the terrible decision to be made (doubly difficult according to the orthodox Jewish faith) with the recognition that adequate opiate analgesia would inevitably shorten her life by a few days. She died at the age of 67.

Twenty years later her youngest child, my sister, then in her 50th year, became aware of a 1 cm nodule in the upper central portion of her left breast. Prompt referral to a specialist and triple assessment by clinical examination, ultrasound scan and fine needle aspiration cytology, confirmed the early breast cancer. She underwent wide local excision and axillary lymph node clearance. The tumour was of intermediate grade, oestrogen and progesterone receptor positive, and axillary lymph node negative. Following surgery she had a radical course of radiotherapy to the breast and was maintained an adjuvant Tamoxifen for five years.

These two anecdotes, although of a very personal significance, strikingly demonstrate the progress that has been made in the sociology, understanding, diagnosis and management of carcinoma of the breast. Also, as I will demonstrate towards the end of the Forward, these narratives provide the necessary insights and directions for future progress.

My mother's generation was probably the last to treat the diagnosis of breast cancer as a taboo. Furthermore, she was probably of a generation and culture whose modesty resulted in a failure to detect or sufficient self-denial, that led to significant delays in the presentation with the disease. I am, of course, well known for my scepticism about the correlation between delay and outcome as far as survival is concerned, yet I have to believe that there is a significant minority where prompt diagnosis will lead to a prolongation of life that is above and beyond that of lead time bias. I also believe that diagnosis when the tumour is small and operable, provides a much better chance for local control with breast preservation. It is also possible that my mother would have stood an additional small chance of 'cure', had there been a mammographic screening programme around at the time.

Her symptom control during her terminal illness was very inadequate, and I can now take some pride in the British-led movement of palliative care and symptom control. These days she would not have suffered so terribly. At the same time, the chemotherapy contributed little to improvement in the quality of her life, and her alopecia was devastating. Sadly I have witnessed little improvement in this field of treatment over the last 25 years. As a pointer to the future, I must re-emphasise that the diagnosis of metastatic breast cancer today is still a death sentence. The chemotherapy is still cruel, and outside its use for specific symptom control it is still of questionable value for prolongation of life.

Coming now to my sister, with the sociological changes and breast cancer awareness, there were no delays in her diagnosis. She was the beneficiary of a one-stop clinic where triple assessment was performed, and a diagnosis established within a few hours. Her surgery was minimal but sufficient to achieve local clearance and pathological staging of the disease, allowing breast preservation and a good cosmetic result, with radiotherapy to the breast using modern tangential fields via a linear accelerator. Over this 25-year period the nature and function of steroid receptors have been worked out, and the immuno-histochemistry techniques have allowed prompt and accurate estimates of the steroid receptor characteristics of all breast cancers. Throughout the last 25 years many collaborative groups have organised themselves to recruit large numbers of patients in randomised controlled trials. This in itself is an achievement worthy of note, and since 1985 we have known with confidence the benefits of adjuvant Tamoxifen, witnessing at last the 30% relative reduction in breast cancer mortality in the population at large that would have been predicted from the results of the individual trials.[1]

I think it is fair to suggest that the results of adjuvant chemotherapy, and in particular high dose therapy, have been less good than predicted, whereas the results of adjuvant endocrine manipulation have been better than predicted. To me, this is indirect evidence to suggest that the non-specific cytocidal effects of chemotherapy are not the way to go, but what this subtle disease needs is the subtle approaches of specific biological therapies of which Tamoxifen and ovarian suppression are exemplars, more by chance than by design.

The final sign post for the future emerging from my family history concerns genetic predisposition. I suspect, although cannot confirm, that there have been three generations of women affected with breast cancer, in a family of Ashkenazi Jewish descent. If that is the case, then there is a significant probability of there being a germ line mutation in the BRCA1/BRCA2 domains. My sister has four daughters aged between 30 and 18. On balance of probabilities, therefore, one or two of them should have inherited the mutant gene if in fact it does exist. I therefore have a profound personal interest in the development of knowledge that will lead to the accurate prediction of genetic predisposition in parallel with the development of knowledge of techniques for monitoring or preventing the disease.

In conclusion therefore, I look upon this volume as an exercise in futurology. A serious reading of the text will demonstrate how we are indeed looking to the future of biological therapies and a better understanding of the genetic predisposition of breast cancer. I am sure my family is in no way unique, although I have the dubious privilege of having an exceptional insight into their problems. However, to make real progress it is necessary to learn from the lessons of the past that the major rate limiting factor for progress is received wisdom in place of an enquiring mind.

Michael Baum

REFERENCE

1   Early Breast Cancer Trialists' Collaborative Group. Tamoxifen for early breast cancer: an overview of the randomised trials. *Lancet* 1998; **351**: 1451–67.

From laboratory to clinic: breast cancer at the turn of the century

Trends in mortality from breast cancer

CAROL HERMON AND VALERIE BERAL

INTRODUCTION

Breast cancer mortality rates have generally been increasing over the past decades, but more recently rates have levelled off or started to decline in many western countries.[1] That conclusion was based largely on an analysis of trends for all ages combined. This paper describes trends in mortality for breast cancer considered separately for women aged 30–49, 50–69 and 70–79 years in 20 countries from 1950 to 1992.

METHODS

Breast cancer mortality data were obtained from the World Health Organization for 20 countries. Data were provided as age-specific numbers of deaths from breast cancer and as population data. Initially mortality rates were derived and age-standardized against the world standard[2] in eight 5-year calendar periods from 1950–1954 to 1985–1989 and the most recent period, 1990–1992 spanning a 3-year interval. Age-specific mortality rates were derived for three age groups, namely 30–49, 50–69 and 70–79 years. In addition, within each of these age groups the age-specific rates were standardized to ensure compatibility across time periods. Data were not examined for women aged under 30 years because of the rarity of the disease in that age group, or for those aged 80 years or above due to the possible non-reliability of death certification data.

RESULTS

Trends for all ages combined

The trends in age-standardized mortality rates are shown in Figure 1.1 for 20 countries, arranged in alphabetical order of country. Generally, breast cancer mortality rates had been increasing, but many countries now show stabilizing or declining rates (e.g. Australia, Canada and the UK).

Trends for women aged 30–49 years

There has been a clear decline in breast cancer mortality over the last 10 years in about one-third of the 20 countries for women aged 30–49 years (Figure 1.2) (e.g. Australia, Austria, Canada, Greece, Switzerland, UK and USA). The earliest and most striking decline in mortality occurred in Canada and the USA, beginning during the period 1965–1969 where previously rates were fairly constant. Mortality rates for Switzerland and the UK showed a decline 10 years later, beginning during the period 1975–1979. Four countries (Germany, Italy, Spain and Hungary) show a similar pattern of breast cancer mortality in that the rates have been increasing until very recently, and have not stabilized or slightly declined until the 1990s. In several countries (e.g. Belgium, Denmark, Finland and New Zealand), breast cancer rates have fluctuated although overall they have remained fairly constant, and this may be a reflection of the small populations of women in this age group. In none of the 20 countries examined (except perhaps Spain) was there clear evidence of a continuing increase in breast cancer mortality rates up to 1990–1992.

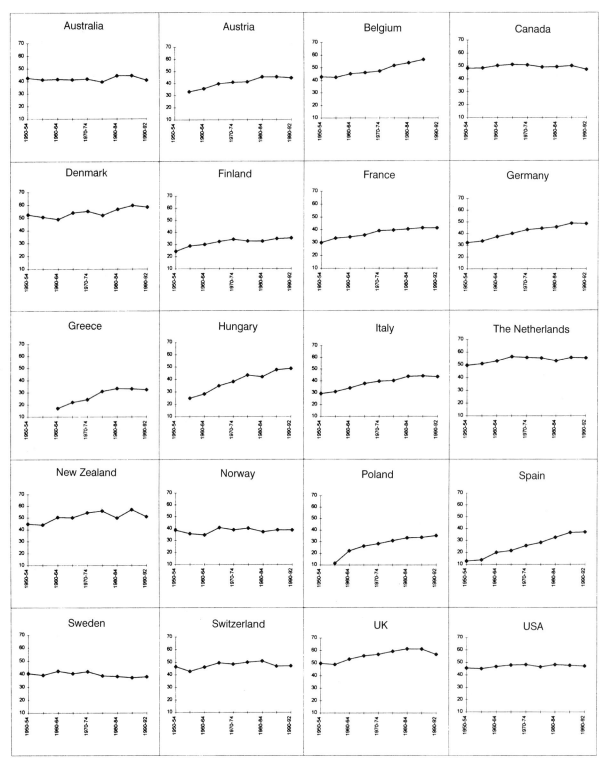

Figure 1.1 *Trends in age-standardized mortality rates per 100 000 women aged 30–79 years (standardized by age to the world standard population) from 1950–1954 to 1990–1992 in 20 countries in Europe, North America, Australia and New Zealand.*

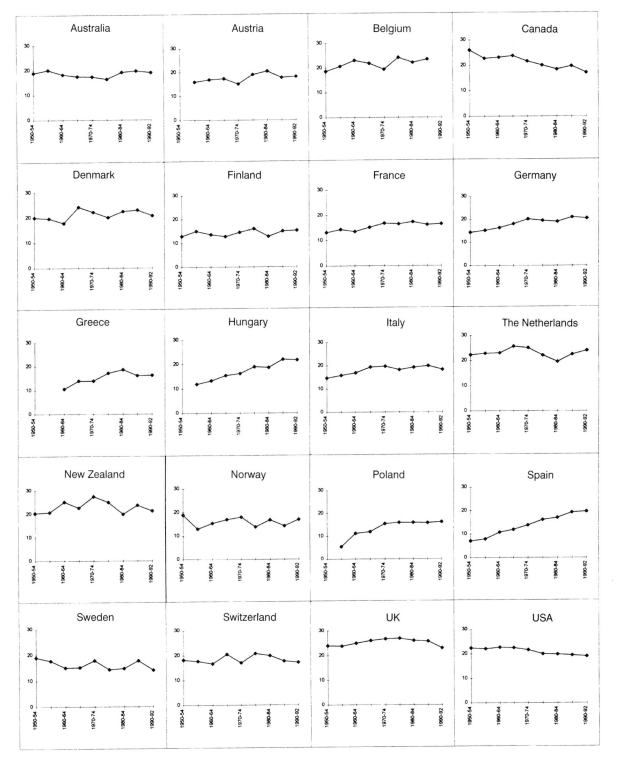

Figure 1.2 *Trends in age-specific mortality rates per 100 000 women aged 30–49 years from 1950–1954 to 1990–1992 in 20 countries in Europe, North America, Australia and New Zealand.*

Trends for women aged 50–69 years

Age-standardized rates for the 20 countries are shown in Figure 1.3. Only Belgium and Poland (and perhaps Spain) show a continued trend of increasing breast cancer mortality rates throughout the period 1950–1992 for women aged 50–69 years. For about half of the countries breast cancer mortality had been increasing until the most recent calendar period, 1990–1992, when rates then appeared to level off or decline (e.g. Austria, France, Greece and Spain). In other countries (e.g. Canada, The Netherlands, Switzerland and the USA) the rates have remained fairly uniform for the first four decades of the study period. In New Zealand, Norway and Sweden, the rates have fluctuated, reflecting the small populations of women aged 50–69 years in these countries.

Trends for women aged 70–79 years

For most countries, the mortality rates are increasing for women aged 70–79 years (Figure 1.4). None of the countries show clear evidence of a recent decline in rates, although in several countries the rates have remained relatively stable in recent years (e.g. Australia, Sweden, Switzerland and the USA).

DISCUSSION

The main conclusion to be drawn from examination of breast cancer mortality trends in Europe, North America, Australia and New Zealand for all ages is that breast cancer mortality rates generally increased during the 1950s and 1960s, but that more recently the rates have stabilized or declined. These results confirm other reports that breast cancer mortality rates may have been declining in recent years.[1, 3–5] This analysis of age-specific mortality rates shows that the change in mortality has occurred primarily in women aged under 50 years, to a lesser degree among women aged 50–69 years, and not at all among women in their seventies. Indeed, there was some evidence of a decline or levelling off of mortality in every country (except perhaps for women aged 30–49 years). Thus the number of countries that continue to show an increase in breast cancer mortality rates progressively increases with increasing age group.

Reports of analyses of breast cancer mortality trends by age and country and over shorter time periods have concluded that these rates vary in different age groups. Geddes and colleagues concluded that, in Europe, the rates were generally increasing for all age groups, but that this increase was less marked in the younger age groups.[6] Others have reported a recent decrease in rates

in the USA among young women.[3,7,8] Hoel et al. have described a similar pattern of declining rates in young women in Finland and Norway,[7] and Ursin et al. reported the same pattern in Norway and the UK.[8] Mortality rates can be influenced by changes in death certification and coding practices, changes in breast cancer incidence, and changes in survival of women with breast cancer.

Changes in death certification and coding practices

Changes and improvements in the coding of breast cancer on death certificates can produce artefactual increases or decreases in mortality rates, and these effects are difficult to quantify. Excluding women of older age groups will minimize the effect of any alterations. However, increases in breast cancer among these older age groups are important issues with regard to the demographic ageing of the population.[9]

Differences in the coding of death certificates may also explain some of the varying levels of mortality across countries. In all of the countries we have considered, diseases have been classified according to the World Health Organization International Classification of Diseases (ICD). There have not been any changes in the ICD coding of breast cancer over the period of study. In the UK there was a local revision in the coding rule in 1984 which resulted in an artefactual increase in breast cancer mortality rates, affecting mainly the older age groups.[10] This revision was later cancelled in 1993.[11] Beral et al. have reported a recent fall in breast cancer death rates in England and Wales.[12] The rates have been declining since 1989, with the greatest decline occurring in 1993. The changes in the coding rules could not account for the declining mortality rates since 1989. The analysis by Beral et al. was restricted to women aged 20–79 years, thus reducing these artefactual effects.

Similar changes in coding practices have been reported in Scandinavia. The National Central Bureau of Statistics in Sweden instituted additional rules in 1981 that produced an artefactual lowering of mortality, the effect being greatest among the older age groups.[13] In Denmark in 1966 information from autopsies was included on death certificates.[14] Consequently, other more common causes of death were coded for older people, resulting in an artificial decline in breast cancer mortality rates for these women. Bolumar et al. reported that an improvement in the quality of death certificates in Spain in the early 1950s could partially explain the increase in cancer mortality during the period 1951–1990.[15] An indication of the potential effect of miscoding on cancer trends is provided by the changes in the residual ill-defined categories. In Spain, the mortality rate assigned to ill-defined causes declined from 16% in 1955 to 3% in 1985.

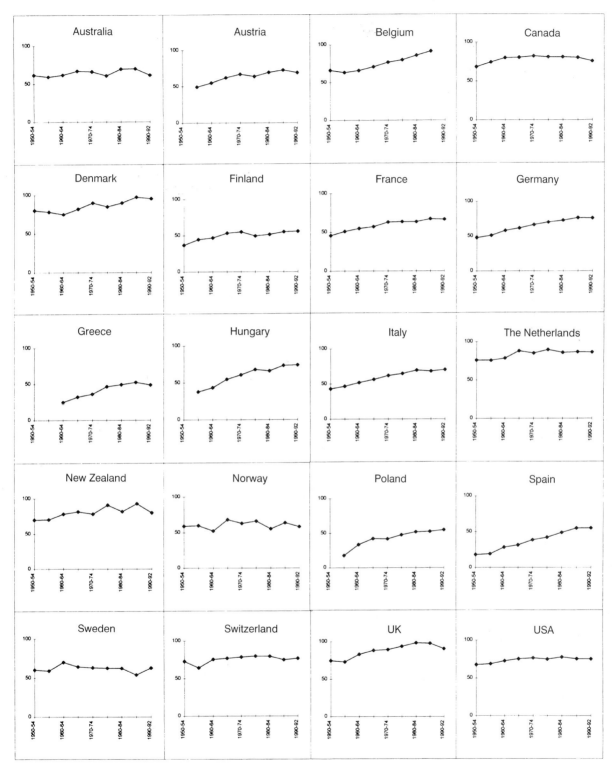

Figure 1.3 *Trends in age-specific mortality rates per 100 000 women aged 50–69 years from 1950–1954 to 1990–1992 in 20 countries in Europe, North America, Australia and New Zealand.*

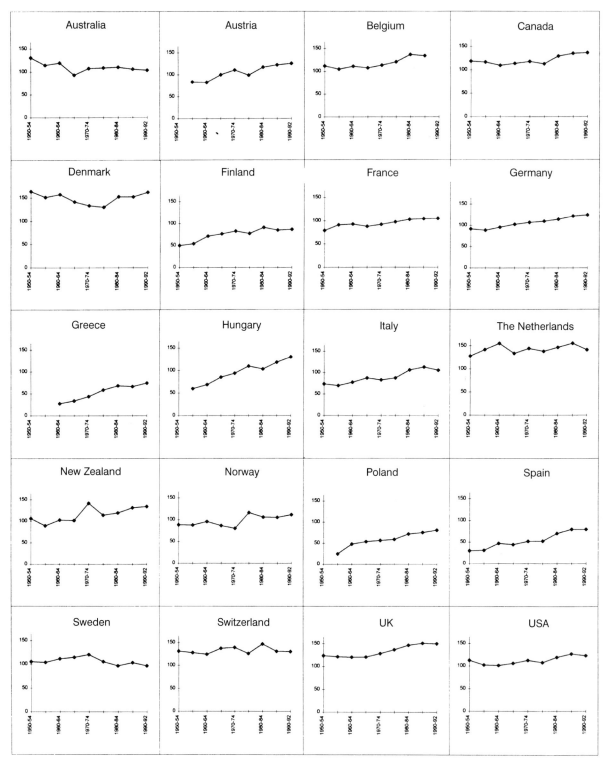

Figure 1.4 *Trends in age-specific mortality rates per 100 000 women aged 70–79 years from 1950–1954 to 1990–1992 in 20 countries in Europe, North America, Australia and New Zealand.*

By limiting our analyses to women aged 30–79 years, the effect of changes in coding of cause of death should be minimized.

Changes in breast cancer incidence

Changes in incidence may influence breast cancer mortality data. This may be due to changes in the occurrence of underlying risk factors for breast cancer, and to changes in the rate of detection of tumours. It is widely accepted that the childbearing pattern of a woman (childlessness, late age at first birth and low parity) influences the risk of her developing breast cancer.[16] Blot et al.[3] and Tarone et al.[17] have demonstrated that in the USA age-specific breast cancer mortality rates parallel changes in childbearing practices for American women aged 40–59 years. This decline in breast cancer mortality has been linked to an increase in fertility during the post-war years. Beral et al. have reported a similar finding in the UK.[5] Among women in England and Wales who were born in 1920, 21% had no children and their average age at first birth was 28.5 years, but for women born in 1945, 10% had no children and the average age at first birth was several years younger. Breast cancer rates have been falling among the generations of women for whom childlessness and the average age at first birth have declined. An analysis of international breast cancer trends has shown a relationship between the decrease in the percentage of women remaining childless by the age of 40 years and a recent decline in breast cancer mortality rates.[1] Hermon et al. have suggested that, internationally, breast cancer rates are converging to a common level,[1] with countries that have high mortality levels experiencing a recent downturn in rates, whilst those countries with low levels of breast cancer mortality continue to show an increase in rates. This may reflect an international convergence of fertility patterns.

Numerous studies world-wide have investigated breast cancer risk and the relationship with oral contraceptives. There is evidence that oral contraceptive use is associated with an increased risk, mainly in young women,[18–20] but that the increased risk does not extend to women of older age groups.[21] However, current users of both oral contraceptives and hormone replacement therapy experience a slightly elevated risk, which decreases again after cessation of use.[22]

Beral et al. have investigated breast cancer trends in Sweden, the UK and the USA in relation to past use of oral contraceptives.[5] In each of the three countries the prevalence of previous oral contraceptive use was similar, namely 80–90% in women aged 40–44 years in 1990, 70–80% for women aged 45–49 years and 50–60% for women in their fifties. The age-specific breast cancer mortality data presented in Figure 1.2 for women aged 30–49 years confirm that rates have been declining in the USA and the UK since 1965–1969 and 1975–1979, respectively, although in Sweden the rates have fluctuated because of the small number of deaths in this age group. Figure 1.3 shows that breast cancer mortality rates for women aged 50–69 years show the same trends for the three countries, with a decline in the USA and the UK occurring later in 1980–1984. Certainly there is no increase in mortality among women in these age groups that could be linked to the introduction of oral contraceptives. In fact, the mortality rates reflect the reverse situation.

Changes in the detection of breast cancer tumours can affect breast cancer mortality. The implementation of a screening programme would result in a decline in the rates of regional and distant breast cancer, which would lag behind an increase in the number of cases of in situ and localized disease. The lag period has been estimated to range from 1 to 5 years depending on the age group of women concerned. Data presented by Miller et al. from the Surveillance, Epidemiology and End Results (SEER) programme of the National Cancer Institute on trends in the age-adjusted incidence of breast cancer among women aged 50 years or over support this concept.[23] National screening programmes have only recently been introduced in many countries, so evidence of a reduction in mortality linked to screening is as yet limited. Blot et al. have attributed part of the reduction in mortality rates among young women (aged < 40 years) in the USA to screening.[3]

Changes in survival

Improvements in survival can be achieved by detection of tumours at an earlier stage and/or by improved treatment. Berrino et al. have recently published a monograph on the survival of cancer patients in Europe.[24] Generally, countries which have shown no change or a slight improvement in relative 5-year survival rates for the period 1983–1985 compared to 1978–1980 have experienced a recent stabilizing of or decline in breast cancer mortality. Evidence from a comparison of mortality rates in the north-eastern USA, which were found to be approximately 25% higher than for women in the south or west, suggested that the difference was due to mortality rates rather than to incidence (which was similar between the areas).[25]

The use of adjuvant chemotherapy during the 1980s has now been shown to be an effective treatment for breast cancer.[26,27] Part of the recent decline in mortality in England and Wales has been attributed to the introduction of such treatment.[5,28] The latest publications from the overview demonstrate that the advantage to patients given adjuvant therapy – whether hormonal or cytotoxic – continues 10–15 years after administration.[29,30] We could therefore expect the present fall in mortality to continue.

CONCLUSION

Breast cancer mortality rates for all ages combined are levelling off or declining in many of the countries examined in Europe, North America, Australia and New Zealand. Data have been presented here on breast cancer mortality trends separately for women aged 30–49, 50–69 and 70–79 years in 20 European and other western countries. For women aged 30–49 years, mortality rates have stabilized or decreased in virtually all 20 countries, and for women aged 50–69 years about half of the countries show evidence of stabilizing or declining rates, whereas for women aged 70–79 years, the mortality rates are generally still increasing in all countries. Thus the recent levelling off or decline in all-age mortality is largely a reflection of the decline or stabilizing of mortality rates for young women.

ACKNOWLEDGEMENTS

The mortality data was provided by the World Health Organization.

REFERENCES

1 Hermon C, Beral V. Breast cancer mortality rates are levelling off or beginning to decline in many western countries. Analysis of time trends, age-cohort and age-period models of breast cancer mortality in 20 countries. *Br J Cancer* 1996; **73**: 955–60.

2 Parkin DM, Muir CS, Whelan SL, Gao YT, Ferlay J, Powell J (eds). *Cancer incidence in five continents. Vol. IV.* Scientific Publications No. 120. Lyon: IARC, 1992.

3 Blot WJ, Devesa SS, Fraumeni JF. Declining breast cancer mortality among young American women. *J Natl Cancer Inst* 1987; **78**: 451–4.

4 Coleman MP, Esteve J, Damiecki P, Arslan A, Renard H. *Trends in cancer incidence and mortality.* Scientific Publications No. 121. Lyon: IARC, 1993.

5 Beral V, Hermon C, Reeves G, Key T. Breast cancer trends in women in Sweden, the UK and the USA in relation to their past use of oral contraceptives. In: Li JJ, Li SA, Nandi A, Gustafsson JA (eds). *Proceedings of the Second International Symposium on Hormonal Carcinogenesis.* Berlin: Springer Verlag, 1996.

6 Geddes M, Balzi D, Tomatis L. Progress in the fight against cancer in EC countries: changes in mortality rates, 1970–90. *Eur J Cancer Prev* 1994; **3**: 31–44.

7 Hoel DG, Davis DL, Miller AB, Sondik EJ, Swerdlow AJ. Trends in cancer mortality in 15 industrialised countries, 1969–1986. *J Natl Cancer Inst* 1992; **84**: 313–20.

8 Ursin G, Bernstein L, Pike MC. Breast cancer. *Cancer Surv* 1994; **19/20**: 241–64.

9 Davis DL, Hoel D, Fox J, Lopez AD. International trends in cancer mortality in France, West Germany, Italy, Japan, England and Wales, and the United States. *Ann N Y Acad Sci* 1990; **609**: 5–48.

10 Office of Population Censuses and Surveys. *Mortality statistics – cause.* Series DH2 No. 11. London: HMSO, 1984.

11 Office of Population Censuses and Surveys. *Deaths in 1993 by cause: provisional numbers.* OPCS monitor DH2 94/2.

12 Beral V, Hermon C, Reeves G, Peto R. Sudden fall in breast cancer death rates in England and Wales (letter). *Lancet* 1995; **345**: 1642–3.

13 National Central Bureau of Statistics. *Dodsorsaker 1981 Official Statistics of Sweden.* Stockholm: Statistics Sweden, 1983.

14 Ewertz M, Carstensen B. Trends in breast cancer incidence and mortality in Denmark, 1943–82. *Int J Cancer 1988*; **41**: 46–51.

15 Bolumar F, Vioque J, Cayuela A. Changing mortality patterns for major cancers in Spain, 1951–1985. *Int J Epidemiol* 1991; **20**: 20–5.

16 Kelsey JL, Gammon MD, John EM. Reproductive factors and breast cancer. *Epidemiol Rev* 1993; **15**: 36–47.

17 Tarone RE, Chu KC. Implications of birth cohort patterns in interpreting trends in breast cancer rates. *J Natl Cancer Inst* 1992; **84**: 1402–10.

18 Pike MC, Henderson BE, Krailo MD, Duke A, Roy S. Breast cancer in young women and use of oral contraceptives. Possible modifying effects of formulation and age at use. *Lancet* 1983; **11**: 926–30.

19 Meirik O, Adami H-O, Christoffersen T, Lund E, Bergstrom R, Bergsjo P. Oral contraceptive use and breast cancer in young women. *Lancet* 1986; **11**: 650–3.

20 UK National Case–Control Study Group. Oral contraceptive use and breast cancer risk in young women. *Lancet* 1989; **1**: 973–82.

21 Wingo PA, Lee NC, Ory HW, Beral V, Peterson HB, Rhodes P. Age-specific differences in the relationship between oral contraceptive use and breast cancer. *Obstet Gynecol* 1991; **78**: 161–70.

22 Alberg AJ, Visuanathan K, Helzlsouer K. Epidemiology, prevention and early detection of breast cancer. *Curr Opin Oncol* 1998; **10**: 492–7.

23 Miller BA, Feuer EJ, Hankey BF. Breast cancer (letter). *N Engl J Med* 1992; **327**: 1756–7.

24 Berrino F, Sant M, Verdecchia A, Capocaccia R, Hakulinen T, Esteve J. *Survival of cancer patients in Europe – the Eurocare Study.* Scientific Publications No. 132. Lyon: IARC, 1995.

25 Goodwin JS, Freeman JL, Freeman D, Nattinger AB. Geographic variations in breast cancer mortality: do higher rates imply elevated incidence or poorer survival? *Am J Public Health* 1998; **88**: 458–60.

26 Early Breast Cancer Trialists Collaborative Group. Systemic treatment of early breast cancer by hormonal, cytotoxic, or immune therapy. *Lancet* 1992; **339**: 1–15.

27 Bonadonna G, Valagussa P, Moliterni A, Zambetti M, Brambilla C. Adjuvant cyclophosphamide, methotrexate, and fluorouracil in node-positive breast cancer: the

results of 20 years of follow-up. *N Engl J Med* 1995; **332**: 901–6.

28 Baum M. Screening for breast cancer, time to think – and stop? (letter). *Lancet* 1995; **346**: 436–7.

29 Early Breast Cancer Trialists Collaborative Group.

Tamoxifen for early breast cancer: an overview of the randomised trials. *Lancet* 1998; **351**: 1451–67.

30 Early Breast Cancer Trialists Collaborative Group. Polychemotherapy for early breast cancer: an overview of the randomised trials. *Lancet* 1998; **352**: 930–42.

FURTHER READING

Peto R, Borham J, Clarke M, Davies C, Beral V. UK and USA breast cancer deaths down 25% in year 2000 at ages 20–69 years. *Lancet* 2000; **355**: 1822.

2

Changing philosophical perspectives in breast cancer

JOHN R BENSON AND MICHAEL BAUM

INTRODUCTION

Advances in medicine have often been dependent upon empirical and serendipitous observations. Whilst a degree of rationality can be applied to empirical approaches, such 'rational empiricism' represents a non-ideal strategy of inconsistent and unpredictable value. The biological underpinning of this methodology may be flawed or indeed non-existent, and therapeutic strategies cannot be targeted and optimized for maximal clinical benefit. Although science is a progression of ideas which often proceeds in a linear fashion, sometimes a 'Knight's Move' can herald a significant advance in understanding of natural phenomena. The enigmatic nature of breast cancer reflects our failure to understand completely the biology of this disease and to appreciate the heterogeneity in behaviour and interactions of cells not only between different tumours, but within the same tumour.

Management of breast cancer over the past century has been governed by defined paradigms of tumour biology. This period has been dominated by two polarized and almost mutually exclusive doctrines. The so-called 'Halstedian paradigm' has been usurped by one of 'biological predeterminism', and each of these paradigms has in turn yielded distinct therapeutic consequences which have dictated popular clinical practice. Limitations of application and tardiness of clinical progress prompt reassessment of the current status quo, and may ultimately precipitate a paradigm shift. The contemporary

paradigm has yielded relatively modest clinical benefits, and it must now be asked whether it is appropriate to persevere with and pursue practices based upon this set of biological tenets, or to effect a doctrinal change and adopt a fresh set of therapeutic strategies based on radically altered perceptions of breast cancer biology.

This chapter outlines these changing philosophical perspectives, and discusses whether the existing paradigm can be refined in the light of recent scientific advances in tumour and molecular biology, or whether further improvements in disease-free and overall survival in breast cancer must await the next paradigm shift. Finally, an alternative and somewhat provocative concept will be proposed which accounts for certain inconsistencies and suggests novel approaches to breast cancer therapy.

THE HALSTEDIAN PARADIGM

The rationale for the Halsted radical mastectomy was based on principles enunciated by Virchow in 1860.[1,2] Following the recognition by Muller in 1810 that cancer was a cellular phenomenon,[3] Virchow proposed that a cancer arose in the breast as a result of a local cellular disturbance. Although it was unknown how or why a group of epithelial cells formed a malignant focus, Virchow presented a treatise on how these cells spread to other sites in the body, thereby establishing more distant foci of disease. His centrifugal theory of dissemination was based on detailed anatomical studies of patients with breast cancer, from which it was concluded that a cancer invaded locally and spread in a progressive and sequential manner along fascial planes and lymphatic channels. At that time, lymph nodes were thought to act as a barrier to various forms of particulate matter, including inorganic particles (e.g. ink),[4,5] bacteria, viruses[6] and blood cells.[7] Virchow added tumour cells to this list, and considered lymph nodes to be mechanical filters which trapped cancer cells and at least temporarily halted more distant spread. The anatomical arrangement of lymph nodes was such as to provide a circumferential line of defence against this centrifugal spread of cancer from a local focus within the breast. Once the filtration capacity of lymph nodes was exhausted, cancer cells could pass through the nodes into the efferent lymphatics and thence to the distal lymphatic system which lay in anatomical continuity.

Such successive encroachment of cancer upon ever more distant structures was the central theme of this paradigm. By implication, surgical treatments which allowed an *en-bloc* resection of the tumour together with associated loco-regional tissues offered the best chance of 'cure'. Such was the underlying rationale for Halsted's radical mastectomy which aimed to remove the tumour, overlying skin and superficial fascia, pectoralis major and minor, lymphatic channels and regional nodes.[8] A corollary of this hypothesis was that the more radical the surgery, the better was the chance of eradicating all tumour. Consequently, super-radical forms of mastectomy, sometimes involving forequarter amputation, were devised and advocated for more advanced tumours.[9]

The Halsted radical mastectomy provided excellent local control, with up to three-quarters of patients being free of loco-regional relapse until they succumbed from distant disease or inter-current illness.[10] It was this excellent local control which created a conceptual mirage which eclipsed the scientific logic of the day and fostered intellectual complacency. This state of affairs was greatly encouraged by ignorance of clinical trials and the variable natural history of breast cancer. Some patients would have survived despite their disease, but also despite surgery which in those earlier years carried a high mortality.[10]

Analysis of early hospital records following introduction of the radical mastectomy revealed no evidence for an improvement in overall survival compared to some of the lesser surgical procedures being performed at the time.[11] Furthermore, Brinkley and Haybittle later reviewed about 700 patients who had undergone radical mastectomy in the late 1940's at a follow-up of 30 years.[12] Fewer than a quarter of these patients showed a similar risk of dying as an age-matched control population. The notorious group of patients at the Middlesex Hospital with untreated breast cancer,[13] together with the occasional anecdotal report, testifies to the fact that breast cancer patients can survive for up to 30 years without treatment. These patients may have uncontrolled locally advanced disease, but growth is indolent and not associated with the development of overt distant metastases. In 1963, Gershon-Cohen estimated from serial mammographic data that tumour doubling times for breast cancer ranged from 23 to 209 days.[14] These data indicate that Halsted's radical mastectomy was not a surgical panacea for breast cancer, and they emphasize the clinical heterogeneity and variable natural history of breast cancer.

The Halstedian paradigm which had been embraced both in philosophy and indeed by the surgical community for over half a century began to falter and appear vulnerable before an emerging body of clinical and laboratory data that supported an alternative biological model. A paradigm shift was both imminent and long overdue.

BIOLOGICAL PREDETERMINISM

It was perhaps ironic that the above Halstedian ethos, which had been staunchly and unquestionably supported by surgeons for so long, was eventually discredited by a small group of surgeons and superseded by a paradigm based on a biological model of breast cancer, in which surgery *per se* figured somewhat less prominently as a component of treatment. In the best traditions of the scientific method, Bernard Fisher proposed an alternative to the Halstedian hypothesis, and then sought to accrue both laboratory and clinical data in support of his theory.[15] The basic tenet of this alternative paradigm was that breast cancer did not spread centrifugally in a predictable and consistent manner determined by anatomical and mechanical dictates. According to the model based on Virchow's teaching, cancer cells within lymph vessels could only travel to the next lymph node, and those which had subsequently invaded the bloodstream would become lodged in the first capillary bed they reached. Thus the pattern of dissemination would be orderly, and distant metastases would be consequent to regional lymph node (RLN) involvement. Instead, Fisher suggested that cancer cells could reach distant sites via the bloodstream at a very early stage of tumour development, irrespective of nodal involvement. Regional lymph nodes were not invariably considered to be instigators of distant disease spread, but rather reflected a situation *in vivo* between tumour and host which favoured dissemination.[15]

Using a perfused rabbit lymphatic popliteal system as a model, the Fisher brothers showed that transnodal passage of tumour cells could occur.[16] They demonstrated passage of cancer cells not only into efferent lymphatics, but also into the bloodstream via lymphatico-venous communications, thus repudiating the concept of nodes as passive filters or barriers to dissemination of tumour cells.[17,18] Furthermore, they also showed that RLNs could destroy tumour cells. Thus negative nodes could be a consequence of tumour cells traversing nodes and/or being destroyed by them, and did not necessarily indicate excision of the primary tumour prior to nodal dissemination. Studies with chromium-labelled cells indicated that during haematogenous dissemination, tumour cells did not always lodge in the first capillary bed they encountered.[19]

These laboratory findings, coupled with the observation that in animal models dormant tumour cells could, after a variable period and on appropriate stimulation, develop into overt metastases, formed the basis for the paradigm of biological predeterminism. The central theme of this paradigm is that breast cancer is predominantly a systemic disease at the outset, with clinical outcome having been predetermined by the extent of micrometastases which have developed during the preclinical phase and are present at the time of diagnosis. Two important therapeutic sequelae arise from this hypothesis. First, the extent of primary surgery does not influence the chances of cure, as it is the subsequent behaviour of these micrometastases which determines survival. The extent of these may be similar in both small and locally advanced tumours, and however radical the loco-regional surgery, it will be of no consequence to these micrometastatic foci. The second implication of this alternative model is that administration of a systemic therapy which counters these putative micrometastases should confer a survival advantage.

At the beginning of the 1970s, clinical trials of breast conservation therapy were initiated by Fisher and others with the primary purpose of testing the first of these predictions. Of interest, some surgeons had advocated less radical forms of surgery for breast cancer prior to this time. Sir Geoffrey Keynes wrote in 1937: 'the treatment of carcinoma of the breast may justifiably be made much more conservative than it usually is, provided that the necessary facilities for irradiation are available'.[20]

In 1972, Hedley Atkins published the results of a clinical trial at Guy's Hospital comparing radical mastectomy (with irradiation of the supraclavicular and internal mammary nodes) to wide local excision (with irradiation of the breast and axillary nodes in addition to the above-mentioned fields) for stage I and II breast cancer.[21] For patients with stage I disease, overall survival was similar in the two arms of this trial and independent of the extent of primary surgery. However, stage II patients had a higher incidence of distant metastases which translated into impaired survival, although this may have reflected suboptimal radiotherapy schedules.

This Guy's trial, together with earlier anecdotal reports of breast-conserving operations, was not conceived on the basis of inferences from the above hypothesis of biological predeterminism. Instead, the rationale for these early forays into breast conservation derived fundamentally from Halstedian principles. The radical mastectomy constituted a rather non-discriminate surgical procedure for a disease which was already recognized as having a broad clinical – if not biological – spectrum. In particular, the Halsted radical mastectomy might represent surgical overkill for some patients with smaller, more locally confined tumours. Depending on the degree of 'centrifugal' spread, individual patients might be 'cured' by lesser surgical procedures such as modified radical mastectomy, simple mastectomy and indeed breast conservation surgery. It was this reasoning, albeit based on a false paradigm, which spurred on the early enthusiasts about breast conservation in an era when to contemplate anything less than a mastectomy for cancer was deemed unorthodox and surgical blasphemy.

In the event, the conclusions of the Guy's trial to some extent supported the new paradigm, although it should be noted that a second trial focusing on stage I patients randomized according to a similar schedule to that described above did reveal both impaired local control and overall survival.[22] None the less, subsequent results from the NSAPB,[23] Milan[24] and smaller trials[25,26] confirmed that breast-conserving techniques did not compromise overall survival. The NSABP-06 trial compared total mastectomy and lumpectomy with or without breast irradiation for tumours 4 cm or less in diameter,[23] whilst Veronesi compared quadrantectomy, axillary dissection and radiotherapy (QUART) with mastectomy for small breast cancers of maximum diameter 2 cm.[24] Despite variation in rates of local breast relapse, overall survival rates were not influenced by the extent of primary surgery, thus supporting the concept that clinical outcome was predetermined by dissemination of micrometastases prior to clinical presentation and primary surgical treatment.

The second therapeutic sequela of this paradigm has also been corroborated by clinical trials, which once again were initiated with the deliberate intent of testing a new hypothesis in accordance with scientific principles and etiquette. To investigate whether adjuvant systemic therapy could provide a survival advantage in patients with putative micrometastases, but with no clinical evidence of metastatic disease, a trial was initiated by the NSAPB in 1971 in which node-positive patients received chemotherapy (L-phenylalanine mustard) as adjuvant treatment.[27] This was the first trial to show that adjuvant systemic therapy could perturb the natural history of breast cancer and improve overall survival. Administration of chemotherapy was restricted to node-positive patients who were considered to have a worse prognosis, and for whom a previous pilot study had revealed a survival advantage.[28] Subsequent trials confirmed that endocrine therapy could also act in an adjuvant capacity to improve both disease-free and overall survival. The 1992 10-year overview by the Early Breast Cancer Trialists' Collaborative Group[29] showed that in unselected patients adjuvant polychemotherapy reduces the annual risk of disease recurrence by 28% and the mortality by 17%, whilst adjuvant tamoxifen reduces the risk of recurrence by 30% and the mortality by 19% in women over 50 years of age.

Therefore unselected adjuvant systemic therapy will reduce the risk of relapse at a constant rate of 20–30% per year, and yields an absolute benefit of approximately 10% reduction in mortality over a period of 10 years. This translates into about 8 to 12 lives being saved per 100 women with stage I and II breast cancer. The most recent overview of adjuvant trials confirms a persistent survival advantage with more prolonged follow-up for both tamoxifen and adjuvant polychemotherapy. Once again, absolute benefits are not dramatic and remain of the order of 5–10%.[30]

Therefore biological predeterminism represents the emergence of a new paradigm based on a scientifically tested hypothesis. The intellectual intransigence which engulfed the Halstedian era should serve as a lesson for future generations of clinicians and scientists, and any tendency towards complacency with the contemporary paradigm must be resisted. Despite the unequivocal benefits of adjuvant systemic therapies, absolute gains remain modest. A 30% reduction in relative risk is much less than would be predicted from the response rates of advanced breast cancer to these same systemic agents.

A PARADIGM IN CRISIS?

Although the underlying premise that most breast cancer is systemic at the outset remains inviolable, it probably has to be acknowledged that a subgroup of patients with early breast cancer exists for whom micrometastatic spread has not occurred prior to either clinical presentation or mammographic detection. It is quite possible for a small tumour to have an established blood supply without infiltration of cancer cells into the tumour vasculature. Similarly, cancer cells can travel to the regional nodes via the lymphatics and remain there without necessarily entering the circulation via lymphatico-venous communications. Treatment of regional nodes which are infiltrated by tumour confers no survival advantage, in accordance with Fisher's precept that positive nodes are indicative of a set of circumstances that favours development of systemic metastases which themselves ultimately determine outcome. Positive nodes are a 'warning of a poor prognosis',[31] and not the 'instigator' of metastatic disease.[15] However, in some node-negative cases there could be cancer cells which have spread along lymphatics from the primary tumour and which remain undetected by the pathologist and do not enter the circulation via lymphatico-venous channels to initiate distant metastases. Indeed, patients with microscopic nodal deposits have a similar prognosis to node-negative patients. Under these circumstances, a patient would theoretically be cured by adequate loco-regional treatment alone. Recent analysis of the long-term follow-up of the Guy's data by Hayward suggests that some patients with stage I

and II disease treated by mastectomy have achieved hazard ratios similar to an age-matched control population.[32] However, data on prolonged follow-up of patients treated for breast cancer has not demonstrated conclusive evidence of statistical cure, with ratios of observed to expected deaths approaching but not reaching unity.[33] Notwithstanding such analytical tools as the Nottingham Prognostic Index,[34] it is impossible to identify this subgroup accurately at the time of diagnosis, and it behoves us currently to offer at least adjuvant tamoxifen therapy to all patients with early invasive breast cancer.

For the majority of patients with breast cancer, the most fundamental and challenging aspect of their disease lies outside the breast and regional tissues. It is from the micrometastatic foci which, after a variable period of dormancy, develop into overt metastases that a patient eventually succumbs. Although local recurrence in the breast following conservation surgery is psychologically disastrous, it does not appear to compromise overall survival though trials hitherto may have insufficient power to detect any real difference in survival rates between these two surgical modalities. Notwithstanding such comments, this is consistent with the hypothesis that such an event is a loco-regional manifestation of a systemic process which was already established at the time of primary loco-regional treatment. The above subgroup of patients who were 'cured' by surgery/radiotherapy alone would not develop local recurrence because no systemic component to their disease exists. However, inadequate loco-regional treatment could result in persistent disease locally, from which systemic dissemination might eventually result.

The above analysis of Guy's data indicates that survival can be adversely affected by suboptimal loco-regional treatment with an excess of axillary recurrences possibly acting as instigators of distant metastases.[35] However, the issue of whether inadequate axillary dissection compromises survival remains controversial. The NSABP-04 trial suggested a 5–6% survival advantage for axillary dissection,[36] and this echoes the philosophy that in patients with disease genuinely confined to the breast and axillary nodes, appropriate loco-regional treatment alone can be curative. Recent results from two randomized trials investigating the value of post-operative radiotherapy in patients undergoing mastectomy and adjuvant chemotherapy have revealed impressive survival advantages for the selective use of radiotherapy in a subgroup of premenopausal node-positive patients.[37,38] Indeed, reductions in mortality (of approximately one-third) attributable to radiotherapy combined with chemotherapy are comparable in magnitude to those which can be achieved by adjuvant systemic therapies alone or breast-screening programmes. These improvements in overall survival are presumably a consequence of more effective eradication of loco-regional disease which, if persistent, becomes the source of distant metastases, a contention supported by the apparent delay in emergence of survival differences even though effects on local recurrence are witnessed at an earlier time period. These loco-regional deposits or so-called 'oligometastases' may be less susceptible to isolated chemotherapy schedules than micrometastases, for which local pharmacokinetics are more likely to favour drug access and penetration to sites of abnormal epithelial proliferation.[39] Interestingly, it is implicit from a breast-screening perspective that a substantial proportion of patients are potentially curable by earlier detection. If it is believed that screening can genuinely reduce mortality, then it probably has to be accepted that all breast cancer is not systemic at the outset. Moreover, it is assumed that the dissemination and establishment of viable micrometastases can occur during the preclinical phase when a breast cancer is mammographically detectable. The crucial question concerns the proportion of tumours that disseminate between the time of radiological detection and clinical presentation. In other words, what proportion of cancers can be successfully detected mammographically *before* any development of micrometastases? Ideally, screening should pick up tumours whilst they are still in the prevascular phase in which growth is very slow and there is no opportunity for haematogenous spread, although it is quite feasible that a tumour can possess an established vasculature without necessarily showing vascular invasion at these early stages of tumour development (see below). A threshold tumour size may exist beyond which dissemination occurs, although as breast cancer is a heterogeneous disease, a range of sizes rather than a single threshold value is likely.[40,41] The magnitude of observed reductions in mortality from screening (25–40%)[42,43] suggests that biological predeterminism is not a universal phenomenon in the natural history of breast cancer. However, phenotypic progression may also account for improved survival rates from screening due to detection of lesions at an earlier, less biologically aggressive stage when the metastatic potential is limited.[40] To some extent, this phenomenon is related to the issue of preclinical dissemination, as tumours with greater malignant potential are more likely to metastasize. The proportion of cells within a tumour with the capacity to invade blood vessels, travel in the circulation and establish viable micrometastases will increase with progression to a more malignant phenotype. The latter may be manifested by enhanced activity at several steps in the process of invasion and metastasis.

Despite the proven efficacy of adjuvant chemotherapy, response rates for early breast cancer are less than half those found in patients with advanced disease. Furthermore, response rates for neoadjuvant therapy appear to be independent of tumour size and correlate weakly with proliferative indices such as Ki67 and percentage S-phase.[44] These clinical observations call into question the applicability of logarithmic cell kill by first-order kinetics and the rationale for dose intensification in chemotherapy schedules. 'More of the same'[45] may not be the answer, and could result in much increased morbidity and a corresponding reduction in quality of life for minor increments in survival.

EVOLUTION OF A PARADIGM OR A PARADIGM SHIFT?

Can the present impasse be overcome by refining the contemporary paradigm, or is it time for a further paradigm shift? Since the basic tenets of biological predeterminism were proposed, there have been great advances in our understanding of regulatory mechanisms in cell growth and differentiation. Clues as to what has gone wrong in neoplastic states have come from studying developmental processes, and it is becoming apparent that cancerous tissues are a kind of caricature of normal tissues.[46] Many tumours are grossly similar to their tissue of origin, this being most evident in well-differentiated lesions. Indeed, less well-differentiated tumours may not represent a degree of de-differentiation *per se*; tumours may arise from malignant stem cells which undergo differentiation like normal stem cells. The proportion of these which have undergone differentiation (and apoptosis) relative to those which continue to proliferate and remain undifferentiated determines the histological grade. Thus a cell may possess the typical features of a malignant phenotype, yet still have gone through a sequential process of differentiation not dissimilar to its non-malignant counterpart.[46] Furthermore, cancer cells display a finite number of aberrant pathways leading to disordered growth patterns, and the alterations in nucleotide sequence and composition which characterize a cancer cell represent only a small fraction of a cell's complete DNA content.

This apparent similarity between normal and malignant cells has been expounded by Schipper,[47–49] who has emphasized that cancer cells are not 'alien' and genetically disparate like exogenous pathogens, but rather they are rogue internal elements which have achieved some degree of autonomy by dislocation of the normal pathways of intercellular communication. However, a cancer cell is not completely autonomous, and some channels of communication persist. In effect, a malignant tumour represents a state of regulatory imbalance in which cancer cells have achieved various degrees of escape from the mechanisms that control normal rates of proliferation and differentiation. A central theme of this proposal is that cancer is a potentially reversible process, and that by correcting abnormal cellular expression and transcriptional patterns, aberrant pathways of communication might be restored and, in turn, 'rogue' cancer cells re-regulated and effectively 'tamed'. Malignant cells would be controlled rather than killed, and survival would be increased by effectively rendering tumour behaviour more benign.

This philosophy of 'cell control' as opposed to 'cell kill' exploits the similarities between cancer and normal cells, in contrast to the cytotoxic model, which relies on presumed qualitative differences between these two cell populations. Cytotoxic therapy is based on the principle of maximal cell kill in a somewhat analogous manner to antimicrobial therapy. However, as mentioned above, cancer cells are not foreign entities but genetic kindreds, and total eradication may be an inappropriate goal. Indeed, as pointed out by Schipper, such a strategy actually provides maximal evolutionary pressure for a deregulated system. Chemotherapy is rather like trying to quell civil disturbance with indiscriminate bombing rather than by negotiation and re-establishing of channels of communication.

Therefore, according to this concept, the therapeutic goal shifts from one of cell kill to re-regulation. As this method exploits the similarities between cancerous and normal tissues, there may be a fundamental advantage over cytotoxic approaches. The latter were derived on the premise that tumours were monoclonal and originated from genetic change within a single cell. It is thus assumed that all cells within a tumour will behave similarly, and that they will respond to a given agent uniformly and consistently. The rationale for combination therapy was based not so much on ideas of separate populations of tumour cells with qualitatively different responses to cytotoxic agents, as on the possibility that the chances of individual cell kill would be maximized by selecting agents which targeted separate biochemical pathways within cells (e.g. abrogation of both protein and DNA synthesis).

It is now recognized that individual tumours are composed of a heterogeneous population of cells with degrees of phenotypic variability based on subtle differences in patterns of gene expression. These result in different rates of proliferation, invasive potential and response to therapeutic agents. Although a particular tumour may be designated as of a certain histological type and grade, these labels are surrogate classifications and represent only the dominant morphological type. Studies have shown that up to one-third of breast cancers have components of more than one histological type,[50] and variation in nuclear grade and degrees of pleiomorphism/number of mitotic figures is common within the same tumour. *In-vitro* thymidine labelling has revealed a considerable spectrum of proliferative potential between cells derived from the same tumour.[51] Functional heterogeneity and response to endocrine therapies are supported by measurements of steroid receptor status. No tumours are strictly oestrogen receptor (OR) negative – in reality they are relatively OR poor and composed of cells which on average have low densities of surface membrane receptors.

It is this biological heterogeneity which underlies the variable natural history of breast cancer, and has hitherto restricted the efficacy of therapies. The potential extent of this cellular heterogeneity within a tumour and its micrometastases has important therapeutic conse-

quences. It is unlikely that even a combination of chemotherapeutic agents will successfully target the majority of cells. Rather, these agents will serve as a therapeutic probe to select subpopulations or clones of cells which have a similar phenotype and response. Depending on the degree of heterogeneity, a particular combination chemotherapy schedule will target a variable proportion of the total cell population, leaving a certain proportion of cells which are unresponsive to any of the agents employed.

It may be more sensible and rational to use therapeutic agents which can exploit the similarities between these differing clones of cells, and that thus have a wider 'cellular appeal'. These could include hormonal and other agents which can accomplish re-regulation through modulation of biological response modifiers and natural cytokines to which most cancer cells can still potentially respond. Such a response will depend upon innate similarities which persist between cancer cells, and is likely to be witnessed in the majority of malignant cells. By contrast, cytotoxic regimens based on a finite number of drugs with specific actions have more limited scope and are likely to influence a smaller proportion of cancer cells. However, as these regulatory strategies largely rely on normal pathways of cellular communication, therapeutic indices may be small. None the less, control of rogue cancer cells by such methods may not be associated with specific deleterious effects on non-neoplastic cells.

Neoplastic progression may result in part from loss of negative growth control through autocrine/paracrine interactions, and agents which can restore inhibitory responses would facilitate re-regulation and 'taming' of rogue cancer cells. Specific mechanisms by which growth control could potentially be re-established will be discussed after the role of the host in tumour evolution and behaviour has been considered.

TUMOUR–HOST INTERACTIONS

The above principle of 'control rather than kill' can be applied within the contemporary paradigm of biological predeterminism. Breast cancer is still considered to be a systemic disease at the outset in the majority of patients. However, a primary cancer together with associated micrometastatic (or macrometastatic) foci could be viewed as local manifestations of a systemic breakdown in growth restraint.

The consistent pattern of metastatic spread of breast cancer argues against chance colonization by autonomous monoclonally-derived malignant breast epithelial cells. Instead, host factors and local tissue components are likely to be major determinants of the detailed phenotypic expression of breast cancer, and to explain why organs such as the liver, lung and brain are affected, but not the kidneys, spleen or muscle.[31]

Furthermore, the response of bone metastases to endocrine therapy differs from that of visceral metastases, yet the malignant epithelial foci within each of these organs ostensibly originate from a common source.

It may be that the current impasse reflects not so much a fault in the current paradigm, as a failure 'to see the forest because of the tree'.[31] In recent years much attention has focused on micrometastases (biological predeterminism) and their progenitor the primary breast tumour (the Halstedian paradigm). These have been viewed as primary epithelial events, with cancer cells themselves ultimately determining proliferative and invasive potential. This is in accordance with the monoclonal theory whereby a tumour arises from primary events within epithelial cells which confer a selective growth advantage. This rather simplistic theory fails to take into account two important concepts. First, neoplastic development is likely to involve multiple genetic events, some of which initiate a tumour, whilst others promote it. Secondly, tumours are composed of several tissue components, of which the dominant proliferative cell type defines the lesion. This convention has tended to undermine any potential importance of 'secondary' tissue elements in the process of carcinogenesis. Epithelial tumours contain not only neoplastic epithelium but also mesenchymal derivatives such as fibroblasts and endothelial cells.

Evidence has now accrued which alludes to a more active role for mesenchymal elements in both the induction and maintenance of the transformed state. Such elements can no longer be considered as merely executing a passive supportive/nutritional role for adjacent neoplastic epithelium. In order to shift attention away from the monoclonal epithelial cell, and to invoke mesenchymal determinants, a unifying hypothesis was proposed to account for certain disparate clinical observations.[52] These include the effects of adjuvant tamoxifen in early breast cancer and the association between gastrointestinal polyps and desmoid tumours. This hypothesis represents an 'innovative look at the forest',[31] and illustrates how novel therapeutic approaches can derive from conceptual shifts.

BREAST CANCER, DESMOID TUMOURS AND FAMILIAL ADENOMATOUS POLYPOSIS COLI – A UNIFYING HYPOTHESIS

The results of adjuvant trials which revealed that the efficacy of tamoxifen in early breast cancer was partially independent of oestrogen receptor (OR) status were counter-intuitive,[29,53,54] as the anti-oestrogen tamoxifen is precluded from acting as a competitive antagonist for the conventional OR. A negative paracrine hypothesis was proposed,[55] and was later corroborated by both experimental[55,56] and clinical data,[57] in which tamoxifen directly stimulates fibroblasts to produce and secrete inhibitory growth factors for neighbouring epithelial cells, be they OR positive or OR negative.

Desmoid tumours are benign proliferative lesions of fibroblasts and may occur in association with familial adenomatous polyposis coli in the condition known as Gardner's syndrome, in which affected individuals develop both ectodermal and mesodermal tumours.[58] In contrast to desmoids, gastrointestinal polyps are composed of a mixture of epithelial and mesenchymal elements. Could fibroblasts within the stroma of polyps share some abnormality with those of desmoids, this contributing to both desmoid formation and epithelial proliferation within polyps?

Mesenchymal elements such as fibroblasts and endothelial cells display important interactions *in vivo* with epithelial cells in both topographical and functional contexts. The precise nature of these stromal–epithelial interactions remain ill-defined and poorly understood, but there is much experimental data to substantiate a role for such interactions in morphogenesis and other developmental processes.[59,60] Furthermore, there is emerging evidence for ongoing stromal–epithelial interactions in the adult organism once morphological and functional maturity has occurred. If such interactions in the adult organism serve to keep abnormal epithelial proliferation in check, then derangements of these may be involved in neoplasia. Moreover, a breakdown in stromal–epithelial interactions could be a consequence not only of primary events within epithelial cells, but also of aberrant function of mesenchymal elements.

Elegant tissue recombination experiments have demonstrated an inductive capacity of mesenchyme on fully differentiated tissues, and revealed how epithelial differentiation and hormonal responsiveness can be determined by mesenchymal characteristics. Adult bladder epithelium when combined with wild-type urogenital mesenchyme (UGM) can redifferentiate into prostatic tissue under the influence of androgens.[59] Bladder epithelium does not contain androgen receptors,[61] which are present exclusively in the UGM, implying that androgens mediate this effect on epithelial cells via mesenchymal elements. Xenograft tumour growth (MCF-7 cells) is influenced by fibroblasts from both benign and malignant breast tumours,[62] and corresponding conditioned medium from these tumours is generally stimulatory to proliferation of MCF-7 breast carcinoma cells *in vitro*,[63–65] whilst that of normal skin fibroblasts can be inhibitory.[66] Further insight into the influence of mesenchyme on its associated epithelium has been provided by experiments in which rodent skin carcinomas were transplanted heterotopically into the uterus and underwent reconversion from a malignant to a benign-appearing epithelium.[67] Dermal mesenchyme may therefore induce a state of immortalization in overlying epidermal cells, which can revert to benign behaviour once freed from this specific 'adverse' stromal influence. Gut epithelium is similar to epidermis in undergoing regular renewal. Could such epithelium, influenced by a local factor, become immortalized by its associated mesenchyme? Co-culture of colonic carcinoma cells with fibroblasts has demonstrated their potential response to mesenchymal factors which stimulate growth and promote differentiation.[68]

To suggest that a mesenchymal abnormality might underlie the development of polyps and desmoid tumours in patients with Gardner's syndrome implies some systemic abnormality of stromal tissue. There is evidence for the pre-existence of aberrant fibroblasts in cancer patients. Skin fibroblasts from patients with a family history of breast cancer display fetal-like migration patterns in collagen gels, whilst those from patients with FAP show abnormal growth characteristics in vitro, with a reduced requirement for serum and a morphology similar to embryonal fibroblasts, with overgrowth and loss of contact inhibition.

These observations allude to a possible systemic abnormality of fibroblasts in cancer patients. Therefore it can be proposed that an intrinsic systemic abnormality of fibroblasts in FAP patients predisposes to both desmoid tumours and gastrointestinal polyps, with local factors initiating tumour formation. What might constitute this intrinsic abnormality of fibroblasts? There is evidence for induction of the negative growth modulator-transforming growth factor β (TGFβ) from stromal cells both in vitro and in vivo in response to tamoxifen. TGFβ represents a family of multi-functional regulatory peptides involved in a range of processes including development, wound healing and carcinogenesis.[69,70] TGFβ has a great diversity of functions, but in general it is inhibitory to a range of epithelial cells,[71–73] and stimulatory to cells of mesenchymal origin.[74] The inhibitory effect of TGFβ on epithelial cells is of paramount interest to anti-cancer strategies, and receptors for TGFβ are widespread, implying that many cells can respond to this negative growth factor. Tamoxifen induces secretion of TGFβ by between 3 and 30-fold in fetal fibroblasts in vitro,[55] and induction of TGFβ occurs in OR-positive and OR-negative breast cancer patients following primary tamoxifen therapy.[57] Furthermore, tamoxifen has recently been shown to increase synthesis of TGFβ1 in primary cultures of breast tumour fibroblasts in vitro.[56]

Thus tamoxifen can directly stimulate fibroblasts to produce and secrete TGFβ which may act in a negative paracrine manner upon neighbouring epithelial cells, irrespective of their OR status. Desmoid tumours can undergo a dramatic clinical response to tamoxifen and the related triphenylethylene toremifene, implying a direct effect of these agents on fibroblasts.[75] Interestingly, in patients with Gardner's syndrome this response may be accompanied by regression of gastrointestinal polyps. These effects could be mediated in a similar manner by induction of TGFβ from component fibroblasts. Therefore if an intrinsic mesenchymal defect exists with a deficiency of TGFβ as a primary fault, this would pro-

duce a local imbalance of growth factors which in conjunction with putative fetal-like characteristics would lead on the one hand to the promotion of fibroblast activity encouraging desmoid formation (desmoid fibroblasts may display an aberrant response and be inhibited by TGFβ), and on the other to disturbance of stromal–epithelial interactions with a reduction in negative stromal paracrine influences resulting in excessive epithelial proliferative activity of the gastrointestinal mucosa.

Colonic adenoma cells in vitro remain sensitive to growth inhibition by exogenous TGFβ,[76] consistent with the hypothesis that failure of a growth inhibitory response to TGFβ results from a change in local levels of growth factor, rather than altered cellular sensitivity.

This intrinsic mesenchymal defect could be a phenotypic manifestation of a genetic abnormality at the 5q21 locus. Both gross constitutional deletions and more discrete genetic lesions focused around this locus have been demonstrated in polyps of FAP patients and desmoid tissue of patients with Gardner's syndrome.[77,78] Such a defect inherited as a germline mutation would be present in all cells, including fibroblasts. In accordance with Knudson's theory,[79] heterozygosity at this locus in epithelial cells predisposes to polyps, whilst a further somatic mutation in the homologous allele would lead to colorectal carcinoma.

It is postulated that heterozygosity at this 5q locus confers an abnormal phenotype characterized by defective secretion of TGFβ by fibroblasts. Such a fault would predispose to both polyps and desmoids. A further somatic mutation of the homologous allele on the cognate chromosome of colonic epithelial cells would trigger actual malignant transformation with development of colorectal carcinoma.

Although abnormalities at the 5q locus are not implicated in breast cancer, certain familial forms could be associated with derangement of stromal–epithelial interactions based on a local imbalance of growth factors. TGFβ is a pre-eminent growth inhibitory signal, upon which several different pathways may ultimately converge. Defective function could result from abnormalities at more than one locus which involve synthesis, secretion or activation of TGFβ. Interestingly, there is an association between breast cancer and non-familial gastrointestinal polyps.[80] This is most probably a consequence of environmental factors, but it could involve a common mechanistic, if not inherited, defect based on deranged stromal–epithelial interactions. Fibroblasts from a subset of breast cancer patients with a strong family history may have significantly lower levels of TGFβ1 secretion, which could be implicated in defective paracrine mechanisms leading to excessive proliferation of breast epithelium. The BRCA-1 gene has recently been cloned,[81] and contains a coding sequence of 22 exons which yields a large protein consisting of 1863 amino acids. This may display functional pleiotropism and possess multiple domains, permitting transcriptional control of disparate genes. BRCA-1 appears to function in a tumour-suppressor capacity, and TGFβ is a possible component of effector pathways leading to growth inhibition, Proximal events may differ for sporadic and hereditary-based carcinogenesis, but more distal events may converge towards a final common growth-inhibitory pathway involving TGFβ and cell-cycle regulatory proteins such as the retinoblastoma protein (pRB),[82,83] and modulators of cyclin-dependent protein kinases (e.g. p15).[84,85]

This intrinsic, inherited mesenchymal defect, which is present in all fibroblasts and is manifested as a primary deficiency of TGFβ production/secretion, represents a breakdown of a systemic growth restraint. TGFβ is a central component of one of the principal negative signalling pathways between cells.[86] The formation of gastrointestinal polyps, desmoid tumours and perhaps some forms of familial breast cancer may be viewed as local manifestations of this systemic disorder. According to the above hypothesis, an epithelial tumour would be initiated by local factors, but a stromal defect would promote epithelial proliferation and immortalization. Although the proposed mesenchymal defect is considered to initiate neither gastrointestinal polyps nor indeed malignant transformation, it none the less has a crucial role in the early promotional phases of neoplasia, where subtle changes in the balance of growth factors in the local tissue milieu can influence rogue proliferative activity. The micro-environment of a primary tumour and its micrometastatic foci contains a pool of polypeptide growth factors and other regulatory cytokines which participate in a co-ordinated network of intracellular communication. Whilst some, such as TGFβ, are inhibitory to epithelial proliferation, others such as insulin-like growth factors (IGF-I and IGF-II) are stimulatory. Furthermore, this pool of positive and negative growth factors can be functioning in either an autocrine or a paracrine capacity. It is the balance of these which determines the polarity and intensity of the effective signal delivered to epithelial cells. There is increasing evidence that the malignant phenotype may be associated with a local tissue imbalance of growth factors. Oncogenic events that promote neoplastic progression could involve either an excess of positive growth factors or a deficiency of negative ones such as TGFβ. It remains unresolved whether altered levels of these growth factors are directly implicated in processes of carcinogenesis. However, the pharmacological manipulation of growth factors is a realistic strategy for both treatment of established tumours and prevention of malignancy. Thus boosting of endogenous levels of TGFβ could correct any pre-existing or acquired deficiency, or compensate for over-production of stimulatory growth factors resulting from activation of cellular proto-oncogenes.[87]

Derangements of mesenchymal–epithelial interactions based on aberrant stromal phenotypes could be expoited clinically if the latter permitted induction of inhibitory paracrine growth factors such as TGFβ, or suppression of positive ones. There is evidence that tamoxifen may have a dual action on stromal cells. It may not only stimulate production of TGFβ, but also inhibit production of insulin-like growth factors I and II which are potent mitogens for breast cancer cells,[88,89] and the levels of which can be modulated both locally and systemically by tamoxifen.[90,91] The development of agents which have more potent and specific effects on synthesis and secretion of growth factors from both epithelial and stromal cells constitutes a rational objective for achieving re-regulation of cancer cells. A pre-existing defect in secretion of a negative growth factor such as TGFβ is not necessarily a pre-condition for efficacy of strategies aimed at augmenting local endogenous levels of TGFβ. However, this phenomenon may be dependent on an aberrant stromal phenotype,[52] which if not inherited and systemic could be acquired by local epigenetic phenomena induced by neighbouring epithelial cells.[92]

The following section will consider how this pharmacological modulation of growth factor levels can be optimally accomplished in relation to the type of agent employed and the timing of administration.

THERAPEUTIC POTENTIAL OF ENDOCRINE MANIPULATION

Endocrine therapies in the adjuvant setting have yielded some surprising and unexpected results. First, the efficacy of adjuvant tamoxifen is partially independent of OR status, and secondly, when confounding influences of combined polychemotherapy are taken into account, the benefits of tamoxifen in post-menopausal patients are twice those of chemotherapy, and are similar in OR-positive and OR-negative patients. Furthermore, ovarian ablation in pre-menopausal node-positive patients yields comparable improvements in disease-free and overall survival to polychemotherapy. A more thorough appraisal of these findings suggests that efficacy could be enhanced and morbidity minimized by modifying the clinical application of agents such as tamoxifen and other hormonal agents.

Thus in contrast to advanced disease, the effects of endocrine manipulation in early breast cancer are highly favourable compared to chemotherapy, and triphenylethylenes such as tamoxifen may more effectively target OR-poor tumours by acting through mechanisms which do not depend on simple competitive antagonism for the ligand-binding site of the OR. Thus tamoxifen can induce TGFβ locally, which can act in a negative paracrine manner on breast carcinoma cells irrespective of their OR status. Conversely, adjuvant tamoxifen therapy is associated with a 30% reduction in circulating levels of IGF-I,[90] an effect which is mediated via modulation of growth hormone levels. Similarly, in a rat model, tamoxifen can reduce the expression of IGF-I in tissues which are targets for breast cancer metastases.[91] This reduction occurs in the stromal compartment of tissues,[93] and is partially independent of pituitary function. Therefore tamoxifen can influence both positive and negative paracrine loops by direct effects on stromal cells which do not possess any OR protein. Some OR-negative patients have essentially been denied tamoxifen therapy because of conceptual rationalization based on a false premise.

As we gain greater understanding of the mechanisms of action of functionally pleiotropic agents such as tamoxifen, together with the biological events underlying disordered growth patterns, further improvements in endocrine therapies may be forthcoming. Ironically, some of these advances may derive from maximal exploitation of OR-independent mechanisms of action of the triphenylethylene group of drugs. These may rely upon the triphenylbutene core and not be a feature of the newer pure anti-oestrogens such as ICI 182,780, whose efficacy in individual tumours may be enhanced at the expense of the number of patients who respond to therapy. Furthermore, any serendipitous clinical benefits of triphenylethylenes on bone and the cardiovascular system might be sacrificed with complete loss of any agonist component. Newer triphenylethylenes such as idoxifene may combine selective attenuation of agonist properties with reduced ureterotrophic activity, yet with preservation of beneficial effects on bone density and lipid profile.[94] The new triphenylethylene, raloxifene, which has minimal effects on the uterus, is currently undergoing phase III trials. Chemotherapy schedules based on cytotoxicity are unlikely to modulate levels of growth factors in any consistent and meaningful manner. Rather than selectively enhancing or suppressing secretory function, the primary action of chemotherapeutic agents is to indiscriminately kill cancer cells by dislocating biochemical pathways, interfering with DNA repair processes and inducing 'cell suicide' (apoptosis).

There are two areas where endocrine therapy could be more appropriately applied in order to exploit natural biological phenomena and in turn improve outcome. Both areas relate to the environment of micrometastases and once again are conceptually contained within the paradigm of biological predeterminism.

There is increasing evidence from hitherto retrospective trials that the timing of surgery within the menstrual cycle affects the long-term prognosis of premenopausal women with breast cancer.[95–99] Surgery during the luteal phase appears to be associated with a more favourable outcome, with initial reports suggesting that the magnitude of this effect might exceed that attainable by the use of current adjuvant regimens.[96] It has been proposed that operating during the follicular phase may compromise outcome because unopposed oestrogen affects the cohesiveness of cells, and surgical manipulation during this phase releases viable clonogenic cells into the circulation. It is questionable whether sufficient numbers of viable cells would be released by such a manoeuvre which could subsequently survive within the circulation, escape immune surveillance and establish distant metastases.

Unopposed oestrogen *per se* may be less important than changes in systemic levels of cytokines such as IGF-I, the levels of which could be linked to the menstrual cycle via pituitary function and growth hormone levels. The micrometastatic foci which exist in most cases of early breast cancer will often remain dormant provided that the primary tumour persists *in situ*.[100] The act of surgery itself is far from biologically neutral, and extirpation of tumour bulk, together with the timing of its removal, could perturb a variety of homeostatic mechanisms which include the delicate balance of growth factors within the micro-environment of micrometastatic foci. There may be a surge of positive, stimulatory growth factors such as IGF-I, FGF and TGFα, accompanied by suppression of inhibitory factors such as TGFβ. Fisher demonstrated that serum obtained from mice following excision of a primary tumour could induce a proliferative response when injected into recipient animals with similar tumours to the donor.[101] Recently Anscher's group have reported a reduction in elevated systemic levels of TGFβ in early breast cancer following primary surgical excision of tumour.[102] Moreover, a primary tumour may produce angiostatin, which inhibits angiogenesis in dormant micrometastases. Therefore the net effect of this local perturbation could be to disinhibit the pre-existing metastatic foci, activate microangiogenesis and 'kick-start' these potential secondary deposits into a growth cycle whereby proliferation exceeds apoptosis and increasing tumour volume is sustained without central necrosis by induction of a malignant microvasculature.[99] The limit of tumour growth without new blood vessel formation is approximately 1 million cells, and further growth is dependent on angiogenesis.[104] Cancer cells produce and secrete angiogenic factors which stimulate new vessel formation from normally quiescent capillaries. Fibroblast growth factor is a potent angiogenic factor, and its local release at the site of micrometastases may be one manifestation of the homeostatic disturbance consequent to surgery upon the primary tumour. When the gene coding for this (FGF-4) is transfected into MCF-7 cells, these become hormone independent and can form tumours in nude mice in the absence of oestrogen.[105] There is a correlation between survival and microvessel density of tumours, implying that angiogenesis is an important determinant of tumour evolution.[106,107] Interactions between new blood vessels and tumour cells are critical for tumour growth and metastatic dissemination, with neovascularization potentially increasing the endothelial surface area through which tumour cells can access the circulation. Moreover, an association has been reported between tumour angiogenesis and the number of breast cancer cells that are shed into the venous circulation during surgery.[108] All tumours share a common dependency on an intact blood supply. The biological sequelae of new vessel leakiness probably varies between tumours in different tissue types, and also between different tumours in a particular tissue. Breast cancer typically spreads via the haematogenous route at an early stage in tumour development compared, for example, to colon cancer. It is interesting to speculate on whether this leakiness of blood vessels *per se* confers any obligate tendency for haematogenous dissemination of tumour cells from the primary focus, or whether a combination of enhanced vessel permeability in conjunction with modified expression of extracellular matrix (ECM) proteins determines metastatic potential. Such ECM proteins can influence both cell adhesion and migration of tumour cells. Recently, an innovative approach to these issues has been proposed involving the development of mathematical models which allow computer simulation of tumour angiogenesis.[109,110] These dynamic models of capillary network formation incorporate various paracrine stimuli acting locally within the tissue micro-environment. These include expression of tumour angiogenic factors (TAFs) and 'matrix angiogenic factors' (extracellular matrix proteins and other polypeptide growth factors). A set of partial differential equations enables estimation of probabilities for endothelial cell migration in response to tissue concentration gradients of TAFs and 'matrix angiogenic factors'.[109] So what would be the consequence of interrupting the 'conversation' between cancer cells and endothelial cells? Would it be possible to abort the angiogenic 'kick-start' which heralds the end of dormancy in a nidus of tumour cells? This mathematical model, in conjunction with an integrated expression profile of growth factors, TAFs and ECM proteins within the primary tumour, may allow prediction of the circumstances and timing of this angiogenic 'kick-start'. Such modelling may be of value not only as a predictive factor for micrometastases, but also as a prognostic factor in primary tumours to determine both disease-free and overall survival. Therapeutic approaches might employ antibodies against fibroblast growth factor[111] or peptide antagonists for FGF and vascular endothelial growth factor (VEGF) receptors such as pentosan polysulphate.[105] These could be used as an adjunct in adjuvant schedules where potential synergistic interactions may occur. For example, tamoxifen induces TGFβ locally, which is also a potent inhibitor of endothelial cell growth.[112,113] Furthermore, tamoxifen has been reported to inhibit angiogenesis in a chick chorio-allantoic membrane model.[114] These potential antiangiogenic effects of tamoxifen could be greatly enhanced by concomitant administration of potent and specific anti-angiogenic agents.

This putative cascade of events, which is triggered by the act of surgery and favours the outgrowth of pre-existing micrometastases, is presumed to be of greater significance when surgery is performed in the follicular phase, although a similar series of events is also likely to occur during the luteal phase. However, the physiological

dictates of the hypothalamo–pituitary–gonadal axis may result in higher systemic levels of positive growth factors (IGF-I) and other stimulatory cytokines during the follicular phase. These could amplify the above cascade and thus impart a worse prognosis when surgery is performed during this phase.

According to this scheme of events, outcome could be improved not only by individually adjusting the timing of surgery for patients, but also by priming the host with systemic therapies prior to surgery. These might include anti-hormones, progestins, anti-angiogenic factors or indeed chemotherapy. If the biological underpinning of neoadjuvant regimens is based on the above considerations, then primary endocrine therapies in conjunction with anti-angiogenic factors may be most appropriate. Exposure of a tumour to a neoadjuvant endocrine regimen may alter the biological potential of cancer cells both within the primary tumour and in any concomitant micrometastases. This modified biological potential could manifest itself as a changed secretory profile of cytokines and angiogenic peptides, and offset any systemic perturbation induced by the act of surgery. Although we cannot prejudge the outcome of current trials on the use of neoadjuvant chemo-endocrine therapies for operable breast cancer, it is difficult to conceive mechanistically how administration of a cytotoxic agent to pre-existing micrometastases could have differential efficacy depending on whether it is used in an adjuvant or neoadjuvant capacity. There is some evidence from animal models that primary tumour removal induces a kinetic response with increased proliferative indices in residual distant tumour foci which were considered to represent 'metastases'.[115] This response is greatest on the day of tumour excision, and falls progressively thereafter. Adjuvant chemotherapy could abrogate this kinetic response in a manner which is a function of the interval between tumour removal and time of administration. Interestingly, chemotherapy was most effective in preventing this flare in proliferative index, suppressing growth of residual tumour foci and improving survival when given prior to surgery. This phenomenon could provide a biological rationale for the use of neoadjuvant chemotherapy in operable breast cancer, but it is unknown whether a similar effect in humans will increase overall survival. However, despite these theoretical advantages, early trials of peri-operative chemotherapy employing brief schedules of thiotepa alone or combined with 5-fluorouracil yielded no overall survival advantage.[116] One study showed some benefit of a single peri-operative cycle of CMF in node-negative patients, but conventional post-operative schedules are superior,[117] and no additional benefit is obtained from a combination of peri-operative and post-operative chemotherapy compared to post-operative therapy alone.[118] Should current trials confirm an improved prognosis with neoadjuvant chemotherapy, then this may represent an underlying mechanism.

However, survival advantages from combined chemo-endocrine schedules could be largely attributable to the endocrine component!

Notwithstanding the potential improvements in overall survival which may result from confining surgery to the luteal phase in premenopausal women, there is some justifiable pessimism apropos of immediate prospects for further significant improvements in absolute benefits for breast cancer patients.

Much of the above discussion has pertained to and been embraced within the paradigm of biological predeterminism. Some of the original concepts have been refined in the light of better understanding of the biology of micrometastases and response to various therapies. The issue of whether we should control or kill is not *per se* a paradigm shift in terms of the biology of breast cancer, although it might be viewed as such with respect to the therapeutic goal. Instead, Schipper's ideas represent an evolved paradigm, with the malignant state depicted as a process rather than a morphological entity. Similarly, it is unclear whether the concept of neoadjuvant therapy demands a new paradigm, or if the scientific tenets of neoadjuvism can be incorporated into the existing paradigm of biological predeterminism. Fisher has recently commented of neoadjuvant therapy that 'uncertainty relates to the fact that no new paradigm has been formulated to govern the use of such therapy and to replace the two independent paradigms that currently govern the treatment of breast cancer'.[119]

Recent studies using the new technique of comparative genomic hybridization have revealed that in some human tumours, including those of breast and prostate, up to a quarter of metastatic lesions do not possess the same amplified chromosomal regions that are typically identified in primary lesions.[120] This alludes to clonal evolution and the potential importance of local host factors in determining the precise cellular expression of metastatic foci. Moreover, this may have important consequences for neoadjuvant programmes in which the response of the primary tumour may not faithfully reflect the behaviour of micrometastases. This could seriously undermine strategies which rely on the prediction of prognosis and clinical outcome from short-term changes in proliferative indices within the primary tumour. As pointed out by Schipper, models based on regulatory strategies do not require complete tumour response to achieve 'functional cure', with the implication that a complete response may not be an accurate predictor of overall survival.[47]

Apart from the limitations of adjuvant systemic therapies, there are other reasons for questioning the validity and applicability of the contemporary paradigm, which fails to account for certain aspects of the natural history of breast cancer. In the final section of this chapter we shall highlight these inadequacies, and predict that any further significant advances in treatment outcome are dependent on a true paradigm shift in which our concepts of the biology of breast cancer undergo a revolutionary reappraisal.

These inadequacies of the contemporary model can be summarized as follows.

Extreme latent intervals

The occurrence of metastases many years after primary management of breast cancer is difficult to reconcile with the biological behaviour of cancer cells and known doubling times. It is traditionally considered that cells which are shed prior to diagnosis remain dormant in the resting (G0) phase of the cell cycle and that, upon reactivation, many cells simultaneously enter G1 and commence cycling.

Significance of cutaneous deposits

If local recurrences arise from dormant cells within the dermis, then these must have persisted essentially unchanged, whilst those around them have been replaced several times over.

Distribution of distant metastases

Early experiments by Fisher with labelled red blood cells confirmed that breast cancer cells do not lodge in the first capillary bed they encounter.[19] Pulmonary metastases are relatively uncommon compared to hepatic and bone secondaries. The contemporary model, for which haematogenous dissemination is a basic tenet, cannot explain this observation.

Mathematical models

Cellular heterogeneity, variable growth rates and clonal evolution tend to preclude the construction of reliable and faithful mathematical models. However, such models based on the natural history of breast cancer suggest that metastatic deposits do not necessarily behave in a manner that would be predicted from the characteristics of the primary tumour. Furthermore, the proliferation of cells within these metastatic foci is not consistent with the doubling times observed within the primary tumour.[121,122]

A REVOLUTIONARY CONCEPT

In order to account for the above inconsistencies together with the disappointments of adjuvant systemic therapies, an alternative model has been proposed which represents a true paradigm shift.[123] Micrometastatic foci are not considered to arise exclusively from the preclinical dissemination of clonogenic cells derived directly from and possessing essentially similar characteristics to the primary tumour. In addition to these cellular mechanisms of metastases which constitute the central doctrine of the contemporary paradigm, an alternative mechanism may exist which could account for some instances of distant metastatic foci and late failures of treatment.

Following death by apoptosis of existing cancer cells, discrete fragments of the cellular genome may be released into the circulation and subsequently taken up by 'scavenger' cells of the reticulo-endothelial (RE) system. These lethal packets of genetic material may be passed on not only to other cells of the RE system, but also to normal differentiated host cells by the process of transfection. The genetic software of these host cells subsequently becomes reprogrammed, leading to expression of integrated oncogenic sequences and a breast cancer cell phenotype.[123]

These fragments of genetic material may contain not only oncogenic sequences, but also latent retroviral elements which impart retroviral-like properties. Thus their presence would be detectable by looking for either retroviral sequence homology or reverse transcriptase (RT) activity, which is a marker for retroviruses. Insertional mutagenesis involving integration of novel genetic sequences has been reported in both rodent models and humans.[124,125] These mobile genetic elements contain promoter sequences under whose influence host transcriptional activity can be modified. Retroviral-like sequences termed retro-transposons are the most likely candidates for these genetic inserts, since the latter encode a functional RT and possess 5′ and 3′ long terminal repeat sequences.[126] The mouse mammary tumour virus (MMTV) inserts close to host proto-oncogenes, which are then up-regulated by enhancer sequences present within this provirus.[127,128]

Although a human homologue of MMTV (HuMTV) which behaves as an infectious agent has never been identified, viral-like particles with RT activity have been reported. For example, retroviral-like particles have been detected in monocytes and cell-free conditioned media of breast cancer patients, but not in extant cancer cells.[129] This is consistent with the hypothesis that such particles are a result and not a cause of breast cancer. Unfortunately, the identity of these particles was inconclusive due to failure to distinguish RT activity from that of cellular DNA polymerase. However, the breast cancer cell line T47-D contains a short sequence (9kb) with homology to MMTV,[130] and the production of particles possessing this sequence and a functional RT is up-regulated on exposure to oestrogen and progesterone. Moreover, these purified particles contain an antigen which cross-reacts with antibodies to the MMTV envelope protein gp52.[131] Therefore T47-D cells may contain a retro-transposon or endogenous retroviral element with distant homology to MMTV, which is up-regulated on hormonal stimulation. Although integration of such a sequence is likely to occur randomly within the genome, insertion close to either a proto-oncogene or a tumour

suppressor might be responsible for some transforming events in human breast cancer, and may influence mechanisms of metastasis. Alternatively, basic retroviral-like sequences may be present in latent form within cancer cells (hitherto undetectable) and subsequently become incorporated into retroviral-like particles on cell death and apoptosis. Such latent integrated retroviral sequences would not have any aetiological significance with regard to the primary tumour *per se*. Incorporation may be an incidental event and only assume significance at a later date with formation of these lethal packets of genetic material.

The phenotypic transformation of normal, differentiated host cells following transfection by these retroviral-like particles which contain oncogenic sequences is a key aspect of this revolutionary concept. All cells contain a complete genetic blueprint, but cellular phenotype is determined by the precise pattern of gene expression (i.e. which genes are switched on and which are switched off). Relatively small changes in gene expression can result in dramatic changes in cell morphology and behaviour. Development itself is a process characterized and dictated by spatial and temporal patterns of gene expression. Nuclei from differentiated tissues can direct embryogenesis when they are transplanted into an enucleated ovum.[132] Pluripotentiality of certain stem-cell lines during development illustrates how patterns of gene expression can be influenced by the particular environment and the precise nature of stimuli converging upon a cell. Teratomas are testimony to the ability of a single cell to differentiate along alternative pathways. Perhaps the most compelling evidence to date that human malignancy might be induced by insertion of alien genetic material is the finding that the human immunodeficiency provirus appears to be integrated within a regulatory domain for the c-fcs/fps oncogene of some lymphomas.[133] Possible mechanisms for malignant transformation include insertional mutagenesis, which could either up-regulate an oncogene or mutate a regulatory gene. Alternatively, the virus may have picked up oncogenes which become incorporated with viral DNA.

The uptake of lethal packets of genetic material by fixed cells of the reticulo-endothelial system may be analogous to the uptake and fixation of ink particles from tattooing. Such particles remain fixed at one anatomical point for many years. Genetic information in the form of a construct might be similarly fixed for prolonged periods until transfection of normal host cells occurs. *In-vitro* studies have demonstrated that monocytes can phagocytose cancer cells,[134] and there is some correlation between grade of tumour and infiltration with monocytes.[135] Thus grade might determine prognosis via this alternative mechanism for development of metastases.

The most likely host targets for this transfection process are stromal cells, which occur in most tissues and for which there is evidence of aberrant phenotypic expression in breast cancer patients.[136,137] This aberrant phenotype may confer upon these cells a degree of 'plasticity' which could facilitate such a transfection process by altering surface membrane properties and rendering cells more receptive to alien DNA constructs. Human lung carcinoma cells introduced into mice can result in transfection of host fibroblasts with expression of human DNA sequences and a phenotype characteristic of the original tumour, yet with retention of a mouse karyotype.[138]

It is not suggested that this revolutionary hypothesis should replace the contemporary paradigm. However, it does partly explain some of the clinical observations which are otherwise inconsistent with the contemporary model. The proposed mechanism for development of distant metastases through subcellular transmission of genetic information offers an explanation for the late failure of current therapies and perhaps some of the shortcomings of adjuvant treatments. Indeed, were these mechanisms to obtain, then micrometastatic foci should be targeted with adjuvant antiviral therapies alongside conventional ones. Curiously, tamoxifen has been reported to have an antiviral effect,[139,140] and part of its action may be either to inhibit transmission of these putative virus-like particles in breast cancer patients or to interfere with transfection of host cells by pre-existing constructs fixed locally in tissues.

CONCLUSION

This chapter has outlined the two dominant paradigms which have formed the basis for the management of breast cancer for much of the twentieth century. Just as science is an evolution of ideas, these premises which constitute the contemporary paradigm represent a variable approximation to the truth. At present we cannot claim to understand fully the biological processes which determine the course and behaviour of any individual breast cancer. However, in striving to improve the treatment outcomes for this disease, strategies are devised based on a set of biological hypotheses which are consistent and consonant with laboratory and clinical observations. It appears that, in the majority of cases of breast cancer, the fundamental problem lies outside the breast. It is paradoxical that the treatment of breast cancer according to the false premises of the Halstedian paradigm was clearly defined in surgical terms, and ostensibly curative procedures based on anatomical dictates were more readily achievable. By contrast, it remains unclear how best to deal with disseminated foci of cells which ultimately determine a patient's clinical fate. There are several areas of uncertainty relating to the systemic component (or nature) of breast cancer. Should the therapeutic goal be to eliminate all cancer cells, or to regulate their behaviour such that they can exist symbiotically and without detriment to the host for longer periods of time? By prolonging disease-free survival, it may be possible to achieve a 'personal' cure in a certain proportion of patients,[33] who would thus remain free of symptoms until they succumbed from causes unrelated to breast cancer. This may constitute a more realistic objective than striving for the elusive 'statistical' or 'clinical' cure. What are the most appropriate groups of anti-cancer agents for early breast cancer, and should these be employed singly or in combination (e.g. tamoxifen plus either an anti-angiogenic agent or an aromatase inhibitor)? What criteria should be used for selecting therapies in individual cases, and can the efficacy of a potential adjuvant be partially assessed on the basis of short-term responses of a primary tumour *in situ*? Predictions about these and the related issue of timing of administration are dependent on generated models of breast cancer behaviour and appropriately designed clinical trials. At present there is no model of universal application which can account satisfactorily for all observations. This, together with the limitations of current therapies, suggests that reassessment of the contemporary paradigm is indicated. The clinico-biological heterogeneity of breast cancer may preclude a mono-paradigmatic scenario. Instead, the behaviour of individual breast cancers may be optimally defined by relative orientation within a set of overlapping, interdependent paradigms. Attempts until now to apply one or other paradigm rigidly to all breast tumours may have frustrated further progress. Thus a variety of different agents, including cytotoxic, anti-hormonal, anti-angiogenic and even antiviral agents may each prove of relevance in particular cases. Furthermore, a subset of patients with localized disease may exist for whom adequate loco-regional treatment is curative, and who are unlikely to benefit from adjuvant systemic therapy.

It is perhaps ironic that as we celebrate the centenary of William Halsted, the most important legacy of breast cancer research over this period is the concept of micrometastatic disease. Let us hope that the conquest of these micrometastases becomes a reality in the early years of this new millenium.

REFERENCES

1 Virchow R. *Cellular pathology* (Chance F, trans.) Philadelphia, PA: Lippincott, 1863.
2 Virchow R. *Die Krankhaften Geschwulste*. Berlin: A. Hirschwald, 1863–1873.
3 Muller J. *Uber den feinern Bau und die Formen der Krankhaften Geschwulste*. Berlin: Reimer, 1838.
4 Gilchrist RK, David VC. Lymphatic spread of carcinoma of the rectum. *Ann Surg* 1938; **108**: 621–4.
5 Drinker CE, Field ME, Ward HK. The filtering capacity of lymph nodes. *J Exp Med* 1934; **62**: 339–405.
6 Buckman CA, Stahl WM Jr. Cell trapping by lymph nodes. *Surg Forum* 1963; **14**: 116–18.
7 Engeset A. Barrier function of lymph glands. *Lancet* 1962; **i**: 324.

8 Halsted WS. The radical operation for the cure of carcinoma of the breast. *Johns Hopkins Hosp Rep* 1898; **28**: 557.

9 Wangensteen OH. Remarks on extension of the Halsted operation for cancer of the breast. *Ann Surg* 1949; **130**: 315.

10 Halsted WS. The results of operations for the cure of cancer of the breast performed at the Johns Hopkins Hospital from June 1889 to January 1894. *Johns Hopkins Hosp Rep* 1894–5; **4**: 297–350.

11 Baum M. The history of breast cancer. In: Forbes JF (ed.) *Breast disease*. Edinburgh: Churchill Livingston, 1986: 95–105.

12 Brinkley D, Haybittle JL. The curability of breast cancer. *Lancet* 1973; **2**: 95–8.

13 Bloom HJG, Richardson WW, Harries EJ. Natural history of untreated breast cancer (1805–1933). Comparison of untreated and treated cases according to histological grade of malignancy. *BMJ* 1962; **i**: 213–21.

14 Gershon-Cohen J, Berger SM, Klickstein HS. Roentgenography of breast cancer moderating concept of 'biological predeterminism'. *Cancer* 1963; **16**: 961–4.

15 Fisher B. Laboratory and clinical research in breast cancer – a personal adventure: the David A. Karnofsky Memorial Lecture. *Cancer Res* 1980; **40**: 3863–74.

16 Fisher B, Fisher ER. Transmigration of lymph nodes by tumour cells. *Science* 1966; **152**: 1397–8.

17 Fisher B, Fisher ER. Barrier function of lymph node to tumour cells and erythrocytes I. Normal nodes. *Cancer* 1967; **20**: 1907–13.

18 Fisher B, Fisher ER. Barrier function of lymph node to tumour cells and erythrocytes II. Effect of X-ray, inflammation, sensitisation and tumour growth. *Cancer* 1967; **20**: 1914–19.

19 Fisher B, Fisher ER. The organ distribution of dissemination of ^{51}C-labelled tumour cells. *Cancer Res* 1967; **27**: 412–20.

20 Keynes G. Conservative treatment of cancer of the breast. *BMJ* 1937; **ii**: 643–7.

21 Atkins H, Hayward JL, Klugman DJ, Wayte AB. Treatment of early breast cancer: a report after 10 years of a clinical trial. *BMJ* 1972; **2**: 423–9.

22 Hayward JL. Prospective studies: the Guy's Hospital trials on breast conservation. In: Harris JR, Hellman S, Silen WJB (eds). *Conservative management of breast cancer*. Philadelphia, PA: J.B. Lippincott.

23 Fisher B, Redmond C, Poisson R *et al.* Eight-year results of a randomised clinical trial comparing total mastectomy and lumpectomy with or without irradiation in the treatment of breast cancer. *N Engl J Med* 1989; **320**: 822–7.

24 Veronesi U, Saccozzi R, Del Vecchio M *et al.* Comparing radical mastectomy with quadrantectomy, axillary dissection and radiotherapy in patients with small cancers of the breast. *N Engl J Med* 1981; **305**: 6–11.

25 Sarrazin D, Dewar JA, Arriagada R *et al.* Conservative management of breast cancer. *Br J Surg* 1986; **73**: 604–6.

26 van Dongen E. *Breast-conserving therapy in operable breast cancer*. EORTC Working Conference on Breast Cancer. 1–3 July 1987, London.

27 Fisher B, Fisher ER, Redmond C. Ten-year results from the National Surgical Adjuvant Breast and Bowel Project (NSABP) clinical trial evaluating the use of L-phenylalanine mustard (L-PAM) in the management of primary breast cancer. *J Clin Oncol* 1986; **4**: 929–41.

28 Fisher B, Slack N, Katrych D, Wolmark N. Ten-year follow-up results of patients with carcinoma of the breast in a co-operative clinical trial evaluating surgical adjuvant chemotherapy. *Surg Gynaecol Obstet* 1975; **140**: 528–34.

29 Early Breast Cancer Trialists' Collaborative Group. Systemic treatment of early breast cancer by hormonal, cytotoxic or immune therapy. 133 randomised trials involving 31 000 recurrences and 24 000 deaths among 75 000 women. *Lancet* 1992; **339**: 1–15, 71–5.

30 Early Breast Cancer Trialists' Collaborative Group. Oxford Meeting, September 1995. *Lancet* (submitted).

31 Devitt J. Breast cancer: have we missed the forest because of the tree? *Lancet* 1994; **344**: 734–5.

32 Hayward J. *Controversies in breast cancer management*. Eighth International Congress on Senology, May 1994, Rio de Janeiro, Brazil.

33 Haybittle JL. Curability of breast cancer. *Br Med Bull* 1990; **47**: 319–23.

34 Todd JH, Dowle C, Williams MR *et al.* Confirmation of a prognostic index in primary breast cancer. *Br J Cancer* 1987; **56**: 489–92.

35 Haywood J, Caleffi M. The significance of local control in the primary treatment of breast cancer. *Arch Surg* 1987; **122**: 1244.

36 Harris J, Osteen R. Patients with early breast cancer benefit from effective axillary treatment. *Breast Cancer Res Treat* 1985; **5**: 17.

37 Overgaard M, Hansen PS, Overgaard J *et al.* Post-operative radiotherapy in high-risk pre-menopausal women with breast cancer who receive adjuvant chemotherapy. *N Engl J Med* 1997; **337**: 949–55.

38 Ragaz J, Jackson SM, Le N *et al.* Adjuvant radiotherapy and chemotherapy in node-positive pre-menopausal women with breast cancer. *N Engl J Med* 1997; **337**: 956–62.

39 Hellman S. Stopping metastases at their source (editorial). *N Engl J Med* 1997; **337**: 996–7.

40 Benson JR. The biology of breast cancer and its relevance to screening and treatment. In: Morgan M, Warren R, Querci Della Rovere U (eds). *Breast screening and management of early breast cancer*.

41 Querci Della Rovere G, Benson JR, Warren R. Screening for breast cancer, time to think – and stop? (letter). *Lancet* 1995; **346**: 437.

42 Shapiro S, Venet W, Strax P, Venet L, Roeser R. Ten- to fourteen-year effect of screening on breast cancer mortality. *J Natl Cancer Inst* 1982; **69**: 349.

43 Tabar L, Fagerberg CJG, Gad A *et al.* Reduction in mortality from breast cancer after mass screening with mammography. *Lancet* 1985; **i**: 829.

44 Makris A, Powles TJ, Dowsett M *et al.* Changes in proliferation in primary breast cancer during chemoendocrine therapy. *Eur J Cancer* 1995; **31A** (**Supplement 5**): 137.

45 Baum M. *The Times*. August 1995.

46 Pierce GB, Spiers WC. Tumours as caricatures of the process of tissue renewal: prospects for therapy by directing differentiation. *Cancer Res* 1988; **48**: 1996–2004.

47 Schipper H, Goh C, Wang TL. Re-thinking cancer: should we control rather than kill ? Part I. *Can J Oncol* 1993; **3**: 207–16.

48 Schipper H, Goh C, Wang TL. Re-thinking cancer: should we control rather than kill ? Part II. *Can J Oncol* 1993; **3**: 220–24.

49 Schipper H. Shifting the cancer paradigm: must we kill to cure ? (editorial). *J Clin Oncol* 1995; **13**: 801–7.

50 Fisher B, Saffer E, Fisher ER. Studies concerning the regional nodes in cancer. IV. Tumour inhibition by regional lymph node cells. *Cancer* 1974; **33**: 631–6.

51 Fisher B, Saffer E, Fisher ER. Studies concerning the regional nodes in cancer. VII. Thymidine uptake by cells from nodes of breast cancer patients. *Cancer* 1974; **33**: 271–9.

52 Benson JR, Baum M. Breast cancer, desmoid tumours and familial adenomatous polyposis coli– a unifying hypothesis. *Lancet* 1993; **342**: 848–50, 1561.

53 Nolvadex Adjuvant Trial Organisation. Controlled trial of tamoxifen as a single adjuvant agent in the management of early breast cancer. *Br J Cancer* 1988; **57**: 608–11.

54 Medical Research Council Scottish Trials Office. Adjuvant tamoxifen in the management of operable breast cancer. *Lancet* 1987; **ii**: 171–5.

55 Colletta AA, Wakefield LM, Howell FV *et al.* Anti-oestrogens induce the secretion of active transforming growth factor beta from human foetal fibroblasts. *Br J Cancer* 1990; **62**: 405–9.

56 Benson JR, Wakefield LM, Baum M, Colletta AA. Synthesis and secretion of TGFβ isoforms by primary cultures of human breast tumour fibroblasts *in vitro* and their modulation by tamoxifen. *Br J Cancer* 1996; **74**: 352–8.

57 Butta A, Maclennan K, Flanders KC *et al.* Induction of transforming growth factor beta₁ in human breast cancer *in vivo* following tamoxifen treatment. *Cancer Res* 1992; **52**: 4261–4.

58 MacAdam WAF, Goligher JC. The occurrence of desmoids in patients with familial polyposis coli. *Br J Surg* 1970; **57**: 618–31.

59 Cunha GR, Donjacour A. Stromal–epithelial interactions in normal and abnormal prostatic development. *Prog Clin Biol Res* 1987; **239**: 259–72.

60 Cunha GR, Bigsby RM, Cooke PS, Sugimura Y. Stromal–epithelial interactions in adult organs. *Cell Differ* 1985; **17**: 137–48.

61 Shannon JM, Cunha GR. Characterisation of androgen binding sites and DNA synthesis in prostate-like structures induced in testicular feminised mice. *Biol Reprod* 1984; **31**: 175–83.

62 Horgan K, Jones DL, Mansel RE. Mitogenicity of human fibroblasts *in vivo* for human breast cancer cells *Br J Cancer* 1987; **74**: 227–9.

63 von Roozendaal CEP, van Ooijen B, Klijn JGM *et al.* Stromal influences on breast cancer cell growth. *Br J Cancer* 1992; **65**: 77–81.

64 Mukaida H, Hirabayashi N, Hirai T, Iwata T, Saeki S, Toge T. Significance of freshly cultured fibroblasts from different tissues in promoting cancer cell growth. *Int J Cancer* 1991; **48**: 423–7.

65 Ryan MC, Orr DJA, Horgan K. Fibroblast stimulation of breast cancer cell growth in a serum-free system. *Br J Cancer* 1993; **67**: 1268–73.

66 Adams EF, Newton CJ, Braunsberg H, Shaikh N, Ghilchick M, James VHT. Effects of human breast fibroblasts on growth and 17β oestradiol dehydrogenase activity of MCF-7 cells in culture. *Breast Cancer Res Treat* 1988; **11**: 165–72.

67 Cooper M, Pinkus H. Intra-uterine transplantation of rat basal cell carcinoma; a model for reconversion of malignant to benign growth. *Cancer Res* 1977; **37**: 2544–52.

68 Richman PI, Bodmer W. Control of differentiation in human colorectal carcinoma lines: epithelial–mesenchymal interactions. *J Pathol* 1988; **156**: 197–211.

69 Roberts AB, Sporn MB. The transforming growth factor betas. In: Sporn MB, Roberts AB (eds). *Peptide growth factors and their receptors. Handbook of experimental pharmacology. Vol. 95*. Heidelberg: Springer Verlag, 1990: 419–72.

70 Massague J. The transforming growth factor β family. *Annu Rev Cell Biol* 1990; **6**: 597–641.

71 Roberts AB, Anzano MA, Wakefield LM, Roche NS, Stern DF, Sporn MB. Type β–transforming growth factor: a bifunctional regulator of cellular growth. *Proc Natl Acad Sci USA* 1985; **82**: 119–23.

72 Tucker RF, Shipley GD, Moses HL, Holley RW. Growth inhibitor from BSC–1 cells is closely related to the platelet type β transforming growth factor. *Science* 1984; **226**: 705–7.

73 Arteaga CL, Tandon AK, Von Hoff DD, Osborne CK. Transforming growth factor β: potential autocrine growth inhibitor of oestrogen receptor negative human breast cancer cells. *Cancer Res* 1988; **48**: 3898–904.

74 Roberts AB, Anzano MA, Lamb LC, Smith JM, Sporn MB. New class of transforming growth factors potentiated by epidermal growth factor: isolation from non-neoplastic tissues. *Proc Natl Acad Sci USA* 1981; **78**: 5339–43.

75 Brookes MD, Ebbs SR, Colletta AA, Baum M. Desmoid tumours treated with triphenylethylenes. *Eur J Cancer* 1992; **28**: 1014–18.

76 Manning AM, Williams AC, Game SM, Paraskeva C. Differential sensitivity of human colonic adenoma and carcinoma cells to transforming growth factor beta: conversion of an adenoma cell line to a tumorigenic phenotype is accompanied by a reduced response to the inhibitory effects of TGFβ. *Oncogene* 1993: **6**: 1471–7.

77 Okamoto M, Sato Ch, Kohno Y *et al.* Molecular nature of chromosome 5q loss in colorectal tumours and desmoids from patients with familial adenomatous polposis. *Hum Genet* 1990; **85**: 595–9.

78 Nishisho I, Nakamura Y, Miyoshi Y *et al.* Mutations of chromosome 5q21 genes in FAP and colorectal cancer patients. *Science* 1991; **253**: 665–9.

79 Knudson AG Jr. Genetics of human cancer. *Annu Rev Genetics* 1986; **20**: 231–51.

80 Jouin H, Baumann R, Derlon A, Varra A *et al.* Is there an increased incidence of adenomatous polyps in breast cancer patients? *Cancer* 1989; **63**: 599–603.

81 Miki Y, Swensen J, Shattuck Eidens D *et al.* A strong candidate for the breast and ovarian cancer susceptibility gene BRCA-1. *Science* 1994; **266**: 66–71.

82 DeCaprio JA, Ludlow JW, Lynch D *et al.* The product of the retinoblastoma susceptibility gene has properties of a cell cycle regulatory element. *Cell* 1989; **58**: 1085–95.

83 Laiho M, De Caprio JA, Ludlow JW, Livingston DM, Massague J. Growth inhibition by TGFβ linked to suppression of retinoblastoma protein phosphorylation. *Cell* 1990; **62**: 175–85.

84 Sherr CJ. Mammalian G1 cyclins. *Cell* 1993; **73**: 1059–65.

85 Hannon GJ, Beach D. p15 INK4B is a potent effector of transforming growth factor β-induced cell cycle arrest. *Nature* 1994; **371**: 257–61.

86 Benson JR, Wells K. Microsatellite instability and a TGFβ receptor: clues to a growth control pathway. *Bioessays* 1995; **17**.

87 Benson JR, Colletta AA. Transforming growth factor β: prospects for cancer prevention and treatment. *Clin Immunotherapeutics* 1995; **4**: 249–58.

88 Myall Y, Shiu RPC, Bhaumick B. Receptor binding and growth-promoting activity of insulin-like growth factors in human breast cancer cells (T47-D) in culture. *Cancer Res* 1984; **44**: 5486–490.

89 Karey KP, Sirbasku DA. Differential responsiveness of human breast cancer cell lines MCF-7 and T47-D to growth factors and 17β-oestradiol. *Cancer Res* 1988; **48**: 4083–92.

90 Pollak M, Huynh HT, Pratt Lefebre S. Tamoxifen reduces serum insulin-like growth factor I (IGF I). *Breast Cancer Res Treat* 1992; **22**: 91–100.

91 Huynh HT, Tetenes E, Wallace L, Pollak M. *In vivo* inhibition of insulin-like growth factor I gene expression by tamoxifen. *Cancer Res* 1993; **53**: 1727–30.

92 Schor SL, Schor AM, Howell A, Crowther D. Hypothesis: persistent expression of fetal phenotypic characteristics by fibroblasts is associated with an increased susceptibility to neoplastic disease. *Exp Cell Biol* 1987; **55**: 11–17.

93 Pollak M. *The challenge of breast cancer*. Lancet Conference, Brugge, 1994.

94 Chander SK, McCaque R, Luqmani Y *et al.* Pyrrolidino-4-iodotamoxifen and 4-iodotamoxifen: new analogues of the antiestrogen tamoxifen for the treatment of breast cancer. *Cancer Res* 1991; **51**: 5851–8.

95 Hrushesky W, Bluming A, Gruber S, Sothern RB. Menstrual influence on the surgical cure of breast cancer. *Lancet* 1989; **2**: 949–52.

96 Badwe RA, Gregory WM, Chaudary MA *et al.* Timing of surgery during the menstrual cycle and survival of premenopausal women with operable breast cancer. *Lancet* 1989; **i**: 1261–4.

97 Senie R, Rosen P, Rhodes P, Lesser ML. Timing of breast cancer excision during the menstrual cycle influences duration of disease-free survival. *Ann Intern Med* 1991; **115**: 337–42.

98 Sainsbury R, Jones M, Parker D, Hall R, Close H. Timing of surgery for breast cancer (letter). *Lancet* 1991; **338**: 392.

99 Veronesi U, Luini A, Mariani L *et al.* Effect of menstrual phase on surgical treatment of breast cancer. *Lancet* 1994; **343**: 1545–7.

100 Folkman J. Angiogenesis in cancer, vascular, rheumatoid and other disease. *Nature Med* 1995; **1**: 27.

101 Fisher B, Gunduz N, Coyle J, Rudock C, Saffer EA. Presence of a growth-stimulating factor in serum following primary tumor removal in mice. *Cancer Res* 1989; **49**: 1996–2001.

102 Kong F-M, Anscher MS, Murase T, Abbott BD, Iglehart JD, Jirtle RL. Elevated plasma transforming growth factor β1 levels in breast cancer decrease following surgical removal of the tumour. *Ann Surg* 1995; **222**: 155–62.

103 Folkman J. Tumour angiogenesis. In: Mendelsohn J, Howley P, Liotta L, Israel M (eds) *The molecular basis of cancer*. Philadelphia, PA: W.B. Saunders Company, 0000: 00–00.

104 Folkman J. What is the evidence that tumours are angiogenesis dependent? *J Natl Cancer Inst* 1990; **82**: 4–6.

105 Lippman ME. *New approaches in diagnosing and treating breast cancer*. Conference organized by Cambridge Healthtech Institute, Philadelphia, PA, November 1994.

106 Weidner N, Semple JP, Welch WR, Folkman J. Tumour angiogenesis and metastasis – correlation in invasive breast carcinoma. *N Engl J Med* 1991; **324**: 1–8.

107 Horak E, Leek R, Klewk N *et al.* Angiogenesis assessed by platelet/endothelial cell adhesion molecule antibodies, as indicator of node metastases and survival in breast cancer. *Lancet* 1992; **340**: 1120–24.

108 McCulloch P, Choy A, Martin L. Association between tumour angiogenesis and tumour cell shedding into effluent venous blood during breast cancer surgery. *Lancet* 1995; **346**: 1334–5.

109 Chaplain M, Baum M, Anderson A, Douek M, Vaidya J. Non-linear mathematical modelling of breast cancer angiogenesis: present and future clinical implications.

110 Bonn D. Bringing numbers to bear in breast cancer therapy. *Lancet* 1997; **350**: 1304.

111 Hori A, Sasada R, Matsutani E *et al.* Suppression of solid tumour growth by immuno-neutralising monoclonal antibody against fibroblast growth factor. *Cancer Res* 1991; **51**: 6180–4.

112 Shultz GS, Grant MB. Neovascular growth factors. *Eye* 1991; **5**: 178–80.

113 Heimark RL, Twardzik DR, Schwartz SM. Inhibition of endothelial regeneration by type-β transforming growth factor from platelets. *Science* 1986; **233**: 1078–80.

114 Gagliardi A, Collins DC. Inhibition of angiogenesis by anti-oestrogens. *Cancer Res* 1993; **53**: 533–5.

115 Fisher B, Gunduz N, Saffer EA. Influence of the interval between primary tumour removal and chemotherapy on kinetics and growth of metastases. *Cancer Res* 1983; **43**: 1488–92.

116 Fisher B, Ravdin RG, Ausman RK *et al*. Surgical adjuvant chemotherapy in cancer of the breast: results of a decade of co-operative investigation. *Ann Surg* 1968; **168**: 337–56.

117 Ludwig Breast Cancer Study Group. Combination adjuvant chemotherapy for node positive breast cancer: inadequacy of a single post-operative cycle. *N Engl J Med* 1988; **319**: 677.

118 Sertoli MR, Pronzato P, Rubagotti A *et al*. Peri-operative polychemotherapy for primary breast cancer: a randomised study. *Proc ASCO* 1991; **10**: 48.

119 Fisher B. Preoperative chemotherapy: a model for studying the biology and therapy of primary breast cancer. *J Clin Oncol* 1995; **13**: 537–40.

120 Kallioniemi O-P. A molecular view of cancer progression (EACR Award Lecture). *Eur J Cancer* 1995; **31A (Supplement 5)**: 95.

121 Henderson IC. Biological variations of tumours. *Cancer* 1992; **69**: 1888–95.

122 Retsky MW, Swartzendruber DE, Wardwell RH *et al*. Is Gompertzian or exponential kinetics a valid description of individual human cancer growth? *Med Hypotheses* 1990; **33**: 95–106.

123 Baum M, Colletta AA. Breast cancer: a revolutionary concept. *Breast Cancer* 1994; **2**: 9–18.

124 Leslie KB, Lee F, Schrader JW. Intracisternal A-type particle-mediated activations of cytokine genes in a murine myelomonocytic leukemia: generation of functional cytokine mRNAs by retroviral splicing events. *Mol Cell Biol* 1991; **11**: 5562–70.

125 Kazazian HH, Wong C, Yousouffian H, Scott AF, Phillips DG, Antonarakis SE. Haemophilia A resulting from *de novo* insertion of L1 sequences represents a novel mechanism for mutation in man. *Nature* 1988; **332**: 164–6.

126 Shimotohno K, Mitzutani S, Temin H. Sequence of retrovirus resembles that of bacterial transposable elements. *Nature* 1980; **285**: 550–4.

127 Nusse R, Van-Ooyen A, Cox D, Fung YK, Varmus H. Mode of pro-viral activation of a putative mammary oncogene (*int*–1) on mouse chromosome 15. *Nature* 1984; **307**: 131–6.

128 Dickson C, Smith R, Brookes S, Peters G. Tumorigenesis by mouse mammary tumour virus: pro-viral activation of a cellular gene in the common integration region *int*-2. *Cell* 1984; **37**: 529–36.

129 Al-Sumidaie AM, Leinster SJ, Hart CA, Green CD, McCarthy K. Particles with properties of retroviruses in monocytes from patients with breast cancer. *Lancet* 1988; **ii**: 5–9.

130 Ono M, Kawakami M, Ushikubo H. Stimulation of expression of the human endogenous retrovirus genome related to the mouse mammary tumour virus. *J Virol* 1987; **61**: 2059–62.

131 Segev N, Hizi A, Kirenberg F, Keydar I. Characterisation of a protein released by the T47-D cell line, immunologically related to the major envelope glycoprotein of mouse mammary tumor virus. *Proc Natl Acad Sci USA* 1985; **82**: 1531–5.

132 Gurdon JB. Nuclear transplantation in eggs and oocytes. *J Cell Sci* 1986; **4 (Supplement)**: 287–318.

133 Shiramizu B, Herndier BG, McGrath MS. Identification of a common clonal immunodeficiency virus integration site in human immunodeficiency virus-associated lymphomas. *Cancer Res* 1994; **54**: 2069–72.

134 Munn DH, Nai-Kong V, Cheung. Phagocytosis of tumour cells by human monocytes cultured in recombinant macrophage colony-stimulating factor. *J Exp Med* 1990; **172**: 231–7.

135 Naukkarinen A, Syrjanen KJ. Quantitative immunohistochemical analysis of mononuclear infiltrates in breast carcinomas: correlation with tumour differentiation. *J Pathol* 1990; **160**: 271–82.

136 Haggie JA, Sellwood RA, Howel A, Birch JM, Schor SL. Fibroblasts from relatives of patients with hereditary breast cancer show foetal-like behaviour *in vitro*. *Lancet* 1987; **i**: 1455–7.

137 Shor SL, Haggie JA, Durning P et al. Occurrence of a foetal fibroblast phenotype in familial breast cancer. *Int J Cancer* 1986; **37**: 831–6.

138 Gupta V, Rajaraman S, Gadson P, Constanzi JJ. Primary transfection as a mechanism for transfection of host cells by human tumour cells implanted in nude mice. *Cancer Res* 1987; **47**: 5194–202.

139 Vennin PH, Gougeon E, Azab M. Antiviral response to tamoxifen. *Lancet* 1992; **340**: 798.

140 Benson JR, Baum M. Antiviral effect of tamoxifen. *Lancet* 1993; **341**: 1288.

3

Biochemical and biological markers of breast cancer progression

ANTHONY LEATHEM, SUSAN A BROOKS AND UDO SCHUMACHER

INTRODUCTION

The behaviour of breast cancer may change during the natural history of the disease, and the tumour heterogeneity allows many factors to influence this.[1] Although numerous predictive and prognostic markers have been described, with the exception of lymph-node status no widely accepted markers for metastasis or progression are available. The Nottingham prognostic index, a product of primary cancer size, grade and node status, continues to have a higher predictive value than any isolated tumour markers, and the addition of more objective measures such as S-phase may help.[2-5] Variation between laboratories makes the value of many biochemical markers (even CEA and CA 15-3) unclear, but biological markers, including racial, geographical, diet and lifestyle factors are likely to have a role in predicting progression and future interventions. They may further identify risks for variable outcome groups – for example, identifying which women with DCIS or with BRCA1/2 mutations will or will not develop invasive cancer. However, because the behaviour of breast cancer can change, a single marker is unlikely to be a reliable long-term predictor, and even accurately predicting metastasis may not predict survival. For example, the number of positive nodes generally relates to outcome,[6] but some patients with 20 or more positive nodes are still alive 10 years later and, conversely, one-third of patients who are histologically node negative develop distant recurrences. Biopsy of the sentinel node (see below) holds great promise for increasing the sensitivity and specificity of detection of metastasis, whilst also being less invasive than axillary dissection.

Biochemical tumour markers mainly reflect tumour mass and differentiation (e.g. CEA and CA 15-3, and other mucin-related markers) or tumour kinetics (e.g. SPF, Ki67, KiS1, PCNA, TK, TPS; see below). Tumour growth is related to differentiation, proliferation and probably apoptosis, and therefore many markers are linked to these processes. An anomaly may result from using many biochemical markers (e.g. those detected by polymerase chain reaction (PCR) and immunohistochemistry in the primary cancer), because patient outcome, particularly response to chemotherapy or hormone therapy and progression, is determined by the metastases. We need to identify new, independent markers directly related to metastases, progression and treatment, or to environmental influences on these. Biological markers (e.g. dietary, socio-economic and geographical factors) are more difficult to identify, and evaluation of these is needed. Some of these markers, while not being of direct benefit to patients, may help us to understand the steps in metastasis and progression. Ideally, markers will help to tailor management of the individual patient. Towards this end, the recent enthusiasm and huge investment in Herceptin® (from Genentech), a promising new monoclonal antibody treatment against the epidermal growth factor receptor HER2 or c-erbB-2,[7-10] highlight the need for a suitable method to identify the 25% of patients whose cancer cells overexpress HER2 or c-erbB-2, and who may benefit from antibody treatment.

Most of the biological, biochemical and pathological markers described here have been developed over the past 5 years, and while many others have been described, few of them show independent value over more reliable standard predictive or prognostic markers.

PATHOLOGY

Apoptosis

Apoptosis, or programmed cell death, is likely to exert a strong influence on tumour progression. Identification of apoptotic cells relies largely on detection of DNA breakdown apoptotic changes, including deoxyribonucleic acid (DNA) laddering patterns on agarose gel electrophoresis and *in-situ* end labelling (ISEL) of fragmented DNA for quantitative apoptotic body determination. Other approaches use antibodies to a protein thought to prevent apoptosis, namely Bcl-2. The death of tumour cells would seem to be an important marker for assessing tumour progression. In a study of apoptosis by DNA strand breaks in fine-needle aspiration biopsies including 11 breast cancers,[11] apoptosis was found to be more common in tumour cells than in normal cells of the same organ, but follow-up studies are needed.

Proliferation

The best single marker (or panel of markers) for cell kinetics has not yet been established. Gasparini et al.,[12] comparing S-phase fraction (SPF), Ki67 and proliferating cell nuclear antigen (PCNA, using PC10 antibody), found the S-phase fraction determined by flow cytometry to be the strongest cell-kinetics marker for overall and disease-free survival. KiS1 is a monoclonal antibody that recognizes a cell-cycle-associated antigen in paraffin sections. A total of 142 cases of stage I and II cancers showed an association between positive staining and poorer prognosis, disease-free survival (P<0.001), overall survival (P<0.001) and post-relapse survival (P=0.008).[13] Semi-quantitative assessment yielded similar results to a more time-consuming quantitative method.

Horiguchi and colleagues[14] found that positive PCNA staining was associated with a significantly worse overall survival. By combining DNA cytometry to assess diploid/aneuploid populations with PCNA, Schimmelpenning found a direct association between PCNA expression and DNA aneuploidy, and reported that tumours which showed a near diploid population with high proliferative activity displayed rapid tumour progression.[15]

Gillett and co-workers compared three cell-cycle-associated antigens using two antibodies to PCNA (PC10 and 19A2) and KiS1 against other established markers,[16] and found that only KiS1 correlated with the S-phase fraction (P<0.001), and that staining by the two PCNA antibodies did not correspond to proliferative activity. Likewise, Betta and colleagues, using PC10 to assess PCNA, were unable to demonstrate prognostic usefulness.[17] Stanton et al., analysing DNA ploidy and the S-phase fraction by flow cytometry of nuclei from paraffin sections of stage I and II patients with at least 8 years of follow-up, were unable to obtain prognostic information.[18] Botti et al., in a study of 25 advanced breast carcinomas, did not find a high PCNA score to be significant in predicting chemosensitivity.[19]

Methodology may also be important. Yuan et al.,[20] in a comparative study of cell image analysis vs. flow cytometry on paraffin blocks from 101 node-negative cancers, found that cell-image analysis gave more sensitive information than flow cytometry on DNA content and detection of aneuploidy, but lacked the specificity of flow cytometry in correlation with clinical outcome.

Angiogenesis

In several cancers, quantification of new vessel growth appears to be a useful independent prognostic factor. However, for breast cancers the value is still uncertain, perhaps due to the heterogeneity of breast cancers added to the difficulties in quantitation and reproducibility. Fox et al. have described a rapid method which they consider gives independent prognostic information,[21] but Siitonen et al. could not find a helpful association between clinical outcome and microvessels (detected by antisera to CD34 and von Willebrand factor),[22] nor could Axelsson et al.[23] or Tynninen et al.[24] Mayers et al.,[25] in a study using an antibody to CD31 on 519 patients with a median 71-month follow-up for node-negative patients, found no association between vascularity, relapse or death. However, they did find an association for node-positive patients, but not an independent one. Kumar et al.,[26] comparing anti CD34 (pan-endothelial) with a new antibody CD105 (to endothelial cells in angiogenic tissue), did not find an association between CD34 and recurrence or survival, but did find such an association for CD105. The value of detecting new vessels, and the best antibodies for this, remain unclear.

Tumour bed biopsy and margins

Objective information on the behaviour of cancers, in addition to lymph-node histology, may be obtained from the breast at the time of initial surgery by examination of the cavity wall or tumour bed after tumour excision for residual cancer. However, this may be more closely related to local recurrence than to survival. Histological examination of bed biopsies taken at lumpectomy[27] showed residual tumour in 27% of 117 patients with early breast cancer. After 3.5 years, 85% of women with negative biopsies were alive, compared to 62% of those with positive biopsies. When evaluating this together with nodal status, a group identified as positive for both risk factors was found to have 35.5% disease-free survival, compared to 95.7% for those with neither risk factor (P<0.01). A significant proportion of patients are likely to have positive margins, and Macmillan et al. reported residual cancer in cavity wall biopsies of 38% of 264 patients following lumpectomy for stage I and II cancers.[28] Presumably positive biopsies show objective evidence of possibly more aggressive biological behaviour. In a study of 289 women, excision margin status appeared to be the most significant determinant of local recurrence following lumpectomy and radiation therapy[29]. In a study of 453 patients with stage I/II cancers,[30] 86 patients (19%) had microscopically positive margins and, comparing negative with positive cases, at 10 years these had 82% vs. 71% disease-free survival and 84% vs. 78% overall survival, suggesting that bed biopsy growth and metastases may behave differently.

S-phase

The S-phase fraction (SPF) provides a useful, if crude, independent estimate of the percentage of cells that are undergoing active cell division, and a high S-phase fraction is generally associated with progression.[31,32] It probably provides a more objective score than nuclear grade, which does require some experience.

In 83 cancers with a median follow-up of 45.6 months, it was closely correlated with KiS1 staining ($P<0.0001$) and recurrence.[33] It appears to be particularly useful for identifying high risk of recurrence in early-stage/node-negative patients.[34–36] However, it is also described as identifying the likely response to chemotherapy in stage II and IIIa patients.[32]

Sentinel lymph-node biopsy

The sentinel node is identified, by injecting dye or radioactive tracer into or around the cancer, as the first node draining a primary invasive cancer. 'Skip' metastases are occasionally noted,[37] in which the sentinel node is negative, and this is particularly disturbing as these may be nodes that have been replaced by cancer. Veronesi et al. found that the sentinel node predicted axillary node status accurately in 97.5% (156 of 160) of patients, and in 38% of cases it was the only positive node.[38] There has been a flood of enthusiasm for this new tool, partly driven by the public, and of publications relating to it.[39–42]

The increased sensitivity of detection of metastasis by concentrating on the sentinel node, with reduced morbidity as a result of avoidance of axillary disection, should increase the value of nodal staging.

BIOCHEMICAL MARKERS OF TISSUE AND SERUM

Carcinoembryonic antigen (CEA)

Carcinoembryonic antigen (CEA) continues its long run in monitoring serum levels, although many papers have shown CA 15-3 to be more sensitive in detecting breast cancer progression than CEA. It is commonly used in tandem with CA 15-3 for follow-up aimed at detection of

relapse (e.g. the studies by Molina et al.,[43] who found a specificity of 99% for both CEA and CA 15-3, and Al-Jarallah et al.[44] The Nottingham group in the UK have used CEA together with CA 15-3 and ESR to evaluate the response to chemotherapy or to a change of therapy,[45] introducing a new index system to select treatment responders.

Tissue polypeptide-specific antigen (TPS)

Tissue polypeptide-specific antigen (TPS) is considered to be particularly suitable for monitoring the response to treatment because of its more specific assessment of proliferation activity.[46] It is probably more specific than the tissue polypeptide antigen TPA described earlier. In a study of 44 different tissues, the highest expression of TPS was found in invasive breast and bladder cancers.[47]

TPS appears to work best in combination with TPA and CEA or CA 15-3.[48,49] As with thymidine kinase (TK) (see below), serum levels of TPS detected systemic recurrence (averaging 2 months' lead time) before clinical diagnosis,[50,51] but levels are affected by liver diseases.[50] Its main use has been in detecting progression,[52] for which it may not be best suited. Nicolini et al. found CA 15-3 and CA 549 levels to be raised more often (92%) than was TPS (85%) during follow-up of 13 metastatic patients,[46] and CA 15-3 (plus β-2 microglobulin and ferritin) was found to be more useful than TPS in diagnosis of bone metastases.[53]

However, its particular value may lie in detecting response to therapy. In a study comparing TPS, CA 15-3 and CEA in 129 women with progressive cancer, van Dalen et al. found TPS (measuring tumour activity) to be a more sensitive (and earlier) marker for measuring treatment response than CEA and CA 15-3 (markers of tumour mass).[49] It has been used to measure efficacy of treatment and detect recurrences in 3000 patients.[54] A faster response to therapy was reported for TPS than for CEA or CA 15-3 by Blijlevens et al.[55] Schuurman et al.[56,57] and Karaloglu et al.[58] chose TPS and CA 15-3, and Cohen et al.[59] chose TPS, CA 15-3 and MCA.

Urokinase-type plasminogen activator (u-PA) and its inhibitor PAI-1

u-PA mediates proteolysis by breaking down the extracellular matrix, and the proteolytic activity is controlled by plasminogen activator inhibitor type 1 (PAI-1). High levels of both compounds have been associated with poor prognosis,[60] and the prognostic value may increase with time to a value of nearly node status.[61] In a study of 247 patients, both u-PA and its type 1 inhibitor PAI-1 were found to be independent prognostic factors for node-negative cancer.[62] In addition, they may predict a poor response to tamoxifen therapy, independent of OR status.[63]

Thymidine kinase (TK)

Thymidine kinase (TK) is a key regulatory enzyme of DNA synthesis. The levels measured in tumour extracts probably reflect tumour activity, but may be of a particular subgroup. Romain,[64,65] in a study of 290 patients with breast cancer, found that tumour cytosol TK status was an independent prognostic factor, and high levels were associated with reduced survival in pre/perimenopausal patients.

Serum levels detected systemic recurrence before clinical diagnosis, with an average lead time of 2 months.[50]

Cathepsin D

Cathepsin D is an acidic lysosomal protease that is expressed in all cells.

The expression of cathepsin D in breast cancers may be related to tumour grade. Several reports have suggested that high cathepsin D levels may be predictive of higher recurrence and lower survival,[50] and show a significant correlation with node status.[66] The association between high cathepsin D levels and poor survival appears to be particularly marked in node-negative breast cancer patients.[67]

However, Ravdin et al.,[68] using monoclonal antibody M1G8, Western blotting and immunohistochemistry, failed to improve the prognostic evaluation of 927 node-negative patients, raising questions about the use of cathepsin D in routine evaluation of node-negative breast cancer patients.[68] More recently, Itoh[69] and Aaltonen et al.[70] did not find cathepsin D to be an independent prognostic factor. The significance of cathepsin D may depend on the method used. Nadji et al.[71] concluded that cathepsin D in stromal cells, but not in cancer cells, as detected by immunohistochemistry, is associated with aggressive behaviour in node-negative patients.

In node-positive patients, Seshadri et al. found an association between high cathepsin D levels and HER-2/neu (c-erbB-2) amplification,[72] suggesting that they may play a combined role in promoting dissemination of metastases.

YKL-40

YKL-40 is a recently described glycoprotein related to chitinase. Serum levels of YKL-40 may be an interesting marker for extent of disease and survival in patients after recurrence of breast cancer. A study which monitored 60 patients with bone or visceral metastases showed that 60% of those with normal serum levels remained alive at 18 months, but only 24% were alive if serum YKL-40 levels were raised.[73]

Epidermal growth factor receptor (EGFR)

Expression of the epidermal growth factor receptor (EGFR) may be associated with oestrogen receptor (OR)-negative tumours and with increased metastasis. Nicholson et al. reported that EGFR expression was associated with loss of endocrine sensitivity in both OR-positive and OR-negative cancers.[74] Gasparini et al. suggested that EGFR might be a significant indicator of recurrence ($P<0.01$ and odds ratio 2.82) but not of death, and that valuable additional information is obtained when combined with S-phase fraction data.[75] In a retrospective study of soluble EGFR in 319 breast cancers, Spyratos et al. indicated that EGFR had a prognostic value,[76] which was not demonstrated by some other studies, and therefore perhaps reflects differences in methodology. The value of EGFR is still unclear despite 10 years of intensive investigations, and this highlights the need for multi-centre standardization and quality control.

pS2

pS2 protein is a polypeptide rich in cysteine, from the pS2 gene, also referred to as BCE1, pNR-2 or Md2, which may predict clinical responsiveness to hormone therapy. The expression is induced by oestrogens, and Motomura et al. reported that pS2 expression in cancer cells was inhibited in patients who were taking tamoxifen.[77] There are some indications that levels may be altered by intake of dietary 'oestrogens'.[78,79] Gion et al., in a study of 267 patients, found pS2 to be the best indicator of overall survival, and useful in a panel consisting of pS2, cathepsin D and TPA in the assessment of risk of relapse.[80] In a study of 319 breast cancers with a median follow-up of 6 years,[76] pS2 positivity was associated with longer survival and was predictive of the response to hormone therapy. An immunoradiometric study of pS2 and OR by Crombach et al. showed high pS2 values correlated with positive OR status and high grade of tumour differentiation, and 85% of pS2-positive tumours were OR-positive.[81]

Both Robbins et al.[82] and Detre et al.[83] found a strong correlation between immunohistochemical and immunoradiometric assessment of pS3, recommending the use of immunohistochemistry for pS2 in paraffin wax-embedded tissue. Ibrahim et al. compared immunoperoxidase for pS2 to 47 FNA and paraffin-embedded breast cancer biopsies and found assessment of FNA expression of pS2 to be reliable and cost-effective, with a sensitivity of 84% and a specificity of 100%.[84]

In a study of node-negative patients who were followed up for 16 months,[85] recurrence was found to be significantly more common in patients with negative OR, PR and pS2 (but it was not associated with cathepsin D levels).

Although the pS2 immunohistochemical study by Dookeran et al. of 178 cancers showed only a weak association with OR, and no association with PR or overall survival,[86] their proposal to classify staining as membrane or cytoplasmic may enable greater precision, as cytoplasmic staining was associated with OR and membrane staining with differentiation.

About 15–30% of OR-negative tumours appear to be positive for pS2,[86,87] and these and the HSP27-positive tumours may represent a subgroup of OR-negative tumours with a good prognosis.

Heat-shock protein 27kD (HSP27), p29 or p24

Heat-shock protein 27kD (HSP27), p29 or p24, may have different roles at different stages of tumour progression. Love and King,[88] in a follow-up study of 361 patients, suggested that high HSP27 levels were associated with a short disease-free interval in node-negative patients, but were also associated with prolonged survival after the first recurrence. This was not confirmed by Tetu et al. in a study of 890 node-positive patients.[89] Detection of HSP27 may help to identify a group of OR-negative tumours with a good prognosis,[90] and may predict failure of doxorubicin treatment.[91]

Heat-shock protein 70kD (HSP70)

Heat-shock protein 70kD (HSP70) is thought to be involved with protein products of the c-myc oncogene and p53 tumour suppressor gene.[92] High levels of expression of HSP70 in node-negative cancers were associated with shorter disease-free survival by uni- and multivariate analysis in 345 tumours ($P=0.006$).[93] Takahashi found a positive correlation between HSP70 and OR, but a negative correlation with p53 and EGFR.[94]

P-glycoprotein (P-gp or P170)

This is the phenotype product of the MDR1 or multidrug resistance gene, and is therefore less a marker of poor prognosis than a marker of poor response to chemotherapy. Over-expression of P-glycoprotein has been associated with a poorer prognosis and with prediction of chemoresistance. In 25 locally advanced breast cancers, P-glycoprotein expression was related to poor response to chemotherapy and a short disease-free interval. P-glycoprotein-negative cases showed the best chemotherapeutic response using the C-219 monoclonal antibody.[19] In 42 previously untreated patients with advanced breast cancer, Gasparini et al. found that P-glycoprotein-positive staining, using antibody JSB-1, significantly predicted the response to chemotherapy only in stage IV patients ($P<0.001$), and significantly predicted a poor response to anthracycline-based chemotherapy ($P=0.03$).[95]

Prostate-specific antigen (PSA)

Prostate-specific antigen (PSA) is produced by prostate epithelial cells and is used as a serum marker for prostate cancer. It has also been reported to be present in 30% of breast cancers and may be associated with OR-negative and/or node-positive cancers.[96] A small study by Melegos and Diamandis suggests that serum PSA might be used for diagnosis of breast cancer and for monitoring patients in remission.[97]

pmn-elastase (PMN-E), the metalloproteinases (MMPs) and tissue inhibitors (TIMP)

Proteolytic enzymes such as metalloproteinases may assist invasion and dissemination to distant sites, and this possibility, largely based on animal models, provided the background for attempts to develop new 'anti-cancer' and 'anti-metastasis' drugs. Yamashita et al. found PMN-E to be a significant prognostic factor in multivariate analysis of 62 cancers.[98] High levels were associated with significantly shortened disease-free survival and overall survival, as were raised levels of the MMP stromelysin-3.[99] Clinically, blocking the MMPs has not been as useful as was anticipated. Interestingly, and contrary to the animal model systems, McCarthy et al. found high levels of metalloproteinase inhibitor, TIMP-1, to be associated with poor survival.[100]

Ring-shaped particles (RSP)

In a study of 120 breast cancers with a median follow-up of 8.7 years, Justice et al. reported that their commercial serum assay for RSP had greater sensitivity and specificity than CEA or CA 15-3 for the presence of active breast cancer,[101] and, as they stated in a subsequent paper, for monitoring lung cancer progression.[102] Such a claim is interesting, but clearly requires independent confirmation.

p53 gene and gene product

p53 (sometimes known as TP53) is possibly the most widely evaluated anti-oncogene or tumour suppressor gene. Its value still remains unclear, although a study of 998 patients indicates its value as an independent predictor of reduced survival.[103] It displays a number of interesting biological features (and of approaches to their analysis) that merit description. p53 gene is mutated in 30–50% of sporadic breast cancers, giving rise to an accumulation of mutated p53 protein. The wild-type gene appears normally to function as a tumour suppressor gene by negatively regulating the cell cycle. Mutations usually occur early in tumour progression, producing a protein known as mutant p53 protein (or mp53), which subsequently seems to be able to induce autoantibody formation. Most p53 mutations occur between exons 5 to 9, and detection of p53 changes has been involved using the following:

- polymerase chain reaction (PCR) to analyse the exon 5–9 by single-stranded conformation polymorphism analysis (SSCP);

- antibodies to different p53 epitopes on the gene product, on p53 in tissues and soluble p53 in serum;
- detection of serum autoantibodies to the p53 protein.

Investigations using antibody specific to the mutant p53 or mp53 and not to the wild-type p53 (antibody 240) would seem to be particularly appropriate in seeking mutant expression. Brief mention should be made of serum measurement of p53 antigen to monitor tumours, and although Micelli et al. detected the antigen in sera of 14 of 75 breast cancer patients (19%),[104] this approach needs to be considered in the context of circulating antibodies against p53 (see section below on autoantibodies) and the possible mechanisms for their development.[105]

Overexpression of p53 is particularly associated with younger age, high histological grade breast cancers.[106] Generally, p53 mutants appear to have only a weak role in predicting survival, although they show a strong association with OR- and PR-negative tumours. Breast cancers that show altered p53 tend to have a poorer prognosis and are more likely to show other features associated with poor prognosis. However, node-negative breast cancer patients with p53 mutations were found to have significantly improved relapse-free survival ($P=0.0007$).[107]

One of the most interesting applications may be the association described by Aas et al. of de-novo resistance to doxorubicin and p53 mutations.[108]

Complete concordance between p53 gene mutation and p53 protein accumulation was found by Thor et al.,[109] and by immunohistochemistry of 295 invasive ductal carcinomas it was shown to be an independent marker for shortened disease-free and overall survival. However, Lohmann et al.,[110] using a combination of immunohistochemistry (antibody 1801), Southern and Northern blotting and direct sequencing of mutation hot spots on 23 frozen cancers, found both mutation without p53 immunoreactivity and immunostaining without mutation. This suggests that p53 accumulation was not such a reliable marker of p53 gene mutation. Similarly, Dunn et al.,[91] using antibody CM1 and PCR-SSCP analysis, found considerable disparity between positive immunohistochemical staining and mutation in 81 tumours.

The methods used vary enormously, and in an attempt to optimize immunohistochemistry for p53, Fisher et al. proposed fixation in phenol formol saline, methacarn or cold formol saline, which in their study resulted in positive staining in 69 of 95 cases (73%).[111] They have advised caution in the interpretation of the different staining patterns, but considered that the latter yielded useful independent prognostic information.

Methodology is clearly important when studying the gene product. Does the p53 protein that is overexpressed in cancer cells differ from the p53 protein of normal cells? Jacquemier et al. stained 106 breast cancers with four different monoclonal antibodies to p53 (1801,

240, DO7 and DO1).[112] They reported that p53 protein was detected with at least one antibody in 40 cancers (38%), but only 15 cancers (14%) were positive with all four antibodies. Despite these discrepancies, positive staining showed a correlation with grade 3 ($P<0.0001$) OR-negative ($P<0.0001$), PR-negative ($P=0.0061$), Ki67-positive ($P=0.0018$) and EGFR-positive ($P=0.0076$), but no correlation with disease-free survival was found in univariate analysis. Thus p53 is perhaps a late marker of recurrence. A study by Hurlimann,[113] using a panel of antibodies M-1801, M-240, M-421 and CM1 on 196 infiltrating ductal carcinomas, obtained positive staining of 71 (36%) ductal carcinomas, rising to 94% of medullary carcinomas. The prognostic value varied with the antibody used. M-1801 was most closely linked to poor prognosis and, curiously, positive M-421 staining was associated with negative M-240. Many other monoclonal antibodies to p53 have been described but have not yet been properly evaluated. Four of them have been compared on paraffin sections by Horne et al.[114] It is clearly necessary to define the epitopes that they recognize.

In a PCR study of 70 cancers,[115] 25% showed an alteration of the p53 gene. This was associated with high histological grade and numerous mitoses, with negative OR and with negative PR, but there was no correlation with nodal status or clinical stage, suggesting this could be a marker of aggressive cancers that might be of possible value in node-negative patients.

In a study of p53 mutations in 47 breast cancers among black women from Michigan, a population that displays particularly high mortality even after adjusting for stage, Blaszyk et al. detected mutations that differed from those in other populations, particularly an excess of A:T → G:C transitions.[116] However, Elledge et al.,[117] in a study comparing white, Hispanic and black breast cancer patients from Texas, did not detect differences in p53 expression, but confirmed that black women had a poorer prognosis, which has also been reported from unrelated studies.

The pattern of p53 protein distribution may be important in identifying likely function and behaviour. Stenmark-Askmalm et al. described nuclear (9%) and cytoplasmic (21%) distribution of protein staining in 164 stage II patients.[118] p53 appeared to be an independent prognostic factor (in addition to node and OR status) and, by this grouping, cytoplasmic p53 was significantly correlated with disease-free survival in patients who were negative for nuclear p53 ($P<0.0001$). Faille observed positive staining with antibody 1801 in 14 of 39 stage III–IV patients (36%) (11 nuclear only, two mixed and one cytoplasmic only).[119] The association with larger tumour size and clinical metastases suggests that p53 mutation could be a late event.

Overall, while some laboratories find p53 to be a helpful independent marker for survival in node-negative patients,[120] others do not.

p53 and Bcl-2 (apoptosis-preventing gene)

An inverse relationship between Bcl-2 and p53 has been described by several authors. Haldar *et al.* found an inverse correlation between the expression of Bcl-2 and p53 gene products,[121] suggesting that mutant p53 might substitute for and down-regulate Bcl-2 expression. Leek *et al.* reported an inverse relationship between Bcl-2 and c-erbB-2 and p53,[122] linking the loss of Bcl-2 as part of an OR-negative, EGFR-positive phenotype.

In 283 node-negative cancers that were followed up for 6 years, Silvestrini *et al.* found bcl-2-positive immunostaining to be associated with small, OR-positive and p53 protein-negative tumours, and they reported that any predictive role of bcl-2 expression was mainly dependent on p53 expression.[123]

Autoantibodies to p53

Autoantibodies to p53 have been detected in the sera of patients with a variety of cancers.[124] The sera of 48 of 182 newly diagnosed breast cancer patients (26%) contained autoantibodies to p53, and their presence correlated with high grade ($P=0.0012$).[125] p53 autoantibodies in these patients also correlated with positive tumour immuno-histochemistry for p53 ($P=0.002$). However, in the seronegative patients, positive tumour staining was strongly associated with a family history of breast cancer, suggesting an immunological difference in heritable breast cancer.

An interesting model for the development of these antibodies has been proposed by Dong *et al.*,[105] and a worsened survival has been linked to p53 autoantibodies,[126] but later papers have been less enthusiastic.[127,128]

Mucins, mucin-related markers and other carbohydrates

Many of the cancer-related antigens have been identified as mucins or as heavily glycosylated proteins bearing O-linked (and N-linked) sugar residues.

MUC1 GENE PRODUCT

This is also known as epithelial membrane antigen (EMA), episialin, mammary-type apomucin and polymorphic epithelial mucin (PEM). It represents a major mucin group which is expressed in many secretory epithelial cells, but particularly in breast tissue. Six kinds of mucin core protein (MUC1 to 6) have been described, consisting of tandem repeats of 20 amino acids, each repeat containing five potential sites for O-glycosylation, allowing carbohydrates to comprise over 50% of the molecular weight.

It is the most immunogenic and widely studied breast mucin, closely related to CA 15-3, Tn and sialosyl-Tn

S-Tn antigens (see below), and is frequently recognized by monoclonal antibodies to these structures. The core protein for MUC appears to undergo aberrant glycosylation in malignancy, the 'cryptic' protein core antigens then becoming recognizable to antibodies such as SM3. Detection of the cryptic core protein may play a role in the diagnosis of cancer. The predominantly O-linked sugars embrace a variety of oligosaccharides, including those of early core glycosylation, Tn and sialyl-Tn which seem likely to yield important prognostic information (see the section below on Tn and S-Tn). Natural antibodies to MUC1 have been described, and attempts are now being made to use synthetic peptides for cancer immunotherapy by Longecker's group in Canada.[129] It seems likely that the value of CA 15-3 in detection of cancer cells lies in its ability to detect a differently glycosylated form to the normal, mature molecule.

MUC2

MUC2 protein, which is present in 19% of invasive breast cancers, has been associated with shortened disease-free survival.[130]

MCA

A related mucin-like carcinoma-associated antigen, MCA, was identified by monoclonal antibodies on breast cancer cell lines. It is raised in progressive disease,[59] and may be of value in identifying patients with liver or bone metastases, as the highest serum values have been reported in patients with liver or bone metastases, and the lowest in those with loco-regional recurrence.[131]

CA 15-3 (OR DF3)

CA 15-3 or CA 15-3 (sometimes known as DF3) antigen appears to indicate tumour mass and may be raised in the sera of up to 80% of patients with metastatic breast cancer. It forms part of a 20-amino-acid glycosylated tandem repeat of the mucin MUC1 gene product or polymorphic epithelial mucin (PEM), and is likely to be closely related to other cancer markers.

Several assays are available, as it has been considered to be the most useful single or combination marker for metastatic breast cancer,[48] and the sensitivity and specificity can be further improved by altering the recommended cut-off points.[132] O'Hanlon *et al.* have suggested that it should be used routinely in pre-operative staging.[52] A survey of follow-up tests by American cancer physicians for women with early breast cancer showed CA 15-3 to be the second most popular serum marker (21% ordered CA 15-3, compared to 38% for CEA).[133] Its expression possibly parallels that of another mucinous marker, namely CA 549[134] (see below).

In a comparison of biochemical markers and clinical disease in 13 relapsed patients, Nicolini *et al.* found that CA 15-3 and CA 549 were more closely related to clinical disease (in 95% of cases) than CEA (46% of cases),[46]

tissue polypeptide antigen (TPA) (60% of cases) and tissue polypeptide-specific antigen (TPS) (85% of cases). Using 1123 sera detections, Busetto et al. found that raised CA 15-3 levels gave a 99.4% positive predictive value for metastasis.[135] To measure the response to treatment, van Dalen et al. have recommended a combination of CA 15-3 (for tumour burden) and tissue polypeptide-specific antigen (TPS) (for tumour activity).[49]

ST-439

This is another related mucin carcinoma-associated antigen. Positive tumours have a better prognosis than negative ones (P<0.01).[136] Serum levels for detection of recurrence showed a greater sensitivity than CEA or CA 15-3, but a lower specificity.[137]

BCA225

BCA225 is a glycoprotein originally secreted by the breast cancer cell line T47D, and its presence in serum may identify the volume of metastatic cells. In recurrent breast cancer, Konishi et al. found raised levels of serum markers CEA, CA 15-3, BCA225 and c-erbB-2 in 32%, 50%, 41% and 27%, of cases, respectively, and selected the mixture of CA 15-3, BCA225 and c-erbB-2 as a combination for detecting progression of breast cancer.[138] In 98 patients with metastases, Iwase et al. did not find serum BCA225 (raised in 44% of cases) to be as sensitive as CEA (55% of cases) or CA 15-3 (68% of cases).[139]

CA 549

This is a mucin-like cancer antigen, probably related to CA 15-3, which may have a similar predictive value.[140] In a multicentre study of sera from patients with benign and malignant conditions, raised levels of CA 549 were reported in 5% of stage I, 14% of stage II, 32% of stage III and 74% of stage IV cancers, and may help to identify stage IV cases.[141] In a study of sera from 59 breast cancer patients, CA 549 gave the highest sensitivity in patients with systemic disease,[142] perhaps associated with metastasis and progression. Similar but not identical results may be obtained with CA 15-3 and MCA.[80] Pavesi et al.,[134] looking at sera from 258 cancer patients, and evaluating CA 549, CA 15-3, CEA and MCA, found that CA 15-3 was similar to CA 549, but overall CA 549 and MCA were the most sensitive indicators of loco-regional relapse, and CA 549 showed the more defined cut-off and specificity. Cazin et al.,[143] comparing CA 15-3 with CA 549 on sera of 95 breast cancer patients and 35 controls, found that CA 15-3 was more effective than CA 549 in detecting disease.

Tn and S-Tn

Tn and its sialic-acid disaccharide sialosyl-Tn (S-Tn) is a small, O-linked sugar that is not expressed on most normal epithelial cell surfaces, but which becomes expressed in cancers where it is associated with aggressive behaviour and poor prognosis. Springer has widely reported an association between Tn and aggressive and metastatic behaviour of breast cancers which has been under-explored,[144] perhaps because the analytical technology has been complex. S-Tn was reported as an independent marker of poor prognosis in 63 breast cancers,[145] although it has been mainly used to identify poor-prognosis groups with gastric cancers.[146–148] Different monoclonal antibodies to Tn may give divergent results as different forms and linkages of Tn can exist (e.g. on erythrocytes and on cancer cells). A likely explanation seems to be that the glycosylation pathway for Tn synthesis in cancers is different to that for normal cells,[149] highlighting the need to select the right antibody in order to unravel a particular problem.

Le(x) or CD15

Le(x), also known as Lewis X or 3-fucosyl-N-acetyl-lactosamine, Galb1–4(Fuca1–3)GlcNAc, SSEA-1 or CD15, is normally expressed as part of the plasma membrane glycoproteins of neutrophils and monocytes. It has been associated with poor prognosis in colorectal[150] and hepatocellular[151] carcinomas, where it appears to be independent of other clinico-pathological features, but it is linked with invasive behaviour in the breast.[152] In 98 breast cancers, Le(x) was frequently associated with the leading edge of invading tumour or with the outer edge of carcinoma in situ, possibly suggesting a role in invasiveness, and associated with cancer cells trapped intravascularly, possibly suggesting a role in metastasis.[153] Narita et al.,[137] found both Le(x) and the sialylated form, S-Le(x), to be markers of poor prognosis in 300 breast cancer patients (P<0.001). Furthermore, Yamaguchi et al.,[154] in a study of 100 patients, found S-Le(x) to be associated with lymph-node spread but an independent significant prognostic factor.

Carbohydrates and changes in glycosylation

An association has become apparent recently, by the use of monoclonal antibodies and lectins, between markers containing the terminal sugars fucose, galactose and/or N-acetyl-galactosamine and metastasis of a variety of tumours, including breast, colorectal, stomach, bladder, prostate and melanoma.[56,57,144,151–161] Part of this association may represent the detection of molecules containing the Tn sugar (GalNAc-O), originally linked to aggressiveness of cancer by Springer.[162] However, polylactosamines and larger related structures have been identified, suggesting that a family of carbohydrate molecules is associated with differing cancer-cell behaviour. The GalNAc-binding lectin from the snail Helix pomatia appears to identify metastatic behaviour in breast,[136,156,163] prostate,[159] melanoma,[164] stomach,[165] oesophagus,[166] and colorectal cancers.[167,168]

The way in which sugars are linked together also seems to be related to progression,[169] particularly the beta 1–6 branching described by Dennis,[170] which is detected by the lectin PHA-L from the kidney bean.

Genes and gene products

Bcl-2 OR BCL2

The Bcl-2 gene encodes for a mitochondrial Bcl-2 protein which is thought to prevent apoptosis of normal cells. The protein has been detected immunohistochemically in hormonally regulated epithelia.

In a study of 283 node-negative cancers which were followed for 6 years, Bcl-2-positive staining was associated with small, OR-positive, slowly proliferating and p53-negative tumours.[123] Bcl-2 failed to maintain prognostic significance in the presence of p53, and relapse-free and overall survival were mainly dependent on p53 expression. In a study of 111 cancers, Leek et al. found a strong positive correlation between Bcl-2 and OR, but a negative association between Bcl-2 and EGFR and between Bcl-2 and the oncogenes c-erbB-2 and p53.[122] No association was found between Bcl-2 and node status, tumour size, differentiation, type or age at excision. These researchers suggested that the loss of Bcl-2 is associated with a range of molecular markers of poor prognosis and may define part of an OR-negative, EGFR-positive phenotype. Intriguingly, in prostate cancers, androgen withdrawal induces apoptosis and in 6 of 13 primary prostate cancers, Bcl-2-containing cells appeared to be intimately associated with neurone-specific enolase-containing tumour neuroendocrine cells,[171] but there was no association in metastatic cancer.

C-MYC

The c-myc gene has been implicated in the development of several animal and human tumours and its amplification is generally associated with decreased survival.[172]

Brandt et al. reported amplification of c-myc in 8–33% of primary breast cancers, and associated it with decreased survival of patients with both primary and secondary cancers,[173] although Watson did not find c-myc amplification present in all metastases.[174] It was also found in 53% of breast cancers that showed over-expression of the proliferation marker KiS1.[175] An interesting study of oncogenes by Berns,[176] comparing c-myc with HER2/neu in 282 patients, with a median follow-up of 74 months, found c-myc to be a useful independent marker, particularly in node-negative and steroid-receptor-positive cancers, while HER2/neu was limited to steroid-receptor-negative disease. Similarly, Pertschuk et al. found c-myc amplification more closely paralleled poor prognosis than did int-2 or c-erbB-2.[177] Roux-Dosseto et al. found c-myc to be an independent prog-

nostic factor, stronger than OR and tumour size, and it could define a subset of node-negative patients with high risk of recurrence.[178] Other authors have reported more limited use, such as amplification only related to metastasis in premenopausal patients by Champeme et al.,[179] and only related to post-menopausal patients by Borg et al.[180] Henry et al. did not demonstrate an association with prognosis,[181] and Pietilainen et al. found it to be a marker associated with the invasive margin ($P=0.0049$) and in axillary lymph-node-negative ($P=0.0028$) tumours, but only weakly independent,[182] so possibly of value in node-negative patients.

C-ERBB-2 (HER2/NEU GENE)

This is more frequently positive in ductal carcinoma in situ (DCIS) than in invasive cancers, although in DCIS there is a close association between c-erbB-2 protein expression and high-nuclear-grade, comedo types, so it may predict future invasiveness. Its value in direct relation to survival is unclear. For example, in paraffin sections of 107 stage I and II breast cancer patients in a randomized trial, 21% of cancers were c-erbB-2 positive and an association was observed with an intraductal component but not with survival or recurrence.[183]

Over-expression of c-erbB-2 may be a useful marker in invasive cancers, for identifying patients who are most likely to benefit from high doses of adjuvant chemotherapy, although other reports contradict this, suggesting that c-erbB-2 expression is associated with failure of response to chemotherapy and hormonal treatment. C-erbB-2 may predict an improved response to doxorubicin,[184] rather than CMF therapy, and has been linked with the response to adjuvant therapy in women with node-positive early breast cancer.[185] In a study of 580 patients in Toronto, Andrulis et al. found that c-erbB-2 or neu identifies a poor-prognosis group among the node-negative patients.[186]

Perhaps the main value of demonstrating c-erbB-2 or HER2/neu gene over-expression, or over-expression of the gene product, will be in the identification of those 25–30% of cancers that may respond to herceptin (or antibody to c-erbB-2/HER2) treatment.

ABNORMALITIES IN THE CYCLIN GENE SUPERFAMILY

These may be associated with tumour development by deregulation of cell-cycle control, leading to progression.

CYCLIN D1

Cyclin D1 is a cell-cycle regulator on the q13 region of chromosome 11, essential for G1 phase progression and a candidate proto-oncogene implicated in the pathogenesis of several human cancers. Over-expression of cyclin D1 may directly result in abnormal mammary cell proliferation in mice and in the development of mouse mammary adenocarcinomas.[187] Over-expressed cyclin D1 has been described in several human cancers, including breast and squamous-cell carcinoma, and up to one-third or half of breast cancers may show high levels of cyclin D1 protein.[188,189] It seems to be particularly interesting, as it may reflect a comparatively early event in cancer, and it is maintained throughout progression to metastasis.[189]

CYCLIN E

Various quantitative and qualitative alterations of cyclin E protein have been described, independent of the S-phase fraction marker of proliferation. Progressively increased expression has been associated with increasing stage and grade, suggesting a potential value for this marker linked to cancer progression.[190]

INT-2/FGF-3 (FIBROBLAST GROWTH FACTOR 3)

Located on chromosome 11, int-2/FGF-3 proto-oncogene was reported to be amplified in 9–14% of invasive breast cancers, which were associated with higher risk of death by Henry et al.[181] but not by Berns.[176] Int-2/FGF-3 has been reported to be a better independent predictor of relapse than c-myc and c-erbB-2.[179] Its value may lie in identifying node-negative and progesterone-receptor-negative patients at higher risk of recurrence.[179]

NM23 (METASTASIS SUPPRESSOR GENE OF MICE)

The nm23 gene was identified from mouse melanoma cells of varying metastatic potential, where it was possibly a metastatic suppressor gene, with two isotypes, H1 and H2, encoding nucleoside diphosphate kinase NDP-K, which was proposed to be a metastasis suppressor. Despite earlier enthusiasm for this marker, its association with breast cancer metastasis or suppression is now less clear. In 130 cancers studied by Tokunaga,[191] the isotype of nm23, H1, but not H2, was inversely associated with lymph-node metastasis (P<0.01), and survival was longer in those tumours which were H1-positive. No relationship was found between expression of the gene nm23-H1 and nodal metastases or other pathological features in 105 patients,[192] and no relationship was seen between the immunohistochemical detection of NDP-K and recurrence or survival in 197 breast cancers.[193] However, Yamaguchi et al.,[154] in a multivariate study of 100 cases, found that nm23-H1 was a significant independent prognostic factor.

BIOLOGICAL AND LIFESTYLE MARKERS

Comorbidity or presence of concurrent diseases

Comorbidity here refers to the presence of other non-malignant disease in patients with breast cancer. Studies

of various cancers, especially those of the prostate, show a higher mortality rate in patients with reported comorbidity. For example, the findings of Albertsen et al. suggest that a comorbidity index provides significant, independent, predictive information concerning patient mortality beyond that provided by histology and clinical stage.[194] Satariano and Ragland, in a longitudinal study of 936 women with breast cancer,[195] found that comorbidity was a strong independent predictor of 3-year survival, and similar results for a larger sample were reported by West et al.[196] The higher morbidity increasingly associated with lower socio-economic status (SES) may go some way towards explaining the higher death rate among those of lower SES. Perhaps, particularly for older patients, trials should include measures of comorbidity, such as the Charlson index.[197]

Familial and hereditary factors

Breast cancers in young women tend to show associations with a family history of breast cancers and to appear histologically more aggressive. However, as decribed below, the overall and recurrence-free survival periods may be longer in this group, and it has been suggested that increased awareness in these families might lead to earlier detection. Ruder et al. observed a better survival rate among breast cancer patients whose maternal relatives had breast cancer.[198] In a Japanese study of 4481 primary breast cancer patients,[199] those with a family history (n=394, or 8.8%) had a longer survival over 15 years compared to those without such a history (72% vs. 60%; P<0.01). A smaller study of North American patients by Israeli found no difference in outcome at 5 years' follow-up, and in a Utah study,[200] younger patients (< 50 years of age at diagnosis) with a family history had a poorer survival. However, in a study of 220 hereditary breast cancer patients (from 58 families) in Omaha, recurrence was lower in the hereditary patients, and stage II hereditary patients were 70% disease-free at 5 years compared to 40% in the case of sporadic cancers.[201] Confusion between familial and hereditary studies may explain such differences, and identification of patients with cancer susceptibility genes (e.g. BRCA1, 2, 3) may clarify this.

Looking for phenotypic markers of family history in a study of 143 Japanese patients, Inada et al. found overexpression of p53 in the primary cancers of 83% of patients with a family history, compared to 34% of patients without a family history, but this was of marginal use as a prognostic marker.[202] However, in a North American study of 192 cancers,[203] while an association was found between younger patients and p53, no significant link with family history was detected.

BRCA1

Paradoxically, although BRCA1 gene mutation has been associated with aneuploid and proliferative features,[204] patients may have lower recurrence and specific death rates.[204,205] In a related study, ovarian cancers associated with BRCA1 mutations appear to have a significantly more favourable clinical course compared to sporadic ovarian cancers.[206]

Diet

Cancer patients frequently supplement or alter their diets. While much advice on diet is available for cancer patients, little objective information exists about dietary effects on cancer progression. Intake of beta-carotene (and vitamin C) was observed to be associated with prolonged survival by Ingram,[207] and in a study of fishermen's wives who were followed from 1970 to 1985, Lund and Bonaa concluded that fish consumption may be associated with lower breast cancer mortality.[208]

Several studies have linked vegetable consumption to a reduced risk of dying from cancers, and many mechanisms for this have been proposed. Of particular relevance to breast and prostate cancers are chemicals that exert a weakly oestrogenic effect and are present in a variety of foods. These are frequently referred to as phyto-oestrogens (phyto = plant), as they are derived from food plants. One large group, related to phenols, with names such as isoflavones and lignans, are derived from different plants by the action of colonic bacteria, and can be readily measured in plasma and urine.[209,210] The phyto-oestrogens can exert different effects on cancer cells, from binding oestrogen ligands to induction of apoptosis and inhibition of tyrosine kinases. Although only weakly oestrogenic, these dietary oestrogens may be ingested in large amounts and might be expected to have some effect. Consequently, there have been attempts to seek a dietary influence of these phyto-oestrogens on breast cancer. The urinary level of these plant oestrogens can vary by 100-fold between populations at high and low risk of breast and prostate cancers.[211] Such measurements in breast cancer patients would seem to be a fertile area for seeking dietary markers that influence cancer progression for both breast and prostate,[212] and for identifying dietary factors that might be readily altered.

Quod ali cibus est aliis fuat acre venenum (what is food to one may be fierce poison to others).

(Lucretius:iv. 637)

Race

The higher mortality observed in black compared to white patients with breast cancer may be more closely related to lifestyle. Ansell *et al.* suggested that this difference might be reduced when adjusted for income, stage and age.[213] A Chicago study of 1518 patients.[214] In a recent study of 439 patients in Florida, Lyman *et al.* found race to be an independent predictor of survival.[215] An intriguing study in Louisiana, which compared the histo-

logical characteristics of 963 white/black invasive breast cancers,[216] matching for factors including socio-economic status and health care, showed that the black women of high socio-economic status had a raised mitotic index and tumour grade, suggesting a more aggressive form of cancer. The increasing incidence and age-adjusted mortality rate in Japan[217] (4.1 deaths per 100 000 members of the population in 1950, which had risen to 6.6 per 100 000 in 1991) may suggest a previously less aggressive type of cancer in the Japanese population. Imaizumi suggests that some environmental factor must have changed to account for this increasing mortality from breast cancer.[218]

Geography

The risk of developing invasive breast cancer may not be directly related to the risk of dying from breast cancer, which varies in different parts of the world. Within Europe, a north–south pattern of survival has been observed for some years,[219,220] unrelated to incidence, and with increasing mortality on moving northwards, but it is still unclear whether this is independent of stage at diagnosis. A similar but smaller difference in mortality has been seen across the USA.[221]

Socio-economic factors

Numerous studies have shown shorter survival times for many diseases in lower compared to higher socio-economic status groups and in black compared to white breast cancer patients. This has been attributed to delay in diagnosis and later stage at presentation.[222] However, after controlling for these prognostic variables, there increasingly seems to be a real association with some factor(s) in lower socio-economic status and perhaps in the cancers of black patients (see section on race above).[216] In a study of 1392 breast cancer patients followed for 5 to 16 years,[223] lower socio-economic status (SES) was significantly related to overall survival, after controlling for stage, age, race, OR and other prognostic factors. The death rates during this period were 29.4% for the lower SES groups compared to 17.9% for higher SES groups ($P<0.001$). Similar findings were reported for affluent compared to deprived populations in south-east England,[224] showing a survival advantage in higher socio-economic groups equivalent to a shift in stage. This presumably results from different factors to those which produce a higher risk of developing breast cancer in higher socio-economic groups. Schrijvers showed a survival advantage for higher socio-economic groups in 3928 patients in The Netherlands,[225] and concluded that stage at diagnosis was the important determinant of these differences. However, a larger study of 29 676 breast cancer patients in south-east England showed a similar survival difference that could not be explained by stage, morphology or treatment.[226] The higher comorbidity frequently observed among lower socio-economic status groups may contribute to this difference.

Psychosocial factors

Many studies have sought to identify the psychosocial factors affecting women at risk of developing breast cancer, and how these factors influence the prognosis.[227] However, more rapid advances may result from seeking factors that influence progression in those women who already have breast cancer. Greer identified patient groups whose psychological disposition in response to cancer may influence the course of the disease.[228,229] The 'helpless, hopeless' succumbed rapidly, while those who exhibited a 'fighting spirit', and even those who displayed denial that they had cancer, would live much longer.

Ramirez et al. suggested a prognostic association between severe life stressors and recurrence of breast cancer in 50 women who had developed their first recurrence compared to 50 women with operable breast cancer in remission (cases and controls were matched for physical, pathological and sociodemographic variables).[230] Severely threatening life events and difficulties were significantly associated with the first recurrence of breast cancer. The relative risk of relapse associated with severe life events was 5.67 (95% confidence interval, 1.57–37.20). However, a study by Barraclough et al. on 204 patients followed for 42 months was unable to find a significant influence of stress or support on disease-free survival.[231]

Spiegel[232–234] and Kogon et al.[235] examined the effect that supportive group therapy might have on survival. Of 86 patients who were followed up for 10 years, the mean survival period following intervention (support for 50 patients) was 36.6 months, compared to 18.9 months in the control group (36 patients). Interestingly, divergence began 20 months after entry to the study, and the survival difference persisted in those with distant metastases. Conversely, Gellert et al.,[236] in a study of psychosocial support therapy for 136 patients with up to a 20-year follow-up, matched 34 participants with 102 non-participants and could not demonstrate a significant favourable increase in survival in the support therapy group.

Patient support by family

In a study of 1011 patients,[237] those women who reported receiving little emotional support from close friends and relatives had a higher death rate during a 5-year follow-up period (relative risk = 1.8). The results of a recent Canadian study of 235 patients over 7 years by Maunsell et al. suggest that women who used confidants had a longer survival (hazard ratio in the range 0.61–0.51, according to the number of confidants).[238]

The types of support that are beneficial have not been identified. Extra support may not increase the survival of patients, but decreased support might contribute to earlier death.

Smoking

An intriguing association was reported by Calle et al. between current smoking and increased risk of death in a 6-year follow-up of a cohort of 604 412 women with 880 breast cancer deaths (adjusted rate ratio = 1.26).[239] It may be linked to comorbidity, but this increase was not seen in former smokers.

Gender of offspring

Janerich,[240] in a study of 2155 parous women with invasive breast cancer in Utah, USA, found that the median survival among women diagnosed under the age of 45 years was 171 months if the first child was female, but only 66 months if the first child was male (hazard rate ratio = 1.66, 95% confidence interval = 1.07–2.57, for male children). This trend disappeared among women who were aged over 45 years at the time of diagnosis.

Time of observation as a factor

The value of individual prognostic factors may vary according to the length of the observation period. An Italian study suggests that long-term relapse (more than 8 years after surgery) is particularly associated with OR-positive cancers.[241] Yoshimoto investigated 11 pathological factors in 462 patients,[242] and found that the influence of nodal involvement and nuclear grade on risk of relapse decreased with time, but that it increased with time for fat infiltration, another odd feature being a possible influence by tumour-infiltrating lymphocytes after 2 years post-operatively. In a study of 786 node-negative patients, the mean nuclear area of cancer cells was the strongest morphological indicator of 5-year survival, but for the next 5 years (after excluding those who had died) only tumour diameter yielded significant prognostic information.[243]

CONCLUSION

Finally, even a large study can produce odd markers. In a report of a study of nearly 33 000 breast cancer patients by Sankila et al.,[244] the adjusted relative excess risk of death was highest among those diagnosed in July and August, and lowest for those diagnosed in March and November (the difference between the lowest and highest risk being 18%). The same pattern was observed in nearly 13 000 colorectal cancers, and the authors consider that this observation may be related more to behaviour and health services than to the stars!

REFERENCES

1 Heimann R, Ferguson D, Gray S, Hellman S. Assessment of intratumoral vascularization (angiogenesis) in breast cancer prognosis. *Breast Cancer Res Treat* 1998; **52**(1–3): 147–58.

2 Ferno M. Prognostic factors in breast cancer: a brief review. *Anticancer* Res. 1998; **18**: 2167–71.

3 Querzoli P, Albonico G, Ferretti S *et al.* Modulation of biomarkers in minimal breast carcinoma: a model for human breast carcinoma progression. *Cancer* 1998; **83**: 89–97.

4 Jansen RL, Hillen HF, Schouten HC. Prognostic and predictive factors in breast cancer. *Neth J Med* 1997; **51**: 65–77.

5 Pinder SE, Ellis IO, Elston CW. Prognostic factors in primary breast carcinoma. *J Clin Pathol* 1995; **48**: 981–3.

6 Fisher B, Bauer M, Wickerham DL *et al.* Relation of number of positive axillary nodes to the prognosis of patients with primary breast cancer. An NSABP update. *Cancer* 1983; **52**: 1551–7.

7 Baselga J, Norton L, Albanell J, Kim YM, Mendelsohn J. Recombinant humanized anti-HER2 antibody (Herceptin) enhances the antitumor activity of paclitaxel and doxorubicin against HER2/neu overexpressing human breast cancer xenografts. *Cancer Res* 1998; **58**: 2825–31.

8 McNeil C. Herceptin raises its sights beyond advanced breast cancer. *J Natl Cancer Inst* 1998; **90**: 822–3.

9 Eiermann W. New antibody for breast cancer therapy. *Fortschr Med* 1998; **116**:18–19.

10 Pegram MD, Lipton A, Hayes DF *et al.* Phase II study of receptor-enhanced chemosensitivity using recombinant humanized anti-p185HER2/neu monoclonal antibody plus cisplatin in patients with HER2/neu-overexpressing metastatic breast cancer refractory to chemotherapy treatment. *J Clin Oncol* 1998; **18**: 2659–71.

11 Gorczyca W, Tuziak T, Kram A *et al.* Detection of apoptosis-associated DNA strand breaks in fine-needle aspiration biopsies by in situ end labeling of fragmented DNA. *Cytometry* 1994; **15**: 169–75.

12 Gasparini G, Boracchi P, Verderio P *et al.* Cell kinetics in human breast cancer: comparison between the prognostic value of the cytofluorimetric S-phase fraction and that of the antibodies to Ki-67 and PCNA antigens detected by immunocytochemistry. *Int J Cancer* 1994; **57**: 822–9.

13 Sampson SA, Kreipe H, Gillett CE *et al.* KiS1 – a novel monoclonal antibody which recognizes proliferating cells: evaluation of its relationship to prognosis in mammary carcinoma. *J Pathol* 1992; **168**: 179–85.

14 Horiguchi J, Iino Y, Takei H *et al.* Expression of proliferating cell nuclear antigen in invasive ductal carcinoma of the breast. *Jpn J Clin Oncol* 1994; **24**: 79–84.

15 Schimmelpenning H, Eriksson ET, Franzen N *et al.* Prognostic value of the combined assessment of proliferating cell nuclea immunostaining and nuclear DNA content in invasive human mammary carcinomas. *Virchows Arch* 1993; **423**: 273–9.

16 Gillett CE, Barnes DM, Camplejohn RS. Comparison of three cell cycle associated antigens as markers of proliferative activity and prognosis in breast carcinoma. *J Clin Path* 1993; **46**: 1126–8.

17 Betta PG, Bottero G, Pavesi M *et al.* Cell proliferation in breast carcinoma assessed by a PCNA grading system and its relation to other prognostic variables. *Surg Oncol* 1993; **2**: 59–63.

18 Stanton PD, Cooke TG, Oakes SJ *et al.* Lack of prognostic significance of DNA ploidy and S phase fraction in breast cancer. *Br J Cancer* 1992; **66**: 925–9.

19 Botti G, Chiappetta G, D'Aiuto G *et al.* PCNA/cyclin and P-glycoprotein as prognostic factors in locally advanced breast cancer. An immunohistochemical, retrospective study. *Tumori* 1993; **79**: 214–18.

20 Yuan J, Hennessy C, Givan AL *et al.* Predicting outcome for patients with node negative breast cancer: a comparative study of the value of flow cytometry and cell image analysis for determination of DNA ploidy. *Br J Cancer* 1992; **65**: 461–5.

21 Fox SB, Leek RD, Weekes MP *et al.* Quantitation and prognostic value of breast cancer angiogenesis: comparison of microvessel density, Chalkley count, and computer image analysis. *J Pathol* 1995; **177**: 275–83.

22 Siitonen SM, Haapasalo HK, Rantala IS *et al.* Comparison of different immunohistochemical methods in the assessment of angiogenesis: lack of prognostic value in a group of 77 selected node-negative breast carcinomas. *Mod Pathol* 1995; **8**: 745–52.

23 Axelsson K, Ljung B-M, Moore D *et al.* Tumor angiogensis as a prognostic assay for invasive ductal breast carcinoma. *J Natl Cancer Inst* 1995; **87**: 997–1008.

24 Tynninen O, von Boguslawski K, Aronen HJ, Paavonen T. Prognostic value of vascular density and cell proliferation in breast cancer patients. *Pathol Res Pract* 1999; **195**: 31–7.

25 Mayers MM, Seshadri R, Raymond W, McCaul K, Horsfall DJ. Tumor microvascularity has no independent prognostic significance for breast cancer. *Pathology* 1998; **30**: 105–10.

26 Kumar S, Ghellal A, Li C *et al.* Breast carcinoma: vascular density determined using CD105 antibody correlates with tumor prognosis. *Cancer Res* 1999; **59**: 856–61.

27 Carpenter R, Cross M, Herbert A *et al. Br J Cancer* 1992; **65**: 14.

28 Macmillan RD, Purushotham AD, Mallon E *et al.* Breast-conserving surgery and tumour bed positivity in patients with breast cancer. *Br J Surg* 1994; **81**: 56–8.

29 Smitt MC, Nowels KW, Zdeblick MJ *et al.* The importance of the lumpectomy surgical margin status in long-term results of breast conservation. *Cancer* 1995; **76**: 259–67.

30 DiBase 1998

31 Dettmar P, Harbeck N, Thomssen C *et al.* Prognostic impact of proliferation-associated factors MIB1 (Ki-67) and

S-phase in node-negative breast cancer. *Br J Cancer* 1997; **75**: 1525–33.

32 Remvikos Y, Mosseri V, Zajdela A *et al.* Prognostic value of the S-phase fraction of breast cancers treated by primary radiotherapy or neoadjuvant chemotherapy. *Ann N Y Acad Sci* 1993; **698**: 193–203.

33 Kreipe H, Alm P, Olsson H *et al.* Prognostic significance of a formalin-resistant nuclear proliferation antigen in mammary carcinomas as determined by the monoclonal antibody Ki-S1. *Am J Pathol* 1993; **142**: 651–7.

34 Merkel DE, Winchester DJ, Goldschmidt RA *et al.* DNA flow cytometry and pathologic grading as prognostic guides in axillary lymph node-negative breast cancer. *Cancer* 1993; **72**: 1926–32.

35 Rosner D, Lane-WW. Predicting recurrence in axillary-node negative breast cancer patients. *Breast Cancer Res Treat* 1993; **25**: 127–39.

36 Stal O, Dufmats M, Hatschek T *et al.* S-phase fraction is a prognostic factor in stage I breast carcinoma. *J Clin Oncol* 1993; **11**: 1717–22.

37 Turner RR, Ollila DW, Krasne DL, Guiliano AE. Histopathologic validation of the sentinel lymph node hypothesis for breast carcinoma. *Ann Surg* 1997; **226**: 271–8.

38 Veronesi U, Paganelli G, Galimberti V *et al.* Sentinel-node biopsy to avoid axillary dissection in breast cancer with clinically negative lymph-nodes. *Lancet* 1997; **349**: 1864–7.

39 Veronesi U. The sentinel node and breast cancer. *Br J Surg* 1999; **86**: 1–2.

40 O'Hea BJ, Hill AD, El-Shirbiny AM *et al.* Sentinel lymph node biopsy in breast cancer: initial experience at Memorial Sloan-Kettering Cancer Centre. *J Am Coll Surg* 1998; **186**: 423–7.

41 Beechey-Newman N. Sentinel node biopsy: a revolution in the surgical management of breast cancer? *Cancer Treat Rev* 1998; **24**: 185–203.

42 McIntosh SA, Purushotham AD. Lymphatic mapping and sentinel node biopsy in breast cancer. *Br J Surg* 1998; **85**: 1347–56.

43 Molina R, Zanon G, Filella X *et al.* Use of serial carcinoembryonic antigen and CA 15.3 assays in detecting relapses in breast cancer patients. *Breast Cancer Res Treat* 1995; **36**: 41–8.

44 Al-Jarallah MA, Behbehani AE, El-Nass SA *et al.* Serum CA-15.3 and CEA patterns in postsurgical follow-up, and in monitoring clinical course of metastatic cancer in patients with breast carcinoma. *Eur J Surg Oncol* 1993; **19**: 74–9.

45 Dixon AR, Jackson L, Chan SY *et al.* Continuous chemotherapy in responsive metastatic breast cancer: a role for tumour markers? *Br J Cancer* 1993; **68**: 181–5.

46 Nicolini A, Ferdeghini M, Colizzi C. Evaluation of CEA, TPA, CA 15-3, CA 549 and TPS in the monitoring of metastatic breast cancer. *J Nucl Biol Med* 1993; **37**: 126–33.

47 Giovagnoli MR, Valli C, Vecchione A *et al.* Immunohistochemical expression of tissue polypeptide specific (TPS) antigen in normal and neoplastic tissues. *Anticancer Res* 1994; **14**: 635–41.

48 Lamerz R, Stieber P, Fateh-Moghadam A. Serum marker combinations in human breast cancer (review). *In Vivo* 1993; **7**: 607–14.

49 van Dalen A, Heering KJ, Barak V *et al. Breast* 1996; **5**: 82–8.

50 Mansour O, Motawi T, Khaled H *et al.* Clinical value of thymidine kinase and tissue polypeptide specific antigen in breast cancer. *Dis Markers* 1993; **11**: 171–7.

51 Giai M, Roagna R, Ponzone R *et al.* TPS and CA 15.3 serum values as a guide for treating and monitoring breast cancer patients. *Anticancer Res* 1996; **16**: 875–81.

52 O'Hanlon DM, Kerin MJ, Kent P. An evaluation of preoperative CA 15-3 measurement in primary breast carcinoma. *Br J Cancer* 1995; **71**: 1288–91.

53 Aydiner A, Topuz E, Disci R *et al.* Serum tumor markers for detection of bone metastasis in breast cancer patients. *Acta Oncol* 1994; **33**: 181–6.

54 Bjorklund B, Einarsson R. *Tumor Diagn Ther* 1996; **17**: 67–73.

55 Blijlevens NMA, Oosterhuis WP, Oosten HR. Clinical value of TPS, CEA and CA 15-3 in breast cancer patients. *Anticancer Res* 1995; **15**: 2711–16.

56 Schumacher U, Stamouli A, Adam E *et al.* Biochemical, histochemical and cell biological investigations on the actions of mistletoe lectins I, II and III with human breast cancer cell lines. *Glycoconj J* 1995; **12**: 250–7.

57 Schumacher U, Adam E, Brooks SA *et al.* Lectin-binding properties of human breast cancer cell lines and human milk with particular reference to Helix pomatia agglutinin. *J Histochem Cytochem* 1995; **43**: 275–81.

58 Karaloglu D, Vasasever V, Erturk N *et al.* The value of TPS in breast cancer. *Eur J Gynaecol Oncol* 1995; **16**: 363–7.

59 Cohen AD, Gopas J, Karplus G *et al.* CA 15-3, mucin-like carcinoma-associated antigen and tissue polypeptide-specific antigen: correlation to disease state and prognosis in breast cancer patients. *Isr J Med Sci* 1995; **31**: 155–9.

60 Solomayer EF, Diel IJ, Wallwiener D *et al.* Prognostic relevance of urokinase plasminogen activator detection in micrometastatic cells in the bone marrow of patients with primary breast cancer. *Br J Cancer* 1997; **76**: 812–18.

61 Schmitt M, Thomssen C, Ulm K *et al.* Time-varying prognostic impact of tumour biological factors urokinase PAI-1 and steroid hormone receptor status in primary breast cancer. *Br J Cancer* 1997; **76**: 306–11.

62 Janicke F, Pache L, Schmitt M *et al.* Both the cytosols and detergent extracts of breast cancer tissues are suited to evaluate the prognostic impact of the urokinase-type plasminogen activator and its inhibitor, plasminogen activator inhibitor type 1. *Cancer Res* 1994; **54**: 2527–30.

63 Foekens JA, Look MP, Peters HA *et al.* Urokinase-type plasminogen activator and its inhibitor PAI-1: predictors of poor response to tamoxifen therapy in recurrent breast cancer. *J Natl Cancer Inst* 1995; **87**: 751–6.

64 Romain S, Christensen IJ, Chinot O *et al.* Prognostic value of cytosolic thymidine kinase activity as a marker of proliferation in breast cancer. *Int J Cancer* 1995; **61**: 7–12.

65 Romain S, Martin PM, Klijn JG *et al.* DNA-synthesis enzyme activity: a biological tool useful for predicting anti-metabolic drug sensitivity in breast cancer? *Int J Cancer* 1997; **74**: 156–61.

66 Gohring U-J, Ingenhorst A, Crombach G *et al.* Cathepsin D expression in primary breast cancer. Comparison of immunohistochemical and biochemical results. *Pathologe* 1993; **14**: 313–17.

67 Ferrandina G, Scambia G, Bardelli F *et al.* Relationship between cathepsin-D content and disease-free survival in node-negative breast cancer patients: a meta-analysis. *Br J Cancer* 1997; **76**: 661–6.

68 Ravdin PM, Tandon AK, Allred DC *et al.* Cathepsin D by western blotting and immunohistochemistry: failure to confirm correlations with prognosis in node-negative breast cancer. *J Clin Oncol* 1994; **12**: 467–74.

69 Itoh T, Nishijima M, Ekimov AI. Polaron and exciton-phonon complexes in CuCl nanocystals. *Phys Rev Lett* 1995; **74**(9): 1645–8.

70 Aaltonen M, Lipponen P, Kosma VM *et al.* Prognostic value of cathepsin-D expression in female breast cancer. *Anticancer Res* 1995; **15**: 1033–7.

71 Nadji M, Fresno M, Nassiri M *et al.* Cathepsin D in host stromal cells, but not in tumor cells, is associated with aggressive behavior in node-negative breast cancer. *Hum Pathol* 1996; **27**: 890–5.

72 Seshadri R, Horsfall DJ, Firgaira F *et al.* The relative prognostic significance of total cathepsin D and HER-2/neu oncogene amplification in breast cancer. The South Australian Breast Cancer Study Group. *Int J Cancer* 1994; **56**: 61–5.

73 Johansen JS, Cintin C, Jorgensen M *et al.* Serum YKL-40: a new potential marker of prognosis and location of metastases of patients with recurrent breast cancer. *Eur J Cancer* 1995; **31A**: 1437–42.

74 Nicholson RI, McClelland RA, Gee JMW *et al.* Epidermal growth factor receptor expression in breast cancer: association with response to endocrine therapy. *Breast Cancer Res Treat* 1994; **29**: 117–25.

75 Gasparini G, Boracchi P, Bevilacqua P *et al.* A multiparametric study on the prognostic value of epidermal growth factor receptor in operable breast carcinoma. *Breast Cancer Res Treat* 1994; **29**: 59–71.

76 Spyratos F, Martin PM, Hacene K *et al.* Prognostic value of a solubilized fraction of EGF receptors in primary breast cancer using an immunoenzymatic assay – a retrospective study. *Breast Cancer Res Treat* 1994; **29**: 85–95.

77 Motomura K, Koyama H, Noguchi S, Inaji H, Kasugai T. Effect of tamoxifen on pS2 expression in human breast cancers. *Oncology* 1997; **54**(5): 424–8.

78 Duda RB, Taback B, Kessel B *et al.* pS2 expression induced by American ginseng in MCF-7 breast cancer cells. *Ann Surg Oncol* 1996; **3**: 515–20.

79 Zava DT, Duwe G. Estrogenic and antiproliferative properties of genistein and other flavonoids in human breast cancer cells in vitro. *Nutr Cancer* 1997; **27**: 31–40.

80 Gion M, Plebani M, Mione R *et al.* Serum CA549 in primary breast cancer: comparison with CA15.3 and MCA. *Br J Cancer* 1994; **69**: 721–5

81 Crombach G, Ingenhorst A, Gohring U-J *et al.* Expression of pS2 protein in breast cancer. *Arch Gynecol Obstet* 1993; **253**: 183–92.

82 Hahnel E, Harvey JM, Royce R. Stromelysin-3 expression in breast cancer biopsies: clinico-pathological correlations. *Int J Cancer* 1993; **55**(5): 771–4.

83 Detre S, King N, Salter J *et al.* Immunohistochemical and biochemical analysis of the oestrogen regulated protein pS2, and its relation with oestrogen receptor and progesterone receptor in breast cancer. *J Clin Pathol* 1994; **47**: 240–4.

84 Ibrahim NBN, Padfield CJH, Rees EJ *et al.* Immunocytochemistry in the assessment of pS2 protein expression in fin aspiration cytology from breast carcinoma. *Cytopathology* 1993; **4**: 323–30.

85 Stonelake PS, Baker PG, Gillespie WM *et al.* Steroid receptors, p52 and cathepsin D in early clinically node-negative breast cancer. *Eur J Cancer* 1994; **30**: 5–11.

86 Dookeran KA, Rye PD, Dearing SJ *et al.* Expression of the pS2 peptide in primary breast carcinomas: comparison of membrane and cytoplasmic staining patterns. *J Pathol* 1993; **171**: 123–9.

87 Pallud C, Le-Doussal V, Pichon M-F *et al.* Immunohistochemistry of pS2 in normal human breast and in various histological forms of breast tumors. *Histopathology* 1993; **23**: 249–56.

88 Love S, King RJB. A 27 kDa heat shock protein that has anomalous prognostic powers in early and advanced breast cancer. *Br J Cancer* 1994; **69**: 743–8.

89 Tetu B, Brisson J, Landery J *et al.* Prognostic significance of heat-shock protein-27 in node-positive breast carcinoma: an immunohistochemical study. *Breast Cancer Res Treat* 1995; **36**: 93–7.

90 Hurlimann J, Gebhard S, Gomez F. Oestrogen receptor, progesterone receptor, pS2, ERD5, HSP27 and cathepsin D in invasive ductal breast carcinomas. *Histopathology* 1993; **23**: 239–48.

91 Dunn DK, Whelan RDH, Hill B *et al.* Relationship of HSP27 and oestrogen receptor in hormone sensitive and insensitive cell lines. *J Steroid Biochem Mol Biol* 1993; **46**: 469–79.

92 Elledge RM, Clark GM, Fuqua SAW *et al.* p53 protein accumulation detected by five different antibodies: relationship to prognosis and heat shock protein 70 in breast cancer. *Cancer Res* 1994; **54**: 3752–7.

93 Ciocca DR, Clark GM, Tandon AK *et al.* Heat shock protein hsp70 in patients with axillary lymph node-negative breast cancer: prognostic implications. *J Natl Cancer Inst* 1993; **85**: 570–4.

94 Takahashi S, Mikami T, Watanabe Y *et al.* Correlation of heat shock protein 70 expression with estrogen receptor levels in invasive human breast cancer. *Am J Clin Pathol* 1994; **101**: 519–25.

95 Gasparini G, Pozza F, Harris AL. Evaluating the potential usefulness of new prognostic and predictive indicators in node-negative breast cancer patients. *J Natl Cancer Inst* 1993; **85**(15): 1206–19.

96 Yu H, Diamandis EP, Sutherland DJA. Immunoreactive prostate-specific antigen levels in female and male breast tumors and its association with steroid hormone receptors and patient age. *Clin Biochem* 1994; **27**: 75–9.

97 Melegos DN, Diamandis EP. Diagnostic value of molecular forms of prostate-specific antigen for female breast cancer. *Clin Biochem* 1996; **29**: 193–200.

98 Yamashita J-I, Ogawa M, Ikei S *et al*. Production of immunoreactive polymorphonuclear leucocyte elastase in human breast cancer cells: possible role of polymorphonuclear leucocyte elastase in the progression of human breast cancer. *Br J Cancer* 1994; **69**: 72–6.

99 Chenard MP, O'Siorain L, Shering S *et al*. High levels of stromelysin-3 correlate with poor prognosis in patients with breast carcinoma. *Int J Cancer* 1996; **69**: 448–51.

100 McCarthy K, Maguire T, McGreal G, McDermott E, O'Higgins N, Duffy MJ. High levels of tissue inhibitor of metalloproteinase-1 predict poor outcome in patients with breast cancer. *Int J Cancer* 1999; **84**: 44–8.

101 Justice G, Guerrero R, Rounds D *et al. Proc Ann Meet Am Soc Clin Oncol* 1992; **12**: A197.

102 Justice G, Rounds D, Guerrero R *et al. Proc Ann Meet Am Soc Clin Oncol* 1993; **12**: A264.

103 Levesque MA, Yu H, Clark GM, Diamandis EP. Enzyme-linked immunoabsorbent assay-detected p53 protein accumulation: a prognostic factor in a large breast cancer cohort. *J Clin Oncol* 1998; **16**: 2641–50.

104 Micelli G, Donadeo A, Quaranta M. The p53 tumor suppressor gene. A preliminary clinical study in breast cancer patients. *Cell Biophys* 1992; **21**: 25–31.

105 Dong X, Hamilton KJ, Satoh M *et al*. Related Articles Initiation of autoimmunity to the p53 tumor suppressor protein by complexes of p53 and SV40 large T antigen. *J Exp Med* 1994; **179**: 1243–52.

106 Ciesielski D, Dziewulska-Bokiniec A, Zoltowska A *et al*. p53 expression in breast cancer related to prognostic factors. *Neoplasma* 1995; **42**: 235–7.

107 Jansson T, Inganas M, Sjogren S *et al*. p53 Status predicts survival in breast cancer patients treated with or without postoperative radiotherapy: a novel hypothesis based on clinical findings. *J Clin Oncol* 1995; **13**: 2745–51.

108 Aas T, Borresen AL, Geisler S *et al*. Specific P53 mutations are associated with de novo resistance to doxoru breast cancer patients. *Nature* 1996; **2**: 811–14.

109 Thor AD, Moore DH II, Edgerton SM *et al*. Accumulation of p53 tumor suppressor gene protein: an independent marker of prognosis in breast cancers. *J Natl Cancer Inst* 1992; **84**: 845–55.

110 Lohmann DR, Brandt B, Hopping W, Passarge E, Horsthemke B. Spectrum of small length germline mutations in the RB1 gene. *Hum Mol Genet* 1994; **3**(12): 2187–93.

111 Fisher CJ, Gillett CE, Vojtesek B *et al*. Problems with p53 immunohistochemical staining: the effect of fixation and variation in the methods of evaluation. *Br J Cancer* 1994; **69**: 26–31

112 Jacquemier J, Moles JP, Penault-Llorca F *et al*. p53 immunohistochemical analysis in breast cancer with four monoclonal antibodies: comparison of staining and PCR-SSCP results. *Br J Cancer* 1994; **69**: 846–52.

113 Hurlimann J. Prognostic value of p53 protein expression in breast carcinomas. *Pathol Res Pract* 1993; **189**: 996–1003.

114 Horne GM, Anderson JJ, Tiniakos DG *et al*. p53 protein as a prognostic indicator in breast carcinoma: a comparison of four antibodies for immunohistochemistry. *Br J Cancer* 1996; **73**: 29–35.

115 Sasa M, Kondo K, Komaki K *et al*. p53 alteration correlates with negative ER, negative PgR, and high histologic grade in breast cancer. *J Surg Oncol* 1994; **56**: 46–50.

116 Blaszyk H, Vaughan CB, Hartmann A *et al*. Novel pattern of p53 gene mutations in an American black cohort with high mortality from breast cancer. *Lancet* 1994; **343**: 1195–7.

117 Elledge RM, Clark GM, Chamness GC *et al*. Tumor biologic factors and breast cancer prognosis among white, Hispanic, and black women in the United States. *J Natl Cancer Inst* 1994; **86**: 705–12.

118 Stenmark-Askmalm M, Stal O, Sullivan S *et al*. Cellular accumulation of p53 protein: an independent prognostic factor in stage II breast cancer. *Eur J Cancer* 1994; **30**: 175–80.

119 Faille A, De-Cremoux P, Extra JM *et al*. p53 mutations and overexpression in locally advanced breast cancers. *Br J Cancer* 1994; **69**: 1145–50.

120 Fresno M, Molina R, Perez-del-Rio MJ *et al*. p53 expression is of independent predictive value in lymph node-negative breast carcinoma. *Eur J Cancer* 1997; **33**: 1268–74.

121 Haldar S, Negrini M, Monne M *et al*. Down-regulation of bcl-2 by p53 in breast cancer cells. *Cancer Res* 1994; **54**: 2095–7.

122 Leek RD, Kaklamanis L, Pezzella F *et al*. bcl-2 in normal human breast and carcinoma, association with oestrogen receptor-positive, epidermal growth factor receptor-negative tumours and in situ cancer. *Br J Cancer* 1994; **69**: 135–9.

123 Silvestrini R, Veneroni S, Daidone MG *et al*. The Bcl-2 protein: a prognostic indicator strongly related to p53 protein in lymph node-negative breast cancer patients. *J Natl Cancer Inst* 1994; **86**: 499–504.

124 Lubin R, Schlichtholz B, Bengoufa D *et al*. Analysis of p53 antibodies in patients with various cancers define B-cell epitopes of human p53: distribution on primary structure and exposure on protein surface. *Cancer Res* 1993; **53**: 5872–6.

125 Mudenda B, Green JA, Green B *et al*. The relationship between serum p53 autoantibodies and characteristics of human breast cancer. *Br J Cancer* 1994; **69**: 1115–9.

126 Peyrat JP, Bonneterre J, Lubin R, Vanlemmens L, Fournier J, Soussi T. Prognostic significance of circulating P53 antibodies in patients undergoing surgery for locoregional breast cancer. *Lancet* 1995 Mar 11; **345**: 621–2.

127 Regidor PA, Regidor M, Callies R *et al.* Detection of p53 auto-antibodies in the sera of breast cancer patients with a new recurrence using an ELISA assay. Does a correlation with the recurrence free interval exist? *Eur J Gynaecol Oncol* 1996; **17**: 192–9.

128 Willsher PC, Pinder SE, Robertson C *et al.* The significance of p53 autoantibodies in the serum of patients with breast cancer. *Anticancer Res* 1996; **16**: 927–30.

129 MacLean GD, Longenecker BM. New possibilities for cancer therapy with advances in cancer immunology. *Can J Oncol* 1994; **4**: 249–54.

130 Walsh MD, McGuckin MA, Devine PL *et al.* Expression of MUC2 epithelial mucin in breast carcinoma. *J Clin Pathol* 1993; **46**: 922–5.

131 Molina R, Jo J, Filella X *et al.* Mucin-like carcinoma-associated antigen (MCA) in tissue and serum of patients with breast cancer: clinical applications in prognosis and disease monitoring. *Int J Biol Markers* 1993; **8**: 113–23.

132 O'Brien DP, Gough DB, Skehill R *et al.* Simple method for comparing reliability of two serum tumour markers in breast carcinoma. *J Clin Path* 1994; **47**: 134–7.

133 Simon MS, Hoff M, Hussein M *et al.* An evaluation of clinical follow-up in women with early stage breast cancer among physician members of the American Society of Clinical Oncology. *Breast Cancer Res Treat* 1993; **27**: 211–19.

134 Pavesi F, Lotzniker M, Scarabelli M *et al.* Circulating CA 549 and other associated antigens in breast cancer patients. *Oncology* 1994; **51**: 18–21.

135 Busetto M, Vianello L, Franceschi R *et al.* CA 15-3 value and neoplastic disease predictivity in the follow-up for breast cancer. *Tumor Biol* 1995; **16**: 243–53.

136 Fukutomi T, Hirohashi S, Tsuda H *et al.* The prognostic value of tumor-associated carbohydrate structures correla gene amplifications in human breast carcinomas. *Jpn J Surg* 1991; **21**: 499–507.

137 Narita T, Funahashi H, Satoh Y *et al.* Serum and immunohistochemical studies of NCC-ST-439 in breast cancer. *J Surg Oncol* 1993; **54**: 5–8.

138 Konishi K, Karaki K, Watanabe K *et al.* Clinical usefulness of tumor markers in breast cancer. *Rinsho Byori* **41**: 1108–15.

139 Iwase H, Kobayashi S, Itoh Y *et al.* Evaluation of serum tumor markers in patients with advanced or recurrent breast cancer. *Breast Cancer Res Treat* 1995; **33**: 83–8.

140 van Krieken L, Heureux F, Longueville J. Longitudinal follow-up of breast cancer patients with the tumor markers and CA 15.3. *Int J Biol Markers* 1995; **10**: 30–4.

141 Chan DW, Beveridge RA, Bhargava A *et al.* Breast cancer marker Ca549. A multicenter study. *Am J Clin Pathol* 1994; **101**: 465–70.

142 Correale M, Abbate I, Dragone CD *et al.* Serum and cytosolic levels of CA549 in breast cancer patients. *Clin Exp Obstet Gynecol* 1993; **20**: 264–7.

143 Cazin JL, Gosselin P, Boniface B *et al.* An evaluation of CA 549, a circulating marker of breast cancer using a procedure for comparison with CA 15.3. *Anticancer* Res 1992; **12**: 719–724.

144 Springer GF. Tn epitope (N-acetyl-D-galactosamine alpha-O-serine/threonine) density in primary breast carcinoma: a functional predictor of aggressiveness. *Mol Immunol* 1989; **26**: 1–5.

145 Castro M, Strauchen J, Mandeli J *et al. Proc Annu Meet Am Soc Clin Oncol* 1991; **10**: A35.

146 Takahashi I, Maehara Y, Kusumoto T *et al.* Combined evaluation of preoperative serum sialyl-Tn antigen and carcinoembryonic antigen levels is prognostic for gastric cancer patients. *Br J Cancer* 1994; **69**: 163–6.

147 Werther JL, Rivera-MacMurray S, Bruckner H *et al.* Mucin-associated sialosyl-Tn antigen expression in gastric cancer correlates with an adverse outcome. *Br J Cancer* 1994; **69**: 613–16.

148 Ma XC, Terata N, Kodama M *et al.* Expression of sialyl-Tn antigen is correlated with survival time of patients with gastric carcinomas. *Eur J Cancer* 1993; **29**: 1820–3.

149 King M-J, Chan A, Roe R *et al.* Two different glycosyltransferase defects that result in GalNAc alpha-O-peptide (Tn) expression. *Glycobiology* 1994; **4**: 267–79.

150 Nakagoe T, Fukushima K, Hirota M *et al.* Immunohistochemical expression of sialyl Lex antigen in relation to sur patients with colorectal carcinoma. *Cancer* 1993; **72**: 2323–30.

151 Torii A, Nakayama A, Harada A *et al.* Expression of the CD15 antigen in hepatocellular carcinoma. *Cancer* 1993; **71**: 3864–7.

152 Nakagoe T, Fukushima K, Hirota M. Immunohistochemical expression of sialyl Lex antigen in relation to survival of patients with colorectal carcinoma. *Cancer* 1993; **72**(8): 2323–30.

153 Brooks SA, Leathem AJC. Expression of the CD15 antigen (Lewis x) in breast cancer. *Histochem J* 1995; **27**: 689–93.

154 Yamaguchi A, Ding K, Maehara M *et al.* Expression of nm23-H1 gene and Sialyl Lewis X antigen in breast cancer. *Oncology* 1998; **55**: 357–62.

155 Langkilde NC, Hastrup J, Olsen S *et al.* Immunohistochemistry and cytochemistry of experimental rat bladder cancer: binding of the lectins PNA and WGA and of a Le(Y) mouse monoclonal antibody. *J Urol* 1989; **141**: 981–6.

156 Brooks SA, Leathem AJC. Prediction of lymph node involvement in breast cancer by detection of altered glycosylation in the primary tumour. *Lancet* 1991; **338**: 71–4.

157 Kojima N, Hakomori S. Cell adhesion, spreading, and motility of GM3-expressing cells based on glycolipid-glycolipid interaction. *J Biol Chem* 1991; **266**: 17552–8.

158 Reese MR, Chow DA. Tumor progression in vivo: increased soybean agglutinin lectin binding, N-acetylgalactosamine-

specific lectin expression, and liver metastasis potential. *Cancer Res* 1992; **52**: 5235–43.

159 Shiraishi T, Atsumi S-I, Yatani R. Comparative study of prostatic carcinoma bone metastasis among Japanese in Japan and Japanese Americans and whites in Hawaii. *Adv Exp Med Biol* 1992; **324**: 7–16.

160 Noguchi M, Thomas M, Kitagawa H *et al.* Further analysis of predictive value of Helix pomatia lectin binding to primary breast cancer for axillary and internal mammary lymph node metastases. *Br J Cancer* 1993; **67**: 1368–71.

161 Noguchi M, Earashi M, Ohnishi I *et al. Int J Oncol* 1994; **4**: 1353–8.

162 Springer GF. T and Tn pancarcinoma markers: autoantigenic adhesion molecules in pathogenesis, carcinoma-detection, and long-term breast carcinoma immunotherapy. *Crit Rev Oncog* 1995; **6**(1): 57–85.

163 Thomas M, Noguchi M, Fonseca L *et al.* Prognostic significance of Helix pomatia lectin and c-erbB-2 oncoprotein in human breast cancer. *Br J Cancer* 1993; **68**: 621–6.

164 Kjonniksen I, Rye PD, Fodstad O. Helix pomatia agglutinin binding in human tumour cell lines: correlation with pulmonary metastases in nude mice. *Br J Cancer* 1994; **69**: 1021–4.

165 Kakeji Y, Maehara Y, Tsujitani S, Baba H, Ohno S, Watanaba A, Sugimachi K. Helix pomatia agglutinin binding activity and lymph node metastasis in patients with gastric cancer. *Semin Surg Oncol* 1994; **10**(2): 130–4.

166 Yoshida Y, Okamura T, Yano K *et al.* Silver stained nucleolar organizer region proteins and Helix pomatia agglutinin immunostaining in esophageal carcinoma: correlated prognostic factors. *J Surg Oncol* 1994; **56**: 116–21.

167 Ikeda Y, Mori M, Adachi Y *et al.* Prognostic value of the histochemical expression of helix pomatia agglutinin in advanced colorectal cancer. A univariate and multivariate analysis. *Dis Colon Rectum* 1994; **37**: 181–4.

168 Schumacher U, Higgs D, Loizidou M *et al.* Helix pomatia agglutinin binding is a useful prognostic indicator in colorectal carcinoma. *Cancer* 1994; **74**: 3104–7.

169 Korczak B, Goss P, Fernandez B *et al.* Branching N-linked oligosaccharides in breast cancer. *Adv Exp Med Biol* 1994; **353**: 95–104.

170 Laferte S, Dennis JW. Purification of two glycoproteins expressing beta 1-6 branched Asn-linked oligosaccharides from metastatic tumour cells. *Biochem J* 1989; **259**(2): 569–76.

171 Segal NH, Cohen RJ, Haffejee Z *et al.* BCL-2 proto-oncogene expression in prostate cancer and its relationship to the prostatic neuroendocrine cell. *Arch Pathol Lab Med* 1994; **118**: 616–18.

172 Garte S. The c-myc oncogene in tumor progression. *Crit Rev Oncol* 1993; **4**: 435–49.

173 Brandt B, Vogt U, Harms F *et al. Proc Annu Meet Am Soc Clin Oncol* 1993; **12**: A237.

174 Watson PH, Safneck JR, Le K *et al.* Relationship of c-myc amplification to progression of breast cancer from in situ to invasive tumor and lymph node metastasis. *J Natl Cancer Inst* 1993; **85**: 902–7.

175 Kreipe H, Feist H, Fischer L *et al.* Amplification of c-myc but not of c-erbB-2 is associated with high proliferative capacity in breast cancer. *Cancer Res* 1993; **53**: 1956–61.

176 Berns EMJJ, Klijn JGM, van Putten WLJ *et al.* c-myc amplification is a better prognostic factor than HER2/neu amplification in primary breast cancer. *Cancer Res* 1992; **52**: 1107–13.

177 Pertschuk LP, Feldman JG, Kim DS *et al.* Steroid hormone receptor immunohistochemistry and amplification of c-myc protooncogene. *Cancer* 1993; **71**: 162–71.

178 Roux-Dosseto M, Romain S, Dussault N *et al.* c-myc gene amplification in selected node-negative breast cancer patients correlates with high rate of early relapse. *Eur J Cancer* 1992; **28**: 1600–4.

179 Champeme MH, Bieche I, Hacene K *et al.* Int-2/FGF3 amplification is a better independent predictor of relapse than c-myc and c-erbB-2/neu amplifications in primary human breast cancer. *Mod Pathol* 1994; **7**: 900–905.

180 Borg A, Baldetorp B, Ferno M *et al.* c-myc amplification is an independent prognostic factor in postmenopausal breast cancer. *Int J Cancer* 1992; **51**: 687–91.

181 Henry JA, Hennessy C, Levett DL *et al.* int-2 amplification in breast cancer: association with decreased survival and relationship to amplification orf c-erbB-2 and c-myc. *Int J Cancer* 1993; **53**: 774–80.

182 Pietilainen T, Lipponen P, Aaltomaa S *et al.* Expression of c-myc proteins in breast cancer as related to established prognostic factors and survival. *Anticancer Res* 1995; **15**: 959–64.

183 Pierce LJ, Merino MJ, D'Angelo T *et al.* Is c-erb B-2 a predictor for recurrent disease in early stage breast cancer? *Int J Radiat Oncol Biol Phys* 1994; **28**: 395–403.

184 Paik S, Bryant J, Park C, Fisher B *et al.* erbB-2 and response to doxorubicin in patients with axillary lymph node-positive, hormone receptor-negative breast cancer. *J Natl Cancer Inst* 1998; **90**: 1361–70.

185 Muss HB, Thor AD, Berry DA *et al.* c-erbB-2 expression and response to adjuvant therapy in women with node-positive early breast cancer. *N Engl J Med* 1994; **330**: 1260–6.

186 Andrulis IL, Bull SB, Blackstein ME *et al.* neu/erbB-2 amplification identifies a poor-prognosis group of women with node-negative breast cancer. Toronto Breast Cancer Study Group. *J Clin Oncol* 1998; **16**: 1340–9.

187 Wang TC, Cardiff RD, Zukerberg L *et al.* Mammary hyperplasia and carcinoma in MMTV-cyclin D1 transgenic m. *Nature* 1994; **369**: 669–71.

188 Gillett CE, Fantl V, Smith R *et al.* Amplification and overexpression of cyclin D1 in breast cancer detected immunohistochemical staining. *Cancer Res* 1994; **54**: 1812–17.

189 Bartkova J, Lukas J, Muller H *et al.* Cyclin D1 protein expression and function in human breast cancer. *Int J Cancer* 1994; **57**: 353–61.

190 Keyomarsi K, O'Leary N, Molnar G *et al.* Cyclin E, a potential prognostic marker for breast cancer. *Cancer Res* 1994; **54**: 380–5.

191 Tokunaga Y, Urano T, Furukawa K *et al.* Reduced expression of nm23-H1, but not of nm23-H2, is concordant with the frequency of lymph-node metastasis of human breast cancer. *Int J Cancer* 1993; **55**: 66–71.

192 Dawkins HJS, Goodall RJ, Hahnel E *et al. Breast* 1993; **2**: 239–245.

193 Sawan A, Lascu I, Veron M *et al.* NDP-K/nm23 expression in human breast cancer in relation to relapse, survival, and other prognostic factors: an immunohistochemical study. *J Pathol* 1994; **172**: 27–34.

194 Albertsen PC, Fryback DG, Storer BE. The impact of co-morbidity on life expectancy among men with localized prostate cancer. *J Urol* 1996; **156**: 127–32.

195 Satariano WA, Ragland DR. The effect of comorbidity on 3-year survival of women with primary breast cancer. *Ann Intern Med* 1994; **120**: 104–10.

196 West DW, Satariano WA, Ragland DR, Hiatt RA. Comorbidity and breast cancer survival: a comparison between black and white women. *Ann Epidemiol* 1996; **6**: 413–19.

197 D'Hoore W, Bouckaert, Tilquin C. Practical considerations on the use of the Charlson comorbidity index with administrative data bases. *J Clin Epidemiol* 1996; **49**: 1429–33.

198 Ruder AM, Moodie PF, Nelson NA *et al.* Does family history of breast cancer improve survival among patients with cancer? *Am J Obst Gynecol* 1988; **158**: 963–8.

199 Fukutomi T, Kobayashi Y, Nanasawa T *et al.* A clinicopathological analysis of breast cancer in patients with a family history. *Surg Today* 1993; **23**: 849–54.

200 Slattery ML, Berry TD, Kerber RA. Is survival among women diagnosed with breast cancer influenced by family history of breast cancer? *Epidemiology* 1993; **4**: 543–8.

201 Lynch H, Salerno G, Watson P *et al. Proc Annu Meet Am Soc Clin Oncol* 1990; **9**: A223.

202 Inada K, Toi M, Imazawa T *et al.* Significance of overexpression of p53 protein in human breast cancer. *Jpn J Cancer Chemother* 1994; **21**: 817–21.

203 Caleffi M, Teague MW, Jensen RA *et al.* p53 gene mutations and steroid receptor status in breast cancer. Clinicopathologic correlations and prognostic assessment. *Cancer* 1994; **73**: 2147–56.

204 Marcus JN, Watson P, Page DL *et al.* Hereditary breast cancer: pathobiology, prognosis, and BRCA1 and BRCA2 gene linkage. *Cancer* 1996; **77**: 697–709.

205 Porter DE, Cohen BB, Wallace MR *et al.* Breast cancer incidence, penetrance and survival in probable carriers of BRCA1 gene mutation in families linked to BRCA1 on chromosome 17q12-21. *Br J Surg* 1994; **81**: 1512–15.

206 Rubin SC, Benjamin I *et al.* Clinical and pathological features of ovarian cancer in women with germ-line mutations of BRCA1. *N Engl J Med.* 1996; **335**: 1413–16.

207 Ingram D. Diet and subsequent survival in women with breast cancer. *Br J Cancer* 1994; **69**: 592–5.

208 Lund E, Bonaa KH. Reduced breast cancer mortality among fishermen's wives in Norway. *Cancer Causes Control* 1993; **4**: 283–7.

209 Adlercreutz H, Mousavi Y, Clark J *et al.* Dietary phytoestrogens and cancer: in vitro and in vivo studies. *J Steroid Biochem Mol Biol* 1992; **41**: 331–7.

210 Lampe JW, Martini MC, Kurzer MS *et al.* Urinary lignan and isoflavonoid excretion in premenopausal women consuming flaxseed powder. *Am J Clin Nutr* 1994; **60**: 122–8.

211 Adlercreutz H, Markkanen H, Watanabe S. Plasma concentrations of phyto-oestrogens in Japanese men. *Lancet* 1993; **342**: 1209–10.

212 Griffiths K, Adlercreutz H, Boyle P *et al. Nutrition and cancer.* Oxford: Isis Medical Media Ltd, 1996.

213 Ansell D, Whitman S, Lipton R *et al.* Race, income, and survival from breast cancer at two public hospitals. *Cancer* 1993; **72**: 2974–8.

214 Heimann R, Ferguson D, Powers C *et al.* Race and clinical outcome in breast cancer in a series with long-term follow-up evaluation. *J Clin Oncol.* 1997; **15**: 2329–37.

215 Lyman GH, Kuderer NM, Lyman SL *et al.* Importance of race on breast cancer survival. *Ann Surg Oncol* 1997; **4**: 80–7.

216 Chen VW, Correa P, Kurman RJ *et al.* Histological characteristics of breast carcinoma in blacks and whites. *Cancer Epidemiol Biomarkers Prev* 1994; **3**: 127–35.

217 Wakai K, Suzuki S, Ohno Y *et al.* Epidemiology of breast cancer in Japan. *Int J Epidemiol* 1995; **24**: 285–91.

218 Imaizumi Y. Longitudinal analysis of mortality from breast cancer in Japan, 1950–1993: fitting Gompertz and Weibull functions. *Mech Ageing Dev* 1996; **88**: 169–83.

219 Smams M, Boyle P, Muir CS. Cancer Mortality Atlas of the European Economic Community. *Recent Results Cancer Res* 1989; **114**: 253–68.

220 Garcia–Arcal MD, Pollan Santamaria M, Lopez-Abente Ortega G. Mortality from breast cancer in the European Community (1970–1985). *Med Clin (Barc)* 1994; **102**(4): 125–8.

221 Sturgeon SR, Schairer C, Gall M *et al.* Geographic variation in mortality from breast cancer among white women in the United States. *J Natl Cancer Inst* 1995; **87**: 1846–53.

222 Richardson JL, Langholz B, Bernstein L *et al.* Stage and delay in breast cancer diagnosis by race, socioeconomic status, age and year. *Br J Cancer* 1992; **65**: 922–6.

223 Gordon NH, Crowe JP, Brumberg DJ *et al.* Socioeconomic factors and race in breast cancer recurrence and survival. *Am J Epidemiol* 1992; **135**: 609–18.

224 Coleman T. Health promotion. Sensitive outcome measures are needed. *BMJ* 1994; **309**(6968): 1581–2.

225 Schrijvers CT, Coebergh JW, van der Heijden LH *et al.* Socioeconomic status and breast cancer survival in the southeastern Netherlands, 1980–1989. *Eur J Cancer* 1995; **31A**: 1660–4.

226 Schrijvers CT, Mackenbach JP, Lutz JM *et al.* Deprivation and survival from breast cancer. *Br J Cancer* 1995; **72**: 738–43.

227 Jensen AB. Psychosocial factors in breast cancer and their possible impact upon prognosis. *Cancer Treat Rev* 1991; **18**: 191–210.

228 Greer S, Morris T, Pettingale KW. Psychological response to breast cancer: effect on outcome. *Lancet* 1979; **2**: 785–7.

229 Greer S. Psychological response to cancer and survival. *Psychol Med* 1991; **21**: 43–9.

230 Ramirez AJ, Craig TK, Watson JP *et al.* Stress and relapse of breast cancer. *BMJ* 1989; **298**: 291–3.

231 Barraclough J, Pinder P, Cruddas M *et al.* Life events and breast cancer prognosis. *BMJ* 1992; **304**: 1078–81.

232 Spiegel D, Bloom JR, Kraemer HC *et al.* Effect of psychosocial treatment on survival of patients with metastatic breast cancer. *Lancet* 1989; **2**: 888–91.

233 Spiegel D. *Br J Psychiatry* 1996; **Supplement 30**: 109–16.

234 Spiegel D. Psychological distress and disease course for women with breast cancer: one answer, many questions. *J Natl Cancer Inst* 1996; **88**: 629–31.

235 Kogon MM, Biswas A, Pearl D, Carlson RW, Spiegel D. Effects of medical and psychotherapeutic treatment on the survival of women with metastatic breast carcinoma. *Cancer* 1997; **80**: 225–30.

236 Gellert GA, Maxwell RM, Siegel BS. Survival of breast cancer patients receiving adjunctive psychosocial support therapy: a 10-year follow-up study. *J Clin Oncol* 1993; **11**: 66–9.

237 Reynolds P, Boyd PT, Blacklow RS *et al.* The relationship between social ties and survival among black and white breast cancer patients. *Cancer Epidemiol Biomarkers Prev* 1994; **3**: 253–9.

238 Maunsell E, Brisson J, Deschenes L. Social support and survival among women with breast cancer. *Cancer* 1995; **76**: 631–7.

239 Calle EE, Miracle-McMahill HL, Thun MJ *et al.* Cigarette smoking and risk of fatal breast cancer. *Am J Epidemiol* 1994; **139**: 1001–7.

240 Janerich DT, Mineau GP, Kerber RA. Gender of the first offspring, age at diagnosis, and survival with breast cancer (Utah, United States). *Cancer Causes Control* 1994; **5**: 26–30.

241 Basso-Ricci S, Coradini D, Bartoli C *et al.* Long-term relapses in breast cancer patients (estrogen receptor status). *Tumori* 1995; **81**: 265–7.

242 Yoshimoto M, Sakamoto G, Ohashi Y. Time dependency of the influence of prognostic factors on relapse in breast cancer. *Cancer* 1993; **72**: 2993–3001.

243 Collett K, Moehle BO, Skioerven R *et al.* Lymph node-negative breast cancer: the prognostic role and time dependency of age, tumor diameter and mean nuclear area. *Oncology* 1994; **51**: 323–8.

244 Sankila R, Joensuu H, Pukkala E *et al.* Does the month of diagnosis affect survival of cancer patients? *Br J Cancer* 1993; **67**: 838–41.

4

Prognostic and predictive factors in invasive breast cancer

HENK-JAN VAN SLOOTEN, JAN HEIN VAN DIERENDONCK AND CORNELIS JH VAN DER VELDE

INTRODUCTION

The ongoing search for new prognostic factors

Over the past fifteen years, only node-positive breast cancer (BC) patients have traditionally been thought to be at sufficiently high risk to justify the toxicities of adjuvant therapy. However, the 1992 update of the Early Breast Cancer Collaborative Trialists' group confirmed that systemic hormonal and cytotoxic treatment improves disease-free survival (DFS) and overall survival (OS), independent of lymph node status.[1] This data strengthened the rationale for adjuvant chemotherapy and hormonal therapy in node-negative BC patients, or in patients whose node status is unknown at the time of starting this treatment (as in trials on pre-operative chemotherapy).

Due to improvements in the detection of early BC, the percentage of node-negative patients has now risen to 70%. The majority of these patients (70–75%) will not experience disease recurrence after local therapy (surgery and/or radiotherapy) alone,[2] suggesting that many node-negative patients are cured by local treatment. Obviously, because of the considerable burden and costs involved, chemotherapy for *all* patients seems inappropriate.

In theory, assessment of risk of recurrence based on tumour size and histopathological classification should be sufficiently compelling to make treatment decisions relatively straightforward in approximately half of the patients with node-negative BC. Almost 30% of patients have tumours either less than 1 cm in diameter or less than 3 cm, but with a favourable histological type. These women have an excellent prognosis (recurrence rate less than 10%) and should not receive additional treatment.[2] The group of 25% of patients with tumours exceeding 3 cm in diameter will very probably recur (> 50%), and therefore almost all of these patients should receive adjuvant therapy. In the remaining group of patients, the recurrence rate is 30%. For this group the decision as to whether or not to treat is difficult and additional prognostic information is needed.

However, it should be stressed that in general it is difficult to assess tumour size accurately in clinical practice. In fact, the decision as to whether a patient should receive adjuvant chemotherapy is usually based on nodal status only, and one can safely state that in order to select high-risk node-negative patients for adjuvant treatment, strong additional prognostic factors are needed.

In order to design optimal treatment strategies for individual patients it is essential to be able to predict a tumour's response to a specific therapy, in both node-negative and node-positive BC. However, factors that predict the risk of recurrence (e.g. node status, tumour size) do not necessarily predict the response to adjuvant therapy. Although some factors that are able to predict response to hormonal therapy are in clinical use or under investigation, at present no clinically useful markers are available that predict response to chemotherapy. Therefore, in particular the development of markers that predict a patient's response to adjuvant chemotherapy will be of great value for the management of both node-positive and node-negative patients.

Thus important clinical questions concerning the treatment of BC patients include the following:

- Which prognostic factors can properly separate the majority of low-risk subsets of node-negative patients from those at high risk?
- What is the minimal level of risk that justifies systemic adjuvant therapy for node-negative patients?
- Which factors predict response to chemotherapy and/or hormone therapy or to novel therapeutic approaches in both node-negative and node-positive patients?[3]

Currently, at least 80 putative BC prognostic factors have been reported, but most of the factors are relatively new, and for many of them their value has not yet been fully established.

Generally accepted prognostic factors

The TNM staging system combines the variables tumour size and local extension (T), regional lymph-node involvement (N) and metastatic spread (M). This system emerged in the 1950s as a response to the need for an accurate system to select patients for clinical trials, to analyse data from these trials and to discuss the prognosis with individual patients.

Histological grade was introduced in the early 1920s by Greenough[4] and Patey and Scarff,[5] and in 1957 Bloom and Richardson reported their improved grading scheme (SBR), which has become widely accepted.[6] Recently, Doussal *et al.* proposed a modified SBR scheme that is more accurate and predictive than the standard SBR grade, especially in node-negative BC patients[7]. The usefulness of combining grade with tumour size and nodal status into a prognostic index[8] is discussed in Chapter 5.

The mitotic index (MI) is probably the most important determinant of the prognostic value of histological grading. However, it is often difficult to discriminate mitotic figures in a tissue section reliably. Moreover, MI is expressed as the number of mitoses per microscope field, and the size of the latter may vary. Finally, the mitotic compartment makes up the smallest portion of cycling cells, thus reducing sampling size.[9] Because human BCs generally show a moderate to low proliferative activity, measurement of a larger part of the cell cycle (e.g. of DNA-synthesizing cells (S-phase) and/or of cells in G2 and G1 phases), would markedly increase the accuracy of measurements.

In recent years, there have been significant improvements in the detection of proliferation rate with the advancement of flow cytometry and the development of a variety of immunohistochemical markers related to cellular proliferation. In this chapter we shall briefly discuss these new applications.

Another generally accepted prognostic factor is the presence of steroid receptors – oestrogen (OR) and progesterone (PgR) – which has found wide application in the selection of (post-menopausal) BC patients for hormonal treatments. A major unresolved issue is why up to 50% of OR-positive tumours are unresponsive, and why eventually all tumours become resistant to these treatments. Conversely, 10% of patients whose tumours do not contain OR respond to treatment with anti-oestrogens. We shall discuss some recent developments that may shed light on this apparent paradox.

Putative prognostic factors

During the past two decades, advances in molecular biology have led to the discovery of a large number of new prognostic factors. Some of these factors were studied in clinical trials, such as markers for tumour cell proliferation, but many factors have only been evaluated in biological and clinical correlative studies, or have been proposed as interesting areas for further research. Many of these new factors are somehow related to established prognostic factors such as histological grade (especially MI) and hormone receptor content, but there are also factors that constitute entirely new aspects, such as factors involved in tumour cell invasiveness and angiogenesis.

As has been stressed by Burke and Henson,[10] any prognostic factor should fulfil the following criteria. It should be statistically significant (i.e. only rarely occurring by chance), independent (i.e. retain its prognostic value when combined with other factors), and clinically relevant (i.e. have a major impact on prognostic accuracy). The ability to measure a prognostic factor reliably and accurately is a prerequisite for its clinical use, but the improvement in accuracy should be balanced against the cost of the analysis which, in addition, should be reproducible and simple to perform.

Unfortunately, the inter-study variability of the majority of new prognostic factors has been shown to be large, and this problem seriously hampers their integration into a predictive system. According to Kennedy,[11] there are a number of arguments why prognostic factors are of limited use in BC.

- Heterogeneity of BC with respect to factors involved in tumour growth and metastasis – no single factor can predict with certainty whether a patient will have a recurrence. Tumours may have good and bad factors, and the number of possible combinations increases with each new factor that is evaluated.
- Many new prognostic factors are not independent but closely interrelated – factors that show significant prognostic value in univariate analysis do not necessarily add significant clinical information. Multivariate analysis of combinations of new and conventional factors is essential to assess the relative

'weight', and to determine which factors are truly independent. The fact is that many studies on new markers have not performed such multivariate analysis.[3]

- Most studies are retrospective and involve insufficient numbers of patients and often insufficient follow-up to allow true determination of the impact of a factor on recurrence or survival.

Prognostic vs. predictive factors

A prognostic factor can be defined as a factor that can provide information at the time of diagnosis or surgery about the possible clinical outcome of the disease (i.e. if the patient would not receive further treatment). A predictive factor is able to predict whether or not a patient is likely to benefit from a specific form of adjuvant treatment. Whereas strong prognostic factors will prevent the (over)treatment of patients with an excellent prognosis, a useful predictive factor may allow the selection for a specific therapy in a patient at high risk, and may prevent the use of a standard treatment in non-responsive high-risk patients.

The above-mentioned hormone receptors can therefore be considered predictive rather than prognostic. Any survival advantage or OR/PgR-positivity is lost after 5 years of follow-up, but the correlation of OR/PgR status with outcome is closely related to responsiveness to hormonal therapy.[1] This example also demonstrates that predictive factors can be the target for a specific type of treatment.

Scope of this chapter

The factors we shall discuss here are mainly of a cellular–molecular–genetic nature, and can be roughly divided into two different categories, namely factors related to uncontrolled cell proliferation and factors related to the interaction between tumour cells and their environment.

In the next section we shall give a brief overview of recent developments in the area of cell-cycle research and regulation of cell survival and cell death. Although this section will probably deter a number of readers with a distinct clinical background, we considered it important to mention some recent discoveries and directions in the molecular biology of BC, because it seems central to understanding the relevance of ongoing research in the field of prognostic/predictive factors and development of new treatment strategies. Important in this context is the explosion in research on cell survival and cell death. Like cell division, cell death can be a fundamental process controlled at genetic and molecular levels, and as such it can be analysed and manipulated.

In a subsequent section we discuss aspects of tumour cell heterogeneity, as it has implications for the evaluation of many factors, as well as technical aspects of estimating proliferative activity and cell death and the significance of these markers as prognostic and predictive factors. We shall then summarize a number of studies that have evaluated the significance of some of the proteins discussed earlier.

As will be discussed later, there have been rapid advances in our understanding of the interaction between tumour cells and their environment. Motility and invasiveness of tumour cells, as well as the capacity of tumour cells to develop tumour stroma and neovascularization, are important signs of malignancy. This area of research may provide important opportunities for the discovery of new molecular factors and targets for control and prevention of BC. We shall then discuss the state of the art with repect to prognosis and treatment.

Finally, we shall briefly discuss how to use a variety of different factors in concert, as well as the recent development of a non-invasive method to analyse metabolism of BCs *in vivo*, which may be especially relevant in the context of monitoring the effects of neoadjuvant therapies.

REGULATION OF CELL NUMBER

Proteins involved in cell-cycle regulation

A great deal of BC research has focused on hormones, growth factors (GFs) and (proto)oncogenes involved in the regulation of cell proliferation. In recent years, cell-cycle research has begun to uncover the complicated programme of events which regulate entrance into the cell-cycle, progression through the cycle, and the mechanisms through which 'checkpoints' operate to maintain cell-cycle integrity and fidelity.

Hormones and polypeptide GFs are important for the induction of proliferation and/or differentiation of human mammary epithelial cells, and these factors can play a significant role in the pathogenesis of BC. In general, BC cells show a reduced requirement for exogenously supplied GFs, due in part to their ability to synthesize and respond to proteins that can regulate their proliferation through intracellular, autocrine, juxtacrine and/or paracrine pathways. BC cells may also express higher levels of specific GF receptors, thereby becoming hypersensitized to certain GFs.[12,13]

Several families of GFs and their receptors are important in BC:

- the epidermal GF (EGF)-related family of peptides.[14] The effects of EGF, transforming GFα (TGFα), and amphiregulin are mediated by the EGF receptor (EGFR), belonging to a family which includes HER-2, HER-3 and HER-4. HER-2, a product of the c-*erb*B-2 (*neu*) oncogene, shows greatest homology to EGFR, and several ligands have been described, including HRG, p75, and gp30;[15]

- insulin and insulin-like GFs (IGF-I and IGF-II), which bind to their own receptors, as well as to IGF-binding proteins present in extracellular fluids;[16]
- the neuroendocrine hormone prolactin (PRL).[17]

The recent elucidation of the steps involved in signal transduction from these receptors to the nucleus is one of the major achievements of molecular biology, and may have considerable implications for cancer research. These signals involve sequences of phosphorylation (i.e. 'activation') by a complex interplay of protein kinases. In short, upon ligand-binding, EGFR family members tend to homo- or even heterodimerize, and one receptor molecule then phosphorylates the other.[18] Insulin and IGF-I receptors have an intrinsic kinase activity that leads to autophosphorylation, whereas the PRL receptor is a non-kinase receptor. PRL-receptor binding activates a JAK kinase, which in turn activates a specific nuclear transcription factor.[19]

In the case of the other GF families, the signalling pathway is much more complex. Phosphorylated EGFR binds to a complex of two cytoplasmic proteins, called GRB2 and SOS respectively,[20] and in the case of IGFR first the insulin receptor substrate IRS-1 is phosphorylated, which subsequently activates GRB2.[21]

The active SOS protein activates Ras, a product of the *ras* proto-oncogene, which in turn activates a kinase known as Raf-1. The latter phosphorylates another kinase, MEK, which then activates MAP kinase.[18]

This Ras-Raf-1-MEK-MAP kinase phosphorylation sequence finally culminates in the activation of nuclear transcription factors, such as the products of members of the c-*myc*, *jun* and *fos* proto-oncogene families. Jun and Fos proteins can form Jun homo- and Jun/Fos heterodimers (the latter is known as AP-1), whereas Myc dimerizes with its homologue Max. These dimers act as potent transcription factors for so-called delayed-response genes, the products of which are essential components of the cell-cycle control system. The role of *myc* is crucial in this context – prevention of its expression prevents cell division in the presence of GFs.[22]

Sex steroid hormones bind to specific intracellular receptors belonging to a superfamily of hormone-dependent transcription factors. The oestrogen–OR complex induces transcription of the *myc*, *fos* and/or *jun* genes by binding to oestrogen response elements of these genes. In human BC cells, oestrogen was reported to have relatively minor effects on *jun* expression, whereas insulin and IGF-1 (and TGFα) seem to induce *jun* rather than *fos*, a finding that would suggest a mechanism for synergy between oestrogen and GFs. Indeed, the reponse to oestrogen is enhanced by the presence of the insulin/IGF family.[23] Another study indicated that the pathway via EGFR induces both *fos* and *jun* family members, but that the primary effect of oestradiol is to induce *myc*.[24] There is also evidence that OR can modulate AP-1 activity, that AP-1 can inhibit OR-induced transcription, and that GFs can mimic or increase oestrogenic effects, even in the absence of oestrogens.[25]

For proliferation, a cell needs to phosphorylate a variety of proteins, including the products of so-called tumour suppressor genes. A crucial event in this process is the activation of complexes between members of the cyclin and cyclin-dependent kinase (CDK) families.[26] Evidence is accumulating that D-type cyclins (notably cyclin D1) and CDK4 are important during the transition from a 'resting' (G0) to a 'cycling' (G1) phase. Cyclin D1 represents a frequent target of oncogenic abnormalities in BC.[27]

The retinoblastoma tumour suppressor gene product (pRb) is a substrate for the cyclin D1/CDK4 complex.[28] Unphosphorylated Rb is able to block cells in G1 phase and it binds a bewildering variety of proteins, in contrast to the phosphorylated form of pRb.[29] These target proteins include the family of transcription factors, collectively known as E2F and believed to be responsible for transcribing a variety of genes, including *myc*, genes encoding enzymes required for DNA synthesis, and several cyclin genes.[30]

A key mechanism in regulation of the activity of cyclin-CDK complexes involves a group of recently defined cyclin-CDK inhibitors (CDIs). One important member of this class of cell-cycle inhibitors is p21 (WAF1, CIP1). The gene of this CDI is transcriptionally regulated by the product of the p53 tumour supressor gene.[31,32]

As early as 1984 it was discovered that irradiation of cells induces metabolic stabilization of p53 protein, leading to its accumulation and G1 arrest.[33] This observation was extended to other genotoxic agents, establishing p53 as a cell-cycle checkpoint protein in response to DNA damage.[34] The p53 gene is induced in response to DNA strand breaks, and a major function of p53 seems to be to guard the integrity of the genome. By inducing p21 protein, p53 may enable cells to repair the DNA damage before they undergo DNA synthesis.[35]

Proteins involved in regulation of cell death

Tumour growth is a balance between the rate of proliferation and the rate of cell death. Consequently, a high MI does not necessarily translate into rapid tumour growth, and a relatively low MI may only lead to an expansion of the tumour cell population if there is also a decreased rate of cell loss.

Many factors traditionally classified as GFs may in fact provide survival signals rather than forcing cells to enter the cell cycle. Without proper survival signals, cells may die by a process that is now generally referred to as apoptosis – a form of cell death in which the cell actively participates by providing the cellular machinery as well as the energy for the process to proceed. It is predominantly defined by morphological characteristics, including cell shrinkage, cytoplasmic membrane blebbing, chromatin condensation, nuclear fragmentation, and ultimately fragmentation of the cell into apoptotic bodies.[36,37]

Apoptotic cells are rapidly phagocytosed by neighbouring cells, without eliciting an inflammatory reaction. The speed of the whole process means that the identification of only a few apoptotic cells within a tissue can represent a considerable degree of cumulative cell loss. Numerically small differences in the percentage of cells with apoptotic morphology ('apoptotic index') can therefore reflect significant differences in tumour growth rates.[38]

Beyond cell death that occurs as a programmed feature of development or adult tissue homeostasis (including the involution of hormone-dependent tissues such as normal and malignant breast epithelium),[39,40] apoptotic deaths can be induced by ionizing radiation, most anticancer drugs, cytokines (TNF-α, FAS ligand, TGF-β), etc.[41] It is now believed that these different stimuli converge on a final common intracellular pathway, as may be reflected in the ability of anti-apoptotic genes, such as Bcl-2, to protect against apoptosis triggered by a large variety of stimuli.[42]

Bcl-2 is the founding member of an expanding gene family, which includes bax.[43] The Bcl-2 homologue Bax dimerizes with itself or with Bcl-2. The ability of Bcl-2 to counter cell death seems to require heterodimerization with Bax, but Bax/Bax homodimers seem to accelerate apoptosis. Therefore the ratio of Bcl-2 to Bax may be an important determinant of the cell's susceptibility to a given apoptotic stimulus.[44]

Members of the Bcl-2 gene family that are potentially relevant to BC include bax, bcl-X, mcl-1, A1, bad and bak, and also a number of proteins that can physically interact with Bcl-2 (but which do not share homology with Bcl-2 family members).[45]

Future research will have to establish the prognostic and predictive value of these proteins. The elucidation of other components involved in the induction of apoptosis downstream of Bcl-2, such as interleukin I-converting enzyme (ICE)-like proteases,[46] may further improve the ability to estimate and modulate the cellular threshold for induction of apoptosis by chemotherapy.

Dependence on both growth and survival factors may be a key method of regulation of cell population size. Survival signals are not necessarily provided only by soluble factors, but also by specific cell–cell interactions (through cadherin-like receptors) or interactions between cells and the extracellular matrix. Indeed, contact of surface integrin receptors with basement membrane proteins seems to be an important survival signal for differentiated epithelial cells. As a result, these cells cannot survive out of position, and it is tempting to speculate that reduced dependence on these 'positional' survival factors might be an important determinant of tumour progression. Apoptosis related to anchorage dependency has recently been termed 'anoikis' ('homelessness').[47]

Molecules contained at the intracellular–extracellular border of focal adhesions include cytoskeletal proteins, products of the src proto-oncogenes, and a recently described focal adhesion kinase (FAK), activity of which is directly linked to the product of src, and involves a signalling pathway that activates MEK.[48] In this context it is interesting that increased levels of FAK have been found to be strongly associated with invasive and metastatic BC.[48]

Although it is debatable whether all cells need this type of signalling to survive, it is likely that all proliferating cells do need survival factors. In fact, the regulation of prolife-ration and cell death may be intimately linked, and it seems that certain key factors in cell number regulation play a double role here. For example, transfection with myc increases the frequency of cycling cells, but this is balanced by increased incidence of apoptosis. Thus, Myc/Max functions to open a pathway not only to cell proliferation, but to cell death as well. The decision as to which pathway to take depends upon additional signals.[49]

It has been found that, in vivo, Myc-induced apoptosis is prevented by IGF-I (but not by EGF), and that a decrease in the number of IGFRs can cause massive apoptosis in several transplantable tumour systems. These data, in addition to other findings, suggest that signalling via IGFR constitutes a very important survival pathway.[50]

Another protein that is relevant in this context is p53, and some forms of apoptosis induction require the action of this protein. This apoptosis-facilitating property of p53 seems to be separable from its growth-suppressing activity and, like the case of myc, the outcome depends on the 'cellular context'.[51] Not only does this activity appear to involve apoptotic responses due to 'unrepairable' DNA damage, but p53 is also implicated in some examples of apoptotic responses due to growth/survival factor withdrawal or to deregulation of cell-cycle progression. The mechanisms involved here have not yet been elucidated, but an intriguing recent finding is that p53 down-regulates Bcl-2 expression and up-regulates bax. Moreover, the 5′ untranslated region of the bax gene also contains a number of motifs that are potential binding sites for the myc gene family.[52,53]

Conclusions

Each cell in a complex multicellular animal is bombarded with signals that determine whether or not it should divide, and signals that dictate whether it will live or die. The function of kinase cascades linking signals initiated by receptor kinases to transcriptional targets is not merely to amplify a signal. It also markedly increases the number of targets for both positive and negative cross-regulation by other signalling pathways. Moreover, the cell-specific patterns in which the numerous elements of phosphorylation cascades are expressed determine the response to both 'upstream' and 'cross-talking' signals.

A consequence of this complexity is that a specific signalling pathway can be deregulated by a variety of different genetic changes. Therefore, if in BC compared to other tumour types a certain component of a signalling pathway shows a low mutation frequency, it does not exclude the possibility that the same signalling pathway is deregulated by other genetic changes.

These genetic changes may lead to an increased tendency to proliferate, but if proliferative signals are perceived 'out of the proper context', this will simultaneously trigger apoptosis. Moreover, as it has become clear that epithelial cells may need contact with basement membranes (and possibly with their neighbouring cells) in order to survive, mutations that lead to constitutive activation of survival signals may be an absolute requirement for multi-layered and metastatic outgrowth of BC cells.

Survival pathways may protect cells from cytotoxic insults, and therefore impact upon the success or failure of anticancer treatment. The molecular mechanisms responsible for the induction and inhibition of apoptosis are now rapidly being unravelled. As a more complete picture emerges, it is hoped that this may not only be relevant to the prediction of treatment response, but also lead to the development of more sophisticated treatment strategies.

DETECTION OF CLONAL HETEROGENEITY, PROLIFERATIVE ACTIVITY AND CELL DEATH

Implications of heterogeneity

It has been postulated that most tumours arise from a single cell of origin, and that tumour progression results from acquired genetic instability within the original clone, allowing sequential selection of more aggressive sublines.[54] BC is a very heterogeneous disease, and it has become clear that this heterogeneity is also present at a genetic level. Flow-cytometric DNA-ploidy analysis has revealed that two-thirds of primary BCs have multiple DNA aneuploid stemlines.[55] However, the results of restriction fragment length polymorphism analysis on 9 advanced BCs suggested that, irrespective of pronounced DNA index heterogeneity, BCs at the time of diagnosis consist of a clonal cell population with an established complement of allelic imbalances, and that the generation of these imbalances generally precedes the clonal outgrowth of tumour cell populations with altered DNA ploidy (which in turn precedes metastasis).[56] Thus different prognostic/predictive factors may vary considerably with respect to their intra-tumour heterogeneity.

With respect to DNA ploidy, Beerman et al. found that, on average, four samples per tumour are needed for a reliable flow-cytometric DNA-ploidy analysis.[57] Other investigators studied intra-tumour variability in DNA index, proliferative activity and glutathione content, and it was found that the likelihood of identifying an aneuploid tumour clone (when present) in a single sample was only 60%, and that analysis of 3–7 samples was needed to

achieve a 90% probability that the test results were representative of the whole tumour. Similar broad variability was observed for the other factors investigated.[58]

Ideally, to avoid conflicting results, all single-site analyses should be abandoned, and instead treatment decisions should be made on the basis of analysis of three or more sites. However, this would result in a large increase in costs, making routine use of multi-site testing unlikely. Some researchers have suggested that samples taken from different sites may be pooled in the laboratory before analysis. Although this may dilute the results obtained from single testing, it is likely to provide a more accurate representation of the whole tumour. Another option may be to take multiple samples during surgery when a tumour is more than 1 cm in diameter, but to analyse only one at first. Only if the result of this single-site analysis would lead to the decision not to treat a patient with adjuvant therapy should the other samples be analysed in order to justify this treatment decision. Tumours less than 1 cm in diameter should be sampled as a whole.[58]

Detection of DNA content and proliferative activity

FLOW CYTOMETRY (FCM)

With FCM, for every cell in a population of (usually 10 000) cells, one or more parameters can be rapidly evaluated. By staining DNA with a fluorescent dye and measuring the amount of DNA in each cell, the ploidy status can be estimated together with the percentage of S-phase cells. Both frozen and paraffin-embedded tissue can be used.

Despite numerous studies, the value of DNA ploidy status as an independent prognostic factor has not been established.[59] In multivariate analysis, aneuploidy is associated with higher histologic grade, higher proliferative activity, and absence of hormone receptor expression. The risk of recurrence of multiploid tumours (more than one tumour stem line present) is not significantly different from that for tumours with one aneuploid stem line, but a rare fraction of breast tumours containing less DNA than normal cells appears to have a poorer prognosis.[59]

Whereas it is relatively easy to measure DNA ploidy from flow-cytometric DNA content distributions, determination of the fraction of S-phase (and/or G2/M) phase cells in a primary or metastatic BC encounters several technical problems. Because histological information is lost after dispersal of solid tissue, which may consist of lymphocytes, macrophages, fibroblasts and tumour cells, it is difficult to discriminate the cell population of interest (unless these cells can be discriminated on the basis of DNA content or cell type-specific antigens detectable by immunofluorescence, or they can be physically isolated prior to the measurement). The results of analysis of aneuploid tumour cell populations are often unreliable due to the presence of debris or multiple stem-cell lines in one tumour with different ploidy. Estimation of S-phase fractions (SPFs) is thus strongly dependent on applied computer-modelling programs that are able to correct for both debris and multiploidy.

In both node-negative and node-positive BC patients SPF seems to be of greater prognostic value than DNA ploidy. A high SPF has been shown to be significantly associated with decreased DFS and OS, and it was concluded that SPF contributes independent prognostic information for predicting the risk of recurrence in node-negative patients.[59,60]

Because many anticancer agents interfere with cell-cycle activities, one would expect SPF to be a good predictor of response to chemotherapy, but the results of studies on this subject have been conflicting. For example, Hedley et al. were unable to identify a subgroup in whom adjuvant chemotherapy was especially beneficial,[61] whereas Stål et al. recently concluded that there is a greater benefit from chemotherapy among patients with a high S-phase fraction.[62]

A recent consensus review of the clinical utility of DNA-FCM in BC makes a number of important recommendations.[63]

- Tissue selected for analysis should contain at least 20% malignant cells.
- Because of intra-tumour heterogeneity, several samples should be analysed.
- As SPF is a continuous variable, and because diploid tumours tend to have a lower SPF than aneuploid tumours, each laboratory should assess its own distribution of SPF values, rather than using published SPF cut-off points.

IN-SITU DETECTION OF PROLIFERATIVE ACTIVITY

The 'gold standard' of cell-cycle analysis is the use of labelled DNA-precursors that are incorporated into the DNA of cycling cells during S-phase. ^{3}H-dThymidine can be detected in tissue sections by autoradiography, whereas the more recently developed halogenated pyrimidines, such as bromodeoxyuridine (BrdUrd), are detected immunohistochemically. Microscopic evaluation of tissue sections generally allows a fairly accurate estimate of the fraction of labelled (S-phase) cells.

Although the potential mutagenic properties of these compounds prevent administration to patients with early BC, some investigators have succesfully applied *in-vitro* labelling of small tumour biopsies. In an extensive study on 1800 node-negative BC patients, Silvestrini et al. recently demonstrated that the ^{3}H-dThymidine-labelling index (TLI) was a significant predictor of OS and the most important factor predicting locoregional recurrence. However, for distant metastases, tumour size was a stronger prognostic factor.[64]

A method that is more suitable for routine clinical application may be the immunohistochemical detection

of 'cell-cycle-related antigens'. The (nuclear) expression of a 395–345 kD polypeptide protein recognized by the Ki-67 antigen is decreased in cells that have entered a non-cycling state and, despite the wide range of nuclear staining intensities during the cell cycle,[65] counting the fraction of Ki-67-positive tumour cells is thought to give a fairly good estimate of the so-called growth fraction of a tumour.

Using the MIB1 monoclonal antibody (MoAb), which was raised against recombinant parts of the Ki-67 antigen and can be used on routinely fixed and processed material, Pinder et al. concluded that computerized image analysis of MIB1-stained BC sections may provide important prognostic information.[66] In a series of 441 node-negative, premenopausal BC patients, we recently found that a high Ki-67 index remained a significant predictor of poor prognosis after multivariate analysis, together with age <43 years and OR negativity (Clahsen et al., unpublished results).

Another marker that has aroused much interest is the proliferating cell nuclear antigen (PCNA), a 36-kD auxiliary protein of DNA-polymerase-δ. During S-phase this protein is tightly bound to the DNA replication machinery, and the typical granular staining patterns observed in S-phase nuclei are identical to that obtained after BrdUrd labelling.[67,68] However, the protein is also present in the nucleoplasm of non-S-phase cells, and cell kinetic studies have indicated that in conditions of unperturbed growth, PCNA positivity (as detected by the widely used PC10, a MoAb suitable for formalin-fixed material) can be used as an operational marker for the growth fraction.[69]

However, there are both technical and biological reasons to be cautious when interpreting PC10-staining results. We and others have observed that immunoreactivity is progressively lost after prolonged fixation in formaldehyde, and antigen-retrieval methods (e.g. heating tissue sections prior to immunohistochemistry) are strongly recommended.[70] Another problem is that PCNA can be induced in non-cycling cells, either by genetic defects in the PCNA gene,[71] by abnormal expression of GFs,[72] or as a result of the involvement of polymerase-δ in DNA repair. Furthermore, different cell types may show intrinsic differences in PCNA mRNA and protein half-life.[69,71]

Gasparini et al. recently compared SPF (FCM), Ki-67 (frozen sections) and PC10 (paraffin sections) in human BCs. A significant correlation was only observed between SPF and Ki-67, and PCNA had no prognostic value for either RFS or OS.[73]

MARKERS FOR APOPTOSIS

In conventional histopathological sections, identification of apoptotic cells is even more difficult than identification of mitotic figures, and few studies have been reported on the significance of apoptosis as a prognostic factor in BC. Using marked condensation of chromatin as a criterion to identify apoptotic cells and bodies, Lipponen *et al.* recently correlated the number of apoptotic events with various histopathological features and patient survival in BC.[74] A high apoptotic index (AI) was associated with tumour necrosis, high grade, lack of sex steroid receptors, accumulation of p53 protein and high proliferative activity. However, multivariate analysis showed MI to be a more accurate prognostic parameter than AI. MI was the only explanatory factor for AI, and both factors gave similar survival estimates.

As yet, no data on the relevance of AI in relation to response to therapy are available.

In order to improve the detection of apoptotic events, our group and others have developed an *in-situ* method to stain DNA breaking points,[75,76] based on the idea that in apoptotic nuclei, DNA is broken down into small segments due to specific cleavage between nucleosomes. However, only the degradation of DNA into relatively large fragments seems to be a prerequisite for chromatin consensation (and therefore for the typical apoptotic morphology), whereas excessive internucleosomal cleavage is probably cell-type specific.[77] Moreover, prolonged treatment with formaldehyde results in a strong decrease in the number of positively staining apoptotic cells. However, it is our experience that, by pre-heating tissue samples, good staining results can be obtained on routinely fixed material,[78] including BC specimens.

SIGNIFICANCE OF PROGNOSTIC AND PREDICTIVE FACTORS INVOLVED IN CELL NUMBER REGULATION

Hormone and growth factor receptors

OR/PGR

Several large patient series have shown a significant difference in DFS and OS between patients with OR-positive and OR-negative tumours. However, the magnitude of this difference is of the order of 8–10%[79], so too small to be of use for a treatment decision on adjuvant therapy. Moreover, the value of PgR (which depends for its expression on the action of oestrogen) is disputed in that respect.[80] A recent large study on node-negative BC patients demonstrated that both OR and PgR failed to predict the 8-year incidence of loco-regional recurrence, and although they were significant predictors of distant metastasis and OS, this information was not independent of other clinico-pathological factors.[81]

However, as was mentioned previously, OR (with or without PgR) is a classical example of a predictive factor that is now widely used to predict response to adjuvant endocrine therapy. Response rates are about 10% in OR-negative tumours, 50% in OR-positive tumours and 75% in OR-positive/PgR-positive tumours. Based on a large prospective study, Ravdin *et al.* concluded that PgR is an

independent predictive factor for response to the anti-oestrogen tamoxifen, and might be a useful predictive factor for treatment with antiprogestins.[82]

False-negative testing of OR has been inherent to the biochemical method used for its detection. Commercially available monoclonal antibodies to OR and PgR have now greatly improved the reliability and sensitivity of immuno-histochemical evaluation, even with regard to formalin-fixed, paraffin-embedded tissues, and the results of a variety of studies indicate that immunohistochemistry will eventually replace biochemical assays.

In view of the finding that 25% of the patients with OR-positive/PgR-positive tumours do not respond to endocrine therapy, it has been suggested that assessment of the co-expression of markers such as EGFR, HER-2, the oestrogen-regulated protein pS2,[83] and also Bcl-2[84] could improve the predictive value. EGFR and HER-2 expression is associated with insensitivity to hormone therapy, whereas pS2 and Bcl-2 are correlated with a response to therapy. The latter markers may be useful for identifying in both OR-positive and OR-negative subgroups those patients who are most likely to respond.

Recently it was discovered that in many OR-negative BCs the reduction of OR gene expression is not due to mutations, but to abnormal DNA methylation causing a strong reduction in gene transcription. It has been suggested that treatment with demethylating agents may render these OR-negative BC cells responsive to hormonal therapy.[85]

EGFR

From a large variety of studies (on over 10 000 patients) it can be deduced that half of the BC patients are positive for EGFR, and that a negative association exists between EGFR and OR. Moreover, higher EGFR levels tend to correlate with higher proliferative activity.[86] Despite extensive research, there is no agreement on the subgroup of patients in whom EGFR may have a discriminative prognostic effect.[87] With regard to its predictive value, in metastatic BC less than 10% of EGFR-positive tumours respond to tamoxifen, whereas one-third of EGFR-negative tumours respond. Because almost none of the EGFR-positive/OR-negative tumors were reported to show an objective response to tamoxifen, evaluation of EGFR may indeed be helpful in selecting patients for this treatment modality.[88]

HER-2

HER-2 can be detected in about 20–30% of BCs and, in contrast to EGFR, in the majority of cases this seems to be caused by gene amplification. As with EGFR, HER-2 over-expression correlates negatively with OR-positivity, and HER-2-positive tumours respond poorly to endocrine therapy.[89] Over-expression/gene amplification is associated with poor prognosis in node-positive BC,[90] and could be an independent factor in predicting haematogeneous spread in BC.[91]

With regard to node-negative BC patients the prognostic value of HER-2 has been more controversial. Press *et al.* have suggested that, because the majority of these studies have been on archival tissue samples, antibody sensitivity might be an important confounding factor.[92] Using a sensitive antibody they were able to show that in this patient group, too, HER-2 correlates with poor prognosis.

Because HER-2 abnormalities are found in 10–15% of node-negative BC patients and 20–30% of node-positive BC patients, it was originally proposed to be a marker of late-stage disease, but this view was contradicted by the finding that 50–60% of ductal-type carcinomas *in situ* are HER-2 positive,[93] with at least 50% showing gene amplification.[94] Current data suggest that HER-2 defines a subset of BCs with a common origin. When other genes critical to the process of invasion are activated as well, the behaviour of HER-2-positive tumours becomes more malignant than that of their HER-2-negative counterparts. BCs that develop through non-HER-2 pathways tend to be less virulent once the invasive cancer has been established.[48]

Recently, the value of HER-2 as a predictive factor has been extensively discussed by Klijn *et al.*,[89] who concluded that most of the evidence indicates that HER-2-positive tumours respond poorly to endocrine therapy, but that there is no consensus on the response to chemotherapy. One of the most convincing studies has shown that in node-positive patients randomized to receive high-dose polychemotherapy (CAF), patients with HER-2-positive tumours had a significantly better DFS and OS.[95]

Because GF receptors have extracellular domains, they are excellent potential targets for treatment. Interesting preclinical results have been obtained with EGFR-specific EGF-diphtheria toxin fusion proteins,[96] as well as with MoAbs directed against EGFR,[97] which have now entered phase I trials.

HER-3

Few studies have been reported on other type I family GFRs. Lemoine *et al.* reported that HER-3 is over-expressed in 29% of node-positive BC patients and in 15% of node-negative BC patients. No association was found with tumour size, grade, OR, EGFR or HER-2.[98] In contrast, Gasparini *et al.* found HER-3 to be correlated significantly with HER-2, but whereas HER-2 was mainly expressed in ductal cancers, HER-3 was present in all histological types. In their analysis, neither HER-3 nor HER-2 was useful as a predictor of DFS and OS.[99]

IGF-IR

In contrast to EGFR, HER-2, and HER-3, the receptor for IGF-I is expressed in the majority of primary human BCs.[89] Very high levels of IGF-IR may predict poor survival,[100] but no data are yet available on IGF-IR levels and response to therapy.

Factors involved in signal transduction and DNA transcription

RAS

Ras mutations are infrequent (approximately 5%) in BC, but from the three human *ras* proto-oncogenes, H-*ras* is over-expressed in 60–70% of the tumours. These high levels cannot be linked to an amplification or rearrangement of the gene.[101] Benign lesions show a similar expression to invasive carcinoma.[102] A strong correlation has been found between *ras* and HER-2 expression.[103]

There is extensive experimental evidence that deregulated Ras function can contribute to uncontrolled growth of breast epithelial cells and, because tyrosine receptor kinases mediate their signal via Ras signal transduction pathways, it is plausible that deregulated function of components upstream or downstream of Ras (see above) may be highly relevant in BC development.[104]

MYC

Amplification of *myc* occurs in 20% of BC patients and is highly predictive of short-term DFS and OS, especially among patients with node-negative or OR-positive tumours.[89] *Myc* does not appear to predict the response to endocrine therapy. As mentioned above, *myc* is required for the effects of oestrogen, and *myc* over-expression and/or *myc* mRNA stabilization may reduce oestrogen dependency.

On the other hand, Klijn *et al.* observed that 64% of patients without *myc* amplification responded to C, F and methotrexate (M) combination chemotherapy, in contrast to only 29% of patients with *myc*-amplified tumours.

Cyclins, Rb and p53

CYCLINS

Amplification of chromosome 11q13, which harbours the PRAD1 gene, encoding for cyclin D1, occurs in 15–20% of BCs and is associated with the presence of lymph-node metastases and significantly shorter DFS and OS.[105] Inappropriate expression of cyclin D1 may result in increased hyperphosphorylation or down-regulated transcription of p53 and pRb.[106] Because the CDK4/cylin D1–complex binds to PCNA which is, as mentioned above, involved not only in DNA replication but also in DNA repair, it may also alter the control of genetic stability.

Recently it was reported that cyclin E is over-expressed in the majority of BCs, and that cyclin E alteration is even more consistent than over-expression of HER-2, cyclin D1 or PCNA positivity.[107]

PRB

Loss of heterozygosity of the Rb gene occurs in about 25% of BC patients and decreased expression in 10–20% of such patients.[89] Abnormal expression of Rb protein has been found to be related to grade, DNA ploidy and nuclear polymorphism, as well as to high proliferative activity.[108] However, no prognostic value has been shown for this protein, and no data are available on the relationship between loss of heterozygosity and response to treatment.[89]

P53

Mutation of p53 has been reported to occur in 15–50% of BCs, depending on the stage of the disease and the method of detection.[108] DNA-based methods mostly make use of the principle that DNA strands containing a mutation in one or more base pairs migrate differently on a polyacrylamide gel, resulting in an abnormal band. Immunohistochemical staining of p53 protein detects an abnormal nuclear accumulation of stabilized p53 protein, which can be due to either a mutation of wild-type p53 or to a stabilization of the protein due to either DNA damage or disregulation of the cell cycle.

In BC, p53 expression has been reported to be strongly associated with high proliferation rate, DNA ploidy, OR and PgR negativity and poor nuclear and histological grade.[109] Most studies have reported a poorer DFS and OS in the case of p53 accumulation, in both node-positive and node-negative BC patients. In a number of studies, multivariate analysis has demonstrated p53 protein accumulation to be an independent prognostic factor in node-negative patients.[110–113] However, in line with data from at least three studies,[114–116] including one on 440 node-negative patients,[116] data from our own study of a series of 441 BCs obtained from EORTC Trial 10854, which evaluated peri-operative chemotherapy (FAC) in premenopausal node-negative patients, did not provide any evidence that p53 accumulation can be used as a prognostic factor in untreated node-negative early BC patients. We also observed that in the chemotherapy arm, patients with p53-positive tumours had a poorer survival than those with p53-negative tumours, indicating that p53 might be useful as a predictive factor.

Whereas experimental data have indicated that loss of p53 function increases resistance to irradiation and adriamycin, the opposite finding has been reported with cisplatin.[117] This drug differs from other DNA-damaging agents in that it causes damage that is primarily repaired through nucleotide excision repair. Cell death as a result of impaired (p53-facilitated) DNA repair may then counterbalance an increase in the apoptosis threshold. Future studies will need to determine for which anti-cancer drugs treatment resistance is mediated by loss of p53 function.

The Bcl-2 gene family

Bcl-2 is expressed in normal breast epithelium, and it seems likely that in this tissue its expression is under hormonal control.[118] Bcl-2 was shown to be expressed in about 70% of breast tumours. A positive correlation was found between high Bcl-2 expression and OR and PgR positivity and low tumour grade, whereas high Bcl-2 expression was negatively correlated with p53 and c-erbB-2 positivity, high Ki-67 index, MI and large tumour-size.[119–121] Patients with tumours expressing high levels of Bcl-2 had a significantly better DFS and OS. However, all of the studies demonstrated that in a multivariate model this association no longer remained significant.

In a similar manner to p53, the effect of Bcl-2 expression on responsiveness to chemotherapy was evaluated in BC material from EORTC Trial 10854. At a median follow-up of 49 months, there was a similar effect of polychemotherapy (FAC) on DFS for patients with Bcl-2-positive and Bcl-2 negative tumours, indicating that Bcl-2 expression does not predict response to FAC in this patient series (Van Slooten, unpublished results).

We and others have also observed that in human BC cells *in vitro*, Bcl-2 is down-regulated by anti-oestrogen treatment or oestrogen depletion, but up-regulated by oestradiol. Because patients with high Bcl-2 levels appear to derive the greatest benefit from treatment with tamoxifen,[122] it is tempting to speculate that this compound may not only inhibit proliferative activity, but may also, by reducing Bcl-2 levels, increase apoptotic activity.

TUMOUR CELL INVASIVENESS AND ANGIOGENESIS

Role of proteases in cellular invasiveness

The degree of malignancy of a tumour is reflected by the interaction between neoplastic cells and the tumour stroma, which in some tumours can comprise up to 90% of the total mass.[123] As was first proposed by Folkman,[124] the development of blood vessel-containing connective tissue is a rate-limiting factor in the growth of both primary tumours and metastases. Increased understanding of the molecular mechanisms involved in tumour cell invasiveness and angiogenesis may therefore not only provide us with a set of powerful prognostic markers, but is also basic to the development of new strategies to control this devastating disease.

A basement membrane (BM) separates epithelial cells effectively from interstitial stroma. During the transition from *in-situ* to invasive carcinoma, tumour cells acquire the capacity to penetrate this BM, thereby gaining access to lymphatics and blood vessels. The extravasation of disseminating tumour cells at distant sites may depend on their ability to penetrate sub-endothelial BMs.

Because epithelial cells themselves are largely responsible for the formation of BMs, and because the interaction between BM and epithelial cells may in fact be an important determinant of cellular differentiation, one would expect that reduced BM formation contributes to a malignant phenotype. Interestingly, over-expression of the nm23-H1 gene in human BC cells *in vitro* leads to the formation of BM and growth arrest.[125] Nm-23 encodes for a nucleoside diphosphate kinase, and was originally identified by screening of cDNA libraries from murine melanoma cell lines of varying metastatic potential.[126] In human BC, reduced expression of nm23 was reported to correlate with comedo-type ductal carcinoma *in situ*, poor differentiation, lymph-node metastasis and poor survival in patients with invasive ductal carcinoma,[127] but the possible role of this gene as a metastasis suppressor gene in BC has been disputed.[128]

BM penetration is a complicated process involving binding via surface receptors, lysis of BM by secretion of degradative enzymes, and migration. Lysis of the extracellular matrix (ECM) should take place in highly localized regions close to the tumour cell surface. Lysis of all ECM components around a cell would seriously hamper cell traction.[123] In invasive cancer cells, various membrane-associated proteases are localized on special membrane protrusions, thereby directing localized ECM degradation.

In BC, representatives from several major classes of proteases are involved, including the aspartyl protease cathepsin D,[129] several members of the family of matrix metalloproteases (MMPs),[130] and the serine proteases urokinase-type plasminogen activator (uPA) and plasmin.[131]

Cathepsin D (cath-D), a 52-kD glycoprotein that is produced in response to oestrogens,[132] has captured the interest of BC researchers for many years. Because of its proteolytic activities, a role in ECM degradation was suggested.[133] However, cath-D is secreted by BC cells in its inactive pro-form, and a low pH (within the pH range measured in lysosomal vesicles) is required for enzyme activity.[134] Moreover, recent *in-vitro* studies have indicated that cath-D secretion by tumour cells is probably not an important determinant of invasiveness *per se*.[135]

Matrix metalloproteases (MMPs) constitute a zinc-binding endopeptidase family which is subdivided into three categories based on substrate preference, namely interstitial collagenases, type IV collagenases (gelatinases) and stromelysins. They are secreted as inactive zymogens, and activated by (enzymatic) disruption of the zinc–protein interaction. There are multiple-step activation and inhibition processes to control protease action. Two specific MMP inhibitors have been identified, which have been designated TIMP-1 and TIMP-2.[130]

Tumours may produce both MMPs and TIMPs, and each can be produced by tumour and stromal cells. With the possible exception of MMP-1, MMPs important in BC appear to be of stromal origin.[136] In the normal breast they probably mediate tissue resorption during post-lactational regression of the gland.[137]

Urokinase-type plasminogen activator (uPA) is a protein capable of pleiotropic functions through distinct and independent mechanisms and its activity is strongly enhanced by binding to its receptor (uPAR). This allows the appropriate orientation to multiple substrates, including plasminogen, hepatocyte growth factor precursor (pro-HGF), fibronectin and other ECM proteins.[138]

Plasminogen is an abundant proenzyme which is converted by uPA into plasmin, a serine protease that can cleave ECM proteins and activate type IV procollagenase and latent transforming growth factor β1 (TGF-β1).[139] The latter eventually shuts off uPA activity by inducing a specific inhibitor of uPA (PAI-1). Binding of PAI-1 to uPA results in an internalization of the uPA–PAI-1–uPAR complex, and it has been suggested that PAI-1 secretion may direct cell migration by enabling cells to displace the proteolytic active sites of uPA on their cell surface.[138]

HGF is a mesenchymally-derived factor involved in stromal–epithelial interactions in various tissues.[140] The HGF-receptor, encoded by the *met* proto-oncogene, is predominantly expressed on epithelial cells.[141] Interestingly, HGF is abundantly expressed by fetal fibroblasts and women with peripheral fibroblasts, expressing a fetal-like phenotype have been reported to have a greater risk of developing BC.[142]

Factors involved in angiogenesis

Long latency periods (sometimes more than 30 years) may occur between apparent curative resection of a primary tumour and detection of recurrent disease,[143] indicating that micrometastases can remain in a 'dormant' state.[144] An interesting explanation for this condition is that the outgrowth beyond a diffusion-limited size of dormant metastases (or of carcinomas *in situ*) depends on their capacity to induce neovascularization.[144,146]

Angiogenesis shows some striking similarities to tumour cell invasion, as endothelial cells must breach the BM that surrounds the existing blood vessel, move from the vascular wall through perivascular connective tissue and parenchyma towards the source of the angiogenic stimulus, and proliferate.[123] The process is strongly dependent on the nature of the ECM,[147] (e.g. capillary tube formation is promoted by laminin and collagen IV, proteins which the endothelial cells themselves can secrete). Attachment of endothelial cells to the ECM occurs through the integrin αvβ3 (vitronectin receptor), which recognizes vitronectin, fibronectin, fibrin, factor VIII and laminin.[148] As was mentioned earlier, integrin-mediated signal transduction constitutes a very important survival signal.[149]

Migration of endothelial cells involves the action of ECM-degrading enzymes in a manner that is functionally indistinguishable from cancer cell invasion of the ECM. In both cases this proteolysis represents a highly controlled dynamic equilibrium.

Tumour cells can induce a variety of GFs that may elicit some or all of the components of this complex process. Basic fibroblast GF (bFGF), EGF and vascular endothelial growth factor (VEGF) stimulate endothelial cells directly to migrate, proliferate and/or form tubes, while platelet-derived VEGF, TNFα, or TGF-β1 may act indirectly by mobilizing host cells (e.g. macrophages, mast cells, fibroblasts) to release angiogenic factors.[150] There is mounting evidence that VEGF (also known as vascular permeability factor) is a crucial factor, induced in many cell types by various stimuli, including hypoxia, differentiation, GFs and tumour promotors.[151] These inductive pathways comprise kinases, oncogenes, tumour suppressor genes, and steroid hormone transcription factors, many of which seem to converge to AP-1. Remarkably, p53 protein constrains the expression of the VEGF gene,[152] whereas it stimulates the expression of a gene encoding for the anti-angiogenic factor trombospondin-1 (TSP-1).[153] This supports the concept that loss of p53 function may have a significant impact on tumour vascularization patterns. It has recently been reported that VEGF has high prognostic value for overall survival in node-negative breast cancer, particularly in OR-positive cases.[154]

Conversion of plasminogen leads to activation of TGF-β1, which stimulates angiogenesis, but plasminogen can also be cleaved by elastase-like enzymes into fragments that either stimulate or strongly inhibit endothelial cell growth. The inhibitory fragment angiostatin was isolated from serum and urine from Lewis lung (LL) carcinoma-bearing mice, and appears to be responsible for the growth inhibition of lung metastases (or secondary implants) by 'primary' LL tumours.[155] Inhibition of metastatic growth by the presence of a primary tumour mass has been observed in a variety of experimental tumour models,[156–158] and this fuelled the concern that in patients, too, the growth rate of occult residual disease may transiently increase after surgical removal of the primary tumour.[159]

Conclusions

The switch to the angiogenic phenotype depends on a net balance of positive and negative angiogenic factors. Both positive and negative factors may be directly produced by tumour cells and/or by neighbouring stromal cells after paracrine stimulation. Although most of the factors involved are relatively short-lived, acting only in the vicinity of the site of production/activation, some factors (e.g. plasminogen, angiostatin and a 16-kD fragment of prolactin) are components of plasma and serum.

The process of angiogenesis has much in common with tumour cell invasiveness, and both the angiogenic and invasive phenotype may occur by an increase in stimulators, a decrease in inhibitors, or a combination of both. Because certain proteases and their inhibitors may reflect metastatic potential, they may be useful as prognostic factors to select node-negative BC patients for adjuvant treatment. Moreover, the complexity of these processes provides an array of targets for pharmaceutical intervention that can be used to prevent metastatic spread as well as the transition from dormancy to aggressive growth. Gasparini and Harris have summarized the biological and pharmacological bases for antiangiogenic therapy of BC as follows.[160]

- The fact that in normal tissues endothelial cells are quiescent and in tumours they are activated/proliferating confers specificity on such treatment.
- Endothelial cells are more directly accessible targets than tumour cells.
- Several angiogenic inhibitors have been discovered with different mechanisms of action, most of which appear to have a low toxicity and favourable therapeutic index.
- Because normal cells are the target, they are unlikely to develop resistance to anti-angiogenic drugs. Furthermore, tumour cells and intratumoural neovessels may constitute two distinct targets for anticancer therapy. A therapeutic approach to both of these targets may lead to a synergistic antitumour effect.

PROGNOSTIC AND PREDICTIVE SIGNIFICANCE OF MARKERS FOR TUMOUR CELL INVASION AND ANGIOGENESIS

Proteases

CATHEPSIN D

In a number of retrospective studies, the level of cathepsin D (cath-D) in the cytosol of primary BC biopsies was found to be an independent factor in predicting relapse.[161–163] Using Western blotting to detect cath-D, Tandon et al. showed that it predicted reduced DFS and OS in node-negative patients only.[164] The result was confirmed by immunohistochemistry.[165] Kute et al. concluded from immunoassays and enzymatic assays in node-negative patients that cath-D was even more useful than tumour size, grade and S-phase.[166] However, other studies have failed to confirm this.[167–169] The lack of reproducibility is illustrated by the recent failure to replicate and improve the 'Tandon study', replacing a polyclonal antiserum by a MoAb.[170] A possible explanation could be that the ratio between active and inactive enzyme is more important than the absolute level of cath-D and that current commercial assays fail to discriminate between those isoforms.[171] Possible explanations for the mechanism by which cathepsin D exerts its prognostic effect have been discussed by Westley and May.[172]

METALLOPROTEASES

Few data are yet available on the prognostic significance of MMPs in BC. Recently it was reported that MMP-11 (stromelysin-3), which is exclusively expressed in fibroblasts associated with invasive carcinoma,[173] is significantly correlated with fatal metastatic disease. However, this factor did not reach the level of significance in node-negative patients.[174]

Immunohistochemical staining of MMP-2 predicted local recurrence, but not DFS and OS.[175] As with cath-D, it may well be that overall levels are less relevant than the degree of activation.[176]

Several studies have used zymography to evaluate the expression of both MMP-2 and MMP-9 in BC biopsies.[177,178] Only activated MMP-2 and the proform of MMP-9 were associated with malignant progression. Increased levels of MMP-9 were also detected in the plasma and serum of BC patients.[179]

UROKINASE PATHWAY OF PLASMINOGEN

Duffy et al. noted that the enzymatic activity of uPA is associated with a shorter relapse rate,[180] and various pre- and prospective studies confirmed that uPA is an independent prognostic factor for relapse in both node-positive and node-negative patients.[181–183] In a large series of 671 BC patients, uPA concentrations in tumour cytosol were found to be significantly associated with increased rates of relapse and death.[182] Surprisingly, a similar prognostic value was found for the uPA inhibitor PAI-1.[184–186] Could PAI-1 play a crucial role in protecting the tumour from degrading itself, or is PAI-1 a strong marker for tumour angiogenesis?[184]

Preclinical studies are in progress aimed at inhibition of uPA activity by antibodies, by saturation of uPARs by uPA fragments, or by constructing hybrid uPA molecules with much longer half-lives.[138] A randomized phase III trial has been initiated in which node-negative patients with high levels of PAI-1 and/or uPA are selected for adjuvant chemotherapy.

Growth factors and receptors

HEPATIC GROWTH FACTOR

As mentioned above, plasmin can activate pro-HGF, and human mammary epithelial cells are very sensitive to this factor.[140] A recent immunohistochemical study of BC specimens from 258 Japanese women showed that HGF is a strong and independent predictor of recurrence and survival.[187]

BASIC FIBROBLAST GROWTH FACTOR

In normal tissues, bFGF is mainly cell associated, but in a transgenic mouse model for dermal fibrosarcoma it was demonstrated that without a change in bFGF production there was a marked change to extracellular release.[188] Nguyen et al. measured bFGF levels in urine from 143 BC patients, and among the 40 patients with elevated bFGF levels, 35 individuals had local or distant 'active' BC.[189]

The development of compounds that either specifically block the binding of bFGF to its receptor or tightly bind to bFGF and thereby inhibit its activity is now in progress.[190]

LAMININ RECEPTOR (LREC)

Laminin is a major component of ECM, and its interaction with endothelial cells plays a critical role during angiogenesis, tumour invasion and metastasis. The ability of cancer cells to bind laminin has been correlated with their metastatic potential.[123] Marques et al. demonstrated in a series of 235 BC patients that the immunostaining of the 67-kD LRec significantly predicted DFS and OS,[191] and a large retrospective study established that LRec is an independent prognostic factor.[192]

A prospective multi-parameter study in 171 node-negative BCs revealed a weak positive association of LRec expression with high levels of neovascularization, but not with hormone receptors, p53 expression or conventional prognostic factors. The joint variable of LRec and microvessel density was the strongest independent prognostic factor for DFS.[193]

Microvessel density (MVD)

Brem et al. were the first to develop a microscopic angiogenesis grading system based on an index incorporating vascular density, endothelial cell hyperplasia and endothelial cytology.[194] More recently, Weidner et al. developed a protocol to quantitate in tissue sections the density of immunostained capillaries and venules. From a series of 49 BCs, they analysed tissue sections immunostained with factor VIII, and found that the number of microvessels per 200 magnification field (counted in the areas of most intensive neovascularization) predicted metastatic disease.[195]

Although several groups subsequently confirmed a relationship between MVD and risk of nodal and/or distant metastases,[196,197] this finding has not been universal.[198,199] It has been argued that staining for factor VIII (von Willebrand factor) is suboptimal, as it is mainly present in large blood vessels and in the endothelial cells of lymph vessels.[200] Using an antibody to platelet/ endothelial cell adhesion molecule (PECAM-1; CD31), which has been found consistently to stain more vessels than any of the endothelial cell markers tested, Horak et al. performed a prospective study in 103 BC patients and observed that MVD increased with tumour size and with poor differentiation, and that it correlated strongly with lymph-node status.[201] Toi et al. described a strong relationship between factor VIII and CD31 staining,[197] and recently confirmed in a large series of patients the value of MVD as an independent prognostic indicator for recurrence-free survival.[85] In addition, MVD correlated strongly with VEGF expression, suggesting an important role for this GF in BC angiogenesis.[202]

Using CD31, Gasparini *et al.* determined in 250 node-negative BC patients the absolute and relative value of MVD, p53, HER-2, peritumoural lymphatic vessel invasion (PLVI), and conventional prognostic indicators. MVD, p53 accumulation, tumour size and PLVI were all significant and independent prognostic factors for RFS, but only tumour size and MVD were also independent predictors of OS.[203]

In contrast, using the protocol outlined by Weidner and anti-CD31 to highlight microvessels in a series of 441 tumours from node-negative BC patients, investigators at our own institution were unable to demonstrate a significant correlation between MVD and histological grade or tumour size. There was also no significant difference in 4-year DFS between patients with a density of less than 75 vessels/mm² and patients with a higher MVD (P.C. Clahsen *et al.*, unpublished results).

It appears therefore that at present MVD measurements are not universally reproducible, and it will be difficult to validate this method in prospective studies performed in many different centres by many different pathologists. Apart from the problems involved in the reliable detection of microvessels, a major bias factor may be related to difficulties in selecting representative invasive tumour and in localizing the neovascular 'hot spot'. Moreover, antibodies to factor VIII or CD31 may not be specific for proliferating or 'activated' endothelial cells. Recently it was found that CD105 (endoglin), a receptor for TGF-β1/3, is selectively expressed in blood vessels in and around tumours,[204] and that tumour-associated endothelial cells that are immunostained for CD105 tend to be negative for factor VIII and CD31.[205]

Conclusions

There are sound theoretical arguments why the degree of (primary) tumour vascularization relates to the probability of metastatic disease:

- there is increased opportunity for tumour cells to enter the circulation;
- new, proliferating capillaries have fragmented BMs and are leaky, making them more accessible to tumour cells;
- degradative enzymes involved in the invasive chemotactic behaviour of endothelial cells may facilitate the escape of tumour cells into the circulation;
- highly angiogenic tumours are more likely to seed distant sites with highly angiogenic clones.

Determination of MVD is increasingly being applied, and improved immunohistochemical procedures and the use of multiparametric computerized image-analysis systems will hopefully improve accuracy, feasibility and reproducibility. Alternatively, the expression and levels of uPA, bFGF, VEGF, etc., would appear to be interesting markers of angiogenic activity. Because this activity represents a net balance between stimulation and inhibition factors such as PAI-1, TSP, angiostatin, etc., are relevant, too. Some of these peptides can be measured in serum or urine, providing an opportunity to monitor the disease after primary surgery.

A wide range of angiogenic inhibitors are currently being evaluated for their efficacy in the treatment of various types of tumours and a number of these agents have already entered phase I/II trials.[150] Soluble receptors or MoAbs to angiogenic factors such as VEGF, compounds such as suramin that bind to and inactivate heparin-binding GFs, strategies aimed at blocking the integrin αvβ3 and compounds such as AGM-1470 (TNP-470) which inhibit endothelial cell proliferation may offer interesting possibilities.[206]

Angiogenesis inhibitors may be used not only to maintain 'dormancy' in micrometastatic disease or in tumours that are resistant to further cytotoxic treatments (i.e. as an adjuvant after debulking surgery or chemo-, radio- or endocrine therapy), but also to increase the antitumour effects of these treatment modalities. For example, preclinical studies have shown that the combination of AGM-1470 with various cytotoxic drugs significantly enhanced their efficacy.[207]

FINAL REMARKS – PROGNOSTIC INDEXES AND NEW WAYS TO MONITOR TREATMENT RESPONSE

Integration – the emergence of new prognostic systems

It is clear from the above account that, as a result of the increase in knowledge of tumour biology, the number of prognostic factors that reach the level of significance in univariate analysis is still growing rapidly. When working with a limited number of factors, relatively simple staging systems (e.g. the TNM classification and the Nottingham Index) have proved useful, but the inclusion of various new markers requires more sophisticated approaches (see Chapter 25).

Basically, three different mathematical methods are being explored for that purpose.

- The standard method for performing multivariate analysis of censored survival data is the Cox proportional hazards model. For this model, putative factors are usually dichotomized (i.e. a cut-off value is determined which assigns the patient to one of two categories). However, Cox models can also include variables measured on a continuous scale, and it has been demonstrated that the use of the latter variables may significantly increase the power of these models.[208] One drawback of Cox models is the need to have each variable measured, because missing data values cannot be incorporated.

- Tree-structured regression models are based on the construction of binary classification trees in which cases are split into subsets based on the values of their predictor variables (recursive partitioning). They are easy to use in clinical decision-making, but can only be applied to complete data sets, and validation of the final tree is required before the results are generalized. It has been emphasized by Clark *et al.* that, although recursive partitioning is very useful for examining previously unknown interactions in subgroups, it should be considered to be an exploratory adjunct to other models rather than a definitive analytical method.[209]

- Neural networks were developed as pattern recognition systems to discriminate between different classes of events. Ravdin *et al.* have demonstrated that neural networks can indeed be used to predict the clinical outcome of BC patients[210] Neural networks are probably as accurate as Cox models when applied to large sets of patients with relatively few prognostic factors. Because they are useful for finding optimal solutions to very complex problems involving multiple parameters, it is expected that they will prove superior to standard multivariate analysis methods in integrating information about multiple prognostic and predictive factors.

Monitoring the treatment response – the emergence of positron emission tomography

Initiation of chemotherapy prior to surgery ('neoadjuvant chemotherapy') is used to make inoperable tumours technically operable, or to reduce the size of relatively large tumours to the extent that breast-conserving treatment becomes an allowable option (see Chapter 15). An additional advantage of this approach is the possibility of evaluating treatment responses of primary tumours, and it is hoped that these responses may reliably predict possible effects on DFS and OS.

Positron emission tomography (PET) appears to be a valuable new tool for making assessments of treatment responses. It is a non-invasive technique, using tracer compounds labelled with short-lived radionuclides, which allows measurement of tissue metabolism *in vivo*. Although its role in oncology is underdeveloped at present, a limited number of studies have shown substantial promise for its use in the management of BC. Using either radioactively labelled glucose or methionine to monitor tumour glycolytic metabolism and protein synthesis respectively, PET was reported to be a sensitive and specific method for detecting the presence of primary BCs and lymph-node metastases.[211]

Moreover, there is mounting evidence that PET can be used to assess treatment response at a very early stage. Treatment-induced metabolic changes in the primary tumour appear to precede detectable changes in tumour size and to be a specific predictor of clinical response.[212] Although further research is needed, PET scanning has potential for:

- identification at an early stage of patients who will not benefit from adjuvant therapy;
- tailoring of adjuvant therapy to the individual patient;
- pre-operative staging of BC patients and prevention of unnecessary biopsies and lymph-node dissections.[213]

REFERENCES

1 Early Breast Cancer Trialists' Collaborative Group Systemic treatment of early breast cancer by hormonal, cytotoxic, or immune therapy. *Lancet* 1992; **339**: 1–15, 71–85.
2 Rosen PP, Groshen S, Kinne DW, Norton L. Factors influencing prognosis in node-negative breast carcinoma: analysis of 767 T1N0M0/T2N0M0 patients with long-term follow-up. *Journal of Clinical Oncology* 1993; **11**: 2090–100.
3 Gasparini G, Pozza F, Harris AL. Evaluating the potential usefulness of new prognostic and predictive indicators in node-negative breast cancer patients. *Journal of the National Cancer Institute* 1993; **85**: 1206–19.
4 Greenough RB. Varying degrees of malignancy in cancer of the breast. *Journal of Cancer Research* 1925; **9**: 452–63.
5 Patey DH, Scarff RW. The position of histology in the prognosis of carcinoma of the breast. *Lancet* 1928; **i**: 801–4.
6 Bloom HJG, Richardson WW. Histological grading and prognosis in breast cancer. *British Journal of Cancer* 1957; **11**: 359–77.
7 Doussal LE, Tubiana-Hulin M, Friedman *et al.* Prognostic value of histological grade nuclear components of Scarff-Bloom-Richardson (SBR). An improved score modification based on a multivariate analysis of 1262 invasive ductal breast carcinomas. *Cancer* 1989; **64**: 1914–21.
8 Galea MH, Blamey RW, Elston CE, Ellis IO. The Nottingham Prognostic Index in primary breast cancer. *Breast Cancer Research and Treatment* 1992; **22**, 207–19.
9 Simpson JF, Dutt PL, Page DL. Expression of mitoses per thousand cells and cell density in breast carcinomas: a proposal. *Human Pathology* 1992; **23**: 608–11.
10 Burke HB, Henson DE. Criteria for prognostic factors and for an enhanced prognostic system. *Cancer* 1993; **72**: 3131–5.

11 Kennedy MJ. Systemic adjuvant therapy for breast cancer. *Current Opinions in Oncology* 1994; **6**: 570–7.

12 Dickson RB, Lippman ME. Estrogenic regulation of growth and polypeptide growth factor secretion in human breast carcinoma. *Endocrine Reviews* 1987; **8**: 29–43.

13 Osborne CK, Arteaga CL. Autocrine and paracrine growth regulation of breast cancer: clinical implications. *Breast Cancer Research and Treatment* 1990; **15**: 3–11.

14 Normanno N, Ciardiello F, Brandt R, Salomon DS. Epidermal growth factor-related peptides in the pathogenesis of human breast cancer. *Breast Cancer Research and Treatment* 1994; **29**: 11–27.

15 Rajkumar T, Gullick WJ. The type I growth factor receptors in human breast cancer. *Breast Cancer Research and Treatment* 1994; **29**: 3–9.

16 Yee D, Rosen N, Favoni R.E, Cullen KJ. The insulin-like growth factors, their receptors, and their binding proteins in human breast cancer. In: Lippman M, Dickson R (eds). *Regulatory mechanisms in breast cancer*. Kluwer Academic Publishers, 1991: 93–106.

17 Ginsburg E, Vonderhaar BK. Prolactin synthesis and secretion by human breast cancer cells. *Cancer Research* 1995; **55**: 2591–5.

18 Earp HS, Dawson, TL, Li X, Yu H. Heterodimerization and functional interaction between EGF receptor family members: a new signaling paradigm with implications for breast cancer research. *Breast Cancer Research and Treatment* 1995; **35**: 115–32.

19 Karin M, Hunter T. Transcriptional control by protein phosphorylation: signal transmission from the cell surface to the nucleus. *Current Biology* 1995; **5**: 747–57.

20 Chrysogelos SA, Dickson RB. EGF receptor expression, regulation, and function in breast cancer. *Breast Cancer Research and Treatment* 1994; **29**: 29–40.

21 White MF, Kahn CR. The insulin signaling system. *The Journal of Biological Chemistry* 1994; **269**: 1–4.

22 Shiu RPC, Watson PH, Dubik D. c-myc oncogene expression in estrogen-dependent and independent breast cancer. *Clinical Chemistry*, 1993; **39**: 353–5.

23 Van der Burg B, De Groot RP, Insbucker L *et al*. Direct stimulation by estrogen of growth factor signal transduction pathways in human breast cancer cells. *Journal of Steroid Biochemistry and Molecular Biology* 1992; **43**: 111–15.

24 Davidson NE, Prestigiacomo LJ, Hahm HA. Induction of jun gene family members by transforming growth factor α but not 17β-estradiol in human breast cancer. *Cancer Research* 1993; **53**: 291–7.

25 Chalbos D, Philips A, Rochefort H. Genomic cross-talk between the estrogen receptor and growth factor regulatory pathways in estrogen target tissues. *Seminars in Cancer Biology* 1994; **5**: 361–8.

26 Pines J. Cyclins, CDCs and cancer. *Seminars in Cancer Biology* 1995; **6**: 63–72.

27 Bartkova J, Lukas J, Müller H. Cyclin D1 protein expression and function in human breast cancer. *International Journal of Cancer* 1994; **57**: 353–61.

28 Bates S, Peters G. Cyclin D1 as a cellular proto-oncogene. *Seminars in Cancer Biology* 1995; **6**: 73–82.

29 Kouzarides T. Transcriptional control by the retinoblastoma protein. *Seminars in Cancer Biology* 1995; **6**: 91–8.

30 Whyte, P. The retinoblastoma protein and its relatives. *Seminars in Cancer Biology* 1995; **6**: 83–90.

31 El-Deiry WS, Tokino T, Velculescu VE *et al*. WAF-1, a potential mediator of p53 tumour suppression. *Cell* 1993; **75**: 817–25.

32 Harper JW, Adami, GR, Wei N. The p21 Cdk-interacting protein Cip-1 is a potent inhibitor of G1 cyclin-dependent kinases. *Cell* 1993; **75**: 805–16.

33 Malzman W, Czyzyk L. UV irradiation stimulates levels of p53 cellular tumour antigen in nontransformed mouse cells. *Molecular Cell Biology* 1984; **4**: 1689–94.

34 Deppert W. The yin and yang of p53 in cellular proliferation. *Seminars in Cancer Biology* 1994; **5**: 187–202.

35 Lane DP. Cancer: p53, guardian of the genome. *Nature* 1992; **358**, 15–16.

36 Kerr JFR, Winterford CM, Harmon BV. Apoptosis; its significance in cancer and cancer therapy. *Cancer* 1993; **73**: 2013–26.

37 Majno G, Joris I. Apoptosis, oncosis, and necrosis. *American Journal of Pathology* 1995; **146**: 3–14.

38 Wyllie AH. Apoptosis and the regulation of cell numbers in normal and neoplastic tissues: an overview. *Cancer and Metastasis Reviews* 1992; **11**: 95 103.

39 Walker NI, Bennet RE, Kerr JFR. Cell death by apoptosis during involution of the lactating breast in mice and rats. *American Journal of Anatomy* 1989; **185**: 19–32.

40 Wijsman JH, Cornelisse CJ, Keijzer R *et al*. Effect of hormone depletion on cell survival in the EMR-86 rat mammary carcinoma. *British Journal of Cancer* 1995; **73**: 1210–15.

41 Hickman JA. Apoptosis induced by anticancer drugs. *Cancer and Metastasis Reviews* 1992; **11**: 121–39.

42 Reed JC. Bcl-2 and the regulation of programmed cell death. *Journal of Cell biology* 1994; **124**: 1–6.

43 Nuñez G, Clarke MF. The Bcl-2 family of proteins: regulators of cell death and survival. *Trends in Cell Biology* 1994; **4**: 399-403.

44 Oltvai ZN, Korsmeyer SJ. Checkpoints of duelling dimers foil death wishes. *Cell* 1994; **79**: 189–92.

45 Häcker G, Vaux DL. A sticky business. *Current Biology* 1995; **5**: 622–4.

46 Los M, Van de Craen M, Penning LC *et al*. Requirement of an ICE/CED-3 protease for Fas/APO-1-mediated apoptosis. *Nature* 1995; **375**: 81–3.

47 Ruoslahti E, Reed JC. Anchorage dependence, integrins, and apoptosis. *Cell* 1994; **77**: 477–8.

48 Cance WC, liu ET. Protein kinases in human breast cancer. *Breast Cancer Research and Treatment* 1995; **35**: 105–14.

49 Green DR, Bisonnette RP, Cotter TG. Apoptosis and cancer. In: de Vita VT, Hellman S, Rosenberg SA (eds). *Important advances in oncology*. Philadelphia, PA: Lippincott Company, 1994: 37–52.

50 Resnicoff M, Abraham D, Yutanawiboonchai W *et al*. The insulin growth factor I receptor protects tumour cells from apoptosis *in vivo*. *Cancer Research* 1995; **55**: 2463–9.

51 Canman CE, Kastan MB. Induction of apoptosis by tumour suppressor genes and oncogenes. *Seminars in Cancer Biology* 1995; **6**: 17–25.

52 Miyashita T, Harigai M, Hanada M, Reeds JC. Identification of a p53-dependent negative response element in the bcl-2 gene. *Cancer Research* 1994; **54**: 3131–5.

53 Miyashita T, Reed JC. Tumour suppressor p53 is a direct transcriptional activator of the human bax gene. *Cell* 1995; **80**: 293–9.

54 Nowell PC. The clonal evolution of tumour cell populations. *Science* 1976; **194**: 23–8.

55 Cornelisse CJ, Van de Velde CJH, Caspers RJC *et al*. DNA ploidy and survival in breast cancer patients. *Cytometry* 1987; **8**: 225–34.

56 Bonsing BA, Devilee P, Cleton-Jansen A-M *et al*. Evidence for limited molecular genetic heterogeneity as defined by allelotyping and clonal analysis in nine metastastic breast carcinomas. *Cancer Research* 1993; **53**: 3804–11.

57 Beerman H, Smit VTHBM, Kluin PM *et al*. Flow cytometric analysis of DNA stemline heterogeneity in primary and metastatic breast cancer. *Cytometry*; **12**: 147–54.

58 Barranco SC, Perry RR, Durm ME *et al*. Intratumour variability in prognostic indicators may be the cause of conflicting estimates of patient survival and response to therapy. *Cancer Research* 1994; **54**: 5351–6.

59 Hedley S, Clark GM, Cornelisse CJ *et al*. Consensus statement on the utility of DNA cytometry in carcinoma of the breast. *Cytometry* 1993; **14**: 482–5.

60 Camplejohn RS, Ash CM, Gillet CE *et al*. The prognostic significance of DNA flow cytometry in breast cancer: results from 881 patients treated in a single centre. *British Journal of Cancer* 1995; **71**: 140–5.

61 Hedley DW, Rugg CA, Gelber RD. Association of DNA index and S-phase fraction with prognosis of node-positive early breast cancer. *Cancer Research* 1987; **47**: 4729–35.

62 Stål O, Skoog L, Rudqvist LE, Carstensen JM *et al*. S-phase fraction and survival benefit from adjuvant chemotherapy or radiotherapy of breast cancer. *British Journal of Cancer* 1994; **70**: 1258–62.

63 Shankey TV, Rabinovitch PS, Badwell B *et al*. Guidelines for implementation of clinical DNA cytometry. *Cytometry* 1993; **14**: 472–7.

64 Silvestrini R, Daidone MG, Luisi A *et al*. Biological and clinicopathologic factors as indicators of specific relapse types in node-negative breast cancer. *Journal of Clinical Oncology* 1995; **13**: 697–704.

65 Van Dierendonck JH, Keijzer R, Cornelisse CJ, Van de Velde CJH. Nuclear distribution of the Ki-67 antigen during the cell cycle: comparison with growth fraction in human breast cancer cells. *Cancer Research* 1989; **49**: 2999–3006.

66 Pinder SE, Wencyk P, Sibbering DM *et al*. Assessment of the new proliferation marker MIB1 in breast carcinoma using image analysis: associations with other prognostic factors and survival. *British Journal of Cancer* 1995; **71**: 146–9.

67 Van Dierendonck JH, Keijzer R, Van de Velde CJH, Cornelisse CJ. Subdivision of S-phase by analysis of nuclear 5-bromodeoxyuridine staining patterns. *Cytometry* 1989; **10**: 143–50.

68 Van Dierendonck JH, Wijsman JH, Keijzer R *et al*. Cell cycle-related staining patterns of anti-proliferating cell nuclear antigen monoclonal antibodies. *American Journal of Pathology* 1991; **138**: 1165–72.

69 Wijsman JH, Van Dierendonck JH, Keijzer R *et al*. Immuno-reactivity of proliferating cell nuclear antigen compared with bromodeoxyuridine in normal and neoplastic rat tissue. *Journal of Pathology* 1992; **168**: 75–83.

70 Siitonen SM, Kallioniemi O-P, Isola JJ. Proliferating cell nuclear antigen immunohistochemistry using monoclonal antibody 19A2 and a new antigen retrieval technique has prognostic impact in archival paraffin-embedded node-negative breast cancer. *American Journal of Pathology*, 1993; **142**: 1081–9.

71 Baserga, R. Growth regulation of the PCNA gene. *Journal of Cell Science* 1991; **98**: 433–6.

72 Hall PA, Coates PJ, Goodlad RA *et al*. Proliferating cell nuclear antigen expression in non-cycling cells may be induced by growth factors *in vivo*. *British Journal of Cancer* 1994; **70**: 244–7.

73 Gasparini G, Boracchi P, Verderio P, Bevilacqua P. Cell kinetics in human breast cancer: comparison between the prognostic value of the cytofluorimetric S-phase fraction and that of the antibodies to Ki-67 and PCNA antigens detected by immunohistochemistry. *International Journal of Cancer* 1994; **57**: 822–9.

74 Lipponen P, Aaltomaa S, Kosma V-M, Syrjänen K. Apoptosis in breast cancer as related to histopathological characteristics and prognosis. *European Journal of Cancer* 1994; **30A**: 2068–73.

75 Wijsman JH, Jonker RR, Keijzer R *et al*. A new method to detect apoptosis in paraffin sections: *in-situ* end-labelling of fragmented DNA. *Journal of Histochemistry and Cytochemistry* 1993; **41**: 7–12.

76 Gavrieli Y, Sherman Y, Ben-Sasson SA. Identification of programmed cell death *in situ* via specific labelling of nuclear DNA fragmentation. *Journal of Cell Biology* 1992; **119**: 493–501.

77 Oberhammer F, Wilson JW, Dive C *et al*. Apoptotic death in epithelial cells: cleavage of DNA to 300 and/or 50 kb fragments prior to or in absence of internucleosomal fragmentation. *EMBO Journal* 1993; **12**: 3679–84.

78 Lucassen PJ, Chung WCJ, Vermeulen JP *et al*. Microwave-enhanced *in situ* end-labelling of fragmented DNA: parametric studies in relation to postmortem delay and fixation of rat and human brain. *Journal of Histochemistry and Cytochemistry* 1995; **43**.

79 Mansour EG, Ravdin PM, Dressler L. Prognostic factors in early breast carcinoma. *Cancer* 1994; **74**: 381–400.

80 Elledge RM, McGuire WL, Osborne CK. Prognostic factors in breast cancer. *Seminars in Oncology* 1992; **19**: 244–53.

81 Silvestrini R, Daidone MG, Luisi A, Boracchi P. Biologic and clinicopathologic factors as indicators of specific relapse

types in node-negative breast cancer. *Journal of Clinical Oncology* 1995; **13**: 697–704.

82 Ravdin PM, Green S, Melink Dorr T *et al.* Prognostic significance of progesterone receptor levels in estrogen-positive patients with metastatic breast cancer treated with tamoxifen: results of a prospective Southwest Oncology Group Study. *Journal of Clinical Oncology* 1992; **10**: 1284–91.

83 Predine J, Spyratos F, Prud'homme JF *et al.* Enzyme-linked immunosorbent assay of pS2 in breast cancers, benign tumours, and normal breast tissues: correlation with prognosis and adjuvant hormonal therapy. *Cancer* 1992; **69**: 2116–23.

84 Gasparini G, Barbareschi M, Doglioni C *et al.* Expression of bcl-2 protein predicts efficacy of adjuvant treatments in operable node-positive breast cancer. *Clinical Cancer Research* 1995; **1**: 189–98.

85 Ferguson AT, Lapidu RG, Baylin SB, Davidson NE. Demethylation of the estrogen receptor gene in estrogen-negative breast cancer cells can reactivate estrogen receptor gene expression. *Cancer Research* 1995; **55**: 2279–83.

86 Harris AL. What is the biologic, prognostic, and therapeutic role of the EGF receptor in human breast cancer? *Breast Cancer Research and Treatment* 1994; **29**: 1–2.

87 Klijn JGM, Berns PMJJ, Schmitz PIM, Foekens JA. The clinical significance of epidermal growth factor receptor (EGF-R) in human breast cancer: a review on 5232 patients. *Endocrine Reviews* 1992; **13**: 3–18.

88 Nicholson S, Sainsbury JRC, Halcrow P *et al.* Expression of epidermal growth factor receptors associated with lack of response in recurrent breast cancer. *Lancet* 1989; **i**: 182–4.

89 Klijn JGM, Berns EJM, Foekens JA. Prognostic factors and response to therapy in breast cancer. *Cancer Surveys* 1993; **18**: 165–97.

90 Slamon DJ, Godolphin W, Jones LA *et al.* Studies of the HER-2/neu proto-oncogene in human breast and ovarian cancer. *Science* 1989; **244**: 707–12.

91 De Potter CR, Beghin C, Makar AO *et al.* The *neu*-oncogene protein as a predictive factor for haematologous metastases in breast cancer patients. *International Journal of Cancer* 1990; **45**: 55–8.

92 Press MF, Pike MC, Chazin VR *et al.* Her-2/neu expression in node-negative breast cancer: direct tissue quantitation by computerized image analysis and association of overexpression with increased risk of recurrent disease. *Cancer Research* 1993; **53**: 4960–70.

93 Van de Vijver MJ, Peterse JL, Mooi WJ *et al.* Neu protein overexpression in breast cancer: association with comedo-type ductal carcinoma *in situ* and limited prognostic value in stage II breast cancer. *New England Journal of Medicine* 1988; **391**: 1239–45.

94 Liu ET, He M, Barcos M *et al.* High frequencey of HER-2/neu amplification in *in situ* carcinoma of the breast: analysis using differential polymerase chain reaction. *Oncogene* 1992; **7**: 1027–32.

95 Muss H, Thor A, Kute T *et al.* c-erbB-2 expression and S-phase activity predict response to adjuvant therapy in women with node-positive early breast cancer. *New England Journal of Medicine* 1994; **330**: 1260–6.

96 Lemaistre CF, Meneghetti C, Howes L, Osborne CK. Targeting the EGF receptor in breast cancer treatment. *Breast Cancer Research and Treatment* 1994; **32**: 97–103.

97 Baselga J, Mendelsohn J. The epidermal growth factor receptor as a target for therapy in breast carcinoma. *Breast Cancer Research and Treatment* 1994; **29**: 127–38.

98 Lemoine NR, Barnes DM, Hollywood DP. Expression of cerbB3 gene product in breast cancer. *British Journal of Cancer* 1992; **66**: 1112–16.

99 Gasparini G, Gullick WJ, Maluta S. c-erbB3 and c-erbB2 gene expression in node-negative breast carcinoma. *European Journal of Cancer* 1995.

100 Berns PMJJ, Klijn JGM, Van Staveren IL. Sporadic amplification of the insulin-like growth factor receptor 1 gene in human breast tumours. *Cancer Research* 1992; **52**: 1036–9.

101 Theillet C, Lidereau R, Escot C. Loss of a c-H-ras-1 allele and aggressive human primary breast carcinomas. *Cancer Research* 1986; **46**: 4776–81.

102 Going JJ, Anderson TJ, Wyllie AH. Ras p21 in breast tissue: associations with pathology and cellular localization. *British Journal of Cancer* 1992; **65**: 45–50

103 Dati C, Muraca R, Tazartes O. c-erbB-2 and ras expression levels in breast cancer are correlated and show a co-operative association with unfavorable clinical outcome. *International Journal of Cancer* 1991; **47**: 833–8.

104 Clark GJ, Der CJ. Aberrant function of the Ras signal transduction pathway in human breast cancer. *Breast Cancer Research and Treatment* 1995; **35**: 133–44.

105 Schuuring E, Verhoeven E, Van Tinteren H, Peterse JL. Amplification of genes within chromosome 11q13 region is indicative of poor prognosis in patients with operable breast cancer. *Cancer Research* 1992; **52**: 5229–34.

106 Bates S, Peters G. Cyclin D1 as a cellular proto-oncogene. *Seminars in Cancer Biology* 1995; **6**: 73–82.

107 Keyomarsi K, O'Leary N, Molnar G *et al.* Cyclin E, a potential prognostic marker for breast cancer. *Cancer Research* 1994; **54**: 380–5.

108 Pietiläinen T, Lipponen P, Aaltomaa S *et al.* Expression of retinoblastoma gene protein (Rb) in breast cancer as related to established prognostic factors and survival. *European Journal of Cancer* 1995; **31A**: 329–33.

109 Elledge RM, Fuqua SAW, Clark GM *et al.* The role and prognostic significance of p53 gene alterations in breast cancer. *Breast Cancer Research and Treatment* 1993; **27**: 95–102.

110 Isola J, Visakorpi T, Holli K, Kallioniemi OP. Association of overexpression of tumour suppressor protein p53 with rapid cell proliferation and poor prognosis in node-negative breast cancer patients. *Journal of the National Cancer Institute* 1992; **84**: 1109–14.

111 Thor AD, Moore II DH, Edgerton SM *et al.* Accumulation of p53 tumour suppressor gene protein: an independent marker of prognosis in breast cancers. *Journal of the National Cancer Institute* 1993; **84**: 845–55.

112 Silvestrini R, Benini E, Daidone MG. p53 as an independent prognostic marker in lymph node-negative breast cancer patients. *Journal of the National Cancer Institute* 1993; **85**: 965–70.

113 Stenmark-Askmalm M, Stal O, Sullivan S *et al.* Cellular accumulation of the p53 protein: an independent prognostic factor in stage II breast cancer. *European Journal of Cancer* 1994; **30A**: 175–80.

114 Ostrowsky JL, Sawan A, Henry L. p53 expression in human breast cancer related to survival and prognostic factors: an immunohistochemical study. *Journal of Pathology* 1991; **164**: 75–81.

115 Hanzal E, Gitsch G, Kohlberger P *et al.* Immunohisto-chemical detection of mutant p53-suppressor gene product in patients with breast cancer: influence on metastasis-free survival. *Anticancer Research* 1992; **12**: 2325–30.

116 Rosen PP, Lesser ML, Arroyo CD. p53 in node-negative breast carcinoma: an immunohistochemical study of epidemiologic risk factors, histologic features, and prognosis. *Journal of Clinical Oncology* 1995; **13**: 821–30.

117 Fan S, Smith ML, Rivet II DJ *et al.* Disruption of p53 function sensitizes breast cancer MCF-7 cells to cisplatin and pentoxifylline. *Cancer Research* 1995; **55**: 1649–54.

118 Sabourin JC, Martin A, Barouch J. Bcl-2 expression in normal breast tissue during the menstrual cycle. *International Journal of Cancer* 1994; **59**: 1–6.

119 Leek RD, Kaklamanis L, Pezzella F *et al.* Bcl-2 in normal breast and carcinoma, association with oestrogen-receptor-positive, epidermal growth factor-negative tumours and *in situ* cancer. *British Journal of Cancer* 1994; **69**: 135–9.

120 Joensuu H, Pylkkanen L, Toikkanen S. Bcl-2 protein expression and long-term survival in breast cancer. *American Journal of Pathology* 1994; **145**: 1191–8.

121 Silvestrini R, Veneroni S, Daidone MG. The bcl-2 protein: a strong prognostic indicator strongly related to p53 protein in lymph node-negative breast cancer patients. *Journal of the National Cancer Institute* 1994; **86**: 499–504.

122 Gee JMW, Robertson JFR, Ellis IO *et al.* Immunohisto-chemical localization of Bcl-2 protein in human breast cancers and its relationship to a series of prognostic markers and response to endocrine therapy. *International Journal of Cancer* 1994; **59**: 619–28.

123 Liotta LA, Steeg PS, Stetler-Stevenson WG. Cancer metastasis and angiogenesis: an imbalance of positive and negative regulation. *Cell* 1991; **64**: 327–36.

124 Folkman J. Tumour angiogenesis: therapeutic implications. *New England Journal of Medicine* 1971; **385**: 1182–6.

125 Howlett AR, Petersen OW, Steeg PS, Bissell MJ. A novel function of the nm23-H1 gene: overexpression in human breast carcinoma cells leads to the formation of basement membrane and growth arrest. *Journal of the National Cancer Institute* 1994; **24**: 1838–44.

126 Steeg PS, Bevilacqua G, Kopper L *et al.* Evidence for a novel gene associated with low tumour metastatic

potential. *Journal of the National Cancer Institute* 1988; **80**: 200–4.

127 Steeg PS, De La Rosa A, Flatow U *et al.* Nm23 and breast cancer metastasis. *Breast Cancer Research and Treatment* 1993; **25**: 175–87.

128 Sawan A, Lascu I, Veron M *et al.* NDP-K/nm23 expression in human breast cancer in relation to relapse, survival, and other prognostic factors: an immunohistochemical study. *Journal of Pathology* 1994; **172**: 27–34.

129 Rochefort H, Capony F, Garcia M. Cathepsin D: a protease involved in breast cancer metastasis. *Cancer Metastasis Reviews* 1990; **9**: 331.

130 Woessner JF. Matrix metalloproteinases and their inhibitors in connective tissue remodelling. *FASEB Journal* 1991; **5**: 2145–54.

131 Dano K, Andreasen PA, Grondahl-Hansen J *et al.* Plasminogen activators, tissue degradation, and cancer. *Advances in Cancer Research* 1985; **44**: 139–266.

132 Westley B, Rochefort H. A secreted glycoprotein induced by estrogen in human breast cancer cell lines. *Cell* 1980; **20**: 353–62.

133 Rochefort H, Capony F, Garcia M *et al.* Estrogen-induced lysosomal proteases secreted by breast cancer cells. A role in carcinogenesis? *Journal of Cellular Biochemistry* 1987; **35**: 17–29.

134 Montcourrei P, Mangeat PH, Salazar G *et al.* Cathepsin D in breast cancer cells can digest extracellular matrix in large acidic vesicles. *Cancer Research* 1990; **56**: 6045–54.

135 Dickson RB, Shi YE, Johnson MD. Matrix-degrading proteases in hormone-dependent breast cancer. *Breast Cancer Research and Treatment* 1994; **31**: 167–73.

136 Basset P, Bellocq JP, Wolf C *et al.* A novel metalloproteinase gene specifically expressed in stromal cells of breast cancer. *Nature* 1990; **348**: 699–704.

137 Alexander CM, Wei Z. Extracellular matrix degradation. In: Hay ED (ed.) *Cell biology of extracellular matrix.* New York: Picnum Press, 1991, 255–302.

138 Fazioli F, Blasi F. Urokinase-type plasminogen activator and its receptor: new targets for anti-metastatic therapy? *Trends in Pharmaceutical Sciences* 1994; **15**: 25–9.

139 Sato Y, Rifkin DB. Inhibition of endothelial cell movement by pericytes and smooth muscle cells: activation of a latent transforming growth factor-β1-like molecule by plasmin during co-culture. *Journal of Cell Biology* 1989; **109**: 309–15.

140 Rubin JS, Chan AM, Bottaro DP *et al.* A broad-spectrum human fibroblast-derived mitogen is a variant of hepatocyte growth factor. *Proceedings of the National Academy of Sciences USA* 1991; **88**: 415–19.

141 Byers S, Park M, Sommers C, Seslar S. Breast carcinoma: a collective disorder. *Breast Cancer Research and Treatment* 1994; **31**: 203–15.

142 Schor SL, Schor AM, Howell A, Crowther D. Hypothesis: persistent expression of fetal phenotype characteristics by fibroblasts is associated with an increased susceptibility to neoplastic disease. *Experimental Cell Biology* 1988; **55**: 11–7.

143 Brinkley D, Haybittle JL. Long-term survival of women with breast cancer. *Lancet* 1984; **i**: 1118.

144 Meltzer A. Dormancy and breast cancer. *Journal of Surgical Oncology* 1990; **43**: 181–8.

145 Folkman J. What is the evidence that tumours are angiogenesis dependent? *Journal of the National Cancer Institute* 1990; **82**: 4–7.

146 Holmgren L, O'Reilly MS, Folkman J. Dormancy of micrometastases: balanced proliferation and apoptosis in the presence of angiogenesis suppression. *Nature Medicine* 1995; **1**: 149–53.

147 Madri JA, Pratt BM. Endothelial cell-matrix interactions: *in vitro* models of angiogenesis. *Journal of Histochemistry and Cytochemistry* 1986; **43**: 85–91.

148 Brooks PC, Clark RAF, Cheresh DA. Requirement of vascular integrin $\alpha v\beta 3$ for angiogenesis. *Science* 1994; **264**: 569–71.

149 Brooks PC, Montgomery, AMP, Rosenfeld M *et al.* Integrin $\alpha v\beta 3$ antagonists promote tumour regression by inducing apoptosis of angiogenic blood vessels. *Cell* 1994; **79**: 1157–64.

150 Fan T-PD, Jaggar R, Bicknell R. Controlling the vasculature: angiogenesis, anti-angiogenesis and vascular targeting of gene therapy. *Trends in Pharmaceutical Sciences* 1995; **16**: 57–66.

151 Klagbrun M, Soker S. VEGF/VPF: the angiogenesis factor found? *Current Biology* 1993; **3**: 699–702.

152 Kolch W, Martiny-Baron G, Kieser A, Marmé D. Regulation of the expression of the VEGF/VPS and its receptors: role in tumour angiogenesis. *Breast Cancer Research and Treatment* 1995; **36**: 139–55.

153 Volpert OV, Stellmach V, Bouck N. The modulation of thrombospondin and other naturally occurring inhibitors of angiogenesis during tumour progression. *Breast Cancer Research and Treatment* 1995; **36**: 119–26.

154 Linderholm B, Tavelin B, Grankvist K, Henriksson R. Vascular endothelial growth factor is of high prognostic value in node-negative breast carcinoma. *Journal of Clinical Oncology* 1998; **16**: 3121–8.

155 O'Reilly MS, Holmgren L, Shing Y *et al.* Angiostatin: a novel angiogenesis inhibitor that mediates the suppression of metastases by a Lewis lung carcinoma. *Cell* 1994; **79**: 315–28.

156 Gorelik E, Segal S, Feldman M. Growth of a local tumour exerts a specific inhibitory effect on progression of lung metastases. *International Journal of Cancer* 1978; **21**: 617–25.

157 DeWijs WD. Studies correlating the growth rate of a tumour and its metastases providing evidence for tumour-related systemic growth-retarding factors. *Cancer Research* 1983; **32**: 138–45.

158 Simpson-Herren L, Sanford AH, Homquist JP. Effects of surgery on the cell cycle kinetics of residual tumour. *Cancer Treatment Reports* 1976; **60**: 1749–60.

159 Van Dierendonck JH, Keijzer R, Cornelisse CJ, Van de Velde CJH. Surgically induced cytokinetic responses in experimental rat mammary tumour models. *Cancer* 1991; **68**: 759–67.

160 Gasparini G, Harris AL. Clinical importance of tumour angiogenesis in breast carcinoma: much more than a new prognostic tool. *Journal of Clinical Oncology* 1995; **13**: 765–82.

161 Thorpe SM, Rochefort H, Garcia M *et al.* Association between high concentrations of Mr52,000 cathepsin D and poor prognosis in primary human breast cancer. *Cancer Research* 1989; **49**: 6008–14.

162 Foekens JA, van Putten WLJ, Portengen H *et al.* Prognostic value of PS2 and cathepsin D in 710 human primary breast tumours: multivariate analysis. *Journal of Clinical Oncology* 1993; **11**: 899–908.

163 Foekens JA, Loop MP, Bolt-de Vries J, Meijer-van Gelder ME, van Putten WLJ, Klijn VGM. Cathepsin D in primary breast cancer: prognostic evaluation involving 2810 patients. *British Journal of Cancer* 1999; **79**: 300–7.

164 Tandon AK, Clark GM, Chamness GC *et al.* Cathepsin D and prognosis in breast cancer. *New England Journal of Medicine* 1990; **322**: 297–302.

165 Isola J, Weitz S, Visakorpi T *et al.* Cathepsin D expression detected by immunohistochemistry has independent value in axillary node-negative breast cancer. *Journal of Clinical Oncology* 1993; **11**: 36–43.

166 Kute TE, Shao Z-M, Sugg NK *et al.* Cathepsin D as a prognostic indicator for node-negative breast cancer patients using both immunoassays and enzymatic assays. *Cancer Research* 1992; **52**: 5198–203.

167 Namer M, Ramalole A, Fontana X *et al.* Prognostic value of total cathepsin D in breast cancer. *Breast Cancer Research and Treatment* 1991; **19**: 89–93.

168 Granata G, Coradini D, Cappelletti V, Di Fronzo G. Prognostic relevance of cathepsin D versus oestrogen receptors in node-negative breast cancers. *European Journal of Cancer* 1991; **27**: 970–2.

169 Winstanly JH, Leinster SJ, Cooke TG *et al.* Prognostic significance of cathepsin D in patients with breast cancer. *British Journal of Cancer* 1993; **67**: 767–72.

170 Ravdin PM, Tandon AK, Allred C *et al.* Cathepsin D by Western blotting and immunohistochemistry: failure to confirm correlations with prognosis in node-negative breast cancer. *Journal of Clinical Oncology* 1994; **12**: 467–74.

171 Lury-Kleintop LD, Coronel EC, Lange MK *et al.* Western blotting and isoform analysis of cathepsin D from normal and malignant human breast cell lines. *Breast Cancer Research and Treatment* 1995; **35**: 211–20.

172 Westley, BR, May FEB. Prognostic value of cathepsin D in breast cancer. *British Journal of Cancer* 1999; **79**; 189–90.

173 Wolf C, Rouyer N, Lutz Y *et al.* Stromelysin 3 belongs to a subgroup of proteinases expressed in breast carcinoma fibroblastic cells and possibly implicated in tumour progression. *Proceedings of the National Academy of Sciences of the USA* 1993; **90**: 1843–7.

174 Engel G, Heselmeyer K, Auer G *et al.* Correlation between stromelysin-3 mRNA level and outcome of human breast cancer. *International Journal of Cancer* 1994; **58**: 830–5.

175 Tryggvason K. Type IV collagenase in invasive tumours. *Breast Cancer Research and Treatment* 1993; **24**: 209–18.

176 Thompson EW, Yu M, Bueno J et al. Collagen induced MMP-2 activation in human breast cancer. *Breast Cancer Research and Treatment* 1994; **31**: 357–70.

177 Brown PD, Bloxidge RE, Anderson Howell A. Expression of activated gelatinase in human invasive carcinoma. *Clinical and Experimental Metastasis* 1993; **11**: 183–9.

178 Davies B, Miles DW, Happerfield LC et al. Activity of type IV collagenases in benign and malignant breast disease. *British Journal of Cancer* 1993; **67**: 1126–31.

179 Zucker S. Mr92,000 type IV collagenase is increased in plasma of patients with colon cancer and breast cancer. *Cancer Research* 1993; **53**: 140–6.

180 Duffy MJ, O'Grady P, Devaney D et al. Urokinase-type plasminogen activator, a marker for aggressive breast carcinomas: preliminary report. *Cancer* 1988; **62**: 531–3.

181 Duffy MJ, Reilly D, O'Sullivan et al. Urokinase-plasminogen activator, an independent prognostic marker in breast cancer. *Cancer Research* 1990; **50**: 6827–9.

182 Foekens JA, Schmitt M, van Putten WLJ et al. Prognostic value of urokinase-type plasminogen activator in 671 primary breast cancer patients. *Cancer Research* 1992; **52**: 6101–5.

183 Janicke F, Schmitt M, Pache et al. Urokinase (uPA) and its inhibitor PAI-1 are strong and independent prognostic factors in node-negative breast cancer. *Breast Cancer Research and Treatment* 1993; **24**: 195–208.

184 Grøndahl-Hansen J, Christensen IJ, Rosenquist C et al. High levels of urokinase-type plasminogen activator and its inhibitor PAI-1 in cytosolic extracts of breast carcinomas are associated with poor prognosis. *Cancer Research* 1993; **53**: 2513–21.

185 Foekens JA, Schmitt M, van Putten WLJ et al. Plasminogen activator inhibitor-1 and prognosis in primary breast cancer. *Journal of Clinical Oncology* 1994; **12**: 1648–58.

186 Bouchet C, Spyratos F, Martin PM et al. Prognostic value of urokinase-type plasminogen activator (uPA) and plasminogen activator inhibitors PAI-1 and PAI-2 in breast carcinomas. *British Journal of Cancer* 1994; **69**: 398–405.

187 Yamashita J, Ogawa M, Yamashita S. et al. Immunoreactive hepatocyte growth factor is a strong and independent predictor of recurrence and survival in human breast cancer. *Cancer Research* 1994; **54**: 1630–3.

188 Kandel J, Bossy-Wetzel E, Radvanyi F et al. Neovascularization is associated with a switch to the export of bFGF in the multistep development of fibrosarcoma. *Cell* 1991; **66**: 1095–104.

189 Nguyen M, Watanabe H, Budson AE et al. Elevated levels of an angiogenic peptide, basic fibroblast growth factor, in the urine of patients with a wide spectrum of cancers. *Journal of the National Cancer Institute* 1994; **86**: 356–60.

190 Fan T-PD. Angiosuppressive therapy for cancer; meeting report. *Trends in Pharmaceutical Sciences* 1995; **15**: 33–6.

191 Marques LA, Franco ELF, Torloni H et al. Independent prognostic value of laminin receptor expression in breast-cancer survival. *Cancer Research* 1990; **50**: 1479–83.

192 Martignone S, Menard S, Bufallino R et al. Prognostic significance of the 67-kiloDalton laminin receptor expression in human breast carcinomas. *Journal of the National Cancer Institute* 1993; **85**: 398–402.

193 Gasparini G, Barbareschi M, Boracchi P et al. 67-kDa laminin-receptor expression adds prognostic information to intra-tumoural microvessel density in node-negative breast cancer. *International Journal of Cancer* 1995; **60**: 604–10.

194 Brem SS, Gullino PM, Medina D. Angiogenesis: a marker for neoplastic transformation of mammary papillary hyperplasia. *Science* 1977; **195**: 880–2.

195 Weidner N, Semple JP, Welch WR, Folkman J. Tumour angiogenesis and metastasis-correlation in invasive breast carcinoma. *New England Journal of Medicine* 1991; **324**: 1–8.

196 Bosari S, Lee AKC, DeLellis RA et al. Microvessel quantitation and prognosis in invasive breast carcinoma. *Human Pathology* 1992; **23**: 755–61.

197 Toi M, Kashitani J, Tominaga T. Tumour angiogenesis is an independent prognostic indicator in primary breast carcinoma. *International Journal of Cancer* 1993; **55**: 371–4.

198 Hall NR, Fish DE, Hunt N et al. Is the relationship between angiogenesis and metastasis in breast cancer real? *Surgical Oncology* 1992; **1**: 223–9.

199 Van Hoef MEHM, Knox WF et al. Assessment of tumour vascularity as a prognostic factor in lymph-node-negative invasive breast cancer. *European Journal of Cancer* 1993; **29A**: 1141–5.

200 Kuzu I, Bicknell R, Harris AL et al. Heterogeneity of vascular endothelial cells with relevance to diagnosis of vascular tumours. *Journal of Clinical Pathology* 1992; **45**: 143–8.

201 Horak ER, Leek R, Klenk N et al. Angiogenesis, assessed by platelet/endothelial cell adhesion molecule antibodies, as indicator of node metastases and survival in breast cancer. *Lancet* 1992; **340**: 1120–4.

202 Toi M, Inada K, Suzuki H, Tominaga T. Tumour angiogenesis in breast cancer: its importance as a prognostic indicator and the association with vascular endothelial growth factor expression. *Breast Cancer Research and Treatment* 1995; **36**: 193–204.

203 Gasparini G, Weidner N, Bevilacqua P et al. Tumour microvessel density, p53 expression, tumour size, and peritumoural lymphatic vessel invasion are relevant prognostic markers in node-negative breast carcinoma. *Journal of Clinical Oncology* 1994; **12**: 454–66.

204 Cheifetz S, Bellon T, Cales C et al. Endoglin is a component of the transforming growth factor-β receptor system in human endothelial cells. *Journal of Biological Chemistry* 1992; **267**: 19027–30.

205 Wang JM, Kumar S, Pye D et al. Breast carcinoma: comparative study of tumour vasculature using two

endothelial markers. *Journal of the National Cancer Institute* 1994; **86**: 386–8.

206 Ingber D, Fujita T, Kishimoto S *et al.* Synthetic analogues of fumagillin that inhibit angiogenesis and suppress tumour growth. *Nature* 1990; **448**: 555–7.

207 Teicher BA, Holden SA, Ara G *et al.* Potentiation of cytotoxic cancer therapies by TNP-470 alone and with other anti-angiogenic agents. *International Journal of Cancer* 1994; **57**: 920–5.

208 Clark GM, Wenger CR, Beardslee S *et al.* How to integrate steroid hormone receptor, flow cytometry, and other prognostic information for primary breast cancer? *Cancer* 1993; **71**: 2157–62.

209 Clark GM, Hilsenbeck SG, Ravdin PM *et al.* Prognostic factors: rationale and methods of analysis and integration. *Breast Cancer Research and Treatment* 1994; **32**: 105–12.

210 Ravdin PM, Clark GM, Hilsenbeck SG *et al.* A demonstration that breast cancer recurrence can be predicted by neural network analysis. *Breast Cancer Research and Treatment* 1992; **21**: 47–53.

211 Adler LP, Crowe JP, Al-Kaisi NK, Sunshine JL. Evaluation of breast masses and axillary lymph nodes with [F-18] 2-deoxy-2-fluoro-D-glucose PET. *Radiology* 1993; **187**: 743–50.

212 Wahl RL, Zasadny K, Helvie M *et al.* Metabolic monitoring of breast cancer chemohormonotherapy using positron emission tomography: initial evaluation. *Journal of Clinical Oncology* 1993; **11**: 2101–11.

213 Jansson T, Westlin JE, Ahlstrom H *et al.* Positron emission tomography studies in patients with locally advanced and/or metastatic breast cancer: a method for early therapy evaluation? *Journal of Clinical Oncology* 1995; **13**: 1470–7.

5

How do anti-oestrogens work?

MICHAEL POLLAK

INTRODUCTION

Anti-oestrogens have well-established indications in the adjuvant and palliative treatment of breast cancer.[1,2] They are currently among the most widely prescribed therapeutic agents in oncology, and if ongoing studies of their efficacy in breast cancer prevention and/or post-menopausal hormone replacement therapy demonstrate efficacy, they will be even more widely prescribed,[1,3] Although the prototype non-steroidal anti-oestrogen was discovered in 1958,[4] tamoxifen, the anti-oestrogen most widely used today, did not become widely used until the late 1970s. Initial approval in the USA was for metastatic breast cancer, and approval for post-operative adjuvant therapy followed almost a decade later.

Despite their extensive clinical use, the mechanism of action of anti-oestrogens is incompletely understood, and remains an active area of research. This is not surprising given the fact that many pharmacological actions of anti-oestrogens are related to the physiology of oestrogens, an area which itself remains incompletely documented. Steroid hormones in general and oestrogens in particular have very long evolutionary histories which can be traced back millions of years to insects and perhaps even to plants.[5–7] It is now recognized that oestrogens have complex integrative roles in regulating physiological processes such as cellular proliferation and differentiation in many organs, as well as their initially described roles in the female reproductive system, and it is therefore not surprising that anti-oestrogens have been found to have actions in organs such as lung, liver and bone, as well as in breast and uterus.

Well-known aspects of the clinical experience with tamoxifen therapy provide important clues to its mechanism of action. When used as post-operative adjuvant treatment, tamoxifen has a significant impact on disease-free survival. The benefit is most apparent in patients with oestrogen-receptor-positive tumours, although an absence of benefit in oestrogen-receptor-negative patients has not been demonstrated, and is the subject of ongoing clinical studies. However, the magnitude of the benefit is modest, indicating that failure of adjuvant tamoxifen to prevent the development of metastases is not a rare event. Tamoxifen usage is associated with an increased incidence of uterine cancer,[8] but this is insignificant relative to the beneficial effect on breast cancer behaviour. Beneficial effects on lipids and bone density have been reported.[9,10] In metastatic breast cancer, clinical experience with anti-oestrogen therapy again indicates clinical efficacy, but non-response is the rule among patients with oestrogen-receptor-negative tumours, and it is also seen in approximately 25% of patients with oestrogen-receptor-positive tumours. Taken together, these data suggest that actions of tamoxifen:

- affect tissues besides the classic targets of breast and uterus;
- vary in a tissue-specific manner with respect to oestrogen agonist vs. antagonist effects;
- are predominantly cytostatic rather than cytocidal;
- are frequently limited by the development of resistance to anti-oestrogen action;
- involve the oestrogen receptor (or, strictly speaking, if they do not involve the oestrogen receptor itself, require some feature of cellular physiology that is highly correlated with expression of oestrogen receptors).

This review will outline for the clinician current knowledge concerning the mechanism of action of anti-oestrogens, and will also indicate some of the areas of active research. Uncovering new information concerning mechanisms of action is not merely an intellectual exercise. It is hoped that such information may provide important insights relevant to proposed applications of anti-oestrogens in postmenopausal hormone replacement therapy and in cancer prevention, and also suggest novel approaches to the important problem of the development of anti-oestrogen resistance in breast cancer patients.

Actions of anti-oestrogens can be analysed at the molecular, cellular and whole organism level. Over the past few decades, direct effects of anti-oestrogens on neoplastic cells have received more attention than systemic effects. It is clear that direct effects are important, as evidenced by the antiproliferative actions of anti-oestrogens seen using *in-vitro* breast cancer cell-culture systems, where systemic effects are excluded. However, there is an impression that, in general, the magnitude of the antineoplastic effect of anti-oestrogens at clinically relevant concentrations is greater when assayed using *in-vitro* compared to *in-vivo* models. This suggests the possibility of additional actions of anti-oestrogens on the host that may lead to an environment which is less conducive to the growth and/or metastasis of breast cancer cells. Just like the 'classic' direct actions on neoplastic cells, such actions may result from interactions between antioestrogens and oestrogen receptors, except that the relevant oestrogen receptors here are not those present on neoplastic cells, but rather those expressed elsewhere in the host (e.g. in the pituitary gland).

ANTI-OESTROGEN – OESTROGEN-RECEPTOR INTERACTIONS

Oestrogens and various anti-oestrogens affect gene expression and cellular behaviour in different directions, but there is a consensus that all of these compounds are ligands for the oestrogen receptor.

There are data to support the view that, in the absence of ligands, the oestrogen receptor forms part of an intracellular complex that includes heat shock proteins, while the presence of a ligand (oestrogenic or anti-oestrogenic) leads to dissociation of the oestrogen receptor from this complex.[11] Oestrogen receptors then mediate the effects of ligands on cellular physiology by modulating gene expression. This occurs by the interaction of specific sites on the oestrogen receptor molecule with oestrogen response elements, which are specific recognition sequences in the promotor sequences of target genes. The influence of anti-oestrogens on the expression of oestrogen-receptor-regulated gene transcription varies and is not identical in all oestrogen-receptor-positive tissues. This may be related to the effects of cell-type-specific transcription factors that act in concert with the oestrogen receptor to modulate gene expression.

Furthermore, the magnitude and direction of the oestrogen receptor effect on gene expression are profoundly influenced by the nature of the ligand bound. An anti-oestrogen – oestrogen-receptor complex will frequently affect gene expression to a different extent or even in the opposite direction to an oestrogen – oestrogen-receptor complex. In addition, there is evidence for an interaction between the modulating effects of tissue-specific transcription factors and the modulating effects of different ligands.[12] This probably underlies important clinical observations concerning the tissue-specific nature of antagonist vs. agonist actions of certain oestrogen-receptor ligands (e.g. tamoxifen), in contrast to the apparent universal antagonist actions of others (e.g. ICI 182780).

Not all genes whose expression is modulated by oestrogens or anti-oestrogens have classic oestrogen response elements. This suggests that there are uncharacterized oestrogen response elements in addition to those already described, or that some genes are indirectly regulated by oestrogens and anti-oestrogens. An oestrogen receptor–ligand complex may bind to a response element and thereby affect the expression of an intermediate gene, whose product in turns acts to up-regulate expression of the gene lacking an oestrogen response element. Such a system makes physiological sense, as it allows for an additional level of physiological control of certain oestrogen-regulated genes. No 'critical' oestrogen-regulated gene that mediates all of the effects of oestrogenic or anti-oestrogenic stimulation has been described. It is likely that the phenotypic changes induced by oestrogens result from the aggregate effects of a change in the pattern of expression of dozens of genes of target cells.

Not all of the experimental data suggest that the oestrogen receptor resides in a protein complex remote from DNA in the absence of ligand. Some results suggest that 'empty' oestrogen receptors can bind to specific oestrogen response elements of target genes.[13] It is unclear whether such 'empty' oestrogen receptors modulate gene expression, as research to date has emphasized comparisons of levels of expression of oestrogen-regulated genes in the presence or absence of various oestrogen-receptor ligands, rather than comparing target gene expression in the presence of 'empty' oestrogen receptors with expression in the absence of oestrogen receptors. Such experiments would have to be conducted by experimentally interfering with expression of the oestrogen receptor in cells that have all of the other machinery for responding to oestrogens.

In view of the mitogenic effects of oestradiol on breast cancer cells, it is somewhat counterintuitive that neoplastic progression is associated with the *loss* of oestrogen receptors. This is in contrast to the findings reported for epidermal growth factor (EGF) receptors. An increase in expression of EGF receptors is associated with more aggressive proliferative and neoplastic behaviour.[14] This is consistent with the simple model in which, in the clonal evolution of neoplastic cells, derangements that result in over-expression of a mitogen receptor confer a growth advantage by increasing responsiveness to extracellular mitogens.[15] One possible explanation for the fact that oestrogen-receptor levels decline with neoplastic progression and that oestrogen-receptor-negative cells exhibit a higher rate of baseline proliferation than oestrogen-receptor-positive cells is that the phenotypic change is mediated by cellular pathophysiology 'downstream' from the oestrogen receptor that completely bypasses the need for oestrogen-receptor action. Another interesting possibility is that unoccupied oestrogen receptors actually act to constrain the expression of genes that are needed for proliferation, and that this constraint is relaxed when oestrogen binds, and is intensified when anti-oestrogens bind. This model would predict that loss of expression of the oestrogen receptor (or an oestrogen-receptor mutation that results in loss of function) in a neoplastic cell would confer a proliferative advantage by removing the constraint imposed by the 'empty' oestrogen receptor on expression of genes needed for proliferation. This model can be viewed as one that regards the 'empty' oestrogen receptor as a gene with tumour suppressor function that is regulated by ligand binding. The model is consistent first with data concerning the well-documented neoplastic proliferation of cells from an oestrogen-receptor-positive to an oestrogen-receptor-negative phenotype, secondly with the selective advantage of oestrogen-receptor-negative over oestrogen-receptor-positive cells, and thirdly with the higher baseline proliferation of oestrogen-receptor-negative cells. However, it is not consistent with separate data which suggests that anti-oestrogens reduce cellular oestrogen-receptor content,[16,17] and there has been little experimental investigation of this model to date.

The phenomenon of neoplastic progression from an anti-oestrogen-responsive phenotype to a non-responsive phenotype occurs frequently. The multiple pathways by which this change can occur at the molecular level,[8,18–20] and some of the mechanisms involved, may even lead to a phenotype characterized by a mitogenic response by neoplastic breast epithelial cells to anti-oestrogens such as tamoxifen.[21] Regardless of the mechanism involved at the molecular level, the consequences at the cellular level are clear. Anti-oestrogen-non-responsive cells will have a proliferative advantage, particularly in the presence of anti-oestrogens, but also in their absence. The descendants of the single cell in which the change initially occurs will comprise an increasing precentage of the tumour with time, and will eventually determine the characteristics of the neoplastic disease of the patient.

There have been reports of so-called 'anti-oestrogen-binding sites' that provide mechanisms for anti-oestrogens to act independently of the oestrogen receptor, and to influence other signal transduction pathways, including those involving histamine,[22] protein kinase C[23] and calmodulin.[24] However, this remains an area of some controversy, as the expression of oestrogen receptors remains a more accurate predictor of response to anti-oestrogens than the expression of any other 'anti-oestrogen-binding site'.

CELLULAR BIOLOGY OF ANTI-OESTROGEN ACTION

The behaviour of oestrogen-receptor-positive cells is regulated by oestrogens and anti-oestrogens. There is evidence that anti-oestrogens do not act merely in a passive fashion to antagonize oestrogen-stimulated actions by blocking oestrogen effects, but rather that they act to directly alter gene expression and cellular behaviour in a direction opposite to oestrogens. The most direct data in this context concerns the growth-inhibitory actions of anti-oestrogens seen in the complete absence of any oestrogenic stimuli.[25–28] These data demonstrate that the hypothesis that 'anti-oestrogens' simply act by blocking oestrogen action is incomplete.

There is considerable interest in the mediation of certain actions of anti-oestrogens by peptide growth factors. One of the earlier observations in this area concerned transforming growth factor beta, which acts as a growth inhibitor for many breast cancer cell lines. Anti-oestrogens up-regulate the expression of transforming growth factor beta by oestrogen-receptor-positive breast cancer cells in tissue culture, and media conditioned by anti-oestrogen-treated cells have been shown to have an inhibitory effect even on oestrogen-receptor-negative cells in some experimental systems.[29–31] More recent reports have documented increased levels of transforming growth factor beta in human breast tumours following treatment with tamoxifen,[32] and tamoxifen administration has also been noted to be associated with an increase in serum transforming growth factor beta levels.[33] However, transforming growth factor beta physiology is complex, and under some circumstances this peptide can act as a growth stimulator or immunosuppressant. Furthermore, anti-oestrogens in many experimental systems inhibit proliferation to a greater extent than the inhibition that can be achieved by optimal concentrations of transforming growth factor beta, indicating that modulation of transforming growth factor beta can at best account for a subset of the antiproliferative effects of anti-oestrogens. There is also evidence to suggest that anti-oestrogens may down-regulate the autocrine production of transforming growth factor alpha, which serves as a ligand for the epidermal growth factor receptor and stimulates proliferation of breast cancer cells under most conditions.[34,35]

More recently described pathways of anti-oestrogen action at the cellular level concern insulin-like growth factor physiology. Insulin-like growth factors are potent breast cancer mitogens.[36,37] The mitogenic effects of both IGF-I and IGF-II are thought to be mediated by the

IGF-I receptor.[38] There is a positive correlation between oestrogen-receptor level and IGF-I-receptor level,[39] but many oestrogen-receptor-negative cell lines exhibit IGF-I receptors and responsivity to IGFs. There are interrelationships between IGF responsiveness and oestrogen responsiveness. *In-vitro* experiments suggest that oestradiol increases the IGF-I receptor level and mitogenic responsivity to IGFs,[40] while anti-oestrogens have the opposite effect.[41,42] This may contribute to the ability of anti-oestrogens to induce apoptosis in susceptible cells, because stimulation of IGF-I receptors provides an important anti-apoptotic signal.[36]

The anti-oestrogen ICI 182780, and to a lesser extent tamoxifen, have been shown to up-regulate autocrine production of insulin-like growth factor binding protein 3 (IGFBP-3) in tissue culture.[26] IGFBP-3 acts as a growth inhibitor in most experimental systems.[43] It is thought to do this mainly by competing with IGF-I receptors for IGF-I and IGF-II, but recently evidence has been presented for a direct growth-inhibitory effect of IGFBP-3 mediated by an as yet incompletely characterized cell-surface IGFBP-3 receptor.[44] The potential importance of this action, particularly in the early cellular response to anti-oestrogens, was suggested by experimental manipulations that involved interfering with anti-oestrogen-induced IGFBP-3 expression by the use of an IGFBP-3 antisense oligodeoxynucleotide.[26] This oligodeoxynucleotide blocked ICI 182780-induced IGFBP-3 expression, and in the presence of this oligo, the antiproliferative action of ICI 182780 was significantly attenuated.

These examples suggest that modulation of peptide growth factor autocrine growth-inhibitory and growth-stimulatory loops represents an important component of anti-oestrogen action. These effects may be modulated by the cellular environment, via paracrine pathways. For example, anti-oestrogen-induced transforming growth factor beta or IGFBP-3 secretion may modulate the production of IGF-II or fibroblast growth factor production by neighbouring fibroblasts in a manner that results in reduced stimulation of proliferation of neoplastic epithelial cells by factors originating in the stroma.

WHOLE-ORGANISM BIOLOGY OF ANTI-OESTROGEN ACTION

Apart from their specific effects on oestrogen-responsive tissues, anti-oestrogens have a number of actions that affect the hormonal milieu systemically. Some of these actions may contribute to their antineoplastic actions.

Effects on gonadotrophins, sex steroid-binding protein and oestradiol

In premenopausal women, tamoxifen can cause a rise in gonadotrophin levels and circulating oestradiol levels by interfering with the normal feedback inhibition pathway by which oestrogens suppress gonadotrophin levels.[45,46] However, it is unclear whether such increases result in elevation of the oestrogenic bioactivity of serum, because sex steroid-binding hormone levels are also elevated by tamoxifen.[47,48] In post-menopausal women, the minor oestrogenic activity of tamoxifen is more evident than in premenopausal women, in whom such activity is rendered insignificant by high levels of oestrogens. This oestrogenic activity can result in decreased gonadotrophin levels.[49]

Effects on the growth hormone–IGF-I axis

The first randomized, placebo-controlled trial demonstrating that tamoxifen suppresses circulating IGF-I levels was reported in 1990, more than a decade after the clinical use of tamoxifen had become widespread.[50] This observation has now been confirmed in a number of other studies,[51] and is of potential significance as IGF-I is a potent breast cancer mitogen.[52] It has now been established that tamoxifen acts to suppress IGF-I levels by at least two mechanisms. First, it acts to inhibit release of growth hormone by the pituitary gland, as shown by both *in-vivo* and *in-vitro* studies.[53,54] This would be expected to have an impact on circulating IGF-I levels, as in many organs IGF-I expression is growth hormone dependent. Secondly, tamoxifen has a separate growth hormone-independent inhibitory effect on IGF-I gene expression.[55] The inhibitory effect of tamoxifen on serum IGF-I levels is strongly correlated with its inhibitory effects on IGF-I gene expression in the liver (the major source of circulating IGF-I), and is also correlated with inhibition of IGF-I expression in other target organs for breast cancer metastasis, such as lung.[55] Most studies have indicated a suppression of serum level to approximately 70% of pretreatment values. It is unlikely that this degree of suppression of serum IGF-I levels directly contributes to the antineoplastic effect of tamoxifen, but it is possible that the decline in serum levels serves as a surrogate for a decline in tissue IGF-I bioactivity in target organs for metastasis, which might well contribute to an antineoplastic effect by rendering the target organs less hospitable for IGF-4-responsive metastatic cells. It has been shown that growth of human breast cancer xenografts is reduced in mice that are genetically deficient in IGF-I, compared to that in IGF-I-replete hosts.[56]

It has yet to be shown to what extent the effect of anti-oestrogens on IGF-I physiology contributes to their antineoplastic action, but recent studies of the correlations between the effects of anti-oestrogens on the uterus and their effects on uterine IGF physiology justify further research in this area. The uterotrophic action of tamoxifen is well known, and is often cited as the prototypical example of the tissue specificity of the agonist vs. antagonist actions of the compound. It has been found that while tamoxifen generally suppresses IGF-I expression, as described above, the uterus is an exception. Here, where tamoxifen stimulates growth, it up-regulates IGF-I expression. In contrast, ICI 182780, an anti-oestrogen which causes uterine involution, down-regulates uterine IGF-I expression.[57] Furthermore, tamoxifen down-regulates the uterine expression of insulin-like growth factor binding protein 3, a protein which interferes with IGF action, while ICI 182780 up-regulates IGFBP-3 expression.[58] These correlations between the actions of various anti-oestrogens on the uterus and their effect on IGF physiology focuses interest on the possibility that the antineoplastic actions of anti-oestrogens are also correlated with effects on IGF physiology, and both clinical and laboratory studies are currently addressing this issue.

Effects on prolactin

Anti-oestrogens are well-recognized inhibitors of oestrogen-stimulated prolactin secretion by the pituitary gland,[59] but the importance of this action in humans is uncertain, as most studies to date suggest that prolactin has effects on human breast cancer that are minor relative to the effects of other peptides such as fibroblast growth factor, epidermal growth factor or the insulin-like growth factors. However, there are data to suggest that the effect of tamoxifen on prolactin secretion may be important in certain rodent breast cancer models.[60]

Effects on angiogenesis

It is recognized that angiogenesis is necessary for primary or metastatic lesions to reach a significant size, and that anti-angiogenic strategies represent an important direction in cancer research.[61] Primary tumour angiogenesis is a correlate of metastasis in breast cancer.[62] Evidence has been presented to support the view that tamoxifen acts as an anti-angiogenic agent,[63] but the mechanisms involved remain unclear. In general, endothelial cells have not been shown to exhibit oestrogen receptors. Therefore, the avenues currently under investigation include the possibility that angiogenesis is reduced by anti-oestrogens via their effects on IGF-I, which is an angiogenic factor,[64] or that anti-oestrogens block oestrogen-dependent secretion of angiogenic factors by oestrogen-receptor-positive breast cancer cells.

APPLICATION OF KNOWLEDGE OF MECHANISM OF ACTION OF ANTI-OESTROGENS

During the last 20 years, anti-oestrogens have been recognized as useful therapeutic agents, and they are now widely used. Tamoxifen, the most extensively used anti-oestrogen at the present time, is of value in the adjuvant management of early breast cancer and in the palliative management of macrometastatic disease. However, in both of these set-

tings, treatment failure due to the emergence of anti-oestrogen resistance is a common problem. Further understanding of the mechanisms of anti-oestrogen action and the mechanisms of the development of resistance may lead to strategies that improve the clinical utility of anti-oestrogens in breast cancer treatment.

For example, the hypothesis that co-administration of a somatostatin analogue with an anti-oestrogen will enhance anti-oestrogen efficacy[65,66] was suggested in part by the findings of recent research concerning the mechanism of action of anti-oestrogens. The previously discussed observations concerning the inhibitory effects of tamoxifen on IGF bioactivity, both at the organism level (reduction of serum IGF-I levels and reduction of IGF-I expression in target organs for metastases) and at the cellular level (down-regulation of IGF-I receptors and up-regulation of IGFBP-3 secretion) motivated research to examine the effects of combining tamoxifen with other agents that target the growth hormone–IGF-I axis. There are many possible approaches, including the use of growth hormone antagonists,[67] growth hormone-releasing hormone antagonists[68] and somatostatin analogues.[69,70] Somatostatin analogues were selected for examination in this context because compounds such as octreotide were known to reduce IGF-I levels,[71] and had well-known long-term toxicity profiles, as they have been extensively used in the management of acromegaly. It was initially observed that co-administration of the agents resulted in enhanced suppression of IGF-I gene expression compared to use of either agent alone.[72] Subsequently it was shown that the octreotide–tamoxifen combination exhibited enhanced antineoplastic activity in the rat DMBA mammary tumour model compared to single-agent tamoxifen.[66] This result contributed to the rationale for a clinical trial programme, which began in 1997, to compare the efficacy and safety of tamoxifen combined with octreotide to that of single-agent tamoxifen in the management of breast cancer in both the adjuvant and palliative settings. In the USA, the NSABP group will compare tamoxifen with octreotide plus tamoxifen in the adjuvant treatment of approximately 3000 stage I breast cancer patients, while the NCIC is studying this issue in a broader cross-section of stage I and II breast cancer patients.[73]

New information concerning the molecular basis of anti-oestrogen action may permit the development of new 'anti-oestrogens' that have optimum profiles with regard to the tissue-specific agonist–antagonist properties for specific clinical applications. The ideal 'anti-oestrogen' for post-menopausal hormone replacement therapy and prevention of post-menopausal breast cancer would be anti-oestrogenic in the breast, oestrogenic with respect to effects on bone density and lipid profile, and neutral or anti-oestrogenic in the uterus. Tamoxifen has a profile quite close to this ideal. This was fortuitous rather than the result of deliberate drug development.[1] Raloxifene has beneficial effects on bone and lipids, but a less uterotrophic effect than tamoxifen.[74] If raloxifene or other 'anti-oestrogens' with comparable profiles are shown to have anti-neoplastic activity that is comparable to or greater than that of tamoxifen, such compounds may prove to have a role in hormone replacement therapy for post-menopausal women, in a way that would lower the incidence of breast cancer, lower lipid-related cardiovascular morbidity and increase bone density. There is controversy as to whether the menopause should be regarded as a hormonal deficiency state that requires treatment, or as a normal physiological stage of development. An evolutionary perspective gives some support to the former viewpoint, as there clearly was no evolutionary selection pressure to optimize quality of life after the childbearing years. For the vast majority of human existence, post-menopausal life was the exception rather than the rule. This situation has been reversed very recently in terms of evolutionary history as a consequence of cultural evolution and improved living conditions. It should therefore come as no surprise that the 'normal' hormonal milieu in post-menopausal women is not an optimum one for preventing cardiovascular morbidity, osteoporosis or breast cancer. Many feel that the potential application of current research with regard to agents such as raloxifene in improving the quality of life of post-menopausal women is entirely appropriate.

Droloxifene[75] and toremifene[76] have antineoplastic activity comparable to that of tamoxifen. Their toxicity profiles differ somewhat from those of tamoxifen in preclinical model systems, but it is not yet clear whether these differences are large enough to result in major differences for patients.

Toremifene exhibits considerably less hepatic carcinogenicity than tamoxifen in the rat,[77] but to date an excess of hepatocellular carcinomas has not been observed in humans on long-term tamoxifen therapy,[78] so the clinical relevance of this result remains uncertain.

On the other hand, pure anti-oestrogens such as ICI 182780 (reviewed by Howell et al.)[79] are very different agents from tamoxifen. They are reported to exhibit more potent anti-oestrogenic effects in breast, and also to be anti-oestrogenic in the uterus. It is anticipated that the beneficial oestrogenic effects of tamoxifen on bone and lipids will not be seen with agents of this class. Complete anti-oestrogens may therefore have limited utility in long-term adjuvant treatment of breast cancer patients with a relatively good prognosis, but may have important roles in the management of metastatic disease. Early reports suggest that some neoplasms that are resistant to tamoxifen are responsive to ICI 182780.[79]

There is considerable interest in optimizing well-tolerated non-cytotoxic treatments for the treatment of certain patients with solid tumours such as breast cancers that are rarely cured by chemotherapy.[80] The clinical results currently obtainable with agents such as tamoxifen provide evidence of the potential of this approach, and justify the use of anti-oestrogens for many groups of breast cancer patients. On the other hand, these same results also point to the need for further research and development, as it has yet to be determined whether tamoxifen as currently used represents the best that can be achieved with anti-oestrogen therapy, or whether new strategies can be devised to meet the urgent clinical need to enhance efficacy.

REFERENCES

1 Lerner L, Jordan VC. Development of antiestrogens and their use in breast cancer: Eighth Cain Memorial Award Lecture. *Cancer Res* 1990; **50**: 4177–89.

2 Jordan VC, Murphy CS. Endrocrine pharmacology of antiestrogens as antitumor agents. *Endocr Rev* 1990; **11**: 578–611.

3 Jordan VC. Studies on the estrogen receptor in breast cancer – 20 years as a target for the treatment and prevention of cancer. *Breast Cancer Res Treat* 1995; **36**: 267–85.

4 Lerner LJ, Holthaus FJ Jr, Thompson CR. A nonsteroidal estrogen antagonist 1-(*p*-2-diethylaminoethoxyphenyl)-1-phenyl-2-*p*-methoxyphenylethanol. *Endocrinology* 1958; **63**: 295.

5 Baker ME. Evolution of regulation of steroid-mediated intercellular communication in vertebrates: insights from flavonoids, signals that mediate plant–rhizobia symbiosis (review). *J Steroid Biochem Mol Biol* 1992; **41**: 301–8.

6 Gerwin N, La Rosee A, Sauer F *et al*. Functional and conserved domains of the *Drosophila* transcription factor encoded by the segmentation gene knirps. *Mol Cell Biol* 1994; **14**: 7899–908.

7 Baker ME. Endocrine activity of plant-derived compounds: an evolutionary perspective (review). *Proc Soc Exp Biol Med* 1995; **208**: 131–8.

8 Jordan VC. Molecular mechanisms of antiestrogen action in breast cancer (review). *Breast Cancer Res Treat* 1994; **31**: 41–52.

9 Love RR, Wiebe DA, Newcomb PA *et al*. Effects of tamoxifen on cardiovascular risk factors in postmenopausal women. *Ann Intern Med* 1991; **115**: 860–4.

10 Love RR, Mazess RB, Barden HS *et al*. Effects of tamoxifen on bone mineral density in postmenopausal women with breast cancer (see comments). *N Eng J Med* 1992; **326**: 852–6.

11 Smith DF, Toft DO. Steroid receptors and their associated proteins (review). *Mol Endocrinol* 1993; **7**: 4–11.

12 McDonnell DP, Clemm DL, Herman T, Goldman ME, Pike JW. Analysis of estrogen receptor function *in vitro* reveals three distinct classes of antiestrogens. *Mol Endocrinol* 1995; **9**: 659–69.

13 Reese JC, Katzenellenbogen BS. Examination of the DNA-binding ability of estrogen receptor in whole cells: implications for hormone-independent transactivation

and the actions of antiestrogens. *Mol Cell Biol* 1992; **12**: 4531–8.

14 Filmus J, Trent J, Pollak M, Buick RN. EGF receptor gene amplified MDA-468 breast cancer cell line and its non-amplified variants. *Mol Cell Biol* 1987; **7**: 251–7.

15 Pollak M, Boyarsky A, Gora P. A mathematical model describing consequences of abnormally high levels of epidermal growth factor receptor on the proliferation of neoplastic cells. *Cancer Invest* 1991; **9**: 513–20.

16 Gibson MK, Nemmers LA, Beckman WC Jr, Davis VL, Curtis SW, Korach KS. The mechanism of ICI 164,384 antiestrogenicity involves rapid loss of estrogen receptor in uterine tissue. *Endocrinology* 1991; **129**: 2000–10.

17 Dauvois S, Danielian PS, White R, Parker MG. Antiestrogen ICI 164,384 reduces cellular estrogen receptor content by increasing its turnover. *Proc Natl Acad Sci USA* 1992; **89**: 4037–41.

18 Osborne CK, Coronado E, Allred DC, Wiebe V, DeGregorio M. Acquired tamoxifen resistance: correlation with reduced breast tumor levels of tamoxifen and isomerization of trans-4-hydroxytamoxifen (see comments). *J Natl Cancer Inst* 1991; **83**: 1477–82.

19 Horwitz KB. How do breast cancers become hormone resistant? (review.) *J Steroid Biochem Mol Biol* 1994; **49**: 295–302.

20 Katzenellenbogen BS. Antiestrogen resistance: mechanisms by which breast cancer cells undermine the effectiveness of endocrine therapy (editorial; comment). *J Natl Cancer Inst* 1991; **83**: 1434–5.

21 Horwitz KB. When tamoxifen turns bad (editorial). *Endocrinology* 1995; **136**: 821–3.

22 Brandes LJ, Macdonald LM, Bogdanovic RP. Evidence that the antiestrogen binding site is a histamine or histamine-like receptor. *Biochem Biophys Res Commun* 1985; **126**: 905–10.

23 O'Brian CA, Housey GM, Weinstein IB. Specific and direct binding of protein kinase C to an immobilized tamoxifen analogue. *Cancer Res* 1988; **48**: 3626–9.

24 Lam HY. Tamoxifen is a calmodulin antagonist in the activation of cAMP phosphodiesterase. *Biochem Biophys Res Commun* 1984; **118**: 27–32.

25 Pratt SE, Pollak M. Estrogen and antiestrogen modulation of MCF7 human breast cancer cell proliferation is associated with specific alterations in accumulation of IGF binding proteins in conditioned media. *Cancer Res* 1993; **53**: 5193–8.

26 Huynh HT, Yang X, Pollak M. Estradiol and antiestrogens regulate a growth inhibitory insulin-like growth factor binding protein 3 autocrine loop in human breast cancer cells. *J Biol Chem* 1996; **271**: 1016–21.

27 Wakeling AE, Dukes M, Bowler J. A potent specific pure antiestrogen with clinical potential. *Cancer Res* 1991; **51**: 3867–73.

28 Vignon F, Bouton MM, Rochefort H. Antiestrogens inhibit the mitogenic effect of growth factors on breast cancer cells in the total absence of estrogens. *Biochem Biophys Res Commun* 1987; **146**: 1502–8.

29 Knabbe C, Lippman ME, Wakefield LM *et al.* Evidence that transforming growth factor-β is a hormonally regulated negative growth factor in human breast cancer cells. *Cell* 1987; **48**: 417–28.

30 Jeng MH, ten Dijke P, Iwata KK, Jordan VC. Regulation of the levels of three transforming growth factor beta mRNAs by estrogen and their effects on the proliferation of human breast cancer cells. *Mol Cell Endocrinol* 1993; **97**: 115–23.

31 Arteaga CL, Tandon AK, Von Hoff DD, Osborne CK. Transforming growth factor beta: potential autocrine growth inhibitor of estrogen receptor-negative human breast cancer cells. *Cancer Res* 1988; **48**: 3898–904.

32 Butta A, MacLennan K, Flanders KC *et al.* Introduction of transforming growth factor in human breast cancer *in vivo* following tamoxifen treatment. *Cancer Res* 1992; **52**: 4261–4.

33 Kopp A, Jonat W, Schmahl M, Knabbe C. Transforming growth factor beta 2 (TGF-beta 2) levels in plasma of patients with metastatic breast cancer treated with tamoxifen. *Cancer Res* 1995; **55**: 4512–15.

34 Dickson RB, Lippman ME. Estrogenic regulation of growth and polypeptide growth factor secretion in human breast carcinoma. *Endocr Rev* 1987; **8**: 29–43.

35 Bates SE, Davidson NE, Valverius EM *et al.* Expression of transforming growth factor alpha and its messenger ribonucleic acid in human breast cancer: its regulation by estrogen and its possible functional significance. *Mol Endocrinol* 1988; **2**: 543–55.

36 Resnicoff M, Abraham D, Yutanawiboonchai W *et al.* The insulin-like growth factor I receptor protects tumor cells from apoptosis *in vivo*. *Cancer Res* 1995; **55**: 2463–9.

37 Baserga R. The insulin-like growth factor I receptor; a key to tumor growth? *Cancer Res* 1995; **55**: 249–52.

38 Ellis MJC, Leav BA, Yang Z *et al.* Affinity for the insulin-like growth factor- II (IGFAI) receptor inhibits autocrine IGF-II activity in MCF-7 breast cancer cells. *Mol Endocrinol* 1996; **10**: 286–97.

39 Peyrat JP, Bonneterre J, Beuscart R, Djiane J, Demaille A. Insulin-like growth factor I receptors in human breast cancer and their relation to estradiol and progesterone receptors. *Cancer Res* 1988; **48**: 6429–33.

40 Stewart AJ, Johnson MD, May FEB, Westley BR. Role of insulin-like growth factors and the type I insulin-like growth factor receptor in the estrogen-stimulated proliferation of human breast cancer cells. *J Biol Chem* 1990; **265**: 21172–8.

41 Nickerson T, Yang XF, Pollak M, Huynh HT. *Post-transcriptional regulation of insulin-like growth factor I receptor by the pure antiestrogen ICI 182,780*. American Association for Cancer Research Annual Meeting, Washington DC, 1996.

42 Nickerson T, Yang X, Pollak M, Huynh HT. Regulation of insulin-like growth factor I receptor gene expression by the pure antiestrogen ICI 182,780 (abstract) 1996.

43 Cohen P, Lamsor G, Okajima T, Rosenfeld RG. Transfection of the human insulin-like growth factor binding protein-3

gene into Balb/c fibroblasts inhibits cellular growth. *Mol Endocrinol* 1993; **7**: 380–6.

44 Oh Y, Muller HL, Lamson G, Rosenfeld RG. Insulin-like growth factor (IGF)-independent action of IGF-binding protein-3 in Hs578T human breast cancer cells. *J Biol Chem* 1993; **268**: 14964–71.

45 Sherman BM, Chapler FK, Crickard K, Wycoff D. Endocrine consequence of continuous antiestrogen therapy with tamoxifen in premenopausal women. *J Clin Invest* 1979; **64**: 398–404.

46 Sawka CA, Pritchard KI, Paterson AH *et al*. Role and mechanism of action of tamoxifen in premenopausal women with metastatic breast carcinoma. *Cancer Res* 1986; **46**: 3152–6.

47 Sakai F, Cheix F, Clavel M *et al*. Increases in steroid-binding globulins induced by tamoxifen in patients with carcinoma of the breast. *J Endocrinol* 1978; **76**: 219–26.

48 Jordan VC, Fritz NF, Tormey DC. Long-term adjuvant therapy with tamoxifen: effects on sex hormone binding globulin and antithrombin III. *Cancer Res* 1987; **47**: 4517–19.

49 Jordan VC, Fritz NF, Tormey DC. Endocrine effects of adjuvant chemotherapy and long-term tamoxifen administration on node-positive patients with breast cancer. *Cancer Res* 1987; **47**: 624–30.

50 Pollak M, Costantino J, Polychronakos C *et al*. Effect of tamoxifen on serum insulin-like growth factor I levels in stage I breast cancer patients. *J Natl Cancer Inst* 1990; **82**: 1693–7.

51 Pollak M. Effects of adjuvant tamoxifen therapy on growth hormone and insulin-like growth factor I (IGF-I) physiology. In: Salmon SE (ed.) *Adjuvant therapy of cancer VII*. Philadelphia, PA: J.B. Lippincott Company, 1993.

52 Arteaga CL, Kitten LJ, Coronado EB *et al*. Blockade of the type 1 somatomedin receptor inhibits growth of human breast cancer cells in athymic mice. *J Clin Invest* 1989; **84**: 1418–23.

53 Tannenbaum GS, Gurd W, Lapointe M, Pollak M. Tamoxifen attenuates pulsatile growth hormone secretion: mediation in part by somatostatin. *Endocrinology* 1992; **130**: 3395–401.

54 Malaab SA, Pollak M, Goodyer CG. Direct effects of tamoxifen on growth hormone secretion by pituitary cells *in vitro*. *Eur J Cancer* 1992; **28A**: 788–93.

55 Huynh HT, Tetenes E, Wallace L, Pollak M. *In vivo* inhibition of insulin-like growth factor-I gene expression by tamoxifen. *Cancer Res* 1993; **53**: 1727–30.

56 Yang XF, Beamer W, Huynh HT, Pollak M. Reduced growth of human breast cancer xenografts in hosts homozygous for the 'lit' mutation. *Cancer Res* 1996; **56**: 1509–11.

57 Huynh HT, Pollak M. IGF-1 gene expression in the uterus is stimulated by tamoxifen and inhibited by the pure antiestrogen ICI 182780. *Cancer Res* 1993; **53**: 5585–8.

58 Huynh HT, Pollak M. Uterotrophic actions of estradiol and tamoxifen are associated with inhibition of uterine IGF binding protein 3 gene expression. *Cancer Res* 1994; **54**: 3115–19.

59 Lieberman ME, Jordan VC, Fritsch M, Santos MA, Gorski J. Direct and reversible inhibition of estradiol-stimulated prolactin synthesis by antiestrogens *in vitro*. *J Biol Chem* 1983; **258**: 4734–40.

60 Manni A, Trujillo JE, Pearson OH. Predominant role of prolactin in stimulating the growth of 7,12-dimethyl-benz(a)anthracene-induced rat mammary tumor. *Cancer Res* 1977; **37**: 1216–19.

61 Folkman J. The influence of angiogenesis research on management of patients with breast cancer (review). *Breast Cancer Res Treat* 1995; **36**: 109–18.

62 Weidner N, Semple JP, Welch WR, Folkman J. Tumor angiogenesis and metastasis – correlation in invasive breast carcinoma. *N Eng J Med* 1991; **324**: 1–8.

63 Gagliardi A, Collins DC. Inhibition of angiogenesis by antiestrogens. *Cancer Res* 1993; **53**: 533–5.

64 Nakao-Hayashi J, Ito H, Kanayasu T, Morita I, Murota S. Stimulatory effects of insulin and insulin-like growth factor I on migration and tube formation by vascular endothelial cells. *Atherosclerosis* 1992; **92**: 141–9.

65 Pollak M, Ingle J, Suman V, Kugler J. Rationale for combined antiestrogen–somatostatin analogue therapy of breast cancer. In: Salmon SE (ed.) *Adjuvant therapy of cancer VIII. Proceedings of the Eighth International Conference on the Adjuvant Therapy of Cancer.* Philadelphia, PA: J.B. Lippincott, 1996.

66 Weckbecker G, Tolcsvai L, Stolz B, Pollak M, Bruns C. Somatostatin analogue octreotide enhances the antineoplastic effects of tamoxifen and ovariectomy on 7,12-dimethylbenz(a)anthracene-induced rat mammary carcinomas. *Cancer Res* 1994; **54**: 6334–7.

67 Cunningham BC, Wells JA. Rational design of receptor-specific variants of human growth hormone. *Proc Natl Acad Sci USA* 1991; **88**: 3407–11.

68 Lumpkin MD, Mulroney SE, Haramati A. Inhibition of pulsatile growth hormone (GH) secretion and somatic growth in immature rats with a synthetic GH-releasing factor antagonist. *Endocrinology* 1989; **124**: 1154–9.

69 Schally AV. Oncological applications of somatostatin analogues. *Cancer Res* 1988; **48**: 6877–85.

70 Weckbecker G, Raulf F, Stolz B, Bruns C. Somatostatin analogs for diagnosis and treatment of cancer. *Pharmacol Ther* 1993; **60**: 245–64.

71 Pollak M, Polychronakos C, Guyda H. Somatostatin analogue SMS 201-995 reduces serum IGF-I levels in patients with neoplasms potentially dependent on IGF-I. *Anticancer Res* 1989; **9**: 889–92.

72 Huynh HT, Pollak M. Enhancement of tamoxifen-induced suppression of insulin-like growth factor I gene expression and serum level by a somatostatin analogue. *Biochem Biophys Res Commun* 1994; **203**: 253–9.

73 Schally AV, Pollak M. Mechanisms of antineoplastic action of somatostatin analogues (invited review). *Proc Soc Exp Biol Med* 1998; **217**: 143–52.

74 Black LJ, Sato M, Rowley ER *et al*. Raloxifene (LY139481 HCl) prevents bone loss and reduces serum cholesterol without causing uterine hypertrophy in ovariectomized rats. *J Clin Invest* 1994; **93**: 63–9.

75 Roos W, Oeze L, Loser R, Eppenberger U. Antiestrogenic action of 3-hydroxytamofen in the human breast cancer cell line MCF-7. *J Natl Cancer Inst* 1983; **71**: 55–9.

76 Robinson SP, Mauel DA, Jordan VC. Antitumor actions of toremifene in the 7,12-dimethylbenzanthracene (DMBA)-induced rat mammary tumor model. *Eur J Cancer Clin Oncol* 1988; **24**: 1817–21.

77 Hard GC, Iatropoulos MJ, Jordan K *et al*. Major difference in the hepatocarcinogenicity and DNA adduct forming ability between toremifene and tamoxifen in female Cr1: CD(BR) rats. *Cancer Res* 1993; **53**: 4534–41.

78 Muhlemann K, Cook LS, Weiss NS. The incidence of hepatocellular carcinoma in US white women with breast cancer after the introduction of tamoxifen in 1977. *Breast Cancer Res Treat* 1994; **30**: 201–4.

79 Howell A, DeFriend D, Robertson J, Blarney R, Walton P. Response to a specific antiestrogen (ICI 182780) in tamoxifen-resistant breast cancer. *Lancet* 1995; **345**: 29–30.

80 Schipper H, Goh CR, Wang TL. Shifting the cancer paradigm: must we kill to cure? *J Clin Oncol* 1995; **13**: 801–7.

6

Novel chemotherapy agents for treatment of breast cancer

GIUSEPPE GIACCONE AND HERBERT M PINEDO

INTRODUCTION

A number of drugs have substantial antitumour activity in advanced breast cancer, including anthracyclines, vinca alkaloids, 5-fluorouracil, methotrexate, mitomycin C and alkylating agents among others. Objective response rates (complete plus partial responses) of 20–30% are achieved by several anticancer agents. However, doxorubicin is still considered to be the most active agent, with a response rate of 40% in previously untreated patients.[1]

The use of combination chemotherapy yields a higher objective response rate than single agents, often above 50%, although generally at the cost of increased toxicity. Despite the use of combination chemotherapy, the percentage of complete responses remains lower than 20%, the duration of responses is less than 1 year, and the overall median survival of metastatic breast cancer is approximately 2 years. In general, patients with metastatic breast cancer cannot be cured by chemotherapy, although very long-lasting remissions can sometimes be obtained with hormonal therapy and/or chemotherapy.

Investigation of new agents in advanced breast cancer is certainly very important, in order to develop more effective treatments, which should produce a higher complete response rate and a longer duration of responses. In prospective studies the new drugs will probably be applied in combination chemotherapy regimens, aimed at avoiding the emergence of broad cross-resistance, by combining drugs with non-overlapping mechanisms of action and side-effects. The subsequent introduction of regimens shown to be active in advanced disease into the adjuvant setting probably represents the most efficient way of reducing mortality due to breast cancer. 'High-risk' patients who have been radically operated in fact have a smaller tumour burden and the likelihood of their already having drug-resistant tumour cell clones is lower than in far advanced disease.

After about a decade in which only a few new active drugs for the treatment of cancer were discovered, in the last few years a number of anticancer agents have entered the clinic, which show striking *in-vitro* and *in-vivo* activity. Some of them have already demonstrated remarkable efficacy in the treatment of advanced breast cancer, as recently reviewed.[1–4] Given the substantial activity of combination chemotherapy in advanced breast cancer, not everyone agrees that new drugs should also be investigated in patients who have not received prior chemotherapy for their metastatic disease. However, most investigators are more confident if some hint of activity of the new drug has already been reported in advanced breast cancer. It is well known that most drugs display a significantly lower activity in previously treated patients. This is probably due to the larger tumour volume in patients with more advanced disease (who will already have undergone one or more series of treatment) and to a higher incidence of drug resistance among tumour cell clones. As combination chemotherapy does not substantially improve the median survival time of patients with metastatic breast cancer, it is considered ethical to postpone the use of conventional treatment after the investigation of a new agent. Here we shall provide an update of the most recent trials of new active agents for the treatment of breast cancer. A summary of active agents investigated in the last few years is given in Table 6.1. A number of new agents display a response rate of more than 20% in previously untreated patients, and some of them have given responses in the range of those reported for doxorubicin, or even higher.

Table 6.1 *New active agents in the treatment of advanced breast cancer investigated in the last 5 years*[*]

Paclitaxel
Docetaxel
Vinorelbine
Anthrapyrazole
Oral etoposide
Edatrexate
Ifosfamide
Menogaril

[*] At least 20% response rate in $\geq$ 2 phase II studies.

NEW MICROTUBULE-INTERACTING AGENTS

The traditional microtubule assembly inhibitors with antitumour activity are the vinca alkaloids, which are derived from the periwinkle plant. They arrest cell mitosis in metaphase by preventing tubulin polymerization to form microtubules, and by inducing depolymerization of microtubules. Several vinca alkaloids have been in clinical use for years, including vinblastine, vincristine, and vindesine, and have activity in advanced breast cancer.[1]

Vinorelbine

Small changes in the structure of the vinca alkaloid molecule are able to modify its toxicity profile substantially and even to abolish its antitumour activity completely. Vinorelbine (5′-nor-anhydrovinblastine) is a new synthetic vinca alkaloid antitumour agent, with myelotoxicity as limiting toxicity, and reduced neurotoxicity. It has been developed with changes brought into the catharanthine nucleus of the vinca alkaloid molecule, and it differs from the other vinca alkaloids in that it has an eight-membered catharantine ring instead of a nine-membered ring (Figure 6.1).[5] Its structure has been designed in order specifically to inhibit the non-assial microtubular system, avoiding neurotoxic effects while preserving antimitotic activity. This drug, like the other vinca alkaloids, has shown definite activity in breast cancer and non-small-cell lung cancer, and its apparently superior therapeutic index might play a role in further development of this drug.[6,7]

The activity of vinorelbine in breast cancer has recently been reviewed.[8] Major objective responses are seen in patients who have not previously been exposed to standard chemotherapy, whereas 20–30% response rates are obtained in patients previously treated by chemotherapy.[8]

Two phase II trials have been published so far in which vinorelbine was employed as a single agent in advanced breast cancer.[9,10] Both studies enrolled patients not previously treated by chemotherapy and employed an intravenous schedule of 30 mg/m^2/week. In a French study,[9] a total of 157 patients were enrolled, of whom 145 patients were evaluable for response. The response rate was 41% (33–49%, 95% confidence interval), with a complete response rate of 7%. Interestingly, visceral sites also responded significantly. The other study enrolled 45 patients, of whom 44 individuals were evaluable for response, and the response rate was 41% (26–56%, 95% confidence interval), with a complete response rate of 7%.[10] Both studies confirmed non-cumulative leucopenia as the dose-limiting toxicity, with 72% of patients developing grade 3–4 neutropenia in the French

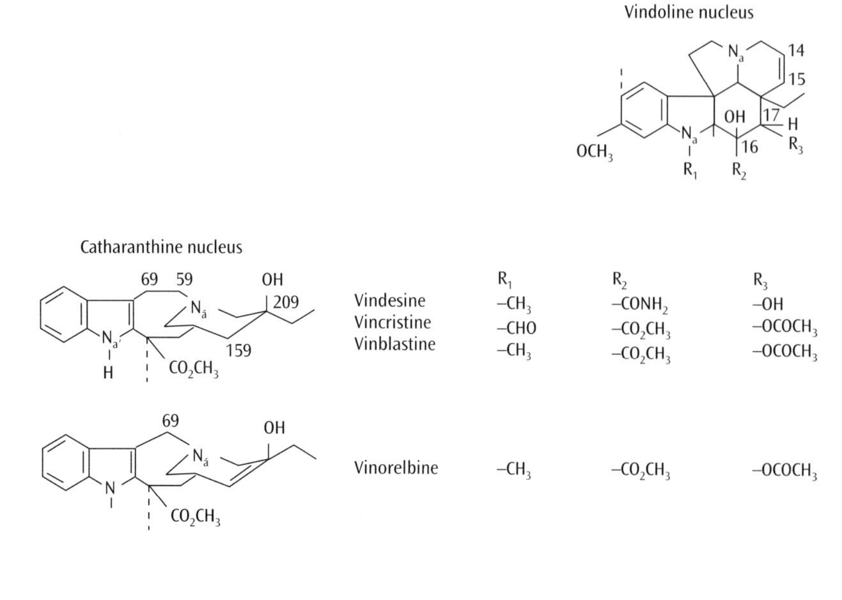

Figure 6.1 *Chemical structure of vinca alkaloids and vinorelbine.*

study.[9] Grade 2–3 peripheral neurotoxicity developed in less than 5% of patients in both studies. However, constipation (sometimes severe), and myalgia were also reported as important side-effects.[9,10] Nausea and vomiting were easily handled with standard anti-emetic medication, and infection did not constitute a problem, despite the severity of neutropenia, which was of short duration.

A phase I study has been performed with vinorelbine administered as a continuous infusion over 94 h in patients previously treated by chemotherapy for advanced breast cancer.[11] The maximum tolerated dose (MTD) was found to be 8 mg/m²/day, neutropenia being the dose-limiting toxicity, and severe mucositis being observed at higher dose levels. In this study a 36% response rate was obtained, and there was evidence of a dose–response relationship and a dose-intensity/activity correlation.

Vinorelbine can also be administered orally, although its bioavailability via this route is relatively low, probably due to a high first-pass effect. In patients who had already been treated with chemotherapy for metastatic disease, oral vinorelbine was given at 80 mg/m² or 50 mg/m² weekly in patients with a maximum of one prior regimen or who had been heavily pretreated, respectively.[12] In 98 elderly breast cancer patients who had been untreated or treated with only one regimen, a response rate of 24% was obtained, whereas in 131 heavily pretreated patients a response rate of 11% was found. Neutropenia and neurotoxicity were less frequent when the oral route was used than with the intravenous administration route, but nausea, vomiting and diarrhoea were definitely more common.

Recently, a study of vinorelbine in combination with doxorubicin has been published.[13] In that study of non-pretreated patients, doxorubicin was given at 50 mg/m² on day 1 and vinorelbine was administered at 25 mg/m² on days 1 and 8 of a 3-weekly cycle. A remarkable response rate of 74% was achieved in 89 assessable patients, of which 21% were complete responses. The response rate was equally good in visceral sites of metastases and superficial metastases. Neutropenia was the dose-limiting toxicity, as expected, with 41% of patients developing grade 3–4 toxicity. Although probably not related to the use of vinorelbine, the rate of cardiac toxicity was impressively high in this series, with 10% of the patients developing signs of cardiac toxicity, and cardiac-related deaths were recorded in three other patients. Peripheral toxicity and constipation were observed in about one-third of treated patients.

In another study of the same schedule, a response rate of 57% was obtained in previously untreated patients, with a complete response rate of 16%.[14] In this study one patient developed congestive heart failure. The remaining toxicity consisted mainly of neutropenia – three patients required hospitalization due to febrile neutropenia, and one patient died of sepsis.

New combinations of vinorelbine with other active agents are currently under investigation.[15] Interesting activities were reported preliminarily in combination with mitoxantrone.[16] In view of its relatively low toxicity as a single agent, vinorelbine might be an attractive treatment for elderly patients with breast cancer. However, one recent study of escalating doses of vinorelbine in combination with doxorubicin, fluorouracil with or without folinic acid showed unacceptable toxicity if the vinorelbine dose was raised too high,[17] with a final dose recommendation of vinorelbine 20 mg/m² for use in combination. A recent study from Germany used G-CSF to ameliorate myelotoxicity in a group of patients with advanced breast cancer using vinorelbine 40 mg/m² (30 min infusion on days 1 and 14) together with fluorouracil and leucovorin.[18]

After six courses of treatment, 5 complete and 17 partial responses were seen in 53 patients, of whom 37 individuals had received no prior chemotherapy.

TAXANES

Taxanes are mitotic inhibitors like the vinca alkaloids and colchicine, but possess a different mechanism of interaction with tubulin. Taxanes in fact stabilize the polymerized microtubules, thereby blocking the disassembly of tubulin polymers. In taxol-treated cells the equilibrium between dimers and microtubules is changed and bundles of microtubules are recovered.[19]

Two major taxanes have entered clinical trials so far, namely paclitaxel (taxol®) and docetaxel (taxotere®). Paclitaxel is isolated from the bark of the Pacific yew (*Taxus brevifolia*), which is a slow-growing tree native to the forests of the Pacific Northwest of North America. In an attempt to solve the supply problem, extensive research on synthetic analogues was initiated. As a result of this effort, a semi-synthetic compound, taxotere, has been developed, the precursor of which can be derived from the renewable source of needles of the European yew (*Taxus baccata*) (Figure 6.2). Both taxanes have remarkable activity in advanced breast cancer.

Paclitaxel

The *in-vitro* activity of taxol was first reported in 1971.[20] However, only when its unique mechanism of action was discovered, was development at the National Cancer Institute pursued in 1977. Paclitaxel development was rather slow, despite its remarkable experimental activity, due to various obstacles including limited drug supply, low solubility and severe hypersensitivity reactions observed in phase I trials. In fact, because of its limited aqueous solubility, paclitaxel for intravenous administration has to be dissolved in a vehicle consisting of Cremaphor and ethanol, which by

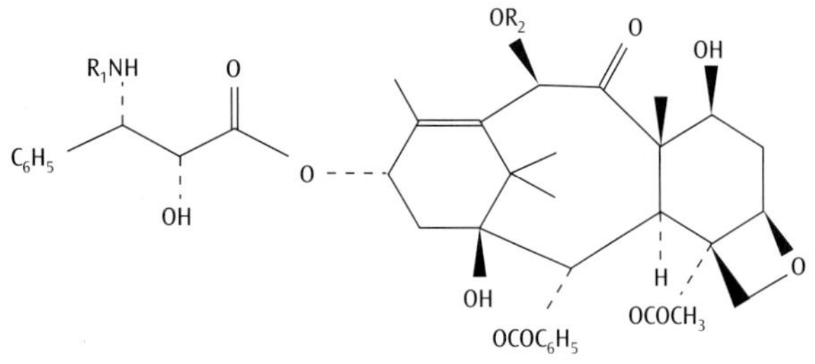

Taxotere: $R_1 = -COOC(CH_3)_3$; $R_2 = H$
Taxol: $R_1 = -COC_6H_5$; $R_2 = -COCH_3$

Figure 6.2 *Chemical structure of paclitaxel (Taxol®) and docetaxel (Taxotere®).*

itself has been associated with bronchospasm and hypotension. It remains unclear whether the hypersensitivity reactions, frequently observed after administration of paclitaxel (plus its vehicle), consisting of dyspnoea, hypotension, bronchospasm, urticaria and erythematous rash, are caused by paclitaxel itself or its vehicle, or both. However, prophylactic premedication including dexamethasone, diphenhydramine and cimetidine dramatically reduced the incidence of hypersensitivity reactions to less than 10% of patients, most of whom experienced only mild-intensity hypersensitivity reactions. This improvement in paclitaxel administration allowed the rapid development of the drug thereafter. Prolonging the duration of infusion, another manoeuver used to reduce the frequency of hypersensitivity reactions, may also be marginally successful.

The dose-limiting side-effect of paclitaxel in 8 phase I trials was neutropenia, but diarrhoea, stomatitis, myalgia/arthralgia, neuropathy and alopecia were also commonly observed. Mucositis was the dose-limiting toxicity in a phase I trial in leukaemic patients where neutropenia did not prevent further dose escalation. The recommended phase II trial dosage in patients with solid tumours is in the range 135–250 mg/m² by 24-hour infusion every 3 weeks, depending on the extent of prior treatment.

A number of phase II studies have been performed in several malignancies, and paclitaxel was shown to have significant antitumour activity in advanced ovarian cancer refractory to cisplatin,[21] non-small-cell lung cancer,[22,23] and breast cancer (see Table 6.2). Several doses and infusion times were investigated, repeated every 3 weeks. For breast cancer these results have recently been summarized and updated.[24]

The first published study on advanced breast cancer used a schedule of 250 mg/m² administered by 24-hour infusion in 25 patients who had received previous chemotherapy either adjuvant to surgery or for metastatic disease.[25] In all but two patients previous chemotherapy included doxorubicin. An objective response rate of 56% was obtained (35–76%, 95% confidence intervals). However, only 6 patients fulfilled the criteria for doxorubicin-refractoriness (i.e. no response while on doxorubicin-containing chemotherapy for metastatic disease, or progressive disease after adjuvant chemotherapy containing doxorubicin), and of these patients two responded to paclitaxel. This finding is interesting, as paclitaxel belongs to the classical MDR_1 phenotype of multi-drug resistance, which includes cross-resistance to anthracyclines, vinca alkaloids and epipodophyllotoxins.[26] As expected, neutropenia was the main toxicity. However, it was accompanied by infection in only 5% of courses. A chronic glove-and-stoking neuropathy developed in most patients at this dose level, but no hypersensitivity reactions were observed.

Another study specifically investigated the activity of paclitaxel in doxorubicin- and mitoxantrone-resistant patients with advanced breast cancer, as doxorubicin is the mainstay of first-line treatment in several institutions.[27] In this study, paclitaxel was given in a continuous infusion over a period of 96 h every 3 weeks, based on the preclinical findings of a higher efficacy of paclitaxel with

Table 6.2 *Paclitaxel in advanced breast cancer*

Reference	Dose schedule	Evaluable patients (n)	Prior CT*	Response rate (CR%)
21	250 mg/m²–24 h	25	11	56% (12%)
23	140 mg/m²–96 h	33	33	48% (0%)
28	200 mg/m²–24 hª	51	51ᶜ	33% (3%)
	250 mg/m²–24 hª	25	25ᵈ	
27	250 mg/m²–24 hª	26	0	62% (12%)
31	135/175 mg/m²–24 h	172	172	23% (2%)
26	135 vs. 175 mg/m²–3 h	111	111	27% (3%)
29	250 mg/m²–3 h	25	0	32% (4%)
	175 mg/m²–3 h	24	24	21% (0%)
30	175/225 mg/m²–3 h	50ᵇ	50	38% (14%)

CT, chemotherapy; CR, complete response.
* Chemotherapy for metastatic disease.
ª G-CSF 5 μg/kg/day from day 3 to day 10 after paclitaxel.
ᵇ Patients progressing 12 months from prior anthracycline-containing chemotherapy.
ᶜ Third or subsequent regimen, prior anthracyclines.
ᵈ Second regimen, prior anthracyclines.

prolonged drug exposures.[28] Twelve patients were entered in the phase I part of the trial, in which the dose of paclitaxel was increased from 120 to 160 mg/m^2 total dose. Dose-limiting mucositis and granulocytopenia prevented further dose escalation of paclitaxel in this schedule. A further 36 patients were then treated at the recommended dose for phase II trials of 140 mg/m^2. Patients enrolled in this phase II part of the study had received a median of two prior regimens for metastatic disease, and 73% had shown no response to prior doxorubicin- or mitoxantrone-containing regimens. Of 33 evaluable patients, 48% showed a partial response, and no difference in response to paclitaxel was observed depending on the extent of prior chemotherapy and on the previous response to doxorubicin or mitoxantrone, possibly suggesting an incomplete cross-resistance to paclitaxel. The authors of this study also suggested that prolonged infusion of paclitaxel might give superior results to shorter infusion times.

The duration of paclitaxel infusion appeared to affect the severity of myelosuppression, without significantly affecting the response rate, in a randomized study with a two-by-two factorial design in advanced ovarian cancer comparing infusion times of 3 vs. 24 h, the 24-h infusion being more myelotoxic than the 3-h infusion. However, in this study, dose appeared to have some impact on response rate (15% with the lower dose of 135 mg/m^2 and 20% with the 175 mg/m^2 dose; $P = 0.2$) and a significant impact on progression-free survival in favour of the higher dose. Neither factor (i.e. infusion duration and dose) had an impact on survival.[29]

A large randomized study investigated the effect of dose on response rate and toxicity in 471 breast cancer patients who had received prior chemotherapy for advanced disease. Paclitaxel was given in a 3-h infusion at 135 or 175 mg/m^2 every 3 weeks.[30] The overall response rate in a preliminary evaluation of 111 patients was 27%, without significant differences depending on previous chemotherapy treatment or anthracycline exposure. Grade 4 granulocytopenia was more frequent in the higher-dose than in the lower-dose regimen (25% vs. 15%).

In a series of studies performed by the same group of investigators, including patients previously untreated for metastatic breast cancer,[31] the activity of paclitaxel was higher in patients not previously exposed to chemotherapy. Patients who were receiving paclitaxel as first-line treatment for advanced disease were given a dose of 250 mg/m^2 in 24-h infusion, whereas patients who had previously been treated received 200 mg/m^2 if paclitaxel was the third or subsequent regimen, and 250 mg/m^2 if paclitaxel was the second-line chemotherapy for advanced breast cancer.[32] All groups of patients received G-CSF, 5 μg/kg/day, on days 3 to 10. The response rate in the first group was 62% of 26 evaluable patients,[31] whereas in the second group it was lower, but not significantly different depending on dose or line of treatment.[32] All of the patients who had previously been treated by chemotherapy received anthracyclines and had either acquired or *de-novo* resistance. G-CSF apparently helped to ameliorate neutropenia, which was the dose-limiting toxicity.

In one study, 3-h infusion doses of 250 mg/m^2 and 175 mg/m^2 were given to chemotherapy-untreated patients and to patients who had received two or more regimens in the past.[33] The response rate was higher in the group that had received the higher dose. However, this was also the group that had received less prior treatment. The group of patients who had received prior treatment included patients who were refractory to anthracyclines, or who had received the maximum cumulative dose of anthracyclines, or who were not candidates for treatment with anthracyclines.

In a study of 50 assessable patients,[34] no significant difference in response rate was observed between 175 mg/m^2 and 225 mg/m^2 as a 3-h infusion, whereas side-effects were increased by raising the dose. These patients had progressed within 12 months from prior chemotherapy (6 adjuvant cases, 19 neoadjuvant cases, and 26 cases of metastatic disease) including anthracyclines.

In a large study of 267 heavily pretreated patients (i.e. who had received at least two prior chemotherapy regimens for advanced disease), two doses of paclitaxel were given. The lower dose of 135 mg/m^2 was administered to patients with prior extensive radiation or mitomycin > 20 mg/m^2.[35] A response rate of 23% was obtained in 172 patients who had measurable disease, irrespective of the number of prior regimens or resistance to anthracyclines. In this study significant febrile neutropenia was observed in 45% of patients, and hospitalization was required in 49% of cases.

Although most of the studies that investigated the activity of paclitaxel in anthracyline-treated patients demonstrated significant activity, in one study in which somewhat stricter eligibility criteria were used, a response rate of only 6% was observed in 36 patients treated with high-dose paclitaxel (250–300 mg/m^2 in a 3-h infusion). Patients were in fact only admitted to this study if they progressed or relapsed while receiving anthracyclines.[36]

Several trials of paclitaxel in combination with other drugs are currently ongoing. In one of these, using paclitaxel in combination with doxorubicin,[37] the dose of doxorubicin was kept fixed at 60 mg/m^2, whereas the dose of paclitaxel was increased in steps of 25 mg/m^2 starting from 125 mg/m^2. Paclitaxel was infused over 3 h, and the sequence of administration of the two drugs was alternated in subsequent cycles in order to evaluate a possible drug–drug interaction. The maximum tolerated dose was identified at 200 mg/m^2 paclitaxel in 34 assessable patients who had never received chemotherapy. The response rate was extraordinarily high, with a complete remission rate of 41% (95% CI 24–59%) and an overall response rate of 94%. However, the median duration of response was not substantially longer than observed in other studies employing similar patient populations (8 months). In this study there was a remarkably high incidence of cardiac toxicity, with 6 patients in fact developing reversible congestive heart failure. The remaining toxicity was as expected. The authors explained the high response rate and cardiac toxicity on the basis of a possible synergistic effect of the combination on both efficacy and toxicity. There was no clear difference in toxicity depending on the sequence of drug administration. In a small study of 25 patients with advanced breast cancer, all pre-treated with chemotherapy, 14 patients achieved a major objective response with median survival of 20 months.[38] Initially these authors used paclitaxel as a single agent, but they subsequently employed it in combination with doxorubicin or vinorelbine.

Another study investigated the combination of a 72-h infusion of paclitaxel with high-dose cyclophosphamide and G-CSF. Of 54 assessable patients, 41 patients had had prior chemotherapy for metastatic disease. The MTD was reached at 160 mg/m[2] paclitaxel in combination with 2700 mg/m[2] cyclophosphamide. The treatment was well tolerated and was mainly administered on an out-patient basis. The response rate was 55%.[39]

Work presented at the Annual American Society of Clinical Oncologists Meeting in 1998 suggested an important additional use for paclitaxel as adjuvant therapy.[40] Paclitaxel was given every 3 weeks for four courses following initial adjuvant therapy with four courses of doxorubicin and cyclophosphamide (AC) combination and found to be superior to not adding treatment after the four courses of AC in a trial involving 3170 patients. At 22 months of median follow-up, the quoted P-values were 0.0077 for disease-free survival and 0.039 for overall survival, but these did not cross the prospectively defined interim analysis boundaries for statistical significance at the 0.05 level. The difference was observed early during follow-up, and was exclusively seen in the 40% of patients who had OR-negative primaries and who therefore did not receive tamoxifen following chemotherapy. One may thus argue that the early difference which was observed was primarily due to differences in the duration of the treatment regimens in the two groups and the early entry into the trial of patients with particularly aggressive neoplasia (e.g. OR-negative primaries), who would have benefited from a longer duration of treatment.

Docetaxel

The semi-synthetic taxane docetaxel has been developed in France, and has demonstrated more potent cytotoxic activity than paclitaxel in several cell lines and experimental tumours.[41,42] In phase I studies, neutropenia was the dose-limiting toxicity and a dose of 100 mg/m[2], given as a 1-h infusion every 3 weeks, has been selected for phase II studies. In contrast to paclitaxel, no apparent schedule dependence has been observed with docetaxel. Besides myelosuppression, the other side-effects of docetaxel were

rather similar to those encountered with paclitaxel (i.e. emesis, diarrhoea, alopecia, neurotoxicity and allergic reactions), while two side-effects seem to be peculiar to docetaxel, namely skin (and nail) toxicity and peripheral oedema. The skin toxicity is in the form of toxic dermatitis with erythema and desquamation, while the peripheral oedema determines weight gain and pleural effusions, and increases as the cumulative dose administered rises.

Antitumour activity of docetaxel was observed during phase I studies in heavily pretreated ovarian and breast cancer patients. Significant antitumour activity has been observed in breast cancer, ovary cancer and non-small-cell lung cancer. Two extensive reviews of preclinical and clinical findings have been published in 1995.[43,44] The results of published studies on breast cancer are summarized in Table 6.3. In the first published study of 32 evaluable patients with breast cancer,[45] a response rate of 58% was achieved in 24 patients who were given docetaxel as second-line chemotherapy, whereas 3 responses were seen in 8 patients who received docetaxel as first-line chemotherapy for metastatic disease. Although no definition of anthracycline resistance was given in this study, 10 of 22 patients who had received anthracyclines previously responded to docetaxel. In this study, grade 4 neutropenia was very frequent (81% of cases), but it was of brief duration and the infection rate was low. Other frequent side-effects included skin reactions, onycholysis and neurosensory toxicity. Of major concern was fluid retention, which was observed in 59% of patients. In this and several other phase II studies in other malignancies no premedication was given, in contrast to the studies performed with paclitaxel. Although premedication has reduced the development of hypersensitivity reactions, its influence on severe skin reactions and fluid retention is less clear,[46] while dose reduction without premedication did not reduce its incidence.[47] Premedication with dexamethasone and antihistamines can slightly reduce and delay the appearance of fluid retention.

In a Japanese study, docetaxel was given at 60 mg/m[2] every 3–4 weeks.[48] Even at this lower dose, an interesting response rate of 44% was observed, and the response rate was apparently higher in previously non-chemotherapy-treated patients than in patients who had received

Table 6.3 *Docetaxel in advanced breast cancer*

Reference	Dose schedule	Evaluable patients (n)	Prior CT*	Response rate (CR%)
39	100 mg/m[2]	32	32	58% (6%)
42	60 mg/m[2]	72	62	44% (7%)
43	100 mg/m[2]	37	0	54% (5%)
44	100 mg/m[2]	31	0	68% (16%)
45	100 mg/m[2]	35[a]	35	57% (9%)
46	100 mg/m[2]	34[a]	34	53% (0%)

CT, chemotherapy; CR, complete response;
  all schedules were given in a 1-h infusion.
* Chemotherapy for metastatic disease.
[a] Resistant to anthracyclines or anthracenedione.

chemotherapy earlier. Within chemotherapy-treated patients, the response rate among anthracycline-treated patients was 32% (out of 28 patients). However, no definition of the refractoriness to anthracyclines was given. In this study, the rate of adverse effects was lower, despite the absence of premedication, than that observed at 100 mg/m². Neutropenia of brief duration was the major toxicity, and peripheral oedema occurred in 21% of patients and was cumulative.

In patients previously untreated by chemotherapy for advanced disease, doxetaxel had a response rate of more than 50%.[49] However, with the 100 mg/m² schedule, 51% of patients required dose reductions due to neutropenic fever, and 81% of patients developed fluid retention after approximately three cycles. This side-effect was so severe that it caused interruption of treatment in 11 patients (30%). In this study, premedication with diphenhydramine hydrochloride and/or corticosteroid was given, after which hypersensitivity-like reactions were observed in the first 6 patients treated. In the study by Chevalier et al.[50] an even higher response rate was observed. However, fluid retention was seen in 26 patients (84%). This side-effect led to treatment discontinuation in 16 of 21 responding patients after a median cumulative dose of docetaxel of 574 mg/m². In this study no routine premedication was administered.

The activity of docetaxel was also investigated in patients refractory to anthracyclines or anthracenedione.[51] The inclusion criteria were that patients must have progressed on that regimen, and that they could not have had more than two different chemotherapeutic regimens in the past. Again, a high response rate of over 50% was obtained in this high-risk group of patients. Interestingly, about one-third of the patients received premedication with diphenhydramine with or without dexamethasone. The patients who received premedication including dexamethasone experienced a later onset of fluid retention than the patients who did not receive dexamethasone (503 mg/m² and 291 mg/m² of median cumulative docetaxel dose at onset, respectively).

In another study of anthracycline-resistant breast cancer patients,[52] a similar response rate was confirmed. Similarly, in this study premedication containing dexamethasone appeared to reduce the incidence of fluid retention and also of skin toxicity.

These results are certainly interesting and compare favourably with those obtained with paclitaxel, although no direct comparisons has been made yet. At present priority is being given to the development of new combination regimens and to reducing side-effects, particularly fluid retention. Docetaxel has been given in combination with doxorubicin or vinorelbine. Dieras et al. reported an overall response rate of 74% (with docetaxel plus doxorubicin) and 67% (with docetaxel plus vinorelbine).[53] Toxicities included neutropenia/infection for the first combination and neutropenia/mucositis for the latter.

NEW ANTIMETABOLITES

Edatrexate

Edatrexate (10-ethyl-10-deaza-aminopterin) is an analogue of methotrexate, an agent with activity in breast cancer. Edatrexate competes for the folate-binding site of the dihydrofolate reductase enzyme, thus inhibiting nucleotide and DNA synthesis. Edatrexate has mucositis as its dose-limiting toxicity, whereas the dose of methotrexate is mainly limited by myelosuppression, and has shown definite activity in previously untreated advanced non-small-cell lung cancer, in which the parent drug does not have much activity.[54]

Two studies have been performed in previously untreated metastatic breast cancer patients with an 80 mg/m² weekly schedule.[55,56] In the first study,[55] 34% of 32 evaluable patients showed a major response. In the second study,[56] 35 patients were enrolled, and in this study prior adjuvant chemotherapy was allowed if at least 12 months had elapsed between completion of treatment and relapse. The objective response rate was 41%. As reported in phase I trials, mucositis was dose-limiting in both studies, and it caused marked dose reductions, resulting in a mean delivered dose intensity of only 57 mg/m²/week in the second study.[56] Other side-effects included myelosuppression, skin rash, pneumonitis and elevated AST.

Further studies of edatrexate in combination with leucovorin, to improve the therapeutic index, are also warranted in breast cancer.[57]

Gemcitabine

Gemcitabine (deoxyfluorocytidine) is a fluorinated derivative of cytosine arabinoside. Among the new antimetabolites, gemcitabine has already reached advanced stages of development and demonstrated activity in a number of solid tumours.[58] In non-small-cell lung cancer it recently produced a 20% response rate in 76 evaluable untreated patients.[59] In a study of 40 assessable patients, of whom 19 patients had received one prior chemotherapy regimen for metastatic disease, gemcitabine gave a response rate of 25% (95% CI, 12.7–41.2%).[60] Gemcitabine was delivered as a 30-min intravenous infusion once a week for 3 weeks followed by a 1-week rest, every 4 weeks. The starting dose was 800 mg/m², and the mean dosage delivered was 725 mg/m². In this study, gemcitabine was confirmed to have a very mild toxicity profile, with infrequent myelosuppression and no alopecia. Flu-like syndrome was reported in 7% of patients, and was readily reversible and treatable with acetaminophen. Given the very mild toxicity of gemcitabine, its combination with other drugs is certainly warranted in breast cancer, although the response rate appears to be lower than that reported with new drugs such as the taxanes.

NEW TOPOISOMERASE II INHIBITORS

A number of new topoisomerase II inhibitors have been synthesized in recent years, and several of them have reached the stage of clinical testing. Two major classes of topoisomerase II inhibitors can be identified, namely drugs which have DNA-cleaving activity, and agents without cleaving activity.[61] Of particular interest among the topoisomerase II inhibitors with cleaving activity are the anthrapyrazoles. These drugs, although structurally related to anthracyclines, lack the paraquinone group and are thus not metabolically reduced to form radicals which are considered to be responsible for the cardiotoxicity of anthracyclines. Among the non-cleaving topoisomerase II inhibitors, merbarone and suramine are undergoing extensive phase II trials.

Losoxantrone

Three anthrapyrazoles (a new class of anticancer agents structurally related to mitoxantrone) have already undergone phase I trials. One of them, namely CI-941, (Losoxantrone) has achieved a remarkable response rate of 63% in a phase II study of 30 assessable patients with advanced breast cancer,[62] 15 of whom had received no prior chemotherapy. The drug was given at 50 mg/m^2 every 3 weeks. Leucopenia was the dose-limiting toxicity, with 75% of patients developing grade 3–4 leucopenia. Alopecia was only seen in 32% of patients, and although no cardiac symptoms were recorded, a slight fall in left ventricular ejection fraction of > 5% was observed in 12 of 15 patients in whom it was investigated.

The preliminary results of a second investigation have recently been reported for 183 patients enrolled in a multicentre study.[63] This study confirmed the positive findings of the first single-centre trial. In fact, patients with no prior exposure to chemotherapy showed a 43% response rate (32–54%, 95% confidence intervals), whereas patients who had received prior chemotherapy showed a 35% response rate. Grade 4 neutropenia developed in 74% of patients, and it was the dose-limiting toxicity. Cardiac toxicity was observed in this study, with 2 patients developing reversible chronic heart failure. Cardiac toxicity was cumulative, with an approximately 50% probability of developing chronic heart failure at a cumulative dose of more than 500 mg/m^2 (corresponding to approximately 13 cycles of treatment). Other toxicities were minor, and alopecia was seen in only 31% of patients.

Iododoxorubicin

Three phase II trials of iododoxorubicin (4′-iodo-4′-deoxydoxorubicin), a doxorubicin derivative, have been published, with conflicting results. All three studies admitted only patients with no prior chemotherapy for metastatic disease. Two of the studies reported a response rate of less than 15% on a total of 34 assessable patients,[64,65] while one study reported a response rate of 35% in 31 evaluable patients.[66] These conflicting results might reflect differences in patient selection. Neutropenia was the major side-effect in all studies, and a decline in left ventricular ejection fraction was reported in two studies.[64,66]

Merbarone

Merbarone, an anthracycline derivative, was recently investigated in 48 evaluable breast cancer patients who had not been pretreated for metastatic disease, with an oral administration schedule. A response rate of 23% was obtained, with substantial haematological toxicity.[67] This response rate was within the range of those in two older studies using the intravenous formulation of menogaril,[68,69] and clearly indicates a lower response rate to this drug compared to doxorubicin.

Prolonged oral administration of etoposide

Etoposide is not a new drug. However, a better understanding of its mechanism of action and pharmacokinetics has stimulated the investigation of new administration routes, such as prolonged oral administration.[70] Etoposide given intravenously has low activity (7% in 383 cumulative patients) in metastatic breast cancer previously treated by chemotherapy.[71] However, it is a highly schedule-dependent anticancer drug, and a 5-day schedule has been shown to be significantly more active than a 24-h infusion in small-cell lung cancer.[72] Recently, chronic administration of low oral doses of etoposide has resulted in activity in several malignancies, including small-cell lung cancer, testicular cancer and lymphomas, even in patients already pretreated with intravenous etoposide.[73] The rationale of this therapeutic approach is the more constant inhibition of the target enzyme, topoisomerase II, that can be achieved by prolonged administration of the drug.

Four studies of chronic oral administration have been published (Table 6.4).[74–77] The majority of the patients in these studies had received prior chemotherapy, and the schedule of oral etoposide administration consisted of a fixed daily dose for 2 or 3 weeks. Interestingly, three studies reported response rates in excess of 20%, which is superior to the figures reported for the intravenous route. In the study by Calvert et al.[74] patients were given 50 mg or 100 mg daily, and there was a clear indication that the response rate was higher with the higher dose (35%) than with the lower dose (10%). Moreover, in this study, patients without prior exposure to chemotherapy had a response rate of 45%, compared to 22% for patients treated with one or more than one prior regimen of chemotherapy. In three of the four studies leucopenia

Table 6.4 *Phase II trials of chronic oral etoposide in advanced breast cancer*

Reference	Dose schedule	Evaluable patients (n)	Prior CT*	Response rate (CR%)
75	50 mg/d×21 q4w	43	21	35% (2%)
76	50 mg/d×21 q4w	18	16	22% (0%)
74	50,100 mg/d×14 q4w	38	24	27% (0%)
77	50 mg/m²/d×21 q4w	21	21	10% (0%)

CT, chemotherapy; CR, complete response.
* Prior chemotherapy for metastatic disease.

was the most frequent side-effect, and although this administration schedule is relatively easy to provide on an out-patient basis and in general it is well tolerated, patients have to be monitored weekly with blood counts, as some of them may develop severe leucopenia. There is in fact wide variation in the bioavailability of oral etoposide, which may explain the large differences in observed toxicity.[74]

Teniposide has been much less extensively tested than its analogue etoposide, but like etoposide it has only minor activity in pretreated advanced breast cancer. In a recent investigation of 27 untreated patients it gave a 37% response rate,[78] with a relatively high dose administration schedule for 5 consecutive days. However, its advantages over etoposide are unclear.

The present data on use of epipodophyllotoxins in breast cancer are still inconclusive, and probably more investigations will be needed in order to determine the proper schedule and patient setting for these drugs. Etoposide is now frequently employed in high-dose chemotherapy regimens with peripheral stem-cell support.

OTHER DRUGS

Carboplatin

Cisplatin is an active agent as first-line chemotherapy in advanced breast cancer.[79] Carboplatin, a cisplatin derivative with a more favourable toxicity profile, has shown low response rates (less than 10%) in patients previously treated by chemotherapy, while in untreated patients a cumulative response rate of 31% was obtained in a total of 85 patients treated in four studies (reviewed by O'Brien *et al.*[80]). Interestingly, a study has been performed with a carboplatin dosage based on glomerular filtration rate to achieve an AUC of 7 mg/mL/min.[81] In 40 patients an overall response rate of 25% was obtained, and 9 of 27 untreated patients (33%) responded. The treatment was well tolerated, with moderate haematological toxicity. This study confirmed the inactivity of carboplatin in pretreated patients and its moderate activity in untreated patients. Carboplatin is the drug of choice for high-dose chemotherapy in breast cancer, with bone-marrow or peripheral stem-cell transplantation, due to its rather selective haematological toxicity.[82] Oxaliplatin, a newer

derivative of cisplatin, also appears to have activity in patients with metastatic breast carcinoma,[83] although it has been more extensively researched in advanced colorectal cancers. This diaminocyclohexane agent appears to belong to a distinct cytotoxic family with a separate and specific intracellular target.

Ifosfamide

Like carboplatin, ifosfamide cannot really be considered a new drug, as it entered clinical trials in the early 1970s. Its development was delayed due to its acute toxicity, but following the development of urothelial protectors (i.e. mesna), haematuria, its major acute side-effect, could be prevented, and clinical trials then resumed. Ifosfamide is clearly active in advanced breast cancer, where its activity in first-line treatment approaches a response rate of 30%. An apparently higher response rate can be obtained with higher-dose ifosfamide with mesna uroprotection.[84,85] Ifosfamide has been used in several combination chemotherapy regimens, with considerable activity. However, the advantage of using ifosfamide instead of cyclophosphamide remains unclear.[1]

NEW TARGETS

Topoisomerases are nuclear enzymes that are important for cell DNA metabolism. Several anticancer drugs in common use are topoisomerase II inhibitors (e.g. doxorubicin, etoposide, amsacrine, mitoxantrone), while only one class of anticancer drugs (i.e. the camptothecins) can specifically inhibit topoisomerase I. In the last few years it has become apparent that topoisomerase I inhibitors are potent anticancer agents.[86] Camptothecin, the first specific inhibitor of topoisomerase I to be discovered, was isolated from the stemwood of *Camptotheca acuminata*, a tree that grows in mainland China. Despite its remarkable potency *in vitro* and *in vivo*, the drug was abandoned in the early 1970s because of its unpredictable toxicity (e.g. haemorrhagic cystitis) and lack of activity. This was partly due to the suboptimal formulation of the compound, which has poor water solubility. Camptothecin analogues, which are water soluble and do not have the unpredictable side-effects of camptothecin, are now undergoing clinical trials. One of them, CPT-11, is at an advanced stage of investigation and has shown definite activity in lung and colon cancers.[86] Studies in advanced breast cancer are ongoing, and the results are eagerly awaited.[87] In a preliminary report one complete response was observed in 12 evaluable patients who had been pretreated for metastatic breast cancer.[88]

In the last decade there have been major advances in our understanding of carcinogenesis processes and the biology of cancer. Cancer is a genetic disease, and it seems likely that the cancer drugs of the future will be designed to attack the abnormalities of cancer genes themselves and/or the protein product which they encode. Some drugs of this type have already been identified and are now undergoing clinical experimentation.

Growth signalling can be inhibited by antagonists which prevent ligand binding. Suramin is one such example, and it inhibits binding of PDGF, TGFβ, EGF and FGF to their receptors. Objective responses have been seen in refractory patients with prostate cancer treated with suramin,[89] and given the interesting *in-vitro* results obtained in breast cancer cells,[90] evaluation in breast cancer patients is now ongoing.[91]

Several inhibitors of tyrosine kinases with anti-proliferative activity have been discovered, and many growth factor receptors and some oncogene products are protein tyrosine kinases. The results of clinical studies of these compounds are awaited. Bryostatins and staurosporins modulate protein kinase C, which is involved in the signal transduction pathway that mediates the effects of growth factors. Phase I trials of bryostatin A have been completed, and further clinical investigations are expected to follow shortly. Bryostatins are protein kinase C agonists which promote nuclear membrane translocation of the enzyme and its degradation following initial activation.

At the 1998 American Society of Clinical Oncologists Meeting two important studies were presented showing the results of a humanized antibody against HER-2 oncogene (Herceptin™) (humanized anti-Her2 antibody)[92] in patients with breast cancer. In the first study,[93] 222 patients with advanced breast cancer, whose tumours over-expressed this oncogene as indicated by immunohistochemistry, were given Herceptin™ 4 mg/kg loading dose and 2 mg/kg weekly thereafter. All of the patients had received prior chemotherapy. Complete responses were noted in 6 patients and partial responses in 25 patients, with an overall response rate of 15%. A reduction in ventricular ejection fraction was recorded in 9 patients, and it was symptomatic in 6 patients, in all cases in patients with prior exposure to anthracyclines. The second study randomized 469 advanced breast cancer patients with tumours over-expressing HER-2 to receive chemotherapy (doxorubicin-cyclophosphamide or paclitaxel) with or without Herceptin™. Both the response rate (36.2% vs. 62%) and the time to progression (5.5 vs. 8.6 months) significantly favoured the combination of chemotherapy with Herceptin™. Furthermore, in this study additional myocardial dysfunction was observed in patients who received Herceptin™.

There is increasing evidence that tumour growth is angiogenesis dependent,[94] including that in breast cancer.[95] New blood vessels enable tumour cells to grow, but also to metastasize. Inhibitors of angiogenesis have now been identified and have recently entered clinical trials.

REFERENCES

1 Clavel M, Catimel G. Breast cancer: chemotherapy in the treatment of advanced disease. *Eur J Cancer* 1993; **29A**: 598–604.

2 Hortobagyi GN. Overview of new treatments for breast cancer. *Breast Cancer Res Treat* 1992; **21**: 3–13.

3 Vanderberg TA. New developments in chemotherapy for metastatic breast cancer. *Anti-cancer Drugs* 1994; **5**: 251–9.

4 Abrams JS, Moore TD, Friedman M. New chemotherapeutic agent for breast cancer. *Cancer* 1994; **74 (Supplement 3)**: 1164–76.

5 Manganey P, Andriamialisoa RZ, Lallehand JY *et al.* 5'-noranhydrovinblastine. Prototype of a new class of vinblastine derivatives. *Tetrahedron* 1979; **35**: 2175–9.

6 Cvictovic E, Izzo J. The current and future plan of vinorelbine in cancer therapy. *Drugs* 1992; **44 (Supplement 4)**: 36–45.

7 Pinedo HM, van Groeningen CJ. Vinorelbine: a horse of a different colour? *J Clin Oncol* 1994; **12**: 1745–7.

8 Hortobagyi GN. Future directions for vinorelbine (navelbine). *Semin Oncol* 1995; **2 (Supplement 5)**: 80–7.

9 Fumoleau P, Delgado FM, Delazier T *et al.* Phase II trial of weekly intravenous vinorelbine in first-line advanced breast cancer chemotherapy. *J Clin Oncol* 1993; **11**: 1245–52.

10 Romero A, Rabinovich MG, Vallejo CT *et al.* Vinorelbine as first-line chemotherapy for metastatic breast carcinoma. *J Clin Oncol* 1994; **12**: 336–41.

11 Toussaint C, Izzo J, Spielmann M *et al.* Phase I/II trial of continuous infusion vinorelbine for advanced breast cancer. *J Clin Oncol* 1994; **12**: 2102–12.

12 Winer EP, Chu L, Spicer DV. Oral vinorelbine (navelbine) in the treatment of advanced breast cancer. *Semin Oncol* 1995; **22 (Supplement 5)**: 72–9.

13 Spielmann M, Dorval T, Turpin F *et al.* Phase II trial of vinorelbine/doxorubicin as first-line therapy of advanced breast cancer. *J Clin Oncol* 1994; **12**: 1764–70.

14 Hochster HS. Combined doxorubicin/vinorelbine (navelbine) therapy in the treatment of advanced breast cancer. *Semin Oncol* 1995; **22 (Supplement 5)**: 55–60.

15 Clemons M, Leahy M, Valle V *et al.* Review of trials of chemotherapy for advanced breast cancer: studies excluding taxanes. *Eur J Cancer* 1997; **33**: 2171–82.

16 Vogel CL. Combination chemotherapy with vinorelbine (navelbine) and mitoxantrone for metastatic breast cancer: a review. *Semin Oncol* 1995; **22 (Supplement 5)**: 61–5.

17 Goss PE, Fine S, Gelnon K *et al.* Phase I studies of fluorouracil, doxorubicin and vinorelbine without (FAN) and with (SUPERFAN) folinic acid to patients with advanced breast cancer. *Cancer Chemother Pharmacol* 1997; **41**: 53–60.

18 Kornek GV, Haider K, Kwasny W *et al.* Effective treatment of advanced breast cancer with vinorelbine, 5-fluorouracil and leucovorin plus human granulocyte colony-stimulating factor. *Br J Cancer* 1998; **78**: 673–8.

19 Roberts JR, Rowinsky EK, Donehower RC *et al.* Demonstration of the cell cycle positions for taxol-induced 'asters' and 'bundles' by sequential measurements of tubulin immunofluorescence, DNA content and autoradiographic labeling of taxol-sensitive and resistant cells. *J Histochem Cytochem* 1989; **37**: 1659–65.

20 Wani MC, Taylor HL, Wall ME *et al.* Plant antitumour agents. VI. The isolation and structure of taxol, a novel antileukemic and antitumour agent from *Taxus brevifolia. J Am Chem Soc* 1971; **93**: 2325–7.

21 McGuire WP, Rowinsky EK, Rosenshein MB *et al.* Taxol: a unique antineoplastic agent with significant activity in advanced ovarian epithelial neoplasms. *Ann Intern Med* 1989; **111**: 273–9.

22 Chang AY, Kim K, Glik J *et al.* Phase II study of taxol, merbarone and piroxantrone in stage IV non-small-cell lung cancer: the Eastern Cooperative Oncology Group experience. *J Natl Cancer Inst* 1993; **85**: 388.

23 Murphy WK, Fossella FV, Winn RJ *et al.* Phase II study of taxol in patients with untreated advanced non-small-cell lung cancer. *J Natl Cancer Inst* 1993; **85**: 384.

24 Clemons M, Leahy M, Valle J *et al.* Review of recent trials of chemotherapy for advanced breast cancer: the taxanes. *Eur J Cancer* 1997; **33**: 2183–93.

25 Holmes FA, Walter RS, Theriault RL *et al.* Phase II trial of taxol: an active drug in the treatment of metastatic breast cancer. *J Natl Cancer Inst* 1991; **83**: 1797–805.

26 van Kalken CK, Pinedo HM, Giaccone G. Multidrug resistance from the clinical point of view. *Eur J Cancer* 1991; **27**: 1481–6.

27 Wilson WH, Berg SL, Bryant G *et al.* Paclitaxel in doxorubicin-refractory or mitoxantrone-refractory breast cancer: a phase I/II trial of a 96-hour infusion. *J Clin Oncol* 1994; **12**: 1621–9.

28 Lopes NM, Adams EG, Pitts TW *et al.* Cell kill kinetics and cell cycle effects of taxol on human and hamster ovarian cell lines. *Cancer Chemother Pharmacol* 1993; **32**: 235–42.

29 Eisenhauer E, ten Bokkel Huinink W, Swenerton K *et al.* European-Canadian randomized trial of paclitaxel in relapsed ovarian cancer: high-dose vs. low-dose and long vs. short infusion. *J Clin Oncol* 1994; **12**: 2654–66.

30 Nabholtz JM, Gelmon K, Bontenbal M *et al.* Randomized trial of two doses of taxol in metastatic breast cancer: an interim analysis. *Proc Am Soc Clin Oncol* 1993; **12**: 60.

31 Reichman BS, Seidman AD, Crown JPA *et al.* Paclitaxel and recombinant human granulocyte colony-stimulating factor as initial chemotherapy for metastatic breast cancer. *J Clin Oncol* 1993; **11**: 1943–51.

32 Seidman AD, Reichman BS, Crown JPA *et al.* Paclitaxel as second and subsequent therapy for metastatic breast cancer: activity independent of prior anthracycline response. *J Clin Oncol* 1995; **13**: 1152–9.

33 Seidman AD, Tiersten A, Hudis C *et al.* Phase II trial of paclitaxel by 3-hour infusion as initial and salvage chemotherapy for metastatic breast cancer. *J Clin Oncol* 1995; **13**: 2575–81.

34 Gianni L, Munzone E, Capri G *et al.* Paclitaxel in metastatic breast cancer: a trial of two doses by a 3-hour infusion in patients with disease recurrence after prior therapy with anthracyclines. *J Natl Cancer Inst* 1995; **87**: 1169–75.

35 Abrams JS, Vena DA, Baltz J *et al.* Paclitaxel activity in heavily pretreated breast cancer: a National Cancer Institute treatment referral cancer trial. *J Clin Oncol* 1995; **13**: 2056–65.

36 Vermorken JB, ten Bokkel Huinink WW, Mandjes IAM *et al.* High-dose paclitaxel with granulocyte colony-stimulating factor in patients with advanced breast cancer refractory to anthracycline therapy: a European Cancer Center trial. *Semin Oncol* 1995; **22 (Supplement 8)**: 16–22.

37 Gianni L, Munzone E, Capri G *et al.* Paclitaxel by 3-hour infusion in combination with bolus doxorubicin in women with untreated metastatic breast cancer: high antitumour efficacy and cardiac effects in a dose-finding and sequence-finding study. *J Clin Oncol* 1995; **13**: 2688–99.

38 Hortobagys GN, Holmes FA, Ibrahim N, Champlin R, Buzdar AU. The University of Texas M.D. Anderson Cancer Center experience with paclitaxel in breast cancer. *Semin Oncol* 1997; **24 (Supplement)**: S30–3.

39 Tolcher AW, Cowan KH, Noone MH *et al.* Phase I study of paclitaxel in combination with cyclophosphamide and granulocyte colony-stimulating factor in metastatic breast cancer patients. *J Clin Oncol* 1996; **14**: 95–102.

40 Goldhirsch A, Coates AS, Castiglione-Gertsch M, Gelber RD. New treatments for breast cancer: breakthroughs for patient care or just steps in the right direction? *Ann Oncol* 1998; **19**: 973–6.

41 Riou JF, Naudin A, Lavelle F. Effects of taxotere on murine and human cell lines. *Biochem Biophys Res Commun* 1992; **187**: 164–170.

42 Bissery M-C, Guenard D, Gueritte-Voegelein F, Lavelle F. Experimental antitumour activity of taxotere (RP 56976, NSC 628503), a taxol analogue. *Cancer Res* 1989; **51**: 4845–52.

43 Pronk LC, Stoter G, Verweij J. Docetaxel (Taxotere): single agent activity, development of combination treatment and reducing side-effects. *Cancer Treat Rev* 1995; **21**: 463–78.

44 Cortes JE, Pazdur R. Docetaxel. *J Clin Oncol* 1995; **13**: 2643–55.

45 ten Bokkel Huinink WW, Prove AM, Piccart M *et al.* A phase II trial with docetaxel (taxotere) in second-line treatment with chemotherapy for advanced breast cancer. *Ann Oncol* 1994; **5**: 527–32.

46 Schrijver D, Wanders J, Dirix L *et al.* Coping with toxicities of docetaxel (taxotere). *Ann Oncol* 1993; **4**: 610–11.

47 Dieras V, Fumoleau P, Chevalier B *et al*. Second EORTC Clinical Screening Group phase II trial of taxotere (docetaxel) as first-line chemotherapy in advanced breast cancer. *Proc Am Soc Clin Oncol* 1994; **13**: 78.

48 Adachi I, Watanabe T, Takashima S *et al*. A late phase II study of RP56976 (docetaxel) in patients with advanced or recurrent breast cancer. *Br J Cancer* 1996; **73**: 210–16.

49 Hudis CA, Seidman AD, Crown JPA *et al*. Phase II study and pharmacologic study of docetaxel as initial chemotherapy for metastatic breast cancer. *J Clin Oncol* 1996; **14**: 58–65.

50 Chevalier B, Fumoleau P, Kerbrat P *et al*. Docetaxel is a major cytotoxic drug for the treatment of advanced breast cancer: a phase II trial of the clinical screening cooperative group of the European Organization for Research and Treatment of Cancer. *J Clin Oncol* 1995; **13**: 314–22.

51 Ravdin PM, Burris HA III, Cook G *et al*. Phase II trial of docetaxel in advanced anthracycline-resistant or anthracenedione-resistant breast cancer. *J Clin Oncol* 1995; **13**: 2879–85.

52 Valero V, Holmes FA, Walters RS *et al*. Phase II trial of docetaxel: a new, highly effective antineoplastic agent in the management of patients with anthracycline-resistant metastatic breast cancer. *J Clin Oncol* 1995; **13**: 2886–94.

53 Dieras V, Fumoleau P, Kalla S, Misset JL, Azli N, Pouillart P. Docetaxel in combination with doxosubicin or vinorelbine. *Eur J Cancer* 1997; **10 (Supplement 7)**: S20–2.

54 Schum KY, Kris MG, Gralla RJ *et al*. Phase II study of 10-ethyl-10-deaza-aminopterin in patients with stage III and IV non-small-cell lung cancer. *J Clin Oncol* 1988; **6**: 446–50.

55 Schornagel JH, van der Vegt S, de Graeff A *et al*. Phase II study of edatrexate in chemotherapy-naive patients with metastatic breast cancer. *Ann Oncol* 1992; **3**: 549–52

56 Vandenberg TA, Pritchard KI, Eisenhauer EA *et al*. Phase II study of weekly edatrexate as first-line chemotherapy for metastatic breast cancer: a National Cancer Institute of Canada Clinical Trials Group study. *J Clin Oncol* 1993; **11**: 1241–4.

57 Lee JS, Libshitz HI, Fossella FV *et al*. Improved therapeutic index by leucovorin of edatrexate, cyclophosphamide and cisplatin regimen for non-small-cell lung cancer. *J Natl Cancer Inst* 1992; **84**: 1039–40.

58 Kaye SB. Gemcitabine: current status of phase I and II trials. *J Clin Oncol* 1994; **12**: 1527–31.

59 Abratt RP, Bezwoda WR, Falkson G *et al*. Efficacy and safety profile of gemcitabine in non-small-cell lung cancer: a phase II study. *J Clin Oncol* 1994; **12**: 1535–40.

60 Carmichael J, Possinger K, Philip P *et al*. Advanced breast cancer: a phase II trial with gemcitabine. *J Clin Oncol* 1995; **13**: 2731–6.

61 D'Incalci M, Capranico G, Giaccone G, Zunino F, Garattini S. DNA topoisomerase inhibitors. In: Pinedo, HM, Chabner, BA, Longo, DL (eds) *The cancer chemotherapy and biological response modifiers annual*. Elsevier Science Publishers, 1993; 61–85.

62 Talbot DC, Smith IE, Mansi JL *et al*. Anthrapyrazole CI-941: a highly active new agent in the treatment of advanced breast cancer. *J Clin Oncol* 1991; **9**: 2141–7.

63 Calvert H, Smith I, Jones A *et al*. Phase II study of losoxantrone in previously treated and untreated patients with advanced breast cancer. *Proc Am Soc Clin Oncol* 1994; **13**: 71.

64 Twelves CJ, Dobbs NA, Lawrence MA *et al*. Iododoxorubicin in advanced breast cancer: a phase II evaluation of clinical activity, pharmacology and quality of life. *Br J Cancer* 1994; **69**: 726–31.

65 Sessa C, Calabresi F, Cavalli F *et al*. Phase II studies of 4'-iodo-4'-deoxydoxorubicin in advanced non-small-cell lung, colon and breast cancers. *Ann Oncol* 1991; **2**: 727–31.

66 Gianni L, Capri G, Greco M *et al*. Activity and toxicity of 4'-iodo-4'-deoxydoxorubicin in patients with advanced breast cancer. *Ann Oncol* 1991; **2**: 719–25.

67 Stewart DJ, Eisenhauer EA, Skillings J *et al*. Phase II study of oral menogaril as first-line chemotherapy for advanced breast cancer: a National Cancer Institute of Canada Clinical Trials Group study. *Ann Oncol* 1992; **3**: 201–4.

68 Eisenhauer EA, Pritchard KI, Perrault DJ *et al*. Activity of intravenous menogaril in patients with previously untreated metastatic breast cancer. A National Cancer Institute of Canada Clinical Trials Group study. *Invest New Drugs* 1990; **8**: 283–7.

69 Sessa C, Gundersen S, ten Bokkel Huinink W *et al*. Phase II study of intravenous menogaril in patients with advanced breast cancer. *J Natl Cancer Inst* 1988; **80**: 1066–9.

70 Hinsworth JD, Greco FA. Etoposide: twenty years later. *Ann Oncol* 1995; **6**: 325–41.

71 Sledge GW Jr. Etoposide in the management of metastatic breast cancer. *Cancer* 1991; **67**: 266–70.

72 Slevin ML, Clarke PI, Joel SP *et al*. A randomized trial to evaluate the effect of schedule on the activity of etoposide in small-cell lung cancer. *J Clin Oncol* 1989; **7**: 1333–40.

73 Greco FA, Johnson DH, Hainsworth JD. Chronic daily administration of oral etoposide. *Semin Oncol* 1990; **17 (Supplement 2)**: 71–4.

74 Calvert H, Lind MJ, Millward MM *et al*. Long-term oral etoposide in metastatic breast cancer: clinical and pharmacokinetic results. *Cancer Treat Rev* 1993; **19 (Supplement C)**: 27–33.

75 Martin M, Lluch A, Casado A *et al*. Clinical activity of chronic oral etoposide in previously treated metastatic breast cancer. *J Clin Oncol* 1994; **12**: 986–91,

76 Palombo H, Estape J, Vinolas N *et al*. Chronic oral etoposide in advanced breast cancer. *Cancer Chemother Pharmacol* 1994; **33**: 527–9.

77 Bontenbal M, Planting AS, Verweij J *et al*. Second-line chemotherapy with long-term low-dose oral etoposide in patients with advanced breast cancer. *Breast Cancer Res Treat* 1995; **34**: 185–9.

78 Nielsen D, Boas J, Engelholm SA *et al*. Teniposide in advanced breast cancer. A phase II trial in patients with no prior chemotherapy. *Ann Oncol* 1992; **3**: 377–8.

79 Smith IE, Talbot DC. Cisplatin and its analogues in the treatment of advanced breast cancer. *Br J Cancer* 1992; **65**: 787–93.

80 O'Brien MER, Talbot DC, Smith IE. Carboplatin in the treatment of advanced breast cancer: a phase II study using a pharmacokinetically guided dose schedule. *J Clin Oncol* 1993; **11**: 2112–17.

81 Calvert AH, Newell DR, Gumbrell LA *et al*. Carboplatin dosage: prospective evaluation of a simple formula based on renal function. *J Clin Oncol* 1989; **7**: 1748–56.

82 Antman K, Ayash L, Elias A *et al*. A phase II study of high-dose cyclophosphamide, thiotepa, and carboplatin with autologous bone-marrow support in women with measurable advanced breast cancer responding to standard-dose therapy. *J Clin Oncol* 1992; **10**: 102–10.

83 Raymond E, Chaney SG, Taamma A, Cvitkovic E. Oxaliplatin: a review of preclinical and clinical studies. *Ann Oncol* 1998; **9/10**: 1053–71.

84 Hortobagyi GN. Activity of ifosfamide in breast cancer. *Semin Oncol* 1992; **19 (Supplement 12)**: 36–42.

85 Gad-El-Mawla N. Use of ifosfamide in the management of breast cancer. *Ann Oncol* 1992; **3 (Supplement 3)**: S21–S23.

86 Burris HA, Rothenberg ML, Kuhn JG, Von-Hoff DD. Clinical trials with the topoisomerase I inhibitors. *Semin Oncol* 1992; **19**: 663–9.

87 O'Reilly S, Kennedy MJ, Rowinsky EK, Donehower RC. Vinorelbine and the topoisomerase I inhibitors: current and potential roles in breast cancer chemotherapy. *Breast Cancer Res Treat* 1995; **33**: 1–17.

88 Bonneterre J, Pion JM, Adenis A *et al*. A phase II study of a new camptothecin analogue CPT-11 in previously treated advanced breast cancer patients. *Proc Am Soc Clin Oncol* 1993; **12**: 94.

89 Stein CA, LaRocca RV, Thomas R *et al*. Suramin: an active anticancer drug with a unique mechanism of action. *J Clin Oncol* 1989; **7**: 499–508.

90 Vignon F, Prebois C, Rochefort H. Inhibition of breast cancer growth by suramin. *J Natl Cancer Inst* 1992; **84**: 38–42.

91 Tkaczuk K, Aisner J, Abrams J *et al*. Suramin pharmacokinetic parameters in women with metastatic breast carcinoma. *Proc Am Soc Clin Oncol* 1994; **13**: 93.

92 Slamon D, Leyland-Jones B, Shak S *et al*. Addition of Herceptin™ (humanized anti-Her2 antibody) for Her2 overexpressing metastatic breast cancer markedly increases anticancer activity: a randomized multinational controlled phase III trial. *Proc Am Soc Clin Oncol* 1998; **17**: 98.

93 Cobleigh MA, Vogel CL, Tripathy D *et al*. Efficacy and safety of Herceptin™ (humanized anti-Her2 antibody) as a single agent in 222 women with Her2 overexpression who relapsed following chemotherapy for metastatic breast cancer. *Proc Am Soc Clin Oncol* 1998; **17**: 97.

94 Folkman J. What is the evidence that tumours are angiogenesis dependent? *J Natl Cancer Inst* 1990; **82**: 4–6.

95 Gasparini G, Harris AL. Clinical importance of the determination of tumour angiogenesis in breast carcinoma: much more than a new prognostic tool. *J Clin Oncol* 1995; **13**: 765–82.

Early detection and prevention

7

Identifying and counselling women at high risk of developing breast cancer

KATHRYN J THIRLAWAY, ANTHONY HOWELL AND D GARETH R EVANS

IDENTIFYING THOSE AT HIGH RISK

Human cancers may follow exposure to particular environmental factors, but it is well established that, at the cellular level, cancer is genetic in origin. Genetic changes associated with initiation and progression are usually acquired 'somatic' events. Occasionally one of these genetic changes may be inherited, resulting in a predisposition to cancer. Almost all types of cancer have been reported in familial clusters, but a site that is commonly involved is the breast.[1] Complex segregation analysis has been applied to breast cancer in order to investigate genetic and environmental models of disease transmission in families, and to determine the most likely explanation for familial aggregation, in view of the fact that breast cancer is probably aetiologically heterogeneous,[2] in that there is more than one gene conferring breast cancer susceptibility in a population. Newman *et al.* found that family analysis of an unselected population-based series of breast cancer patients demonstrated an autosomal-dominant model with an incomplete but highly penetrant susceptibility allele as the explanation for transmission of breast cancer in 4% of all breast cancer cases.[3] They reported that the lifetime risk may be as high as 40–50% in first-degree relatives of those with the gene (equivalent to a 50% risk of inheriting the breast cancer gene). Other workers have similarly found a model of a dominant susceptibility gene to be the best explanation of the pattern of breast cancer in families.[1] It is often difficult to establish that an aggregation of breast cancer in a family is truly hereditary, as the disease is so common. However, early

age at diagnosis, bilaterality and multiple affected family members would be more likely to suggest the presence of a dominant gene.

Inherited cases account for only a small proportion of breast cancer. However, those at risk in families may benefit from screening and early diagnosis, particularly as they are at risk of developing the disease at a much younger age. Studies of families with breast cancer have provided the opportunity to localize and clone two breast cancer genes (BRCA1) on chromosome 17,[4,5] and (BRCA2) on chromosome 13.[6] While genetic testing has only been reported in a few large families until now,[7–10] the onset of mutation studies in BRCA1 and BRCA2 means that many more individuals at risk of breast cancer will have access to predictive diagnosis.

PSYCHOLOGICAL ISSUES ASSOCIATED WITH BEING 'AT RISK'

A family history of breast cancer has been reported to correlate with high levels of psychological distress.[11,12] Population screening for BRCA1/BRCA2 mutations may soon be practicable, and it has been predicted that as many as 1 in 200 women may carry a mutation that confers at least an 85% lifetime risk of developing breast cancer.[7] The psychological implications of genetic testing for breast cancer need to be established, but it might be expected that – similarly to those currently aware of the implications of their family history of breast cancer – informed carriers of BRCA1/BRCA2 mutations will be susceptible to psychological distress.

The availability of a genetic test for breast cancer will involve a three-stage process for many women with a family history of breast cancer, each stage having its own associated psychological implications.

1 The availability of a genetic test for breast cancer will result in women 'at risk' having to decide whether or not to undergo a genetic test. Ensuring informed consent and establishing guidelines for providing information about the benefits and costs of testing are crucial issues which arise.

2 The psychological support needed by women who undergo genetic testing is another unresolved issue. There is some consensus that women who are told they are carriers will need psychological support. It is also possible that being told one is not a carrier or deciding against screening could have adverse psychological consequences.

3 The behavioural consequences of testing, in terms of surveillance or prevention tactics, are unknown. How can we help each individual decide on the management strategy that suits her own physical and psychological condition best?

It is imperative that research is carried out in all of these three areas. However, it will be necessary to provide counselling and support for 'at-risk' women while research is establishing the specific needs of this group. There is a growing body of research from women who have a family history of breast cancer. To some degree, preparation for the advent of screening can be based on information from other areas. It is possible to draw conclusions from the psychological impact of genetic testing for other adult-onset Mendelian diseases, such as Huntington's disease, and from traditional genetic counselling methods developed for such conditions. Finally, there are some large families with many cases of breast cancer and sometimes ovarian cancer who are suitable for linkage analysis for BRCA1/BRCA2 mutations. A few of these families have already been offered the opportunity to learn their genetic status. There is some limited data on psychological distress and behavioural change for these linkage-analysis families. This chapter will discuss the psychological implications and counselling needs of women who are considering genetic testing, at each of the three stages we have defined above, drawing on the literature available from the specified related areas. We shall also consider future research aims.

THE DECISION TO TAKE THE TEST

How many women will request the test? Around 75% of first-degree relatives of women with ovarian cancer said they would take the BRCA1 genetic test if it became available, and a further 20% said they would probably want to be tested.[13] These high rates of interest in testing may grossly overestimate actual uptake. Despite initially similar rates (66%) of interest in testing for Huntington's disease, only 15% of relatives have actually come forward for testing.[13] High uptake of testing should be anticipated, as there is potential for surveillance and prevention tactics to improve morbidity and mortality for breast cancer, whereas the outlook for those who carry the gene for Huntington's disease is near certain premature death. However, Richards et al. suggested that some women with a family history of breast cancer may assume that when a genetic test is developed, a certain cure or prevention strategy will also be available.[14] The realization, with good pre-test information, that the only certain prevention strategy currently available is prophylactic surgery may bias women against testing. Nevertheless, initial uptake of testing in five BRCA1-linked families containing 71 at-risk individuals was found to be 65% for women and 40% for men (Evans, personal communication).

Ethical issues

AGE OF TESTING

Various ethical dilemmas arise from genetic screening for breast cancer. First, at what age should testing be offered? Biesecker et al. have provided information on carrier status to 35 members of a family suitable for linkage analysis;[7] their policy was not to offer the test to children. Similarly, Lynch et al. did not offer testing to minors, despite some requests for testing of children by their parents.[9] This is consistent with pre-symptomatic protocols for Huntington's disease.[7] Breast cancer occurring under the age of 18 years is extremely rare, and this would appear to be a logical stance. However, some consensus among all of these centres participating in genetic testing must be reached.

CONFIDENTIALITY

The issues of confidentiality are complex. Clearly information and counselling should be given individually. Within any family, a high-risk test for one family member has implications for the others. For example, a woman at 25% risk who has a high-risk result and goes on to have prophylactic mastectomy provides her mother, at an original risk of 50%, with information concerning her risk which may or may not be asked for. If an individual does not wish to tell her family that she carries a gene predisposing her to breast cancer, what can be done about any female relatives who may also be at risk? Again there will need to be some consensus about these issues among test centres. The wider issue of confidentiality and health insurance is less problematic in the UK than in the USA. In the UK, women can receive prophylactic surgery on the National Health Service. However, for those wishing to have private health insurance, the genetic test will undoubtedly affect their premiums.

Perception of risk

A number of researchers have reported that perception of risk, not actual risk, is related to intended uptake of genetic screening in breast and ovarian cancer,[13] and also in colon cancer[15] and other inherited disorders.[16] Furthermore, perception of risk in female, but not male, genetic counsellees has been found to be influenced more by psychosocial factors than by statistical considerations.[16] Perception of risk correlates with actual risk in some women attending a breast cancer family history clinic.[17] However, over half of the women attending the clinic still misinterpreted their personal risk. Careful counselling, with regard to their own actual risk only led to moderate improvements in accurate estimates of personal risk.[18]

Despite being told that the BRCA1 gene was responsible for cancer development in only a few families with many members affected with breast or ovarian cancer, 59% of the first-degree relatives interviewed by Lerman et al. believed that they were likely to have inherited this gene.[13] Conversely, Evans et al. found that women who were referred to a breast cancer family history clinic were more likely to underestimate rather than overestimate their own personal risk.

The research on risk perception in women with a family history of breast cancer is not consistent. Lerman et al. have postulated that the higher women perceive their risk to be, the more likely they are to want the test.[17] How closely perception of risk correlates with actual risk is unclear, and therefore how many women who have a realistic chance of carrying a gene mutation will opt for testing is difficult to assess. Ideally, the pre-test counselling and information will ensure that women have an accurate understanding of their likelihood of carrying the gene, on which to base their decision about testing.

Counselling and information needs

The aim of pre-test counselling must be to ensure that women make a choice based on accurate information. Epidemiological data are essential for providing genetic counsellors with accurate figures for selective risk.[19] Lerman et al. reported that women with a family history of ovarian cancer would be interested in BRCA1 mutation screening primarily to learn about their children's risks.[13] The majority were also interested in order to increase their use of screening and improve their personal health care. Pre-test counselling will need to expand on traditional genetic counselling to include information on surveillance and preventative strategies, areas that are not applicable to genetic counselling for Huntington's disease.

This chapter will concentrate on genetic testing for breast cancer in women. Men who carry BRCA1 mutations are not at increased risk of developing breast cancer.

However, there is some evidence of a 3- to 4-fold increased risk of prostate and colon cancer in male carriers.[20] While male carriers do not have such serious issues of personal vulnerability and management to consider, the hereditary nature of the abnormal gene they carry and its consequences for their daughters is an issue which some men may feel that they wish to discuss.

GENETIC INFORMATION

Potential test takers will need some understanding of genetic inheritance in order to make an *informed* decision about testing. Biesecker et al. reported that many members of a family who were suitable for linkage analysis and had been recently informed of their carrier status appreciated an explanation of how BRCA1 mutations were inherited,[7] since prior to this it appeared to the family members that the cases were frequent but random. Richards et al. have suggested nine concepts that should be introduced to a person considering genetic testing.[14] These include fundamental information such as the paired nature of chromosomes, as well as specific issues about BRCA1 mutations. Even the most basic explanation of genetic theory will take considerable time and effort to explain, and use of videotaped material may prove beneficial in helping women towards a more realistic personal risk assessment.[21,22]

Those contemplating genetic testing will also need to be made aware of the incomplete penetrance of the BRCA1/BRCA2 mutations. It is estimated that approximately 15% of carriers may not develop breast cancer. About half of the breast cancer families who have had linkage analysis have been unlinked at the BRCA1 locus.[15] Those who take the test need to be aware that if linkage is not established at the BRCA1 or the BRCA2 locus, there is a chance that genetic inheritance is present but due to another gene.[23] Finally, the possibility of error must be broached. The results given by Biesecker et al. to a linkage analysis family were communicated as 98% likely to be accurate.[7] This level of accuracy may not be possible in smaller families for linkage analysis. Mutation testing in a population setting may be very misleading, and will be highly dependent on the sensitivity of mutation detection techniques. It will also only test for one of five or more genes that cause hereditary breast cancer. Nevertheless, once a causative mutation has been found in a specific family, it will allow 100% accuracy for testing 'at-risk' individuals, although the accuracy of perception following attempts to describe quantitative risk to an individual woman remains uncertain.[24]

CONFIDENTIALITY

The issues of confidentiality were discussed earlier, and will need to be broached with each individual. Guarantees about confidentiality must be made by each testing centre to each person screened.

PSYCHOLOGICAL IMPACT

An important component of pre-test counselling is to identify individuals who are psychologically vulnerable to the negative consequences of learning their career status.[25] Standard psychological instruments or structured interviews could be used to assess psychological status. Lerman and Croyle have argued strongly that pre-test counselling must include some preparation for the psychological impact of test results.[15] Some pre-test assessment of psychological state will enable the pre-test counselling to be directed appropriately. There is evidence from traditional genetic counselling that rehearsing various result scenarios can minimize the likelihood of untoward psychological consequences.[15]

MANAGEMENT STRATEGIES

At the pre-testing stage, all potential management strategies for carriers must be discussed. Currently there are three options available to women who have a strong family history of breast cancer, for whom there is a chance of carrier status. These options are intensive surveillance, participation in the tamoxifen prevention trial (which includes regular screening) or prophylactic bilateral mastectomy. The costs and benefits of each option will need to be presented in turn, and quite possibly some rehearsal of the management decision at the pre-test stage may be useful for some women.

Pre-test counselling aims

It is agreed that pre-counselling for genetic testing for breast cancer should consist of at least two sessions.[7,13–15] To provide the level of information necessary for women to make an informed choice (see Table 7.1), probably a minimum of two sessions are needed for adequate information and counselling. A second session is important because it provides the opportunity to assess the woman's level of understanding from the first session, and to fill in gaps in information, as well as providing the opportunity

Table 7.1 *A summary of pre-test counselling aims*

A To provide information on:
Genetic theory
Incomplete penetrance
Possibility of linkage at other loci
Possibility of error
Available management strategies for carriers

B To assess:
Psychological state
Perception of risk
Level of understanding of all aspects of section A

C To prepare for the psychological impact of the results,
possibly using rehearsal strategies already utilized in
traditional genetic counselling

for a period of reflection. A limited level of understanding in genetic counsellees, even after careful counselling, has been reported.[13,18] Consensus must be reached as to what is an adequate level of information for an individual to give informed consent to testing. If an adequate level of understanding is not achieved, further counselling will need to be provided so that an informed decision is possible. It is likely that many women who are considering testing will require more than two counselling sessions in order to reach what is currently being suggested as necessary understanding. There are various strategies which may assist in information provision. Evans *et al.* have reported that a letter reiterating what was said at a family history counselling session improves estimates of personal risk by women.[18] The possible usefulness of a taped copy of the counselling session needs to be investigated. Finally, if a partner, relative or friend is present, it is possible that a second person, with whom the information could be discussed later, may improve understanding.

PSYCHOLOGICAL IMPACT OF GENETIC TESTING

Carriers

It is established that a significant minority of women with a family history of breast cancer suffer psychological distress to a degree that warrants counselling.[11,12,26] It is reasonable to assume that being informed of carrier status for BRCA1/BRCA2 mutations will have a similar if not more severe impact on psychological functioning. Biesecker *et al.* gave information on carrier status for BRCA1 mutations to 35 members of a family suitable for linkage analysis.[7] At the time of being presented with their test results, many family members were unable to sort out their feelings immediately and discuss them further. Lynch *et al.* gave 181 individuals the results of testing for BRCA1 mutations.[9] A total of 78 individuals were found to be carriers, and of these over one-third reported sadness, anger or guilt. It was apparent to Biesecker *et al.* that follow-up counselling, after the results had been assimilated, would be essential for the members of the linkage analysis family with which they were dealing.[7]

Lynch and Watson performed a linkage analysis for BRCA1 mutations in a suitable extended family and informed them of their carrier status.[8] They discovered from telephone interviews 3–6 weeks subsequent to the disclosure of carrier status that a substantial proportion of women identified as gene-mutation carriers were experiencing some psychological distress, most commonly in the form of persistent worries, depression, confusion and sleep disturbance. It seems that the impact of being informed of carrier status is consistent with the impact of disclosure of carrier status for other traditional genetic disorders.[7,8]

Non-carriers

Biesecker et al. found that many individuals who underwent linkage analysis and who were told that they probably were not carriers of BRCA1 mutations felt guilt and responsibility towards those members of their family who were carrying the mutations.[7] One family member who was scheduled to have prophylactic surgery was able to accept that she was not a carrier and cancelled her surgery, but was 'overwhelmed' with guilt that she had been spared. Similarly, many of those who are told that they do not carry the gene for Huntington's chorea have been reported to suffer guilt and also a certain sense of loss.[27] Having lived with the threat of premature death for many years, some find it difficult to adjust to the prospect of a potentially disease-free normal lifespan.[27] Lynch and Watson reported that several family members who were found to be low-risk on linkage analysis expressed disbelief and wished to continue with intense surveillance, while some were still considering prophylactic surgery.[8] Disbelief and a desire to continue surveillance were also reported in some of the women who were given negative results in the study by Lynch et al.[9] Provision must therefore be made for non-carriers from breast cancer families who may benefit from follow-up counselling.

Individuals who decide against testing

At this early stage of development of genetic counselling for breast cancer, it is impossible to say what the effect of deciding against testing might be. Recent evidence from a prospective study of the impact of genetic testing for Huntington's disease suggests that deciding against testing may be more detrimental psychologically than testing, regardless of the test result.[28] Wiggins et al. reported that those who decided against testing were more psychologically distressed than either non-carriers or carriers at 12 months.[28] Those opting against testing may well appreciate the opportunity for follow-up counselling.

Biesecker et al. informed one member of the linkage analysis family, who had already undergone prophylactic bilateral mastectomy, of her non-carrier status.[7] Although she was very ambivalent about taking the test, she was able to accept that her earlier choice to undergo prophylactic mastectomy was the best decision she could have made given the information available at the time of surgery. Similarly, Lynch et al. reported that several women who received negative BRCA1 results after prophylactic surgery were satisfied that they had made the best choices given the information available to them at the time.[9] Women who have had prophylactic surgery may wish to know their carrier status, and some thought should be given to the best way in which to counsel those individuals who are found to be non-carriers.

Summary

Pre-test and follow-up counselling should be available to all those who have been tested for BRCA1/BRCA2 mutations, regardless of carrier status, and also to those who decided against testing. Early data from linkage-analysis families suggests that individuals are too overwhelmed when they receive their results to benefit from counselling, but they may well require it later.[7] The frequency and type of counselling that should be employed is an area that needs to be investigated. Many of the women who are carriers will also want to discuss their personal management strategy; this could be simultaneous or provided separately. Shiloh and Saxe have suggested that genetic counsellees often interpret non-directive counselling about risk as negative (i.e. the more neutral a counsellor is, the more negatively the counsellee interprets their situation, regardless of actual risk).[16] A non-directive approach may be best for psychosocial support, whereas a less neutral approach may be appropriate in discussions of management strategies.

MANAGEMENT STRATEGIES

At the time of writing, there are three main management strategies available to women with a family history of breast cancer, namely intensive surveillance, joining chemoprevention trials and prophylactic surgery.

Intensive surveillance

The national breast screening programme in the UK starts for women at the age of 50 years. Breast cancer due to mutations of the BRCA1/BRCA2 gene is characterized by an average onset at well below 50 years of age. Women found to be carrying BRCA1/BRCA2 mutations could be offered screening at a much earlier age. Women with a strong family history of breast cancer are already often offered mammography at an earlier age, usually through a breast cancer family history clinic.[18] However, there are no published data which indicate that mammography for those under 50 years of age is effective. Younger breasts tend to be more dense, which makes detection of abnormalities more difficult. There is no consensus on mammographic screening or the interval of screening for women at risk for breast cancer, or indeed on age of onset for screening. Some workers have suggested biennial clinical breast examinations and annual mammography starting 5 years before the earliest onset age in the family.[29] There are concerns about the risks posed by radiation in frequent long-term mammography, although the more modern mammographic methods use very low radiation doses.[30] Until mammography in younger, at-risk women has been properly researched, we are ill equipped to inform women about the effectiveness of intense surveillance, and data in this area are urgently required.

Chemoprevention trials

Women who have a strong family history of breast cancer are currently being offered the opportunity to join the tamoxifen prevention trial in the UK, other European countries, Australia and America. The hypothesis derives from the observation that new tumours in the contralateral breast are reduced if women take tamoxifen after surgery.[31] Women who join the trial are randomly assigned to tamoxifen or a placebo for 5 years, and are then followed up with clinical examinations and mammography. It will be some time before the results are known. If tamoxifen is found to help prevent breast cancer, then it will be a real alternative for women who carry BRCA1/BRCA2 mutations. It would be a less radical intervention than surgery, but would still represent a preventive strategy in addition to surveillance. Regular mammography and clinical examinations could be offered alongside tamoxifen. The psychosocial implications of long-term tamoxifen treatment are currently being investigated, as there are no data available on the effect of long-term tamoxifen as a preventative. Some women experience physical side-effects from tamoxifen (usually hot sweats or vaginal discharge or other menopausal symptoms), and these are known to have a negative impact on quality of life.[32]

Prophylactic surgery

A minority of women in the UK with a strong family history of breast cancer are offered and/or choose to have prophylactic bilateral mastectomy.[7,33] It is possible, when genetic testing for BRCA1/BRCA2 mutations becomes more widely available, that more women will decide to have such surgery. Biesecker et al. reported that, of the female carriers identified in their linkage-analysis family, most opted for prophylactic surgery.[7] In the study by Lynch et al., many of the women who received positive test results had already developed breast cancer or undergone prophylactic surgery prior to genetic testing.[9] However, of the 31 women who were eligible for prophylactic mastectomy, only 35% contemplated prophylactic surgery. It is important that women are informed of all the possible physical and psychological implications of such surgery.[34]

To date there has been very little systematic research on the psychosocial consequences of prophylactic mastectomy. However, it may be possible to gain some insight from women who have had surgical treatment for breast cancer. The impact of mastectomy on psychological functioning has been well researched, but the advent of breast-conserving treatments for breast cancer made it possible to distinguish psychological distress caused by fear of cancer from that caused by loss of the breast. The data indicate that fear of cancer rather than loss of the breast is the major factor involved in psychological morbidity,[35] although there is some protection of body image and feelings of sexual attractiveness to be gained from breast conservation.[36] It is encouraging that breast reconstruction has been reported to reduce the negative impact of mastectomy. Both Schain et al.[36] and Goin and Goin[37] have reported that immediate reconstruction rather than delayed reconstruction has a protective effect against psychological distress.

Women at high risk of developing breast cancer now, as well as those identified as carriers of BRCA1/BRCA2 mutation in the future, face different dilemmas to those diagnosed with breast cancer.[38] Breast cancer is sometimes treated by local excision which conserves the breast. Prophylactic bilateral mastectomy surgery may be more radical than the treatment that would be offered if breast cancer was to develop. BRCA1/BRCA2 mutations have incomplete penetrance, so carriers cannot be certain that surgery is necessary.

The psychological benefits and costs of prophylactic bilateral mastectomy need to be established. It is possible that for women whose quality of life is adversely affected by fear of developing breast cancer, the psychological benefits of such surgery may outweigh any negative consequences. For example, Lerman and Croyle have postulated that prophylactic surgery may reduce chronic uncertainty and worry.[15] Although there may be many potential psychological costs associated with prophylactic mastectomy, women who consider this option and then choose not to have surgery may fare worse. It is essential that prospective research evaluates the consequences of this drastic surgical intervention on subsequent anxiety and quality of life.

Many women who have strong family histories of breast cancer, linked to the BRCA1 and possibly to the BRCA2 locus, also have a risk of ovarian cancer.[23] Some carriers of BRCA1/BRCA2 mutations may well also have to consider prophylactic oophorectomy. Lynch et al. reported that 76% of female carriers of BRCA1 mutations considered prophylactic oophorectomy, compared to only 35% of those considering prophylactic mastectomy.[9] The psychological impact of prophylactic removal of the ovaries is unknown, and while it is a less controversial issue and receives less media attention, it should not be dismissed as less distressing than prophylactic removal of the breasts. Removal of the ovaries has a significant effect on hormonal balance, which has the potential to have an enormous psychological effect on some women. Loss of fertility could have a negative psychological impact, particularly for those women who are childless or who have not yet had all of the children that they wished for.

RESEARCH ISSUES

There are many research issues that arise from genetic testing for breast cancer. Lerman and Croyle have stated that the most important research goal is to understand why two individuals with similar risks can react so differently to similar information regarding breast cancer.[15] Research questions fall into three main categories, namely decision-making, information and psychological categories.

Decision-making issues

Women with a family history of breast cancer have two decisions to make, namely whether to take the test and what management strategy to adopt if they are found to carry BRCA1/BRCA2 mutations. To a greater or lesser extent these decisions are linked. One woman may decide to have a genetic test only if she is happy that there is a management strategy that will suit her. Another may decide to have the test but prefer to leave the decision about management until she has received the results. The variables that moderate the decision process should be identified, and the potential moderators are numerous (see Table 7.2).

Table 7.2 *Potential moderators of the decision-making process*

Sociodemographic characteristics
Psychological state
Personality
Coping style
Attitudes and beliefs about breast cancer and treatment
Perception of personal risk prior to testing
Perception of severity of the disease
Perceived benefits of management strategies
Personal family experience of breast cancer
Family considerations (e.g. risk to daughters)

Information issues

It seems that, both in traditional genetic counselling and also in risk presentation at breast cancer family history clinics, little information is retained from the counselling session. The amount of information that women retain from one session to the next should be monitored. Potential strategies to improve information retention, such as follow-up letters, tapes of interviews, provision of an information helpline and the presence of a partner, relative or friend, need to be investigated.

Psychological questions

What are the psychological consequences of undergoing genetic testing for breast cancer? Do carriers, non-carriers and those who decide against testing fare differently either immediately or in the long term? Are there any pre-counselling strategies that can protect against the negative psychological impact of screening (e.g. rehearsal)? Finally, is a more neutral counselling style interpreted as more negative?

CONCLUSION

Genetic screening for breast cancer offers the chance to reduce mortality in women who have inherited an 85% probability of developing the disease. Those women who are contemplating testing will need reliable information and psychological support so that their decisions are based on unbiased appraisal of the situation, and not on fear or misunderstanding. Initially, guidelines for screening centres will have to be based on information from other related areas. The issues of effective and ethical communications of risk, psychological support, surveillance and prevention strategies can then be addressed in the specific context of breast cancer screening in order to ensure the best possible information and psychological support during the decision-making process.

REFERENCES

1 Claus EB, Risch NJ, Thompson WD. Age at onset as an indicator of familial risk of breast cancer. *American Journal of Epidemiology* 1993; **131**: 961–72.
2 Evans HJ. Genetic predisposition to some common cancers. *MRC News* 1990; **49**: 46–7.
3 Newman B, Austin MA, Lee M, King MC. Inheritance of human breast cancer: evidence for autosomal-dominant transmission in high-risk families. *Proceedings of the National Academy of Sciences of the USA* 1988; **85**: 3044–8.
4 Hall JM, Lee MK, Newman B *et al*. Linkage of early-onset familial breast cancer to chromosome 17q21. *Science* 1990; **250**: 1684–9.
5 Miki Y, Swensen J, Shattuck-Eider D *et al*. A strong candidate for the breast and ovarian cancer gene BRCA1. *Science* 1994; **266**: 66–71.
6 Wooster R, Neuhausen SL, Mangion J *et al*. Identification of a breast cancer gene BRCA2. *Nature* 1995; **378**: 789–91.
7 Biesecker BB, Boehnke M, Calzone K *et al*. Genetic counselling for families with inherited susceptibility to breast and ovarian cancer. *Journal of the American Medical Association* 1993; **269**: 1970–4.
8 Lynch HT, Watson P. Genetic counselling and hereditary breast/ovarian cancer. *Lancet* 1992; **339**: 1181.
9 Lynch HT, Lemon SJ, Durham C *et al*. A descriptive study of BRCA1 testing and reactions to disclosure of test results. *Cancer* 1997; **79**: 2219–28.
10 Watson M, Murdy V, Lloyd S *et al*. Genetic testing on breast/ovarian cancer BRCA2 families. *Lancet* 1995; **346**: 8974.
11 Kash KM, Holland JC, Halper MS, Miller DG. Psychological distress and surveillance behaviours of women with a family history of breast cancer. *Journal of the National Cancer Institute* 1992; **84**: 25–30.
12 Lerman C, Daly M, Sands C *et al*. Mammography adherence and psychological distress among women at risk to breast cancer. *Journal of the National Cancer Institute* 1993; **85**: 1094–80.

13 Lerman C, Daly M, Masny A, Balshem A. Attitudes about genetic testing for breast-ovarian cancer susceptibility. *Journal of Clinical Oncology* 1994; **12**: 843–50.

14 Richards MPM, Hallowell N, Green JM, Munton F, Statham H. Counselling families with hereditary breast and ovarian cancer; a psycho-social perspective. *Journal of Genetic Counselling* 1995; **4**: 219–33.

15 Lerman C, Croyle R. Psychological issues in genetic screening for breast cancer susceptibility. *Archives of Internal Medicine* 1994; **154**: 609–16.

16 Shiloh S, Saxe L. Perception of risk in genetic counselling. *Psychology and Health* 1989; **3**: 45–61.

17 Evans DGR, Burnell LD, Hopwood P, Howell A. Perception of risk in women with a family history of breast cancer. *British Journal of Cancer* 1993; **67**: 612–14.

18 Evans DGR, Blair V, Greenhalgh R, Hopwood P, Howell A. The impact of genetic counselling on risk perception in women with a family history of breast cancer. *British Journal of Cancer* 1994; **70**: 934–8.

19 Pharoah PDP, Day NE, Duffy S, Easton DF, Ponder BAJ. Family history and the risk of breast cancer: a systematic review and meta-analysis. *International Journal of Cancer* 1997; **71**: 800–9.

20 Ford D, Easton DF, Bishop TD, Narod SA, Goldgar DE and the Breast Cancer Linkage Consortium. Risks of cancer in BRCA1-mutation carriers. *Lancet* 1994; **343**: 692–5.

21 Cull A, Miller H, Porterfield T *et al*. The use of videotaped information in cancer genetic counselling: a randomised evaluation study. *British Journal of Cancer* 1998; **77**: 830–7.

22 Cull A, Anderson EDC, Campbell S, Mackay J, Smyth E, Steel M. The impact of genetic counselling about breast cancer risk on women's perceptions and levels of distress. *British Journal of Cancer* 1999; **79**: 501–8.

23 Easton DF, Bishop DT, Ford D, Crockford GP and the Breast Cancer Linkage Consortium. Genetic linkage analysis in familial breast and ovarian cancer: results from 214 families. *American Journal of Human Genetics* 1993; **52**: 678–701.

24 Hallowell N, Richards MPM. Understanding life's lottery: an evaluation of studies of genetic risk awareness. *Journal of Health Psychology* 1997; **2**: 31–43.

25 Bottorff JL, Ratner PA, Johnson JL *et al*. Communicating cancer risk information: the challenge of uncertainty. *Patient Education Counselling* 1998; **33**: 67–81.

26 Thirlaway KJ, Fallowfield L, Nunnerley H, Powles T. Anxiety in women 'at risk' of developing breast cancer. *British Journal of Cancer* 1996; **73**: 1422–6.

27 Nance MA, Leroy BS, Orr HT, Parker T, Rich SS, Heston LL. Protocol for genetic testing in Huntington's disease: three years of experience in Minnesota. *American Journal of Medical Genetics* 1991; **40**: 518–22.

28 Wiggins S, Whyte P, Huggins M *et al*. The psychological consequences of predictive testing for Huntingdon's disease. *New England Journal of Medicine* 1994; **327**: 1401–5.

29 King MC, Rowell S, Love SM. Inherited breast and ovarian cancer. What are the risks? What are the choices? *Journal of the American Medical Association* 1993; **269**: 1975–80.

30 Strax P. Control of breast cancer through mass screening. From research to action. *Cancer* 1989; **63**: 1881–7.

31 Powles T, Davey I, McKinna. Chemoprevention of breast cancer. *Acta Oncologica* 1989; **28**: 865–7.

32 Nayfield SG, Karp JE, Ford LG, Andrew D, Kramer BS. Potential role of tamoxifen in prevention of breast cancer. *Journal of the National Cancer Institute* 1991; **83**: 1450–9.

33 Hartmann LC, Schaid DJ, Woods JE *et al*. Efficacy of bilateral mastectomy in women with a family history of breast cancer. *New England Journal of Medicine* 1999; **340**: 77–84.

34 Eisen A, Weber BL. Prophylactic mastectomy – the price of fear. *New England Journal of Medicine* 1999; **340**: 137–8.

35 Fallowfield U, Hall A, Maguire GP, Baum M. Psychological outcomes of different treatment policies in women with early breast cancer outside of a clinical trial. *British Medical Journal* 1990; **301**: 575–80.

36 Schain WS, Wellisch DK, Pasnau RO, Landsverk J. The sooner the better: a study of psychological factors in women undergoing immediate versus delayed breast reconstruction. *American Journal of Psychiatry* 1985; **142**: 40–6.

37 Goin MK, Goin JM. Psychological reactions to prophylactic mastectomy synchronous with contralateral breast reconstruction. *Plastic and Reconstructive Surgery* 1982; **70**: 355–9.

38 Massie MJ. Prophylactic mastectomy for women at high risk for breast cancer. A reasonable treatment? In: *Psycho-Oncology. V. Psychosocial factors in cancer risk and survival*. Sloan-Kettering, 1993.

FURTHER READING

Armstrong K, Eisen A, Weber B. Primary care: assessing the risk of breast cancer. *New England Journal of Medicine* 2000; **342**: 564–571.

8

Early detection and prevention: benefits, costs and limitations of screening

INGVAR ANDERSSON AND STEFAN RYDÉN

INTRODUCTION

The prognosis of breast cancer is highly dependent on the presence and extent of lymph-node metastases as well as on the size of the primary tumour. There is also a clear relationship between the size of the tumour and the risk of regional lymph-node metastases. It thus seems likely that early detection should be a most important strategy in reducing breast cancer mortality. Mammography is a powerful diagnostic tool which has the potential to detect breast cancer at a non-palpable and sometimes even a pre-invasive stage. The diagnostic usefulness of mammography has been enhanced by numerous technical advances which have also resulted in reduced radiation exposure. It therefore seems logical that early diagnosis by breast screening with mammography should reduce breast cancer mortality.

Reduction of breast cancer mortality is the primary and fundamental objective of breast screening. In addition to this, breast screening should have the potential to reduce breast cancer morbidity by permitting less extensive surgical therapy, with less need for post-operative radiotherapy and adjuvant therapy, all of which may result in an increased quality of life for breast cancer patients.

Studies of breast screening have been conducted for more than three decades. In addition to several case–control and cohort studies, eight major randomized controlled clinical trials have addressed the question of whether screening with mammography can reduce mortality in breast cancer. The results of these studies have been analysed and re-analysed, updated, meta-analysed and subjected to external reviews, all of which have resulted in an overwhelming literature on breast screening and a constant, ongoing debate regarding the interpretation of the presented data. Although some findings are now indisputably established, many others are not.

It is beyond the scope of this chapter to provide full coverage of all aspects of breast screening. However, we shall try to review the results of the major trials and to focus on some of the questions which have been of major concern in the debate on breast screening. Such questions include the reproducibility of trial results in service screening, the cost-effectiveness of breast screening, the possible adverse effects of screening, quality control and screening from a public health perspective.

GENERAL ASPECTS OF SCREENING MODALITIES

Clearly the sensitivity of the screening procedure (i.e. its ability to identify cancer cases correctly) is of great importance. It is perhaps not as apparent that the specificity of a screening procedure (i.e. its ability to identify non-cancerous cases correctly) is even more important. This is due to the fact that the sensitivity is concerned with cancer cases only, which represent a small proportion in the population. However, the specificity has an impact on the vast majority of the screening population.

In many western countries, the annual incidence of breast cancer is approximately 2 cases per 1000 women in the age group 50–70 years. This means that if 1000 women are screened on a biannual basis, four women will have breast cancer and 996 women will be free of disease. In practice, it is a more challenging task to identify the 996 non-cancerous cases correctly than it is to detect the four cancer cases.

Table 8.1 illustrates a screening programme involving 10 000 women with a cancer prevalence of 4/1000 (i.e. there is a total of 40 cancer cases that can be detected). A sensitivity of 95% will imply that two cancer cases are missed.

Table 8.1 *The importance of sensitivity and specificity in a hypothetical screening programme involving 10 000 women with a cancer prevalence of 4/1000*

Sensitivity (%)	False-negatives	Specificity (%)	False-positives
98	1	98	199
95	2	95	498
90	4	90	996

A specificity of 95% would mean that almost 500 false-positive cases would be produced. A sensitivity of 90%, which is probably a common achievement would mean four missed cancers, which although not ideal, is acceptable. However, a specificity of 90% would imply almost 1000 false-positives, which is not acceptable.

Accordingly, it is important to realize that the predictive value of a positive finding (i.e. the likelihood that a woman with a positive mammogram is affected by breast cancer) is dependent on the prevalence of the disease. Screening for a low-prevalence disease such as breast cancer, will produce an unexpectedly high number of false-positive cases as illustrated above. Accordingly, the predictive value will be low. In the programme illustrated in Table 8.2, 3.3% of all of the screenees were recalled for work-up.

Table 8.2 *The positive predictive value for breast cancer at various stages of the work-up of suspicious findings (data from the Malmö Mammographic Screening Trial)*

	Percentage of screenees	Predictive value
Recall	3.3	13
Referral	1.0	43
Recommendation for surgery	0.6	73

The positive predictive value of such a recall was 13%. In other words, 13 of 100 recalled women finally turned out to have breast cancer. It should be stressed that a 3.3% recall rate is lower than the average in most screening programmes.

After radiographic work-up, the majority of those recalled could be classified as non-suspicious for breast cancer and returned to the screening programme, and only 1% of those initially screened remained suspicious.

These women were referred to the breast clinic. The predictive value of such a referral was 42%. After fine-needle aspiration biopsy, 0.6% of those initially screened remained suspicious to such a degree that surgery was recommended. The positive predictive value of such a recommendation was 73%. Thus 3 out of 4 operations resulted in a diagnosis of breast cancer.

This illustrates the requirements of screening modalities, including the quality of the interpretation. In addition, a screening technique must be fast and relatively inexpensive. It should also be acceptable in terms of not producing too much discomfort. Several techniques have been tried for screening for breast cancer, and those that have not fulfilled the prerequisites include thermography, diaphanography (light scanning) and ultrasound.[1–3] Also, it is not clear whether breast cancer mortality can be reduced by screening with physical examination alone or breast self-examination alone. The only techniques that have a well-documented effect are mammography and mammography in combination with physical examination.

This does not mean that some of the above techniques may not be of additional value (e.g. ultrasound). The same applies to magnetic resonance imaging (MRI), although its definitive role has yet to be defined. However, it is not likely to play a role as a screening procedure in the near future.

BREAST SCREENING TRIALS

Randomized controlled trials provide the best method of assessing the efficacy of screening.[4] The first randomized trial on breast screening to provide evidence of a positive effect of breast screening was the Health Insurance Plan of Greater New York (HIP) trial by Shapiro, Strax and collaborators. At 5 and 10 years, a statistically significant reduction in the number of breast cancer deaths was observed in the invited group.[5,6] After 18 years of follow-up, there was a 25% relative reduction in deaths from breast cancer in the 40–49 years age group. The significance of this reduction has been disputed. The mortality reduction in the 50–59 and 60–64 years age groups was 23% and 17% respectively.[7]

In Sweden, Lundgren *et al.* showed in the early 1970s that breast cancer screening with mammography could be performed with a simplified, single-view mammography without concomitant clinical examination.[8,9]

The pioneering work of Shapiro, Strax and Lundgren stimulated a world-wide interest in breast screening, resulting in the introduction of seven additional randomized trials, between 1976 and 1982 in Sweden, Scotland and Canada.[10–21] The major characteristics of these trials are listed in Table 8.3.

The most relevant studies are all randomized controlled trials with death from breast cancer as the study

Table 8.3 *Basic characteristics of the eight randomized trials of breast cancer screening*

Study (start year)	Age at entry (years)	Randomization	Screening modality		Sample size		Attendance at first round (%)
			Views	Interval (months)	Study	Control	
HIP (1963)	40–64	Individual	M+CBE Two	12	30 239	30 756	67
WE (1977)	40–74	Cluster-geographic	M One	24–33	78 085	56 782	89
Malmö (1976)	45–69	Individual	M Two	18–24	21 088	21 195	74
Stockholm (1981)	40–64	Cluster-birth cohort	M One	28	39 164	19 943	81
Gothenburg (1982)	40–59	Individual (<50) Cluster (+ 50)	M Two	18	20 724	28 809	84
Edinburgh (1979)	45–64	Cluster-GP registries	M+CBE Two	12–24	23 226	21 904	61
Canada 1 CNBSS 1 (1980)	40–49	Individual	M+CBE Two	12	25 214	25 216	100
Canada 2 CNBSS 2 (1980)	50–59	Individual	M+CBE Two	12	19 711	19 694	100

M, mammography;
CBE, clinical breast examination.

end-point. The Swedish studies are population based, which means that the entire female population in a defined geographical area and a certain age range was included in the studies. In the Edinburgh study, screening was offered to women registered with general practices in the city. In the Canadian studies, volunteers were recruited by advertising in different media.

Randomization was performed either on an individual basis or on the basis of clusters which could be either geographical, as in the WE study, or general, as in the Edinburgh study.

Two groups were thus created, one of which was invited to screening repeatedly, while the other served as a control group. The two groups should be equal in all other respects, such as age and distribution of risk factors associated with death from breast cancer. Theoretically, the best way to achieve this goal is by randomization on an individual basis. In the case of cluster randomization it should be demonstrated whether and in what respect the two groups differ, and how such a difference should be accounted for. In the Edinburgh trial there is some data indicating that the invited group might a priori have had a lower risk of breast cancer than the control group. An adjustment for this difference was made in the most recent update of the Edinburgh trial.[22]

The status of the control group is another factor which may influence the results. Basically, women in the control groups received ordinary health care, with the exception of the Canadian trial, in which controls underwent a clinical examination at the start of screening. As a result of this procedure, the diagnosis of breast cancer was advanced in time for those control group patients who had a palpable cancer at clinical examination. As a result of this intervention, the reduction in breast cancer mortality may be evident later in this study than in studies without any intervention in the control group. It should also be noted that CNBSS2 compares mammography and clinical breast examination (CBE) in the invited group with CBE only in the control group.

The fact that controls receive normal health care means that the trial results to some extent reflect the standard of care, in particular the availability of regular breast examination, including mammography in the presence of minimal or no symptoms. Furthermore, it may reflect women's attitudes (e.g. their inclination to seek advice early for breast symptoms). The results of screening would thus be more impressive in a population in which women seek advice late, or in which mammography would not be available or the general standard of care is low.

In the Malmö study 24% of the control group women had at least one mammogram during the first 8.8 years of study.[13] It also follows that the impact of a systematic (population-based) screening programme in a society where the majority of eligible women already undergo regular examination, including mammography (e.g. by their gynaecologists), would be minimal. A negative trial result in such a situation does not mean that screening mammography is without effect.

However, it would be an important piece of information for those who have to allocate sparse health-care resources to screening programmes.

The measure of effect in the studies is the incidence of death from breast cancer in the invited groups, including non-attenders, compared to that in the control groups. Thus the aim of the trials has been to assess the effect of offering screening to women rather than assessing the effect among those who actually underwent screening, which is equivalent to an intention-to-treat approach. This also means that compliance is of great importance. Furthermore, there was self-selection within the invited group. It turns out that non-attenders have a greater than average risk of dying from breast cancer (i.e. greater than that for controls), which is in turn due to the fact that these women have an unfavourable staging when their breast cancer is diagnosed.[23] The non-compliers represent a complex group; one subset represents women with socio-economic and psychiatric problems, including alcohol abuse. Some of these women may already have felt a tumour in the breast before being invited, but do not want to have the diagnosis confirmed, or they may even deny the possibility of the existence of a malignant tumour. In the Malmö study about 50% of the breast cancer deaths occurred among non-compliers despite the fact that they represented only about 30% of the population.[13]

This self-selection bias is also of interest in relation to the case–control studies.[24–27] In these studies, women who died of breast cancer were compared with age-matched controls with regard to screening history. The relative risk for those who had a screening mammogram compared to those who did not was calculated. This means that compliers were compared with non-compliers.

According to the above, this implies a risk of overestimating the effect of screening. In fact this has also been demonstrated in a case–control analysis of the invited group in the Malmö trial.[28] The case–control technique resulted in an odds ratio (relative risk) of 0.42 (95% CI, 0.22–0.78), while the trial result was 0.96.

The reason for assessing mortality rather than survival in studies of screening is to keep under control a number of biases which operate in the screening situation. With screening, the diagnosis of breast cancer is advanced in time by about 2–3 years.[29]

Thus survival will always be prolonged in screening-detected cases, even if the course of the disease is not altered by early detection and the following treatment. This is the *lead time* bias.

The *length bias* refers to the fact that, for purely statistical reasons, screening is more likely to detect a slow-growing than a fast-growing tumour. This is because the slow-growing tumour is in a detectable stage for a longer period of time – the so-called sojourn time. The problem of length bias is most pronounced in the first screening round. It should be remembered that breast cancer is a disease with a wide spectrum with regard to outcome, from virtually benign to highly malignant. Studies of tumour characteristics such as S-phase, hormone receptors and labelling index also indicate that screening-detected cancers are, on average, less 'aggressive' than control group cancers.[30,31] Length-biased sampling is also one of the reasons for the 'surplus' of cancers generated by screening.

In a Danish autopsy study of 83 women aged 22–89 years (median 67 years), 6 individuals had been treated for invasive breast carcinoma during their lifetime.[32] Of the remaining 77 women, 15 cases of invasive breast cancer and 14 cases of cancer *in situ* were found. The prevalence of primary malignant breast lesions was 25.4%. The authors concluded that 70% of breast neoplasms may never develop into clinically relevant disease. However, many of these can be detected by mammography.

Finally, there is a *detection bias* which is related to properties inherent to the screening modality (i.e. mammography). In principle, the same would be true for physical examination. From a radiological point of view there are several morphological types of breast carcinoma, some of which are easier to detect at an early stage, such as the spiculated tumour type, compared to the small circumscribed carcinoma, which is more difficult to identify, especially in a glandular breast. If these tumour types have a different prognosis, the screening sample could be skewed. There is some evidence that this could be the case.[33–35]

The primary goal in breast cancer screening is to reduce the mortality caused by the disease. Thus death from breast cancer has been the end-point of all trials. It is critically important that the end-point is correctly defined and assessed.

It is especially critical that the cause of death is validated in the same way in the invited group as in the control group. Ideally, the cause of death should be validated by an independent end-point committee whose members are blinded to the identity of the cases. Such a procedure was adhered to in the Malmö and HIP studies and later in the overview of the Swedish trials.[5,6,13,15] In that overview it was also demonstrated that the results were virtually identical, irrespective of whether the official death statistics or classification by the end-point committee were used.[36] This conclusion is not necessarily valid for other studies in other countries.

RESULTS OF SCREENING TRIALS

Table 8.4 summarizes the effects on breast cancer mortality in the randomized trials. The effect is usually

Table 8.4 *Randomized trials of breast screening: age at entry, follow-up and relative risks for breast cancer death*

Study	Age at entry (years)	Relative risks (95% CI)	
		All ages	Age under 50 years
HIP	40–64	0.71 (0.55–0.93)	0.77 (0.53–1.11)
Kopparberg (W)	40–74	0.68 (0.52–0.89)	0.57 (0.37–1.22)
Östergötland (E)	40–74	0.82 (0.64–1.05)	1.02 (0.59–1.77)
Malmö*	45–69	0.81 (0.62–1.07)	0.64 (0.45–0.89)
Stockholm	40–64	0.80 (0.53–1.22)	1.01 (0.51–2.02)
Gothenburg	40–49	0.86 (0.54–1.37)	0.95 (0.31–0.96)
All Swedish centres	40–74	0.76 (0.66–0.87)	0.71 (0.57–0.89)
Edinburgh	45–64	0.84 (0.63–1.12)	0.88 (0.55–1.41)
Canada 1	40–49	—	1.14 (0.83–1.56)
Canada 2	50–59	0.97 (0.62–1.52)	—

* The under 50 years age cohort in the Malmö trial consists of two groups.[42]

expressed as a relative risk of dying from breast cancer in the invited group compared to the control group, which is the same as the percentage difference in breast cancer mortality between the groups. The meaning of relative risks may be misleading to those who are not familiar with epidemiology.[37] A better way of describing the effect may be in terms of absolute numbers, as will be illustrated below.[38]

Looking at all age groups, it is evident that all trials show a tendency towards a beneficial effect of screening on breast cancer mortality. The magnitude of this effect varies between the studies. Only two of the trials showed a statistically significant effect on breast cancer mortality, namely the HIP study and the Kopparberg part of the two-county trial. In the Östergötland part of this study, as well as in the Malmö trial, the reduction in breast cancer mortality almost reached the level of statistical significance. The other two Swedish studies have a shorter follow-up and fewer events.

The Swedish trials have probably provided the most reliable information regarding the value of mammographic screening. These trials were relatively uniform with regard to screening technique, and they were all population based, which minimizes the risk of selection bias. They had a high attendance rate, with good quality in terms of equipment and organization, and they addressed the single question of the value of mammography without any other screening procedure such as breast self-examination (BSE) or clinical breast examination (CBE).

These studies have also been subjected to an external review with a validation of the causes of death among breast cancer patients by an independent committee.[15] It is therefore appropriate to discuss the results of the Swedish trials in more detail.

MORTALITY REDUCTION IN THE SWEDISH TRIALS

Taking all of the Swedish trials together, a statistically significant reduction of 24% in breast cancer mortality was observed.[15] The 1993 overview was based on a total of 282 777 randomized women, 156 911 in the invited group and 125 866 in the control group. During the time of the study, these women contributed 2 569 000 person-years of follow-up and a total of 843 breast cancer deaths (418 in the invited group and 425 in the control group). In absolute terms the breast cancer mortality in the invited group was 29 per 100 000 person-years of follow-up compared to 37 per 100 000 person-years of follow-up in the control group. The absolute benefit is the difference (i.e. 8 per 100 000 person-years of follow-up).

Table 8.5 illustrates the fact that the effect on breast cancer mortality varied with age. A statistically significant reduction in breast cancer mortality was observed only among women aged 50 to 69 years at entry. In this age group, the Swedish studies showed a 29% relative reduction in breast cancer deaths. Thus the overview provided undisputed evidence of an effect in this age group.

The oldest age group (70–74 years) contained relatively few person-years of follow-up and few events. No significant effect of screening was observed. However, only the WE trial included women in this age group, and

Table 8.5 *Overview of Swedish trials: person-years of follow-up, number of breast cancer deaths and relative risks according to age group*[15]

Age group (years)	Person-years of follow-up (× 1000)		Breast cancer mortality events		RR (95%)
	Study	Control	Study	Control	
40–49	427	350	73	68	0.87 (0.63–1.20)
50–59	540	454	137	162	0.71 (0.57–0.89)
60–69	372	271	121	126	0.71 (0.56–0.91)
70–74	91	64	48	36	0.94 (0.60–1.46)

due to a low attendance rate among these women, entry was closed after two screening rounds. No other trial has included women over 70 years of age. Also, further analysis of the two-county trial argues in favour of screening older women.[39] Perhaps screening in this age group should be offered on an individual basis.

In the age group under 50 years a non-significant 13% reduction in breast cancer deaths was observed. As can be seen in Table 8.5, 777 000 person-years of follow-up did not provide more than 141 events in this age group. In fact, death from breast cancer is a relatively rare event in middle-aged women. According to Statistics Sweden, the annual breast cancer death is 5 per 10 000 women aged 45–64 years.[40]

Further follow-up of the younger age group in the Swedish trials through 1993 showed a 23% reduction (RR 0.77, 95% CI 0.59–1.01). At this point the median trial time (i.e. from the date of randomization until the end of the first screening round of the control group) ranged from 4.4 years in Stockholm to 14.6 years in Malmö with a median of 7 years. The median follow-up time (i.e. from the date of randomization until the end of follow-up) was 12.8 years, ranging from 9.9 years in Gothenburg to 15.5 years in Malmö. The effect on breast cancer mortality was about the same in the 40–44 and 45–49 years age groups at entry, RR 0.74 and 0.79, respectively. In the 40–44 years age group, the vast majority of breast cancer cases had been diagnosed before the age of 50 years, 94% in the invited group and 89% in the control group.[41] Of a total of 83 breast cancer deaths only two in the invited group and five in the control group occurred after the age of 50 years. These and other data indicated that the impact of screening was due mainly to cases detected before rather than after the age of 50 years. According to the updated results, 5 deaths were prevented, which corresponds to a relative risk reduction of 23%. Recent results from an extended study in Malmö as well as from the Gothenburg trial show statistically significant reductions in breast cancer mortality of 36% and 45%, respectively.[42,43]

The Canadian Breast Screening Study (CNBSS) is the only study specifically designed to assess the effect of breast cancer screening in women under the age of 50 years.[20] This study showed no effect after a mean period of 10.5 years of follow-up. In fact, a 14% increase in breast cancer mortality was observed in the mammography group. It is important to remember that the CNBSS had a different design to the Swedish trials. First, it was not a population-based trial but rather a study of the efficacy of screening women who chose to be screened. Theoretically, that might imply a trial population with an a priori lower (or higher) risk of dying from breast cancer. In fact, there is evidence that the survival was superior in the control group of the CNBSS at 7 years compared to the control group of the two-county trial (WE study). Secondly, the control group of the CNBSS was initially screened by physical examination, which

should mean that the diagnosis of breast cancer was advanced in many cases.

A meta-analysis using the most recent data from all randomized trials showed a statistically significant reduction in breast cancer mortality of 18%, (RR 0.82, 95% CI 0.71–0.95).[44] Including data from the Swedish trials only, this resulted in a statistically significant mortality reduction of 29% (RR 0.71, 95% CI 0.57–0.89).

The initial results indicated an age-specific effect of screening. There are several possible explanations for a less marked effect in younger women, including the lower sensitivity of mammography in this age group. Furthermore, more recent data from Dutch and Swedish screening programmes indicate a faster tumour progression in women under 50–54 years of age compared to older women.[45–47] However, the results from the Malmö and Gothenburg trials indicate a similar effect in women under and over 50 years of age.

SERVICE SCREENING

The results obtained in trials conducted by enthusiastic pioneers are not necessarily transferable to a routine screening setting.[16] Moreover, the results obtained from one country or region are not necessarily reproducible in another country or region, due to differences in healthcare systems, women's attitudes, the level of technological

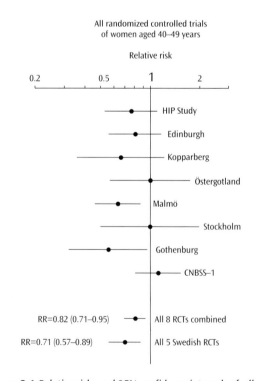

Figure 8.1 *Relative risks and 95% confidence intervals of all randomized controlled clinical trials (RCTs) of screening mammography that included women aged 40–49 years at entry.*[44] *RR, relative risk.* Reprinted from *J Natl Cancer Inst Monogr* 1997; **22**: 87–92 by permission of Oxford University Press.

standards, and so on. However, there are indications from parameters such as stage distribution, detection rates and attendance rate that service screening in Sweden, England and in the USA may result in a reduction in breast cancer mortality rates similar to that observed in the trials.[48–50]

Recent data from a study performed in 17 counties in Sweden based on official statistics has questioned the value in terms of mortality reduction of repeated routine screening for women aged 50 to 69 years.[16] The breast cancer mortality rate from 1970 to 1986 among women aged 50 to 78 years was studied using the official statistics of Sweden. Using a regression analysis, the expected breast cancer mortality rate for the period 1987 to 1996 was calculated. The expected mortality reduction as a result of screening was calculated using data from the WE study, showing a 28% reduction after 5 years of screening.

The actual mortality reduction was found to be non-significant (0.8%). In absolute terms, 55 lives were saved, compared to the expected 739 lives. The study has been questioned for several reasons. There is uncertainty as to whether the slope of the mortality curve, as extrapolated from the mortality experience during the period from 1970 to 1986, really represents the situation without screening. Factors such as therapy and various cohort effects might influence the mortality rate. The results of the WE study may also not be representative of the whole country.

In fact, in the Swedish overview only the WE study reached the level of statistical significance, the remaining studies showing a lower effect.[15] Furthermore, the mortality reduction was observed earlier in the WE study than in the other Swedish studies.

It will probably take several years before a significant mortality reduction can be expected as a result of screening. In this context it is worth noting that the breast cancer mortality rate has been declining in Sweden for many years (since the 1960s, see Table 8.6).[40] This has to be accounted for when evaluating the effect of screening outside controlled trials. A similar trend has been observed in recent years in other countries (e.g. England).[51] There are probably several explanations for this decline, including increased awareness among women resulting in earlier diagnosis, better diagnostic methods and improved treatment. In the last decade it has been shown that adjuvant therapy reduces breast cancer mortality by 20–30%.[52]

Table 8.6 *Age-standardized death rate (per 100 000) according to Statistics Sweden 1993*[40]

	1975	1980	1985	1990
Breast cancer	41.9	40.1	37.2	35.4
Lung cancer	15.9	17.2	19.3	21.1
Cardiovascular disease	777.0	718.5	667.6	575.3

QUALITY CONTROL

To be successful on a national level, a screening programme must have uniform and high standards in all of the specialities involved. To maintain such a standard, a continuous quality control is necessary. In a pilot study of the quality of service screening in Southern Sweden (with a population of 1.6 million residents), a relatively wide variation was observed in the parameters that were studied.[53] The project involved not only the screening procedure itself but also the diagnostic work-up of patients with suspicious findings and surgical procedures. Table 8.7 lists some important parameters. It should be noted that the period of study reflected prevalence screening as well as later screening rounds.

Table 8.7 *Parameters used in the assessment of screening centres in Southern Sweden*[53]

Participation rate	77.1%	(65.0–85.1)
Recall rate	3.7%	(1.3–5.9)
Breast cancer detection rate		
First screening round	7.5%	(4.4–11.4)
Second or later rounds	3.6%	(3.0–4.4)
Proportion of early cancers		
Non-invasive	16%	(6–23)
Invasive ≤ 1 cm	32%	(20–39)
Non-invasive plus stage I	69%	(56–84)
Interval cancers (rate per thousand participants)		
0–12 months	0.5	0.3–0.9
13–24 months	0.8	(0.5–1.1)

It was also found in this quality-control programme that the mean absorbed dose varied with a factor of 4.3, most of which was due to the fact that some centres preferred dark films and very bright light when reading the films. This is an example of a significant finding which can be corrected relatively easily. The dose issue becomes very important when large numbers of healthy women are exposed (e.g. in a screening programme).

Table 8.8 lists some parameters that were used to assess the surgical procedures. There was substantial variation between different surgical departments in the proportion of women undergoing breast conservative surgery.

An unacceptably high proportion of patients (43%) with *in-situ* breast cancer had undergone axillary surgery, with considerable variation between different centres. Most of the morbidity associated with breast surgery comes from operations in the axilla. Moreover, axillary surgery is not considered to be state of the art treatment for carcinoma *in situ*. The reasons for performing the procedure despite this may include inadequate pre-operative evaluation, or a wish to avoid a second procedure, should the primary lesion turn out to be invasive.

Table 8.8 *Parameters used to assess the performance in 11 surgical clinics involved with the treatment of screening-detected breast lesions*[53]

Parameter	Mean	Variance
Pre-operatively established diagnosis of breast cancer by fine-needle aspiration biopsy (% of all breast cancers)	66	42–88
Surgical biopsy* (% of participants)	3.2	0.9–8.4
Positive predictive value of a recommendation for surgical biopsy* (%)	44	14–62
Axillary surgery in patients with carcinoma *in situ*	43	0–75
Breast-conserving surgery	62	35–77

* Includes only patients without a cytologically established diagnosis of breast cancer.

However, this is another example of an important finding in a quality control programme and a faulty routine that could easily be rectified.

Standards of acceptable performance have been defined in many countries. It is important that these standards involve all procedures that might result from screening. Methods for quality control must be built into the organization of service screening, as well as educational programmes for all types of specialities involved in the screening procedure and in the work-up and treatment of patients detected at screening.

COST-EFFECTIVENESS IN BREAST SCREENING

If costs were of no consequence, health-care practitioners would be obliged simply to provide maximally effective care – that is, the kind of care that could be expected to bring about the greatest improvement in health that science and technology can offer.[54]

As health-care resources are limited, allocation of resources and the introduction of new technology or new interventions should be based on some analysis of cost-effectiveness. Several cost-effectiveness (CE) analyses in breast screening have been undertaken.[55-66]

The principal objective of mammography screening is to reduce the risk of dying from breast cancer. The main effect measures are thus the number of breast cancer deaths that are prevented and the number of life-years (LY) gained. As the screening procedure may have both beneficial and detrimental effects on the quality of life of participating women, quality-adjusted years of life saved (QUALY) are also commonly used to assess the net benefit of screening.[62-64] Under all circumstances, service screening will be a costly procedure. In an analysis of cost-effectiveness it is important not only to include direct costs for the screening procedure, but also a direct measure of health-related outcome.

Direct costs are a function of the price of the screening service and the frequency with which it is delivered. Indirect costs include all costs attributable to diagnosis and treatment of screen-detected abnormalities. These will also include expected savings in terms of less aggressive treatment, less treatment for advanced disease, life savings, and also costs for health care in women who have a prolonged survival due to screening. It is obviously a complicated procedure with many hazards, and the published results span a broad range. Computerized simulation programmes have been developed to model screening programmes and effects.[58,67] Such comprehensive programmes probably provide the best method of calculating cost-effectiveness. Another approach is based on calculations on observational studies.[68,69]

These studies are based on observed results from screening programmes collected over a relatively short period of time, and may thus underestimate the value of long-term effects. These latter studies have estimated higher costs per life-year saved than studies based on computerized simulation programmes.

The methods by which CE analyses are performed vary considerably as do the results. In a review of different studies, the cost per life-year saved ranged from US$ 3400 to US$ 83 830 for screening women over the age of 49 years.[70] These considerable differences can be explained to a large extent by differences in programme assumptions (e.g. frequency and price per screening examination, detection rates, biopsy rates, etc.), modelling assumptions (e.g. time period of calculation, inclusion of costs for therapy of primary or advanced disease, etc.), medical care patterns and discounting.

When relatively well-defined programmes are evaluated with corrections for different assumptions about consequences, very similar results have been obtained. In two different major studies of cost-effectiveness, the cost per life-year saved by screening women over 49 years of age was found to be around US$ 7200.[70] It thus seems that breast cancer screening for women aged 50 years or more is cost-effective in countries with relatively high breast cancer incidence and mortality rates, provided with high mammographic quality and attendance.

A good example of a model that covers many aspects of the process is the Dutch model.[59-62] In this model all social costs during the period 1988–2015 of breast cancer assessment and treatment in The Netherlands were calculated in a situation without breast screening compared to different screening polices.[57] It was calculated that about one-third of the additional costs of the screening programme was compensated for by savings in assessment and treatment. The net effect of the addition of screening was a 10% increase in the total costs. With 10 biannual screens per woman between 50 and 70 years of age, with an attendance rate of 70%, the cost per prevented death was calculated to be about US$ 50 000. The cost per life-year gained was about US$ 5000.

An interesting observation that highlights the difficulties of extrapolating the results of cost-effectiveness from one situation to another is a study from the Dutch group.[61] The cost-effectiveness of mass screening for breast cancer by inviting women aged 50–70 years, 2-yearly, in four EC countries (France, Spain, the UK and The Netherlands) was calculated using the Dutch model. The UK and The Netherlands have a high incidence and mortality from breast cancer, whereas France and especially Spain have a much lower incidence. The results revealed large differences in cost-effectiveness between these countries. Compared to The Netherlands and the UK, the cost per life-year gained was almost three times as high in France and almost five times as high in Spain.

The health-care system may also have an impact on costs, as is illustrated by an analysis from the USA showing generally much higher costs than in the corresponding European studies.[66–71] Using the cost-effectiveness ratios for breast cancer screening in women over 50 years of age that were obtained in the UK and The Netherlands, of approximately US$ 4000 per life-year gained, breast screening compares favourably with other health-care measures. Cervical screening, which is well established in most European countries, has been shown to be about three times as costly per life-year gained.[71]

A consistent finding in different studies is that the cost-effectiveness of breast screening deteriorates if women under 50 years of age are included. de Koning and coworkers found that by extending the lower age limit from 50 to 40 years the number of breast cancer deaths prevented during a period of almost 30 years increased by 1.9%, and the number of life-years gained increased by 4.9%. However, the costs per life-year gained increased by 41%.[60]

The low cost-effectiveness of screening women under 50 years of age has also been highlighted in the Forrest report.[56] The message is amplified in several recent reports.[72–75] It should be stressed that the calculations are based on several assumptions, and that they vary accordingly.[76]

SCREENING FROM A PUBLIC HEALTH PERSPECTIVE

It has been demonstrated beyond doubt in several trials that the breast cancer mortality rate was reduced by screening with mammography. The evidence was discussed earlier in this chapter. As a further positive consequence of screening, the need for treatment of advanced disease was reduced, and furthermore less aggressive treatment could be used in many cases. Probably a normal screening result reduced anxiety levels in many women.

Before embarking on a general service screening programme, several issues need to be considered. Can the trial results be transferred to the service screening situation? If so, what is the net benefit of the intervention on women's health? In other words, if advantages are weighed against disadvantages, what is the net result? Finally, are there alternative interventions which have a greater impact on women's health?

In the propaganda in favour of screening, the increasing incidence of breast cancer is often used as an argument for screening. This is not totally relevant. Breast cancer screening represents a secondary prevention, and cannot prevent cancer from occurring. Furthermore, it is worth noting that even a nation-wide programme will detect an unexpectedly low proportion of all cancers in the population. According to official statistics in Sweden, about 60% of all breast cancers occur in women aged 50 to 70 years. Furthermore, screening will only detect a proportion of the cancers in the invited population, due to less than 100% attendance and to the occurrence of interval cancers.

More relevant than the incidence is the mortality of breast cancer. As mentioned above, the mortality from breast cancer has been decreasing in several countries, including Sweden, over the past 30 years.

Table 8.6 shows the age-standardized mortality in Sweden since 1970 for breast and lung cancer and, for comparison, also for cardiovascular disease.

In the USA, lung cancer has overtaken breast cancer as the most frequent cause of cancer death among women. Being mainly smoking related, lung cancer is a disease for which primary prevention would be possible. Compared to cardiovascular disease, breast cancer is a relatively uncommon cause of death. Should the resources be spent on measures against lung cancer and cardiovascular disease, such as anti-smoking propaganda and low-fat diet recommendations? Could mammographic screening be combined with such education?

Experience with regard to service screening from Sweden, England, The Netherlands and the USA indicates that the results of the controlled trials can be duplicated.[48,49] Had there been no side-effects of screening, even a small advantage in terms of prevented deaths would have been acceptable, at least in affluent countries. Unfortunately, however, disadvantages do exist and it is the net benefit that should be taken into account. This means that the advantages of screening should be weighed against the disadvantages.

There are some evident disadvantages, such as the false-positive screening results.[16,77–80] It is known that the recall for work-up of a suspicious mammogram is a cause of substantial trauma to some women, even if they are cleared of the suspicion.[81,82] For this reason it is important to keep the specificity high and the management of these patients on a high professional level.[83,84]

A more serious problem is the detection of biologically insignificant cancer. As a result of screening, some cancers are detected which would otherwise never have become clinically apparent. This is true for many tubular carcinomas and it is even more true for carcinoma *in situ* (CIS). It is not known what proportion of CIS will progress to clinically relevant disease, but it is likely to be less than 50%, and perhaps less than 30%.[32,85]

If 15% of screening-detected cancers are CIS and 50% of these are biologically irrelevant, 3 cases per 10 000 screened (cancer prevalence 4.0/1000) would have a biologically insignificant cancer detected and treated. These women would have to live with the psychological burden of a cancer diagnosis for the rest of their lives.

Another disadvantage is related to the lead time. Through screening the time of diagnosis is advanced by 2 to 4 years.[12,29] This means improved survival and less mutilating surgery for some women. For the remaining women, probably the majority, the course of the disease will be unaffected, the only difference for these women being that they have to live with the knowledge of having been treated for breast cancer for a longer period of time.

The carcinogenic effect of ionizing radiation is well known for moderate and high exposure. For lower doses, such as those used in mammography, the effect is not as well understood. However, most experts agree, that the dose–response relationship can be described by linear extrapolation down to the level of the background radiation. In screening, the exposure is of the order of a few cGy (rads) if screening is performed biannually between the ages of 40 and 70 years. It is known that the carcinogenic effect is age dependent, being highest in childhood and adolescence and decreasing thereafter. There is also a latency period of about 8 to 10 years before any excess cancers will appear in a population that has been exposed to radiation.

The radiation hazard of mammography has been discussed intermittently ever since Bailar drew attention to the problem during the early days of mammographic screening.[86] Since then doses have been reduced substantially by improved techniques, in particular by the introduction of efficient intensifying screens. Furthermore, our knowledge of the carcinogenic effect of low doses has improved, and the data suggest a rather higher risk than was previously assumed.[87]

The risk associated with the low doses used in mammography is negligible in a clinical setting. However, the screening situation is different in that a large population of healthy women are exposed, and also because the favourable events are very few in relation to the number of individuals exposed.

Therefore any risk, even if small, has to be taken seriously. It is generally agreed that screening between the ages of 50 and 70 years is acceptable in terms of radiation exposure. In younger women the situation is less favourable, due to more life-years at risk and a lower effect of screening on breast cancer mortality.

Theoretical calculations by Mattsson et al. have shown that the ratio of avoided/induced deaths in women aged 40 to 49 years was 5 and 21 respectively, using two different hypothetical risk estimates. For women aged 40 to 69 years, the corresponding ratios between avoided and induced deaths were 22 and 104, respectively.[88]

In addition, there is evidence which indicates that the radiation therapy, especially when given to the left breast, may have an unfavourable effect on the heart.[89] It has also been shown that the risk of lung cancer is increased, especially in smokers.[90] Furthermore, an increased incidence of breast cancer in the contralateral breast has been observed after radiotherapy.[91] These effects depend on the radiation technique used and are in all likelihood smaller with modern radiotherapy.[92] These effects are relevant from a screening point of view only in those patients who would not have been treated in the non-screening setting (mainly cases of CIS). However, an earlier diagnosis in some patients due to screening may reduce the need for radiotherapy. Thus the net effect is not easily determined.

In the Malmö trial an attempt was made to quantify the side-effects of screening as well as the benefits among women under 50 years of age.[42] The main findings are summarized in Table 8.9.

Table 8.9 *Assessment of potential harm and benefit from screening women under 50 years of age (per 100 000 person-years*[42]

Positive effects	n	Negative effects	n
Prevented deaths	20	Further examination of false-positives	1260
Prevented cases of metastatic disease	20	Surgery for benign disease	56
Breast-conserving surgery	36	Treatment of clinically insignificant cancer	10
Reassurance	?	Radiation-induced breast cancer death	1
		False reassurance	?

All in all, there is a fine balance between the advantages and disadvantages, and any flaw in the organization or professional operation of a screening programme will jeopardize the overall benefits of the intervention. Quality assessment should therefore be a mandatory part of any screening programme.

REFERENCES

1 Moskowitz M, Milbrath J, Gartside P, Sermeno A, Mandel D. Lack of efficacy of thermography as a screening for minimal and stage I breast cancer. *N Engl J Med* 1976; **295**: 249–52.

2 Alveryd A, Andersson I, Aspegren K *et al.* Lightscanning versus mammography for the detection of breast cancer in screening and clinical practice. A Swedish multicenter study. *Cancer* 1990; **65**: 1671–7.

3 The W, Wilson ARM. The role of ultrasound in breast cancer screening. A consensus statement by the European Group for Breast Cancer Screening. *Eur J Cancer* 1998; **34**: 449–50.

4 Wilson JM, Jungner G. *Principles and practice of screening for disease.* WHO Public Health Papers No. 34. Geneva: World Health Organization, 1968.

5 Shapiro S, Strax P, Venet L. Periodic breast screening in reducing mortality from breast cancer. *J Am Med Assoc* 1971; **215**: 1777–85.

6 Shapiro S. Evidence on screening for breast cancer from a randomized trial. *Cancer* 1977; **39**: 2772–82.

7 Shapiro S, Venet W, Strax P, Venet L. *Periodic screening for breast cancer: the Health Insurance Plan Project and its sequelae, 1963–1986.* Baltimore, MD: Johns Hopkins University Press, 1988.

8 Jacobsson S, Lundgren B, Melander O, Norén T. Mass-screening of a female population for detection of early carcinoma of the breast. *Acta Radiol* 1975; **14**: 424–32.

9 Lundgren B, Jacobsson S. Single view mammography. *Cancer* 1976; **38**: 1124–9.

10 Tabàr L, Fagerberg G, Gad A *et al.* Reduction in mortality from breast cancer after mass screening with mammography. *Lancet* 1985; **i**: 829–32.

11 Tabàr L, Fagerberg G, Day NE, Duffy SW, Kitchin RM. Breast cancer treatment and natural history: new insights from results of screening. *Lancet* 1992; **339**: 412–14.

12 Tabàr L, Fagerberg G, Hsiu-Hsi C *et al.* Efficacy of breast cancer screening by age. *Cancer* 1995; **75**: 2507–17.

13 Andersson I, Aspegren K, Janzon L *et al.* Mammographic screening and mortality from breast cancer: the Malmö mammographic screening trial. *BMJ* 1988; **297**: 943–8.

14 Frisell J, Eklund G, Hellström L, Lidbrink E, Rutqvist LE, Somell A. Randomized study of mammography screening: preliminary report on mortality in the Stockholm trial. *Breast Cancer Res Treat* 1991; **18**: 49–56.

15 Nyström L, Rutqvist LE, Wall S *et al.* Breast cancer screening with mammography: overview of Swedish randomised trials. *Lancet* 1993; **341**: 973–8.

16 Sjönell G, Ståhle L. Mammography screening does not significantly reduce breast cancer mortality in Swedish daily practice. *Läkartidningen* 1999; **96**: 904–13.

17 Mayor S. Swedish study questions mammography screening programmes. *BMJ* 1999; **316**: 621.

18 Murray I. Women urged not to desert cancer testing. *The Times* 12 March, 1999.

19 Roberts MM, Alexander FE, Anderson TJ *et al.* Edinburgh trial of screening for breast cancer: mortality at seven years. *Lancet* 1990; **335**: 241–6.

20 Miller AB, Baines CJ, To T, Wall C. Canadian National Breast Screening Study. 1. Breast cancer detection and death rates among women aged 40 to 49 years. *Can Med Assoc J* 1992; **147**: 1459–76.

21 Miller AB, Baines CJ, To T, Wall C. Canadian National Breast Screening Study. 2. Breast cancer detection and death rates among women aged 50 to 59 years. *Can Med Assoc J* 1992; **147**: 1477–88.

22 Alexander FE, Anderson TJ, Forrest APM, Hepburn W, Kirkpatrick AE. 14 years of follow-up from the Edinburgh randomised trial of breast-cancer screening. *Lancet* 1999; **353**: 1903–8.

23 Lidbrink E, Frisell J, Brandberg I *et al.* Nonattendance in the Stockholm mammography screening trial: relative mortality and reasons for nonattendance. *Breast Cancer Res Treat* 1995; **35**: 267–75.

24 Palli D, Rosselli del Torco M, Buiatti E *et al.* A case–control study of the efficacy of a non-randomized breast cancer screening program in Florence (Italy). *Int J Cancer* 1986; **38**: 501–4.

25 Verbeck ALM, Holland R, Sturmans F *et al.* Reduction of breast cancer mortality through mass screening with modern mammography. *Lancet* 1984; **i**: 1222–4.

26 Collette HJA, Rombach JJ, Day NE *et al.* Evaluation of screening for breast cancer in a non-randomised study (the DOM project), by means of a case–control study. *Lancet* 1984; **i**: 1224–6.

27 Demisse K, Mills OF, Rhoads GG. Empirical comparison of the results of randomized controlled trials and case–control studies in evaluating the effectiveness of screening mammography. *J Clin Epidemiol* 1998; **51/2**: 81–91.

28 Gullberg B, Andersson I, Janzon L, Ranstam J. Letter to the editor. Screening mammography. *Lancet* 1991; **337**: 244.

29 Walter SD, Day NE. Estimation of the duration of a pre-clinical disease. *Am J Epidemiol* 1983; **118**: 865–86.

30 Hakama M, Holli K, Isola J *et al.* Aggressiveness of screen-detected breast cancers. *Lancet* 1995; **335**: 221–4.

31 Klemi PJ, Joensuu H, Toikkanan S *et al.* Aggressiveness of breast cancers found with and without screening. *BMJ* 1992; **304**: 467–9.

32 Nielsen M, Jensen J, Andersen J. Precancerous and cancerous breast lesions during lifetime and autopsy. *Cancer* 1984; **54**: 612–15.

33 Garne JP, Aspegren K, Linell F, Rank F, Ranstam J. Primary prognostic factors in invasive breast cancer with special reference to ductal carcinoma and histologic malignancy grade. *Cancer* 1994; **73**: 1438–48.

34 Ikeda DM, Andersson I, Wattsgård C, Janzon L, Linell F. Interval carcinomas in the Malmö Mammographic Screening Trial. Radiographic appearance and pathological considerations. *Am J Roentgenol* 1992; **159**: 287–94.

35 De Nunzio MC, Evans AJ, Pinder SE *et al.* Correlations between the mammographic features of screen-detected invasive breast cancer and pathological prognostic factors. *Breast* 1997; **a**: 146–9.

36 Nyström L, Larsson LG, Rutqvist LE *et al.* Determination of cause of death among breast cancer cases in the Swedish randomized mammography screening trials. *Acta Oncol* 1995; **34**: 145–52.

37 Fahey T, Griffits S, Peters TJ. Evidence-based purchasing: understanding results of clinical trials and systematic reviews. *BMJ* 1995; **3**: 1056–60.

38 Schmidt JG. The epidemiology of mass breast cancer screening – a plea for a valid measure of benefit. *J Clin Epidemiol* 1990; **43**: 215–25.

39 Chen HH, Tabàr L, Fagerberg G, Duffy SW. Effect of breast cancer screening after age 65. *J Med Screen* 1995; **2**: 10–14.

40 Cancer incidence in Sweden, Stockholm, 1993.

41 Larsson LG, Andersson I, Bjurstam N *et al.* Updated overview of the Swedish randomized trials on breast cancer screening with mammography: age group 40–49 at randomization. *J Natl Cancer Inst Monogr* 1997; **22**: 57–61.

42 Andersson I, Janzon L. Reduced breast cancer mortality in women under age 50. Updated results from the Malmö mammographic screening program. *J Natl Cancer Inst Monogr* 1997; **22**: 63–8.

43 Bjurstam N, Björneld L, Duffy SW *et al.* The Gothenburg breast cancer screening trials. First results on mortality, incidence and mode of detection for women aged 39–49 years at randomisation. *Cancer* 1997; **80**: 2091–9.

44 Hendrick RE, Smith RA, Rutledge III JH, Smart CR. Benefit of screening mammography in women aged 40–49: a new meta-analysis of randomized controlled trials. *J Natl Cancer Inst Monogr* 1997; **22**: 87–92.

45 Tabàr L, Fagerberg G, Chen HH *et al.* Tumour development, histology and grade of breast cancers: prognosis and progression. *Int J Cancer* 1996; **66**: 413–19.

46 Tabàr L, Fagerberg G, Chen HH *et al.* Screening for breast cancer in women aged under 50: mode of detection, incidence, fatality and histology. *J Med Screen* 1995; **2**: 94–8.

47 Peer PGM, van Dijck JAAM, Hendriks JHCL. Age-dependent growth rate of primary breast cancer. *Cancer* 1993; **71**: 3547–51.

48 Baker L. Breast cancer detection demonstration project: five-year summary report. *Cancer* 1982; **32**: 194–225.

49 Thurfjell E. Population-based mammography screening in clinical practice. Results from prevalence round in Uppsala county. *Acta Radiol* 1994; **35**: 487–91.

50 Chu KC, Tarone RE, Kessler LG *et al.* Recent trends in US breast cancer incidence, survival and mortality rates. *J Natl Cancer Inst* 1996; **88**: 1571–9.

51 Beral V, Herman C, Reeves G, Peto R. Sudden fall in breast cancer death rates in England and Wales. *Lancet* 1995; **345**: 1642–3.

52 Early Breast Cancer Trialists' Collaborative Group. Systemic treatment of early breast cancer by hormonal, cytotoxic or immune therapy. *Lancet* 1992; **339**: 1–15, 71–85.

53 Andersson I, Rydén S, Karlberg I. Mammografins kvalitet granskad (quality control of service screening in Sweden). *Läkartidningen* 1995; **35**: 3106–9.

54 Donabedian A. Quality and cost: choices and responsibilities. *Inquiry* 1988; **25**: 90–9.

55 Gravelle HSE, Simpson PR, Chamberlain J. Breast cancer screening and health service cost. *J Health Econ* 1982; **1**: 185–207.

56 Forrest P. *Breast cancer screening. Report to the Health Ministers of England, Wales, Scotland and Northern Ireland.* London: 1986.

57 Knox EG. Evaluation of a proposed breast cancer screening regimen. *BMJ* 1988; **297**: 650–4.

58 van der Maas PJ, de Koning HJ, Ineveld BM *et al.* The cost-effectiveness of breast cancer screening. *Int J Cancer* 1989; **43**: 1055–60.

59 de Koning HJ, van Oortmarssen GJ, van Ineveld BM, van der Maas PJ. Breast cancer screening: its impact on clinical medicine. *Br J Cancer* 1991; **61**: 292–7.

60 de Koning HJ, van Ineveld BM, van Oortmarssen GJ *et al.* Breast cancer screening and cost-effectiveness; policy alternatives, quality of life considerations and the possible impact of uncertain factors. *Int J Cancer* 1991; **49**: 531–7.

61 van Ineveld BM, van Oortmarssen GJ, de Koning HJ, Boer R, van der Maas PJ. How cost-effective is breast cancer screening in different EC countries. *Eur J Cancer* 1993; **12**: 1663–8.

62 Fraser NM, Clarke PR. Cost-effectiveness of breast cancer screening. *Breast* 1992; **1**: 169–72.

63. Mushlin AI, Fintor L. Is screening for breast cancer cost-effective? *Cancer* 1992; **69**: 1957–62.

64 Eddy DM, Hasselblad V, McGivney W *et al.* The value of mammography screening in women under age 50 years. *J Am Med Assoc* 1988; **259**: 1512–19.

65 Tabàr L, Fagerberg G, Duffy SW, Day NE. The Swedish two-county trial of mammographic screening for breast cancer: recent results and calculation of benefit. *J Epidemiol Commun Health* 1989; **43**: 107–14.

65 Kattlove H, Liberati A, Keeler E, Brook R. Benefits and costs of screening and treatment for early breast cancer. *J Am Med Assoc* 1995; **273**: 1512–19.

67 US Congress, Office of Technology Assessment. *Breast cancer screening for Medicare beneficiaries: effectiveness, costs to Medicare and US.* Washington, DC: Government Printing Office, 1987.

68 Gerard K, Salkeld G, Hall J. Counting the costs of mammography screening: first year results from the Sidney Studies. *Med J Austr* 1990; **152**: 466–71.

69 Clarke PR, Fraser NM. *Economic analysis of screening for breast cancer – final report.* Edinburgh: Scottish Home and Health Department, 1991.

70 Brown ML, Fintor L. Cost-effectiveness of breast cancer screening: preliminary results of a systematic review of the literature. *Breast Cancer Res Treat* 1993; **25**: 113–18.

71 van Ballegooijen M, Habbema JDF, van Oortmarssen GJ, Koopmanschap MA, Lubbe JTN, van Agt HME. Preventive Papsmears: striking the balance between costs, risks and benefits. *Br J Cancer* 1992; **65**: 930–3.

72 Glasziou P, Irwig L. The quality and interpretation of mammography screening trials for women aged 40–49. *J Natl Cancer Inst Monogr* 1997; **22**: 73–7.

73 Linver MN, Paster SB. Mammography outcomes in a practice setting by age: prognostic factors, sensitivity, and positive biopsy rate. *J Natl Cancer Inst Monogr* 1997; **22**: 113–17.

74 Frisell J, Lidbrink E, Hellström L, Rutqvist LE. Follow-up after 11 years – update of mortality results in the Stockholm mammographic screening trial. *Breast Cancer Res Treat* 1997; **45**: 263–70.

75 Salzmann P, Kerlikowske K, Phillips K. Cost-effectiveness of extending screening mammography guidelines to include women 40 to 49 years of age. *Ann Intern Med* 1997; **127**: 955–65.

76 Feig SA. Mammographic screening of women aged 40–49 years. Benefit, risk, and cost calculations. *Cancer* 1995; **76**: 2097–106.

77 Gram IT, Lund E, Slenker SE. Quality of life following a false-positive mammogram. *Br J Cancer* 1990; **62**: 1018–22.

78 Elmore JG. Barton MB, Moceri VM, Polk S, Arena PJ, Fletcher SW. Ten-year risk of false-positive screening mammograms and clinical breast examinations. *N Engl J Med* 1998; **338**: 1089–96.

79 Sox HC. Benefit and harm associated with screening for breast cancer. *N Engl J Med* 1998; **338**: 1145–6.

80 Mushlin AI, Kouides RW, Shapiro DE. Estimating the accuracy of screening mammography: a meta-analysis. *Am J Prev Med* 1998; **14**: 143–53.

81 Lidbrink E, Levi L, Pettersson I *et al.* Single-view screening mammography: psychological, endocrine and immunological effects of recalling for a complete three-view examination. *Eur J Cancer* 1995; **31A**: 932–3.

82 Tobias IS, Baum M. False-positive findings of mammography will have psychological consequences. *BMJ* 1996; **312**: 1227.

83 Ellman R, Angeli N, Christians A, Moss S, Chamberlain J, Maquire P. Psychiatric morbidity associated with screening for breast cancer. *Br J Cancer* 1989; **60**: 781–4.

84 Gilbert FJ, Cordiner CM, Affleck IR, Hood DB, Mathieson D, Walker LG. Breast screening: the psychological sequelae of false-positive recall in women with and without a family history of breast cancer. *Eur J Cancer* 1998; **34**: 2010–14.

85 Graversen JP, Blichert-Toft M, Dyreborg U, Andersen J. *In-situ* carcinomas of female breast. Incidence, clinical findings and DBCG proposals for management. *Acta Oncol* 1988; **27**: 679–82.

86 Bailar JC III. Mammography: a contrary view. *Ann Intern Med* 1976; **84**: 77–84.

87 International Commission on Radiological Protection. Recommendations of the International Commission on Radiological Protection. ICRP Publication No. 60. *Ann ICRP* 1991; **21**: 1–3.

88 Mattsson A, Leitz W, Rutqvist LE. Radiation risk and mammographic screening of women from 40 to 49 years of age: effect on breast cancer rates and years of life. *Br J Cancer* 1999.

89 Benjamin W, Corn, Bruce JT, Goodman RL. Irradiation-related ischemic heart disease. *J Clin Oncol* 1990; **8**: 741–50.

90 Neugut AI, Murray BA, Santos J *et al.* Increased risk of lung cancer after breast cancer radiation therapy in cigarette smokers. *Cancer* 1994; **73**: 1615–20.

91 Boice JD, Harvey EB, Blettner M *et al.* Cancer in the contralateral breast after radiotherapy for breast cancer. *N Engl J Med* 1992; **326**: 781–5.

92 Landberg T. The role of radiotherapy in breast-conserving treatment. *Acta Oncol* 1995; **34**: 675–80.

9

Hazards, disadvantages and drawbacks of breast cancer screening

PETR SKRABANEK (with Addendum by JEFFREY S TOBIAS)

INTRODUCTION

Breast cancer screening represents one facet of a 'new' medicine, in which the old tradition of caring for the sick has been replaced, under the slogan 'prevention is better than cure', by emphasis on the surveillance of the healthy. According to the new 'healthist' paradigm, individuals should be responsible for their own health, as most diseases, especially cancer and coronary heart disease, are said to be preventable by a correct lifestyle and regular health-checks.

According to the guidelines for preventive care issued by the American College of Physicians in 1991, a low-risk, healthy woman should attend her physician once a year and, between the ages of 18 and 80 years, have 256 tests, examinations and counselling sessions, including physical examination of her breasts, mammography, and instruction in breast self-examination. This figure does not include recalls for false-positive results. No evidence is provided that such activity would do more good than harm to a healthy woman.

Screening for early disease as a preventive measure only makes sense if early detection and treatment change the natural history of the disease and reduce morbidity and mortality. The screening test should be simple, cheap and accurate. In the case of breast cancer, there is no agreement as to whom to screen, how often, and by what technique. The natural history of breast cancer is poorly

understood, particularly in its early stages, and it is a subject of controversy whether early diagnosis, or delay in diagnosis, is an important determinant of prognosis. There is no agreement on the optimum management of various stages of breast cancer. Randomized controlled trials of breast cancer screening do not provide unequivocal evidence of benefit, and their interpretation hinges upon abstruse statistical 'adjustments'.

Desperate diseases elicit desperate responses. Mass screening programmes have been introduced before critical appraisal of the available evidence, including harm-benefit analysis. As breast cancer is a highly politicized, emotional issue, it is taken for granted that screening must be a good thing. The ethics of offering screening to women without informing them about the uncertainties of benefit and the nature of the risks are not on the agenda of the advocates of screening. As with the rest of preventive medicine, breast cancer screening takes place in an ethical vacuum.[1]

The hazards, disadvantages and drawbacks of breast cancer screening include the following:

- iatrogenic harm caused by over-diagnosis and over-treatment;
- radical treatment of borderline and *in-situ* lesions;
- false-positive results generating false alarms, anxiety and cancerophobia;
- false-negative results providing false reassurance and causing delay in treatment;

- the feeling of guilt in women who did not accept an invitation for screening and who subsequently develop breast cancer;
- early diagnosis adding extra cancer years with benefit of life extension;
- inevitable exploitation of screening hysteria by private business, especially that directed at young women;
- cost-ineffective use of health resources.

THE NATURAL HISTORY OF BREAST CANCER

The crucial element by which the rationale for screening stands or falls is the answer to the following question. Is there an interval in the natural history of breast cancer during which the tumour is large enough to be detectable by screening but can still be in a pre-metastatic stage?

Breast cancer is not a disease, but rather it is a number of different pathological processes with variable course and prognosis. Long-term survival may be determined not by early diagnosis but by the biological nature of the tumour and its intrinsic malignancy. However, 'early' diagnosis in the clinical sense is not 'early' in the biological sense. By the time breast cancer reaches the limit of palpability (about 10 mm in diameter) or detectability by mammography (about 3–5 mm in diameter), the tumour has undergone 28–29 binary divisions. Bauer et al. estimated that by the time the tumour has reached a volume of 125 mL and a diameter of 6mm, 90% of tumours have already metastasized.[2] When the tumour volume reaches 1 mm[3], vasal dissemination of cancer cells has already taken place.[3]

Cancers detected by screening are slower growing and their prognosis is less likely to be affected by a delay in diagnosis, compared to more aggressive tumours that surface between screening sessions. The doubling times of breast cancer growth range from less than 50 to more than 500 days, and an average breast cancer, at the time of being detected 'early', has been growing for 6–10 years.[4] In other words, at the time of detection by screening, the tumour has already passed through 60–70% of its natural history.[5]

As breast cancer is a systematic disease at the time of diagnosis, it is not surprising that loco-regional therapy has no effect on survival. It has been argued for the past 100 years, in the face of contrary evidence, that if patients were diagnosed early, radical mastectomy would cure them all. The refusal to face the reality and the ad-hoc rationalization of therapeutic failure has been compared to the logic adduced by proponents of fringe medicine.[6] According to Baum, chemotherapy seems to provide some benefit for premenopausal women with node-positive disease. For this group, screening has not been shown to have any advantage. The value of chemotherapy for post-menopausal women is questionable, yet it is this group which is invited for screening.

Instead of a vigorous debate about the natural history of breast cancer, the advocates of screening simply ignore the issue. If the premises on which mass screening is based are false, then the promises of such screening only raise false hope. One of the prerequisites of any screening programme is a simple, reliable and accurate test. Mammography fulfils none of these criteria. Hendrick described mammography as 'one of the most difficult forms of radiology'.[7] The architect of the British National Breast Cancer Screening Programme, Sir Patrick Forrest, admitted that 'mammography is not a good screening test. It is not simple and quick to administer, easy to interpret, or cheap'.[8]

These unwelcome observations may be deposited in the professional literature, but tend to be kept away from women invited for screening. Such secrecy is ethically indefensible.

BREAST SELF-EXAMINATION (BSE)

There is something intuitively appealing in promoting BSE, as it costs nothing, and it is widely believed that it causes no harm. Since the beginning of this century, BSE has been recommended by cancer societies as part of their belief that 'early cancer is curable cancer'. For the medical profession, BSE has the additional advantage of placing the responsibility for early diagnosis (and thus the prognosis) on the woman herself.

BSE is a vague term. Most breast cancers are discovered by women themselves accidentally, and even women who adhere to some ritualized form of BSE at regular intervals, a lump may be discovered outside the scheduled BSE. There is no agreement as to the age at which women should start practising BSE, although schoolgirls in their teens are often instructed in BSE as part of their health education. The proportion of false alarms increases sharply with decreasing age.

Frank and Mai pointed out that BSE, far from being harmless, presents three kinds of potential risks,[9] namely anxiety, unnecessary surgical investigations of false-positive findings and false reassurance. The fear that a newly discovered lump is cancer paralyses many women and renders them unable to seek an early appointment with a doctor for further assessment. When the appointment is eventually made, further delays may follow, often weeks or months before a final surgical diagnosis is reached. Even when no lump is found during regular BSE, would the woman's luck hold? To live in fear of death is to fear living.

In women under the age of 30 years, the positive predictive value of BSE is about 1% – that is, out of 100 consecutive biopsies of suspicious lumps, 99 are not cancers. In a randomized trial of BSE in Nottingham, in women aged 45–64 years, the positive predictive value of BSE was 4% – that is, only one in 25 lumps was malignant.[10]

There is no evidence that BSE reduces either morbidity or mortality from breast cancer. As part of the British project for the early detection of breast cancer, two centres (Nottingham and Guildford) used a randomized protocol for BSE. Based on 400 000 woman-years of observation, women randomized to BSE had a slightly higher cumulative breast cancer mortality than the controls (RR 1.04; 95% CI 0.86–1.26).[11] It is now accepted that BSE is an ineffective method of screening and should not be recommended as public health policy.[12]

The force which dogma exerts on common sense is illustrated by a statement in the authoritative Forrest Report which introduced national breast cancer screening in the UK:[13] 'There is no evidence to show that BSE is effective in reducing mortality from breast cancer. Lack of effectiveness should not, however, discourage women from practising BSE.'

In 1991 in the UK, the emotive issues underlying BSE came to the fore again. The outgoing Chief Medical Officer, Sir Donald Acheson, announced that BSE is not a very effective method of detecting breast cancer and could lead to a false sense of security. His successor, Dr Kenneth Calman, agreed 'that there is no convincing evidence that a ritual of monthly BSE reduces deaths,' yet in the same breath he urged women to 'be aware of their breasts in such everyday activities as bathing, showering and dressing.' The Minister of Health, Virginia Bottomley, endorsed Calman's advice and was sure that it would be warmly welcomed by women.[14] Far from being welcomed, the message left many women bewildered and alarmed. They were not told the whole truth, namely that by the time a woman discovers a lump in her breast, the outcome is predetermined by the biological nature of the tumour, which, if it is of metastatic potential, has already metastasized. One journalist pointed out the irrationality of the government's new advice as follows. If BSE does not reduce mortality from breast cancer, and is therefore a waste of time, why should its ritualized form be abandoned only to be replaced by practising it every day?[15]

Even *The Times* entered the fray and devoted an editorial to the controversy (8 October 1991). Abandoning logic, the editorialist attacked Sir Donald Acheson for speaking 'unwisely' and giving 'medically unsound' advice, instead of adhering to the dogma that 'early detection is good medicine – and good medical economics'.

PHYSICAL EXAMINATION (PE)

One of the *ad hoc* explanations for the ineffectiveness of BSE is that women 'do not do it right'. The average diameter of tumours discovered by BSE in two British controlled trials was about 3 cm, the same as that in the controls.[16,17] However, PE by physicians is not much more effective. Even under the best circumstances, when specially trained medical personnel carried out PE, the average size of tumours was 2.5 cm. The National Surgical Adjuvant Breast Project (NSABP) protocols required frequent examinations of contralateral breasts or of ipsilateral breasts (for local recurrence) after surgery, and the average size of tumours discovered by PE was 2.5 cm and 2.4 cm, respectively.[5]

American optimism about the value of mammographic screening is based on their only randomized controlled trial, conducted in the 1960s, namely the Health Insurance Plan of New York (HIP) trial, which claimed a 30% reduction in breast cancer mortality. This result has not been matched since, even using the most sophisticated mammographic technology available. As Forrest admitted, 'if there is any doubt about the HIP study, it is why the results are so good.'[8] Yet, strictly speaking, the HIP trial was not a mammography trial, as PE was part of the protocol, and less than 20% of new breast cancers were detected by mammography alone. As Haagensen and Asch pointed out,[18] the inclusion of mammography would account for the prevention of only 3 deaths per 100 breast cancers.

Some advocates of screening argue that PE is as effective as mammography,[19] without the disadvantages of detecting non-infiltrating lesions with little or no invasive potential. This argument constitutes special pleading, ignores the natural history of breast cancer and begs the question of whether PE is not as ineffective as mammography. The inclusion of PE in the protocol of the Edinburgh randomized controlled trial, in addition to mammography, did not translate into a significant reduction in breast cancer mortality in the screened group.[20]

The confused thinking about the role of PE in breast cancer screening is exemplified by the position taken by A. B. Miller, one of the world experts on breast cancer screening. While admitting that 'early diagnosis has greater prognostic importance than any therapeutic effect', thus implying that the lead time gained by mammography (2–3 years) over PE or BSE gives no extra benefit to screened women, he also maintains that 'there are too few data to indicate whether mammography adds significantly to the benefit yielded by PE or BSE'.[21]

CANADIAN NATIONAL BREAST CANCER SCREENING STUDY (NBSS)

One part of the NBSS study enrolled around 39 000 women, aged 50 to 59 years, for random allocation to either annual mammography and PE, or PE alone. The addition of mammography to PE had no impact on mortality from breast cancer up to 7 years of follow-up.[22] The second part of the NBSS study randomized some 50 000 women aged 40 to 49 years to either annual mammography and PE, or an initial PE alone, while both groups were taught BSE. No benefit of mammography was demonstrated. In fact, the mammography group had more breast cancer deaths than the control group (38 vs. 28 deaths) with 7 years after entry.[23]

These results generated unease among the advocates of screening. The application of Occam's razor would lead to the conclusion that screening, whether by PE, BSE or mammography, does not affect breast cancer mortality. The aftermath of the NBSS trials is illustrative of the entrenched position taken by the advocates of screening, who refuse to accept any evidence which throws doubt on their belief that 'screening is good', while clinging to any flimsy evidence which supports a forgone conclusion. Miller was quoted as follows in the Canadian Cancer Society publication, *Progress Against Cancer*: 'continued follow-up, perhaps to 20 years, may be needed to show reduced mortality'.

The advocates of screening in the USA found the NBSS results completely unacceptable, particularly the suggestion that mammography in women under the age of 50 years is ineffective, and they accused the Canadian trialists of poor standards. Yet far lower standards of mammography in the obsolete HIP trial have never been questioned, as that trial produced the desired results.

An excess of deaths in young women who were offered mammography has been observed on other trials (Malmö, Stockholm and 2-County trials). Various biologically plausible explanations have been put forward to account for this unexpected finding. The fact remains that there is no evidence that mammography in women under the age of 50 years confers any benefit on women who take advantage of it. Many professional bodies, especially in the USA, recommend mammography for younger women, but in the absence of any evidence of its effectiveness, such recommendations are ethically indefensible.[24,25]

To an impartial observer, the advocates of screening are less than honest in the search for truth. For example, B. Goldman, an emergency physician, saw the chorus of criticism of the NBSS results as the wish to destroy the message by shooting the messenger 'indeed the first sound heard following the study's release was the rush of vested-interest groups anxious to attack it', rather than to pause and reflect on it.[26] Similarly, Thomas Chalmers, a pioneer advocate of randomized control trials and of scientific evaluation of medical technologies, noted that 'the vigour of the objections by the clinical experts who are sure that mammography is effective in their hands is reminiscent of the reception received by previous randomized control trials that challenged clinical dogma'.[27]

RANDOMIZED CONTROLLED TRIALS

Of four randomized controlled trials completed by 1990, two did not use individual randomization, but randomization by clusters (the 2-County and Edinburgh trials), and two included PE in addition to mammography (the HIP and Edinburgh trials). The Malmö trial failed to reproduce the optimistic results of the 2-County trial. While the Malmö trial was better planned, executed and reported than another trial, its results were dismissed by the advocates of screening as being based on 'too small numbers'. If 42 000 women followed up for 10 years is too small a number to show clinical benefit, it is legitimate to ask whether the benefit which would satisfy statisticians has any clinical relevance.

It is a well-known phenomenon in medicine that initial claims of therapeutic successes, as reported by enthusiasts, become less impressive with time as more stringent methodological criteria are introduced by unbiased investigators who are attempting to reproduce the original claims. The paradoxical observation of decreasing benefit of screening with increasing sophistication of mammography and better study design would indicate that the initial reports exaggerated the benefit, and raises the question of whether mammography is in any way effective (see Table 9.1). The results of mammography trials are presented in terms of a relative risk reduction in breast cancer mortality. This is a misleading measure of benefit, as it does not take into account the denominator. Thus 50% relative risk reduction is as true for a reduction from 2 per 100 000 to 1 per 100 000 as for a reduction from 2 per 10 to 1 per 10. The respective values for absolute risk reductions are 1:100 000 (i.e. 0.001%) and 1:10 (i.e. 10%).

The reciprocal of the absolute risk reduction provides a practical and easily understandable value, namely the number of patients treated per patient who benefits.[28] Applied to the benefit of screening, the reciprocal is the number of women invited for screening per one breast cancer death prevented or postponed annually. The corresponding numbers for the HIP, 2-County, Edinburgh and Malmö trials are 5000, 13 000, 12 000 and 68 000, respectively.

The HIP and 2-County trials were conducted by enthusiastic advocates of screening and they claimed significant benefits. The Edinburgh and Malmö trials took place in a calmer atmosphere and failed to achieve statistically significant benefits. One of the principals behind the HIP trial was Philip Strax, who believes that 'most women with breast cancer can be saved'. He served as Director of the Guttman Institute which was founded 'primarily to develop methods to stimulate motivation of women to accept the (physical and mammographic) examinations'. Strax has also been a consultant to the Strax Breast Institute. Between them, these two institutes screen 70 000 women annually, 'saving more lives in the process'. Strax feels so strongly about his mission that he has even suggested that 'we must use the hysteria evidenced by the media and exaggerated in the minds of women to stimulate them to accept and even demand mass screening'.[29] Compare these emotive outbursts with the view of Maureen Roberts, Director of the Edinburgh Breast Cancer Screening Project: 'I hope that pressure is not put on women to attend. The decision must be theirs,

Table 9.1 *Results of mammography trials*

	Trial			
	HIP	2-County	Edinburgh	Malmö
Eligible age (years)	40–64	40–74	45–64	45–69
Attendance at first screen (%)	65	89	61	74
Screening interval (years)	1	2–3	1	1.5–2
Screening method	Two-view mammography plus PE	One-view mammography	One-view mammography plus PE	Two-view mammography
Number of screening rounds (%)	4	3–4	7 (mammography in years 1,3,5 and 7; PE in years 2,4 and 6)	6
Woman-years (study)	207 614	545 371	157 946	186 297
Woman years (control)	210 969	389 157	147 854	187 016
Average length of follow-up (years)	7	7	7	9
Deaths from breast cancer (study)	81	124	68	63
Deaths from breast cancer (control)	124	119	76	66
Relative reduction in breast cancer mortality (%)	35	29	17 (NS)	5 (NS)
Absolute reduction in breast cancer mortality (%)	0.02	0.008	0.008	0.001
Number of women invited for screening per one breast cancer death prevented or postponed	5 000	13 000	12 000	68 000

NS, non-significant.

and a truthful account of the facts must be available to the public and the individual patients. It will not be what they want to hear'.[30]

In a recent meta-analysis of five Swedish randomized controlled trials, a significant reduction in breast cancer mortality was achieved in only one trial.[31] All-cause mortality in the pooled mammography groups was 10.0%, compared to 9.4% in the controls. In this sense, not a single life was 'saved'.[32] As mortality from breast cancer in these trials amounted to less than 1% of all deaths, no claims for a reduction in breast cancer mortality can be made before a detailed analysis of the causes of deaths other than breast cancer is performed by an independent death-ascertainment panel. Minor misclassification would annul any claimed benefit (e.g. suicide, car accident, stroke or a second malignancy in a woman with ter-

minal breast cancer classified as breast cancer death in the control group, but as death other than breast cancer in the mammography group).

OVER-TREATMENT

Advanced mammographic techniques are capable of detecting 'cancers' which would not become clinically manifest in the lifetime of a woman. In the 2-County, Edinburgh and Malmö trials, the excess of breast cancer diagnoses in the mammography groups, as compared to the controls, was 40%, 50% and 30%, respectively. The argument put forward by screeners that this is not over-diagnosis, but rather it is early detection prerequisite to a successful screening programme, is gainsaid by the absence of such over-diagnosis in the HIP trial, which was nevertheless the most successful trial.

The scope for over-treatment has been documented by Greenberg and Stevens,[33] who compared the rates of breast surgery in the USA and the UK. Despite the fact that breast cancer mortality is similar in both countries, American women are about twice as likely to have breast surgery as women in the UK, presumably due to enthusiastic promotion of screening mammography in the USA.

Following the introduction of mass screening in Kopparberg County (one of the two counties in the 2-County trial), the rate of breast operations doubled, and it remained about 75% higher than in a neighbouring county, which did not have a screening programme, for the duration of the trial.[34]

'MINIMAL' CANCER (WITH MAXIMAL SURGERY)

Screening mammography has created a new field of breast pathology – a grey area of clinically silent, 'occult', 'minimal', 'precancerous' lesions, including sclerosing and microglandular adenosis, tubular carcinoma, sclerosing duct hyperplasia, juvenile papillomatosis, atypical duct hyperplasia, papillary lesions and carcinoma *in situ*. Interpretation of breast biopsies is a subjective process. When histological slides with ductal carcinoma *in situ* were mixed with various benign proliferative abnormalities and circulated among 18 seasoned histopathologists with a special interest in breast disease, there was a general tendency to over-diagnose and to report benign lesions as malignant. The level of inter-observer and intra-observer agreement was poor.[35] The potential for unnecessary mastectomies is high, and 'even a low over-diagnosis rate can discredit the screening programme'.[36]

While it is true that all large cancers were once small, it does not follow that all small cancers would grow and cause clinical disease. There is a large reservoir of unrecognized disease which can be tapped by special diagnostic techniques, such as mammography, but 'early' diagnosis of this kind, with subsequent therapeutic intervention, is not necessarily beneficial. The true size of the iceberg of breast cancer can be estimated by autopsy studies in women who died of various causes, without any suspicion of breast cancer. A Danish study of 110 consecutive medico-legal autopsies found that about 30–40% of middle-aged women harboured foci of clinically undiagnosed breast cancer or ductal carcinoma *in situ*.[37] With the increasing sensitivity of screening mammography, more such lesions will be detected, ultimately defeating the rationale for screening.[38]

Some American surgeons, impressed by the finding of 'histological' cancer in random biopsies of contralateral breasts in patients with clinical cancer, have performed contralateral 'prophylactic' mastectomies,[39] even though

the clinical incidence of contralateral breast cancer is only about 0.5% annually. The *reductio ad absurdum* of this reasoning would be prophylactic mastectomies in all middle-aged women as a major contribution to the reduction of breast cancer mortality.

The term 'minimal' cancer encompasses both carcinoma *in situ* and invasive cancers less than 0.5 cm (or less than 1 cm) in diameter. The intention behind the coining of this term by Gallagher and Martin was to describe 'breast carcinoma which is readily curable by available means',[40] yet, the term is meaningless, as small invasive cancers are not 'early' in the biological sense. Rosenberg *et al.* found that 40% of clinically occult cancers (less than 1 cm in diameter) were accompanied by positive axillary nodes.[41] On the other hand, carcinoma *in situ* is not a distinct pathological entity. It is arbitrarily defined along a continuous spectrum of progressively more atypical hyperplasia.[42]

CARCINOMA *IN SITU* (DUCTAL)

Before the introduction of screening mammography, carcinoma *in situ* (CIS) (mainly ductal) represented less than 5% of newly diagnosed breast cancers. They were palpable, often very large lesions, in which microinvasion was difficult to exclude. The standard treatment was radical mastectomy.[43] Non-palpable CIS are now common findings in screened women, and in population screening programmes the proportion of CIS lesions among newly discovered breast cancers is of the order of 20–30%. CIS represent about one-third of occult lesions (28%,[44] 38%,[41] 36%[45]).

The discovery of ductal CIS during mass screening creates a serious dilemma for both the surgeon and the patient. As only 25–55% of women with this diagnosis run the risk of developing subsequent invasive cancers,[46] 45–75% of these women will have unnecessary surgery. Total mastectomy is the most likely choice, even though there is no agreement on the optimum management of ductal CIS. Options include observation alone, local resection with or without radiotherapy, and ipsilateral or bilateral total mastectomy.[47]

It is a paradox that pre-malignant lesions are often treated more aggressively than early invasive cancers, for which local excision is now the preferred option. In the absence of reliable data from controlled trials, dogmatic statements are commonplace. For example, Schwartz *et al.* stated categorically that 'we cannot condone any procedure less than total mastectomy for invasive and *in situ* cancer of ductal origin, regardless of the small size of the primary lesion'.[48]

As in the majority of cases, the diagnosis of ductal CIS does not predict the development of clinical cancer in the future. The pathologist is not diagnosing 'cancer', but offering the statistical odds of possible development of cancer in the future. This departure from traditional pathological diagnosis (benign vs. malignant), and its replacement by what might be called 'stochastic pathology,' based on statistical estimates, has profound consequences for the rationale of screening. How many unnecessary mastectomies will be acceptable for one mastectomy which changes the natural history of the disease?

LOBULAR CIS AND PROPHYLACTIC MASTECTOMY

Although both ductal and lobular CIS arise from the same structures, namely the terminal ductules of individual lobules,[42] and some CIS may exhibit the features of both, their histological appearance and natural history are generally quite different. Lobular CIS is not a local precancerous lesion, but a risk marker for the development of ductal or lobular invasive cancer in either breast in about 25% of women with lobular CIS.[46] This makes the dilemma for the surgeon and the patient even more painful than in the case of ductal CIS. Again, therapeutic options range from the wait-and-see policy to mastectomy, although if mastectomy is to be contemplated, it would have to be bilateral.

There is something absurd about trying to prevent cancer by removing organs in which it may arise. Furthermore, it is a poor reward for a woman who has practiced BSE diligently and attended regularly for screening. Lobular CIS is not detected by mammography as such, but it is an accidental finding in 1–3% of breast biopsies, and it is women who practise BSE and participate in screening programmes who have the most unnecessary biopsies. Women who are less health-conscious and who discover breast cancer accidentally are more likely to be treated with breast-conserving surgery.

Some American surgeons are so eager to perform 'prophylactic' bilateral mastectomies that they accept as indications for the operation not only lobular CIS but also benign conditions, such as fibrocystic changes, or even psychological indications, such as cancerophobia.[49]

HARM TO THE PROFESSION

If breast cancer screening is based on false premises and its rationale is incompatible with the natural history of the disease,[4] then mass mammography will have no impact on mortality rates. In the long term, such an outcome would tend to undermine the credibility of the medical profession.

Mass mammography has a deleterious effect on medical practice as it increases the scope for 'defensive' medicine. With a high proportion of false-positive and false-negative mammograms, under-diagnosis or over-diagnosis is inevitable. As the public is led to believe that 'early cancer is curable cancer' and that mammography 'saves lives', dissatisfied patients whose diagnoses were missed on screening will sue their radiologists, pathologists and physicians for malpractice. Similarly, women who suspect that their mastectomy was unnecessary will hire lawyers who will insist on a review of pathological slides and mammograms.

Spratt and Spratt noted that physicians may find themselves involved in lawsuits for causing delays in the diagnosis of breast cancer, even though the natural history of the disease cannot be influenced by 'early' diagnosis.[3] One physician, aware of the fact that to miss breast cancer diagnosis is one of the most expensive mistakes a doctor can make, declared 'I'll continue to screen healthy patients aggressively and pray that nobody slips through the cracks'.[50]

According to the 1988 annual report of an insurance company in St Paul, Minnesota, failure to diagnose cancer was one of the commonest and most costly claims, and 30% of these claims came from breast cancer patients, with an average claim of $100 000.[3]

One form of defensive medicine is the 'defensive' write-up of screening trials. Vital pieces of information are omitted, trials are reported by a 'salami' technique, adverse effects are either not discussed or underestimated, benefits are obfuscated by providing relative percentages, negative trials are dismissed or not cited, criticisms are unanswered and ignored, and the ethical dimension is unacknowledged. Wishful thinking is the bane of medical progress. When invited to testify before the Forrest Committee, I was surprised to hear two of the most eminent public health experts arguing that it was no longer a question of 'if' but of 'what women' and 'how often we should do it'. Yet the evidence available at that time was limited to the HIP trial and the incompletely reported 2-County trial. The committee had recommended mass screening before the negative results of their own trial in Edinburgh were available.

COST-EFFECTIVENESS

Cost-effectiveness is a popular catchcall of our times, but reliable information is difficult to obtain. What is the cost-effectiveness of mammography screening in young women, if more women die in the screened group than in the controls? How do we cost a loss in quality of life? Cost-effectiveness analyses of breast cancer screening range from $14 000 per 'life saved' to $388 000 per extra 10 years of life, and such a range does not inspire confidence in the reliability of the models on which these estimates are based.[51] Eddy calculated that the addition of mammography to physical examination in women aged 50–65 years cost $84 000 for the gain of one extra year of life, and for women aged 40–49 years it was $134 000.[52]

Clearly, mass mammography screening is not an effective use of limited resources. However, any calculations of cost-effectiveness are premature if the fundamental question of whether the benefits of screening outweigh the risks remains unanswered.[53,54]

Rodgers analysed the Edinburgh-Guildford trials and showed that for one breast cancer death prevented or postponed, 14 000 women were invited for screening (of whom 9500 attended), 24 cancers were diagnosed, 700 women were referred for surgical assessment, 24 unnecessary biopsies were performed and 7 cancers were 'interval cancers' (either missed by screening or emerging between subsequent screening rounds).[54]

Schmidt showed that the reduction in risk of dying from breast cancer in women who accepted mammography screening was 10 times less than the annual risk of dying on the road for a car driver driving 14 km a day.[53] Based on the Malmö trial, for each woman whose breast cancer was prevented or postponed, 150 women would have been diagnosed with breast cancer 2–3 years earlier (the lead time of mammography) without any extra benefit. These 'extra cancer years' can be compared to extra time spent on a phantom train which is destined to crash, by boarding it a few stations earlier.

ETHICAL ASPECTS OF MASS BREAST CANCER SCREENING

Mass screening programmes are population experiments in prevention, with uncertain outcomes, otherwise it would be unethical to randomize women in screening trials in such a manner that the controls would be deprived of an established benefit. Furthermore, screened women are not patients but healthy women to whom a promise of an extension of their health is made.[55] For such a promise, much more secure evidence must be available than in the instance of therapeutic medicine when the doctor responds to the patient's request for help and offers whatever is best according to current knowledge, even though many therapies have not been properly assessed.

Experiments[56] on human volunteers are codified, and the individual volunteer is protected by an array of international declarations requiring, among other things, the full disclosure of potential risks and voluntary, competent, informed and understanding consent. Why, then, in mass experiments such as breast cancer screening, is no such protection offered to the women who are invited for screening? Is it due to the fear that, if there was full disclosure of facts, many women would choose not to attend?

It is imperative that women who are invited for breast cancer screening are provided with full information about the magnitude of the expected benefits (in absolute, not relative, terms) and about the nature and likelihood of adverse effects. It is not enough for the advocates of screening to state that the harm-benefit ratio is 'acceptable'. It must also be acceptable to women themselves, when they have had the opportunity to acquaint themselves with the facts.

In an editorial in the *British Medical Journal*, a lawyer and a paediatrician have suggested that 'failure to obtain informed consent for a screening procedure is not only ethically unacceptable but also exposes the health authority to the risk of litigation'.[57]

As it is unlikely that the screening industry will get their house in order, a forum should be set up, at which representatives both of the public and of the medical and legal professions could identify the ethical shortcomings of screening practices and draw up guidelines to protect the public.[58]

CONCLUSION

Good evidence that screening for breast cancer by mammography or physical examination has a major effect on mortality is lacking, and there is therefore no justification for population screening. Morbidity from breast cancer screening is often underplayed.[59] It is ethically indefensible to invite women to attend such examinations without a full and frank discussion of possible harmful effects as well as theoretical benefits. The medical profession does not have sufficient knowledge to reduce mortality from this disease. In particular, its natural history is imperfectly understood.

REFERENCES

1 Skrabanek P. Why is preventive medicine exempted from ethical constraints? *J Med Ethics* 1990; **16**: 187–90.
2 Bauer *et al.* 1980.
3 Spratt JS, Spratt SW. Medical and legal implications of screening and follow-up procedures for breast cancer. *Cancer* 1990; **66**: 1351–62.
4 Skrabanek P. False premises and false promises of breast cancer screening. *Lancet* 1985; **ii**: 316–20.
5 Fisher ER. Pathological considerations in the treatment of breast cancer, In: Grundfest-Broniatowski S, Esselstyn CB (eds). *Controversies in breast disease: diagnosis and management.* New York: Marcel Dekker, 1988: 151–80.
6 Baum M. The epistemology of surgery. In: Dunstan GR, Shine-Gourm EA (eds). *Doctor's decisions.* Oxford: Oxford University Press, 1989; 133–44.
7 Hendrick RE. Mammography quality assurance. Current issues. *Cancer* 1993; **72** (**Supplement**): 1466–74.
8 Forrest P. *Breast cancer: the decision to screen.* London: The Nuffield Provincial Hospitals Fund, 1990.
9 Frank JW, Mai V. Breast self-examination in young women: more harm than good? *Lancet* 1985; **ii**: 654–7.
10 Mant D. Breast self-examination. *Br Med Bull* 1991; **47**: 455–61.
11 UK Trial of Early Detection of Breast Cancer Group. First results on mortality reduction in the UK trial of early detection of breast cancer. *Lancet* 1988; **ii**: 411–16.

12 Clark S. Breast cancer in Europe. *Lancet* 1993; **341**: 429.

13 Forrest P. *Breast cancer screening.* London: The Nuffield Provincial Hospitals Fund, 1987.

14 Gillen D. No need for rituals. *BMJ* 1991; **313**: 876.

15 Grant L. The lump every woman dreads. *The Independent on Sunday,* 6 October 1991.

16 Turner J, Blaney R, Roy D *et al.* Does a booklet on breast self-examination improve subsequent detection rates? *Lancet* 1989; **ii**: 357–9.

17 Philip J, Harris WG, Flaherty C *et al.* Breast self-examination – clinical results from a population-based prospective study. *Br J Cancer* 1984; **50**: 7–12.

18 Haagensen CD, Asch T. Screening for breast carcinoma. In: Haagensen CD, Bodian C, Haagensen DE (eds) *Breast carcinoma: risk and detection.* Philadelphia, PA: WB Saunders, 1981: 501.

19 Mittra I. Breast screening: the case for physical examination without mammography. *Lancet* 1994; **343**: 342–4.

20 Roberts MM, Alexander FE, Anderson TJ *et al.* Edinburgh trial of screening for breast cancer: mortality at seven years. *Lancet* 1990; **335**: 241–6.

21 Miller AB. The role of screening in the fight against breast cancer. *World Health Forum* 1992; **13**: 277–85.

22 Miller AB, Baines CJ, To T, Wall C. Canadian National Breast Cancer Study. II. Breast cancer detection and death rates among women aged 50 to 59. *Can Med Assoc J* 1992; **147**: 1477–88.

23 Miller AB, Baines CJ, To T, Wall C. Canadian Breast Cancer Screening Study. I. Breast cancer detection and death rates among women aged 40 to 49 years. *Can Med Assoc J* 1992; **147**: 1459–76.

24 Jatoi I, Baum M. American and European recommendations for screening mammography in younger women: a cultural divide? *BMJ* 1993; **307**: 1481–3.

25 Elwood JM, Cox B, Richardson AR. The effectiveness of breast cancer screening by mammography in younger women. *Online J Curr Clin Trials* 1993.

26 Goldman B. When considering attacks against the National Breast Cancer Screening Study, consider the sources. *Can Med Assoc J* 1993; **148**: 427–8.

27 Chalmers TC. Editorial: mammography after 30 years. *Online J Curr Clin Trials* 1993.

28 Lampacis A, Sackett DL, Roberts RS. An assessment of clinically useful measures of the consequences of treatment. *N Engl J Med* 1988; **318**: 1728–73.

29 Strax P. Control of breast cancer through mass screening: from research to action. In: Fortner JG, Rhoads JE (eds) *Accomplishments in cancer research (1988) Prize Year. General Motor Cancer Research Foundation.* Philadelphia, PA: Lippincott, 1989: 76–88.

30 Roberts MM. Breast cancer screening: time for a rethink? *BMJ* 1989; **299**: 1153–5.

31 Nystrom L, Rutquist LE, Wall S *et al.* Breast cancer screening with mammography: overview of Swedish randomised trials. *Lancet* 1993; **341**: 973–8.

32 Skrabanek P. Breast cancer screening with mammography. *Lancet* 1993; **341**: 1531.

33 Greenberg ER, Stevens M. Recent trends in breast surgery in the United States and United Kingdom. *BMJ* 1986; **292**: 1487–93.

34 Holmberg DM, Adami H-O, Persson I *et al.* Demands on surgical inpatient services after mass mammography screening. *BMJ* 1986; **296**: 1779–82.

35 Gad A. Ten-years experience from a randomised controlled breast cancer screening programme. II. Diagnostic aspects. In: *Proceedings of a conference on cancer screening.* Florence: Centro per lo studio e la prevenzione oncologica, 1987: 37–8.

36 Dobrossy L. Diagnosing borderline breast cancer (BBC): a public health view – rationale for WHO's involvement in a joint OECI/WHO project. *Arch Geschwulstforsch* 1990; **60**: 227–9.

37 Nielsen M, Thomsen JL, Primdahl S, Dyreborg U, Andersen JA. Breast cancer and atypia among young and middle-aged women: a study of 110 medicolegal autopsies. *Br J Cancer* 1987; **56**: 814–19.

38 Coebergh JWW. Doubts on the future cost-effectiveness and desirability of population-based screening in The Netherlands. *Acta Clin Belg* 1993; **48** (**Supplement 15**): 6–11.

39 Urban JA. Surgical treatment of primary breast cancer – conservative versus radical. In: Lewison EF, Montague ACW (eds) *Diagnosis and treatment of breast cancer.* Baltimore, MD: William & Wilkins, 1981: 119.

40 Gallagher HS, Martin JE. An orientation to the concept of minimal breast cancer. *Cancer* 1971; **28**: 1505–7.

41 Rosenberg AL, Schwartz GF, Feig SA, Patchefsky AS. Clinically occult breast lesions: localisation and significance. *Radiology* 1987; **162**: 167–70.

42 Lagios MD. Human breast precancer: current states. *Cancer Surv* 1983; **2**: 383–402.

43 Gillis DA, Dockerty MB, Clagett OT. Pre-invasion intraductal carcinoma of the breast. *Mayo Clin Proc* 1959; **51**: 521–9.

44 Sickles, EA. Mammographic features of 300 consecutive nonpalpable breast cancers. *Am J Roentgenol* 1986; **146**: 661–3.

45 Meyer JE, Eberlein TJ, Stomper PC, Sonnenfeld MR. Biopsy of occult breast lesions. Analysis of 1261 abnormalities. *J Am Med Assoc* 1990; **262**: 2341–3.

46 Wolmark N. Minimal breast cancer: advance or anachronism? *Cancer J Surg* 1985; **28**: 252.

47 Ketcham AS, Moffat FL. Vexed surgeons, perplexed patients and breast cancers which may not be cancer. *Cancer* 1990; **65**: 387–93.

48 Schwartz GF, Patchefsky AS, Feig SA, Shaker GS, Schwartz AB. Multicentricity of non-palpable breast cancer. *Cancer* 1980; **45**: 2913–16.

49 Dowden RV, Grundfest-Broniatowski S. Prophylactic mastectomy: when and how? In: Grundfest-Broniatowski S, Esselstyn CB (eds) *Controversies in breast disease: diagnosis and management.* New York: Marcel Dekker, 1988: 219–34.

50 Vanzant RC. Screening and informed consent. *N Engl Med* 1993; **329**: 277.

51 Skrabanek P. The cost-effectiveness of breast cancer screening (editorial). *Int J Technol Assess Health Care* 1991; **7**: 633–5.

52 Eddy DM. Screening for breast cancer. *Ann Intern Med* 1989; **111**: 389–99.

53 Schmidt J. The epidemiology of mass breast cancer screening – a plea for a valid measure of benefit. *J Clin Epidemiol* 1990; **43**: 215–39.

54 Rodgers A. To tell or to sell? Informed consent in breast screening. *Cancer Top* 1990; **8**: 27–8.

55 Chamberlain J, Coleman D, Ellmann R *et al*. Sensitivity and specificity in the UK Trial of Early Detection of Breast Cancer. In: Miller AB, Chamberlain J, Day NE *et al*. (eds) *Cancer screening*. Cambridge: Cambridge University Press, 1991: 3–17.

56 Rodgers A. Breast cancer screening – an alternative viewpoint. *West Eng Med J* 1990; **105**: 22–3.

57 Edwards PJ, Hall DM. Screening, ethics and the law. *BMJ* 1992; **305**: 267–8.

58 Skrabanek P. Shadows over screening mammography. *Clin Radiol* 1989; **40**: 4–5.

59 Dixon JM, John TG. Morbidity after breast biopsy for benign lesions in a screened population. *Lancet* 1992; **339**: 128.

ADDENDUM

Although Dr Skrabanek died in 1994, we are honoured to publish what amounted to his final thoughts on a subject to which he had made so many contributions. The world moves on, and Petr Skrabanek would doubtless have been both fascinated by and vocal in his commentary on the emerging evidence on breast screening, particularly the important recent publication from Sweden by Sjönell and Ståhle,[1] which is referred to by Drs Anderssen and Ryden in Chapter 8. This analysis of the 10-year outcome of mammographic screening in daily clinical practice in a large part of Sweden between 1987 and 1996 failed to show a significant reduction in breast cancer mortality.

The study population consisted of women aged 50–69 years, resulting in a total of almost 2 million mammograms, with a participation rate of 79–81% throughout the country. The authors were disappointed by the failure of screening to produce an improvement in mortality over this period, particularly when this was taken together with the substantial anxiety engendered by the studies, in terms of false-positive mammography and, in some cases, months of unresolved uncertainty about whether or not a cancer might be present. The importance of inter-observer variability in breast cancer screening has been recognized for many years.[2] They also pointed out that many thousands of these patients had been unnecessarily exposed to biopsies and even breast surgery, although critics of the Swedish results point out that, in some cases, patients had been diagnosed with cancer prior to the commencement of the screening period and that, in any event, 10 years might not be a long enough period for demonstrating a measurable reduction in mortality. Many critics suggested that the initial screening decade should be regarded as an investment for the future, so further publication of updated data will be of immense importance, particularly as the study population consisted of over 600 000 women, with a high rate of participation (88% for the first invitation to the screening programme and 70–85% for the second and subsequent screening rounds, undertaken at 2-yearly intervals).

Despite the criticisms, Sjönell and Ståhle pointed out that in other screening programmes in the USA, Europe and Sweden, earlier studies had shown a significant reduction in mortality from breast cancer as little as 5–7 years after the introduction of the mammographic programme, and that the trend for a reduction in mortality over this period had been replicated in other studies, although generally it was not as substantial in benefit as the initial studies had predicted. A meta-analysis undertaken in 1993 of all Swedish clinical trials of mammography showed that the mortality in breast cancer was reduced by 28% in women aged 50–69 years, a reduction which was statistically significant from the fifth year onwards, and was seen consistently up until the eighth year.[3] However, it is certainly possible that with increasing awareness about breast cancer, patients with symptomatic or palpable cancers are now presenting at an earlier stage, with correspondingly smaller tumours and better prognosis, and consequently making it more difficult for a further screening benefit to emerge, at least until a point beyond the tenth year of follow-up.

A further recent study from Sweden[4] has shown a substantial concordance between Swedish National Health statistics and the mortality initially reported in the Swedish Clinical Trials of mammographic screening. Indeed, this general agreement made it possible to study whether or not the results of these clinical trials could be reproduced in daily Swedish health-care practice, as pointed out by Sjönell and Ståhle.[1] From the analysis of the annual report of mortality rates, an assessment of the effects of the introduction of screening could reasonably be determined, particularly since the screening programme had commenced in 1989, and therefore a large proportion of the Swedish female population (aged 50–69 years) had undergone a third mammographic assessment by 1994.

It may well be that the maximum benefit from the large study population described and published by Sjönell and Ståhle has not yet been observed. However, the early (10-year) data are clearly at variance with previous results. In view of the high costs and false-positive rates, together with an unacceptable level of negative biopsies, I feel one must conclude that the jury remains firmly out, even allowing for the fact that for a small minority of patients, breast screening can clearly prove to be a life-saving procedure. Many of the current anxieties and concerns were prophetically voiced by Dr Skrabanek as far back as 1985 in his classic critique 'False premises and false promises of breast cancer screening.[5]

REFERENCES

1 Sjönell G, Ståhle L. Mammography screening does not significantly reduce breast cancer mortality in Swedish daily practice. *Läkartidningen* 1999; **96**: 904–13.

2 Howard DH, Elmore JG, Lee CH, Wells CK, Feinstein AR. Observer variability in mammography. *Trans Assoc Am Physicians* 1993: 96–100.

3 Nystrom L, Rutqvist LE, Wall S *et al.* Breast cancer screening with mammography: overview of Swedish randomised trials. *Lancet* 1993; **341**: 973–8.

4 Nystrom L, Larson LG, Rutqvist LE *et al.* Determination of cause of death among breast cancer cases in the Swedish randomised mammography screening trials. *Acta Oncol* 1995; **84**: 145–52.

5 Skrabanek P. False premises and false promises of breast cancer screening. *Lancet* 1985; **ii**: 316–20.

10

The psychological costs of breast screening

STEPHEN SUTTON

INTRODUCTION

Screening programmes, like all medical procedures, have costs as well as benefits. Some costs are relatively easy to assess – for example, the direct financial costs of setting up specialist screening units or the economic cost involved in people taking time off work to attend for screening. Other costs are less tangible but no less important. These are the psychological costs of screening.[1,2] Psychological costs should be included together with financial and other costs when estimating the cost-effectiveness of an existing or proposed screening programme in terms of the gain in quality-adjusted life-years.[3,4] At present, such analyses are precluded by the lack of good data, although on the basis of values assigned by experts, de Haes *et al.* estimated that a programme of biennial mammographic screening for women aged 50–70 years was 8% less effective when an adjustment was made for quality of life.[3] They considered this adjustment to be too small to influence the decision to introduce a large-scale breast cancer screening programme. This chapter will not attempt to assess the cost-effectiveness of breast screening. Its aim is less ambitious, namely to review the evidence concerning the psychological costs of breast screening, focusing particularly on anxiety and distress.

A number of commentators have suggested that anxiety aroused by breast screening, particularly among women with false-positive results, may significantly offset the benefits of reduced mortality and less severe treatment.[5–8] This chapter, which extends and updates an earlier review,[9] will highlight some of the issues relating to anxiety and breast screening, review the findings from the major published studies, and make recommendations for future research. The psychological issues associated with being at high risk for developing breast cancer because of a strong family history or genetic predisposition are discussed in Chapter 7, so will not be addressed here. The present chapter is limited to population screening programmes for breast cancer in which there is no attempt to select women on the basis of risk factors (other than age).

WHAT IS ANXIETY?

The word 'anxiety' is used in many different ways. It may be used to refer to worry or concern about getting breast cancer, to a transient mood state (as might be experienced just prior to undergoing an unfamiliar medical procedure), or to severe anxiety symptomatic of psychiatric morbidity. Related terms encountered in the literature include stress, distress, psychological impact, psychological costs or side-effects, psychological well-being and reassurance. Terms such as psychological costs and quality of life would include other adverse states, emotions or conditions such as anger, resentment, depression and anticipation of pain, as well as fatigue, sexual dysfunction, helplessness, dissatisfaction with social relationships, and inability to work.

In addressing the question of the psychological impact of breast screening, it is useful to consider the various stages in the screening process and the different subgroups of women that it generates. The emotional trauma associated with the diagnosis of breast cancer and all that this entails is well established, but there exists the possibility that psychological disturbance may be more common or more severe among women with screen-detected as opposed to symptomatic cancer. Women who are recalled for further investigation of an abnormal mammogram and who are subsequently declared normal ('false-positives') may be incompletely reassured and may react with feelings of anger as well as anxiety. They may also be less likely to reattend for future mammograms. Women who are placed on early recall may suffer anxiety arising from feelings of uncertainty. Receiving the letter of invitation, undergoing the screening test itself, and waiting for and receiving the letter of results may also arouse anxiety in some women, even among the vast majority who receive a negative result. Other women may gain from the experience through the reassurance conferred by a negative result, while yet others may be inappropriately reassured and conclude that they do not need to undergo further screening. Women who receive a negative result but who subsequently develop symptoms ('false-negatives') may differ in their emotional reactions from other women with symptomatic cancer. It is clear that there are many opportunities for anxiety to be aroused during the screening process. In all of these examples, the immediate family as well as the woman herself may be affected. Finally, publicity about the breast screening programme could raise the level of 'cancerophobia' and general anxiety in the unscreened population.

In trying to assess whether or not anxiety is a significant problem in the context of breast screening, it has to be remembered that anxiety is a normal part of everyday life and an accepted concomitant of routine medical procedures such as going to the dentist. It may have positive as well as negative effects. For example, concern about breast cancer may motivate women to attend for screening, and false alarms may prompt women to examine themselves regularly for lumps and to adopt cancer-preventive actions. The arousal of mild and short-lived anxiety in a proportion of women who participate in the breast screening programme should not be regarded as a problem or as a cost of screening. Anxiety only becomes a problem if it is severe, enduring, or has an adverse impact on other aspects of life and psychological functioning. For instance, if the anxiety aroused by going for a first breast screen was to deter a woman from going again or from having other types of check-up, it would be reasonable to regard this as a cost of screening. It would be useful to compare the levels of anxiety aroused during breast screening with those aroused during other commonplace medical procedures. To my knowledge, no studies have done this to date.

REVIEW OF THE MAJOR PUBLISHED STUDIES

Although a number of studies in the breast screening literature and numerous surveys of user satisfaction have included measures of anxiety, only a handful of studies have attempted systematically to assess the magnitude and duration of changes in anxiety at different stages in the screening process. These studies have used a variety of designs and measuring instruments, and the findings are not amenable to meta-analysis or quantitative synthesis. Each study will therefore be summarized in turn in chronological order of publication. With two exceptions, all of the studies were conducted in the UK, some prior to the introduction of a national screening programme in 1988 and some subsequent to this.

Dean et al.[10] gave a 30-item version of the General Health Questionnaire (GHQ) to 290 first-time attenders at a breast screening clinic while they were waiting to be screened, and again 6 months later.[11] Women who were recalled for further assessment were excluded from the sample. The mean GHQ score was low (around 2.0) and did not differ significantly on the two occasions. The 'case rate' (prevalence of psychiatric morbidity) based on a cut-off score of 3 also remained virtually the same (around 17%). There was no difference in the psychiatric morbidity of the screened sample compared to that of a matched randomly sampled community control group. When questioned at follow-up, 30% of the attenders said that they were made anxious by receiving the first letter of invitation, and 20% said they found the screening procedure itself anxiety-arousing. On the other hand, the procedure was found to be reassuring by 86% of women, and only 9% complained of not feeling reassured by the time they left the clinic. Only 8% of the attenders thought screening had made them more anxious about developing breast cancer.

In a similar study, Ellman et al. administered the GHQ to 302 screening clinic attenders immediately before and 3 months after they were screened.[12] Initially, 25% were classified as probable cases of psychiatric morbidity, but this figure fell significantly to 19% at follow-up. This study was conducted in a well-established annual screening programme, and the great majority of attenders had been screened in previous years. Any increases in anxiety would therefore be expected to be smaller than those among first-time attenders. The case rate in a comparison group of 300 false-positives was initially slightly, but non-significantly higher than among the routinely screened women (30% vs. 25%), and fell to the same level (19%) at 3 months. Scores on the anxiety subscale were initially significantly higher among the false-positives than among the screening clinic attenders but this difference was no longer evident at follow-up.

Bull and Campbell[13] sent the Hospital Anxiety and Depression Scale (HADS)[14] to four groups of women, namely 750 women invited for screening (group A), 420 women who had a normal mammogram (group B), 240 women who were declared normal after further assessment (group C), and 68 women who were declared normal after open biopsy (group D). Women in group A were sent the questionnaire with the invitation, and women in groups B, C and D were sent it six months after a normal result was declared. The HADS results showed no evidence of an increase in anxiety or depression across the four groups, whether this was assessed by comparing mean scores or the percentages showing abnormal levels of anxiety or depression. Indeed, if anything there was a decrease in anxiety and depression. When asked the question 'Has the screening left you more anxious about having breast cancer, less anxious, or unchanged?' (groups B, C and D only), 10% said more anxious and 41% less anxious, i.e. there was a net reduction in anxiety. On the other hand, 10% of women in group D reported examining themselves for lumps more often than once a week, and the authors concluded that this group may require professional counselling.

In a Norwegian study, Gram et al. found a significantly higher prevalence of breast cancer anxiety 6 months after screening among false-positives than among women who received negative results (40% vs. 22%).[15,16] The second figure was significantly lower than in an uninvited population sample, suggesting that the negative screenees had been reassured. The difference between the false-positives and the negative screenees was still evident 1 year later (29% vs. 13%). The 1990 report contains detailed comparisons between these groups on various quality of life measures. The authors summarize the results as follows:

> A false-positive mammogram was described by 7 (5%) of the women as the worst thing they had ever experienced. However, most women with a false-positive result regarded this experience, in retrospect, as but one of many minor stressful experiences creating a temporary decrease in quality of life. They report the same quality of life today as women with negative screening results, and 98% would attend another screening.

Lerman et al. in the USA compared women with high-suspicion mammograms, low-suspicion mammograms and normal mammograms 3 months after screening.[17,18] The three groups differed significantly in the expected direction on a number of questions, including anxiety about the results of future mammograms, current tendency to worry about developing breast cancer, and current impairment of mood and daily activities because of worry about breast cancer. Attendance rates for subsequent screening did not differ.

Important data on the frequency of false-positive results have recently been published for a cumulative 10-year period.[19] This study, from centres in Seattle and Boston, assessed the 10-year risk of false-positive screening mammograms over a 10-year period among 2400 women aged 40–69 years at entry to the study.[19] Mammograms or clinical breast examinations that were interpreted as indeterminate, aroused a suspicion of cancer, or prompted recommendations for additional work-up for women in whom breast cancer was not then diagnosed during the following year were all considered to be 'false-positive' tests. The results showed that of the women who were screened, almost a quarter (23.8%) had at least one false-positive mammogram, and 13.4% had

at least one false-positive breast examination, for a final result of 32% having at least one false-positive result for either test. Over the full interval the estimated cumulative risk of a false-positive result was almost 50% after 10 mammograms, and half this figure (22%) after 10 clinical breast examinations. These false-positive tests led to many hundreds of out-patient appointments, diagnostic mammograms, ultrasound tests and biopsies. The authors estimated that among women who do not have breast cancer, 18.6% will undergo biopsy after 10 mammogram investigations, and for every $100 spent on screening, an additional $33 was spent to evaluate the false-positive result. It was clear from the data that false-positive rates were higher for younger than for older women – just under 8% (for each investigation) for women aged 40–49 years but only 4.4% for women aged 70–79 years.

In the study by Walker et al.,[20] 1635 women completed the HADS at baseline before they knew they were going to receive an invitation to attend for screening and again at screening 6 weeks later. Anxiety and depression scores were significantly *lower* at screening than at baseline, although the changes were quite small in absolute terms. Women who scored in the borderline range at baseline were more likely to move into the normal than the clinically significant range for both anxiety and depression, and women who scored in the clinically significant range for anxiety were more likely to become normal than *vice versa*. Thus there was no suggestion that women with borderline scores at the time of the survey were especially vulnerable. Attenders reported various stress-related changes in their behaviour and feelings during the week prior to breast screening. For example, more women reported that their sleeping habits, ability to stop worrying, ability to relax and concentrate and level of irritability had been 'worse than normal' as opposed to 'better than normal'. However, the majority of women reported that their behaviour and feelings had been 'normal' during this week. It is not possible to tell whether these stress-related 'changes' represent genuine changes in behaviour and feelings related to the impending screening attendance, as the questions were not asked at baseline.

Sutton et al. followed a large cohort of women through the screening process,[21] with anxiety measures at several key points – at baseline (prior to the screening invitation), at the screening clinic (either immediately before or immediately after screening) and at follow-up (about 9 months after baseline). The instruments used included the Spielberger State-Trait Anxiety Inventory (STAI) questionnaire[22] and the anxiety subscale of the GHQ. On average, the women were not unduly anxious at any of the three time-points in the screening process. Among attenders, there was no significant difference between state anxiety levels immediately before and after screening. As in the study by Walker et al.,[20] anxiety was lowest at the clinic and highest at baseline, but the changes were rather small. Again, as in the earlier study, anxiety did not predict attendance – there were no differences in anxiety levels between attenders and non-attenders at baseline. As expected, women who received false-positive results recalled feeling extremely anxious after they had received the referral letter, but their retrospective anxiety was also higher than in the negative screenees at earlier stages in the screening process before they knew their results. They also reported having experienced more pain and discomfort during the X-ray.

A further more recent study was reported by Gilbert et al.,[23] who evaluated the psychological effects of false-positive mammography screening in 124 women who had taken part in the UK National Health Service Breast Screening Programme. In addition, the effects of recall on women with and without a family history were compared. Both at the screening and at recall, these women were asked to complete a health questionnaire which has been validated as demonstrating changes in stress-related behaviour over the previous week. In the week before screening, compared to women who did not have a family history of breast cancer, those with a positive family history had lower scores on the standard depression scales, and also reported fewer stress-related behavioural changes. At recall, regardless of family history, the women were more likely to have a borderline or clinically significant anxiety than at baseline for screening. None the less, for most women their recall-induced anxiety was relatively transient, lasting less than 1 month. Compared to women without a family history, those with a family history were more anxious up to 4 months after recall, although their anxiety scores tended to be somewhat lower than at the baseline evaluation. The view of the authors was that breast screening programmes must ensure that steps are taken to minimize the number of women who are recalled for unnecessary investigations.

SUMMARY AND INTERPRETATION OF FINDINGS

The overall picture that emerges from these studies is that anxiety does not seem to be a serious problem in routinely screened women who receive a negative result. This finding is important from a public health viewpoint because negative screenees are numerically a very large group and represent the vast majority of women who participate in population breast screening programmes. The findings from the two most recent studies were remarkably similar, despite the fact that different questionnaires were used. Using repeated measures on the same women, both studies showed a significant *reduction* in anxiety between baseline and screening, instead of the predicted increase. One interpretation of the observed pattern of change in the study by Sutton et al.[21] is that the baseline questionnaire and covering letter prompted many women to think about the prospect of breast

screening for the first time, and thus produced a slight increase in anxiety. Thus the initial measure of anxiety may not have been a true baseline. It may also have served to prepare the women for the forthcoming invitation for screening, and pre-empted some of the anxiety that this communication might otherwise have aroused. However, this explanation cannot account for the results of the study by Walker et al.,[20] since the women in that study did not know at baseline that they were soon to be invited for screening – the baseline measure of anxiety was uncontaminated by the knowledge of impending screening. An alternative explanation, which could apply to both studies, would postulate a measurement artefact. There is some evidence that a second administration of the GHQ tends to yield lower scores than the first administration,[24] suggesting that the first measure is reactive – completing an anxiety questionnaire for the first time may itself be slightly anxiety-provoking. The same effect may occur with the Spielberger and HADS questionnaires. The existence of such effects would have important implications for any studies that use questionnaires to assess negative mood states. This phenomenon needs to be investigated using a number of different questionnaires. In particular, the effects of varying the time interval between measures and the number of administrations need to be examined.

Not surprisingly, women who receive false-positive results show evidence of anxiety and other negative sequelae. As pointed out in a recent editorial by Sox,[25] false-positive results produce anxiety and complications, and are expensive. Three months after a mammogram regarded as highly suspicious turned out to be falsely positive, worry adversely affected the mood of 26% of women in one study, compared to 9% where the mammogram was normal.[17] The most plausible interpretation of the findings from the study by Sutton et al.[21] is that these women's memories of the earlier stages of screening were tainted by their later experiences. An alternative explanation is that they really were more anxious at these earlier stages than the negative screenees and they really did experience more pain. Gram and Slenker reported a similar finding which they interpreted in terms of possible physical differences between the false-positives and the negative screenees:[16] 'women in the FP (false-positive) group have breasts that are more difficult to examine due to size or density, thus necessitating a stronger and more painful compression of the breasts' (p.251). There is no evidence that bears directly on this suggestion, although Rutter et al. found that pain and discomfort during mammography were unrelated to bust size and physical build.[26]

A number of consistent predictors of attendance for breast screening have been identified, including the practice of other health-related behaviours and beliefs, attitudes and intentions with regard to breast screening.[27,28] Prior to the studies by Walker et al.[20] and Sutton et al.,[21] anxiety and depression had not been investigated as potential predictors of attendance. These studies showed no differences between attenders and non-attenders at baseline on anxiety or depression. Thus there is no evidence that breast screening programmes tend to attract women who are psychologically more or less healthy than average. However, it should be remembered that it is much more difficult to obtain information from non-attenders than from attenders. In studies of breast screening, response rates to questionnaires are consistently lower among non-attenders even when address inaccuracies are taken into account. This may bias the comparison of attenders and non-attenders. It is possible that women who neither return a questionnaire nor attend for screening represent a particularly anxious group.

RECOMMENDATIONS FOR FUTURE RESEARCH

Given the paucity of hard data on anxiety and other potential psychological costs of breast screening, it is important that research continues to investigate these issues. The following section will outline a number of areas for future research.

Most studies to date have used the STAI, GHQ and HADS. These were designed as general measures of anxiety, depression or psychiatric morbidity. However, they were not designed to be specific to breast cancer and breast screening. It is quite possible that a medical procedure may have no detectable effect on general anxiety but a substantial effect on cancer-specific or breast cancer-specific worry or anxiety. The Psychological Consequences Questionnaire (PCQ) was developed by Cockburn et al. specifically to measure the psychological sequelae of mammographic screening.[29] However, it has been used in only one study to date, and requires further psychometric investigation to examine its factor structure.

All of the studies reviewed above used structured self-completion questionnaires. It has been suggested that unstructured personal interviews may give a rather different picture.[30] With cervical screening, adverse effects emerged more strongly in studies in which data were collected via face-to-face interviews.[31,32] In future studies of anxiety and breast screening, an attempt should be made to supplement data from self-completion questionnaires with more qualitative data.

An interesting issue raised by the paper by Sutton et al. concerns the difference between contemporaneous and retrospective measures of anxiety.[21] Contemporaneous measures ask people how they are feeling now (or how they have been feeling very recently), whereas retrospective measures ask people to recall how they were feeling at some time-point in the past. The relationship between the two needs to be studied using comparable measures. This could be extended to other aspects of the experience of mammography. For instance, it is possible that remembered pain differs from pain experienced at the time with regard to intensity or duration. It would also be of interest to study anticipated anxiety and pain.

Apart from the study by Lerman et al., no studies have investigated the behavioural consequences of anxiety. A woman who has a bad experience of screening may be less likely to return for subsequent screening. The factors that predict reattendance for breast screening need to be investigated and the role of anxiety studied in this context. On the other hand, repeated attendance for breast screening may be associated with a reduction in anxiety over time, particularly between the first and second occasions. A similar process may also occur at a societal level. A new screening procedure may arouse anxiety at first, but as it becomes a familiar and accepted part of health service provision it may lose its emotional impact. Another possibility is that screenees still experience anxiety when they are participating in an established programme, but that they tolerate this and the other negative aspects better than they would do in the case of a newly introduced programme.

The issue of individual differences in vulnerability to anxiety has received little attention in the literature on anxiety and breast screening. Some women experience or report more anxiety than others, and some show greater reactivity (i.e. greater changes in anxiety) in response to screening-related events. It is important to investigate the factors that influence and moderate anxiety. Sutton et al. examined demographic correlates of anxiety and found a consistent effect of age.[21] Even within the restricted age range studied (50–64 years), the younger women were significantly more anxious. Further research is needed to explore the basis of this effect. Personality factors may moderate the effects of screening on anxiety. Miller distinguished between *monitoring* and *blunting* styles of coping.[33] In the present context, monitors would be predicted to seek out information about breast cancer and breast screening, while blunters would tend to avoid such information. This distinction has obvious implications for cancer education. Monitoring–blunting is assessed using the Behaviour Style Questionnaire.[33] In studies of ovarian screening and colposcopy using this questionnaire, women with an information-seeking coping style showed higher levels of distress.[34] One might expect to find a similar association in the context of breast screening. In addition, coping style may act as a moderator. Not only may information-seekers be more distressed, but they may also show greater increases in anxiety in response to screening-related events than information-avoiders.

CONCLUSIONS

The studies published to date are generally encouraging in suggesting that anxiety is not a significant problem among women who receive a negative screening result. On the other hand, women who receive false-positive results show more evidence of adverse psychological impact consistent with a temporary diagnosis of breast cancer. However, it should be emphasized, that the evidence base is small and there are many aspects of this complex issue which have not yet been addressed. It is important that research continues to investigate the potential psychological costs, as well as the benefits of breast screening. To the extent that anxiety is shown to be a problem among particular subgroups of women generated by a breast screening programme, we shall then need to focus our attention on evaluating ways of reducing or minimizing psychological distress by modifying the information that is given to women, or by offering additional advice, support and counselling.[35]

ACKNOWLEDGEMENTS

I would like to thank the Imperial Cancer Research Fund for financial support.

REFERENCES

1 Marteau TM. Psychological costs of screening. *British Medical Journal* 1989; **299**: 527.

2 Wardle J, Pope R. The psychological costs of screening for cancer. *Journal of Psychosomatic Research* 1992; **36**: 609–24.

3 De Haes JCJM, de Koning HJ, van Oortmarssen GJ, van Agt HME, de Bruyn AE, van der Maas PJ. The impact of a breast cancer screening programme on quality-adjusted life years. *International Journal of Cancer* 1991; **49**: 538–44.

4 White E, Urban N, Taylor V. Mammography utilization, public health impact, and cost-effectiveness in the United States. *Annual Review of Public Health* 1993; **14**: 605–33.

5 Roberts MM. Breast screening: time for a rethink? *British Medical Journal* 1989; **299**: 1153–5.

6 Schmidt JG. The epidemiology of mass breast cancer screening – a plea for a valid measure of benefit. *Journal of Clinical Epidemiology* 1990; **43**: 215–25.

7 Tobias JS, Baum. False-positive findings of mammography will have psychological consequences. *British Medical Journal* 1996; **312**: 1227.

8 Wright C. Breast cancer screening: a different look at the evidence. *Surgery* 1986; **100**: 594–8.

9 Sutton SR. Experiences of screening: anxiety issues. In: Austoker J, Patnick J (Eds) *Report of UKCCCR/NHSBSP Workshop. Breast screening acceptability: research and practice.* NHSBSP Publication No. 28. Sheffield: NHSBSP, 1993.

10 Dean C, Roberts MM, French K, Robinson S. Psychiatric morbidity after screening for breast cancer. *Journal of Epidemiology and Community Health* 1986; **40**: 71–5

11 Goldberg DP, Williams P. A user's guide to the General Health Questionnaire. Windsor: NFER-Nelson, 1988.

12 Ellman R, Angeli N, Christians A, Moss S, Chamberlain J, Maguire P. Psychiatric morbidity associated with screening for breast cancer. *British Journal of Cancer* 1989; **60**: 781–4.

13 Bull AR, Campbell MJ. Assessment of the psychological impact of a breast screening programme. *British Journal of Radiology* 1991; **64**, 510–15.

14 Zigmond AS, Snaith RP. The Hospital Anxiety and Depression Scale. *Acta Psychiatrica Scandinavica* 1983; **67**: 361–70.

15 Gram IT, Lund E, Slenker SE. Quality of life following a false-positive mammogram. *British Journal of Cancer* 1990; **62**: 1018–22.

16 Gram IT, Slenker SE. Cancer anxiety and attitudes toward mammography among screening attenders, non-attenders, and women never invited. *American Journal of Public Health* 1992; **82**: 249–51.

17 Lerman C, Trock B, Rimer BK, Boyce A, Jepson C, Engstrom PF. Psychological and behavioral implications of abnormal mammograms. *Annals of Internal Medicine* 1991; **114**: 657–61.

18 Lerman C, Trock B, Rimer BK, Jepson C, Brody D, Boyce A. Psychological side-effects of breast cancer screening. *Health Psychology* 1991; **10**: 259–67.

19 Elmore JG, Barton MB, Moceri VM, Polk S, Arena PJ, Fletcher SW. Ten-year risk of false-positive screening mammograms and clinical breast examinations. *New England Journal of Medicine* 1998; **338**: 1089–96.

20 Walker LG, Cordiner CM, Gilbert FJ *et al*. How distressing is attendance for routine breast screening? *Psycho-Oncology.* 1994; **3**: 299–304.

21 Sutton S, Saidi G, Bickler G, Hunter J. Does routine screening for breast cancer raise anxiety? Results from a three-wave prospective study in England. *Journal of Epidemiology and Community Health* 1995; **49**: 413–18.

22 Spielberger CD. *Manual for the State-Trait Anxiety Inventory STAI-Form Y.* Palo Alto, CA: Consulting Psychologists Press, 1983.

23 Gilbert FJ, Cordiner CM, Affleck IR, Hood DB, Mathieson D, Walker LG. Breast screening: the psychological sequelae of false-positive recall in women with and without a family history of breast cancer. *European Journal of Cancer* 1998; **34**: 2010–14.

24 Goldberg DP. Manual of the General Health Questionnaire. Windsor: NFER-Nelson 1978.

25 Sox HC. Benefit and harm associated with screening for breast cancer. *New England Journal of Medicine* 1998; **338**: 1145–6.

26 Rutter DR, Calnan M, Vaile MSB, Field S, Wade KA. Discomfort and pain during mammography: description, prediction and prevention. *British Medical Journal* 1992; **305**: 443–5.

27 Calnan M. Predictors of attendance. In: Austoker J, Patnick J (Eds) *Report of UKCCCR/NHSBSP Workshop. Breast screening acceptability: research and practice.* NHSBSP Publication No. 28. Sheffield: NHSBSP, 1993.

28 Sutton SR, Bickler G, Sancho-Aldridge J, Saidi G. Prospective study of predictors of attendance for breast screening in inner London. *Journal of Epidemiology and Community Health* 1994; **48**: 65–73.

29 Cockburn J, De Luise T, Hurley S, Clover K. Development and validation of the PCQ: a questionnaire to measure the psychological consequences of screening mammography. *Social Science and Medicine* 1992; **34**: 1129–34.

30 Wardle J, Pernet A, Stephens D. Psychological consequences of positive results in cervical cancer screening. *Psychology and Health* 1995; **10**: 185–94.

31 Beresford JM, Gervaize PA. The emotional impact of abnormal pap smears on patients referred for colposcopy. *Colposcopy and Gynecologic Laser Surgery* 1986; **2**: 83–7.

32 Posner T, Vessey M. *Prevention of cervical cancer: the patient's views.* London: King's Fund, 1988.

33 Miller SM. When is a little knowledge a dangerous thing? Coping with stressful events by monitoring versus blunting. In: Levine S, Ursin H (Eds) *Coping and health: Proceedings of a NATO conference. New York: Plenum Press,* 1980.

34 Wardle FJ, Collins W, Pernet AL, Whitehead MI, Bourne TH, Campbell S. Psychological impact of screening for familial ovarian cancer. *Journal of the National Cancer Institute* 1993; **85**: 653–7.

35 Marteau TM. Reducing the psychological costs. *British Medical Journal* 1990; **301**: 26–8.

11

Methodological issues in the design of chemoprevention trials

JACK CUZICK

INTRODUCTION

Interventions aimed at preventing disease offer new scope, but also challenging new problems, for the now cherished randomized clinical trial. Not only are the logistic problems formidable, but the fundamental principles upon which trial methodology is based require adaptation, extension, and further elaboration. In this chapter, the main issues will be discussed in the context of the prevention of breast cancer. The chapter is divided into two main sections. In the first section, fundamental principles are discussed. These include the following:

- interventions aimed at early- vs. late-stage events in carcinogenesis;
- use of high-risk groups vs. volunteers from the general population;
- the balance of beneficial vs. potential adverse effects in a prevention setting;
- the need for long-term follow-up and high compliance over several years of treatment;
- monitoring results from other studies while conducting the trial.

In the second section, these principles will be applied to the design of a chemoprevention trial for breast cancer, and the following specific points are considered:

- the need for randomization;
- the use of a placebo and double-blind trials;
- provision for a run-in period;
- choice of endpoint(s);
- number of patients;
- factorial designs of more than one agent;
- recruitment strategies.

These points are illustrated by considering the design aspects of a trial of the oestrogen agonist tamoxifen. The issues are also relevant to trials of other potential chemopreventive agents, such as retinoids and new oral contraceptives, and also for dietary intervention trials.

FUNDAMENTAL PRINCIPLES

Early- vs. late-stage prevention

Carcinogenesis is a multi-stage process in which several steps must occur, possibly in no particular order, before cancer appears. The time between the early events and clinical cancer may well be 20 to 30 years or more for solid tumours, and this is illustrated in breast cancer by the fact that irradiation during adolescence and in the late teens can increase the risk of breast cancer more than 20 years later,[1-3] and that the age of menarche and age at first childbirth are important risk factors for breast cancer, even in postmenopausal women.[4-5] In addition, early-stage events, which in most cases probably involve mutation or some other fundamental alteration of DNA, are probably very common and are a result of many different sources of exposure. Most of these changes are not destined to progress to cancer, and will spontaneously revert to normal. Thus for an agent to be effective, it will have to have a broad spectrum of activity and be very free of side-effects, since a woman treated in her teenage years or in the following decade will still have all of her reproductive and adult life ahead of her.

Measures aimed at reducing or counteracting early-stage factors are extremely difficult to evaluate because a 30- to 40-year follow-up is required, and a study could well exceed the working career of the investigators who designed and initiated the trial. Thus a provision for such long-term trials to be handed over to the next generation of investigators is essential. The women being studied are also likely to have moved during the follow-up, possibly several times, and to have changed their name if they have married.

Trials aimed at counteracting or preventing late-stage (so called 'promoter') events are logistically more feasible. In breast cancer, there are well-documented risk factors which occur at an age close to that at which the incidence of breast cancer is high, notably age at menopause, certain types of benign breast disease with epithelial proliferation and atypia, and mammographic dysplasia seen in the course of routine screening for breast cancer. These factors may be due to a particular hormonal environment, or they may simply be markers which indicate that a woman is at high risk for some other reason. In any case, the fact that an early age at menopause, either occurring naturally or produced by artificial means, can dramatically reduce breast cancer risk indicates that hormonal changes in women above the age of 40 years can have a marked influence on the subsequent incidence of breast cancer.[6] It can be seen from Figure 11.1 that women who have an artificial menopause before the age of 40 years are at less than half the risk of women whose menopause occurs after the age of 50 years and that a 5-year difference in the age at menopause leads to a difference of about 25% in the breast cancer rates. Moreover, since the incidence of breast cancer is already high by the age of 45 years, much of the protective effect of any planned intervention that is begun after the age of around 40 years is likely to become apparent within the first 10 years of follow-up. It is also

worth noting that a non-toxic cytostatic agent which arrests the growth of preclinical cancerous lesions for 5 to 10 years also represents effective prevention of clinical breast cancer, and from a practical point of view is nearly as effective as true prevention. Thus the goals of a trial to tackle the later stages of carcinogenesis need be less ambitious, and the answers will become available within a shorter time period.

Use of high-risk groups vs. volunteers from the general population

From the perspective of managing a trial, and in the interests of cost, it is very useful to be able to concentrate attention on a high-risk group. This is because the power of a trial depends on the number of end-points (breast cancers), and if the trial could, say, be focused on a population that has a four-fold relative risk of breast cancer, then only a quarter of the number of volunteers would be needed. This is an important consideration when contemplating interventions that will involve tens of thousands of women. It also has advantages in terms of safety, because any untoward side-effects that may occur either during treatment or at a late stage are more favourably balanced by the prospects of a much greater reduction in the absolute incidence of this disease.

However, there are some disadvantages to using a high-risk subgroup.[7] One theoretical problem is that the results obtained from one high-risk group may not be generalizable to the entire population. However, this concern can be overstated, as there is no indication that the clinical course of breast cancer has anything to do with specific risk factors. However, the difference in risk, particularly genetic risk, between the patients in the

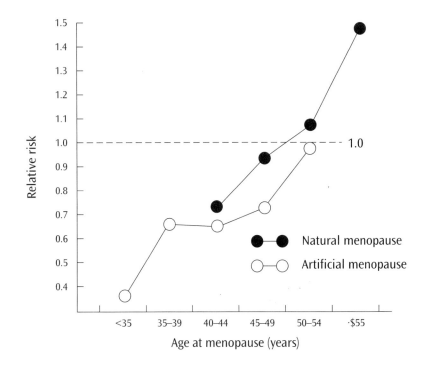

Figure 11.1 *Risk of breast cancer according to age at natural or artificial menopause.*

NSABP–P1 trial[8] and those in the Royal Marsden trial[9] has been suggested as one explanation for the conflicting findings. A further problem relates to the anxiety that could be generated by telling a woman that she is at high risk of breast cancer. This can be especially difficult in a trial situation, as only half of the women can be offered active treatment, and also one has to admit that the efficacy in a prevention setting of the agents under test is unknown (otherwise the trial would be unethical).

Practical concerns in finding and approaching a high-risk group are more important and require careful consideration. The first of these involves finding a truly high-risk group of reasonable size. Most known risk factors have a risk of about twofold and jointly affect up to about 10% of the population. Women at fourfold or higher risk are extremely uncommon with currently available risk factors. Such women have been identified in the following rare circumstances: those women with a mother or sister having bilateral breast cancer before the age of 40 years; women who have two first-degree relatives with premenopausal breast cancer; or women who themselves have had atypical hyperplasia or lobular carcinoma *in situ*. Such women are much too rare for a prevention trial to be based solely on them, but they do form a useful very-high-risk subgroup. Women with a family history of premenopausal breast cancer in a first-degree relative, multiple blood relatives with breast cancer, high-risk mammographic parenchymal patterns, proliferative benign breast disease and/or possibly nulliparity represent a sizeable group with a more than twofold elevated risk, for which a prevention trial is logistically feasible. Given that breast cancer is such a common disease, even a twofold increase translates into a 1 in 6 lifetime risk, and for women aged over 45 years, indicates at least a 1 in 25 risk over the next 10 years.

Mechanisms are needed for identifying and counselling women at increased risk of breast cancer. A national screening programme may be a useful way of identifying such women, and this would seem to be a natural extension of such programmes which currently only detect invasive cancer at an earlier stage, but often still too late for effective treatment. At present, however, it is necessary to consider other sources, including women attending breast clinics and their family members. These sources are likely to remain important for women under the age of 50 years, for whom screening does not appear to be very efficacious, and who are not covered by most national screening programmes. The advent of family history clinics for counselling women at high risk of breast cancer provides an ideal setting for undertaking prevention studies. The needs of women at high risk of breast cancer are different to those of women with breast cancer or other breast symptoms, and separate clinics help to reinforce the important difference between prevention and treatment.

Another approach is to consider volunteers from a group at normal risk, using only age as an entry criterion. Because the incidence of cancer rises rapidly with age, this is a useful concentrating factor. The American prevention trial accepts women aged over 60 years without any risk factors, and the Italian trial accepts hysterectomized women aged 50–60 years without any risk factors. When applied to women under the age of 60 years, this approach requires a much larger sample size. Another concern is compliance, as one is not always dealing with women who have experienced breast cancer in a close family member or who have had a previous biopsy for breast disease, both of which are likely to be strong motivating factors.

Beneficial effects vs. potential adverse effects

The balance between beneficial effects and potential adverse effects needs to be very heavily weighted in the direction of the former for a prevention trial, as we are dealing with healthy women who have no symptoms of disease. It is important to remember that the benefits of a prevention trial do not become apparent immediately, and in fact are impossible to demonstrate or experience on an individual level, as a reduction in the incidence of disease for the entire group is not easily appreciated by the individual participant who simply continues to exist in a disease-free state. However, any adverse effects are more likely to occur early in the treatment phase and are readily attributed to the preventive agent, whether it is to blame or not. For example, in the pilot study of Powles *et al.*,[10] with the exception of hot flushes and other menopausal symptoms, other short-term side-effects which had been attributed to tamoxifen from uncontrolled studies were equally distributed between active treatment and placebo, and led to a similar drop-out rate (see Table 11.1). Furthermore, even a single serious event, such as a liver cancer in a tamoxifen prevention trial, could have serious implications, even though no excess has been observed in more than 1 million women-years of treatment with tamoxifen in an adjuvant setting.

The available evidence suggests that a single case of liver cancer is most likely to be sporadic and unrelated to treatment, but this would be difficult to explain to the woman unfortunate enough to suffer this fate. The risk of possible adverse effects must be even less when an intervention is contemplated on a volunteer group that is at no increased risk of breast cancer. Here the benefits are diluted compared to a high-risk group, so adverse effects must also be reduced if the same benefit-to-risk ratio is to be maintained.

Although difficult to quantify, it is useful to try to put numbers on the likely positive and negative events which will occur, and at what stage in the trial they are likely to occur. Overall, a strong positive ratio should be anticipated, possibly at least 5 to 1, to make it possible to endure any unfortunate early setbacks. Ideally, some beneficial 'side-effect' should exist which guarantees a favourable overall benefit-to-risk ratio. Use of an oral contraceptive which might reduce breast cancer falls into this category, although some would say that the reduction of breast

Table 11.1 *Side-effects in the Royal Marsden Pilot Prevention Trial:*[10] *non-compliance figures indicate that the side-effect was severe enough to lead to cessation of treatment, and are based on all eligible patients (percentage values are shown in parentheses)*

	Tamoxifen	Placebo	Significance
Total number	920	926	
Hormone replacement therapy			
Before randomization	131 (14)	134 (14)	NS
On treatment	126 (14)	119 (13)	NS
Total	257 (28)	253 (27)	NS
Hysterectomy	29 (3)	16 (2)	NS
Ovarian surgery	14 (2)	15 (2)	NS
Not receiving HRT*	507	531	
Nausea	41 (6)	65 (10)	$P = 0.02$
Non-compliance	16	11	NS
Vomiting	3 (<1)	9 (1)	NS
Headache	82 (12)	96 (14)	NS
Non-compliance	10	19	NS
Hot flushes			
Premenopausal	151 (36)	75 (17)	$P < 0.001$
Post-menopausal	66 (29)	54 (25)	NS
Total	225 (34)	134 (20)	$P < 0.001$
Non-compliance	43	8	$P < 0.001$
Weight gain	44 (7)	71 (11)	$P < 0.001$
Non-compliance	9	6	NS
Menstrual irregularities	93 (14)	57 (9)	$P < 0.002$
Non-compliance	14	4	
Mood change	15 (3)	13 (3)	NS
Non-compliance	12	6	NS
Vaginal discharge			
Premenopausal	53 (13)	12 (3)	$P < 0.001$
Post-menopausal	53 (24)	17 (8)	$P < 0.001$
Total	108 (16)	30 (4)	$P < 0.001$
Non-compliance	9	3	NS

* This number is the denominator for the side-effects given below.
NS, non-significant.
Reproduced from Powles TJ, Hardy JR, Ashley SE *et al. The Royal Marsden Hospital pilot tamoxifen chemoprevention trial. Breast Cancer Research and Treatment* 1994; **31**: 73–83, with kind permission from Kluwer Academic Publishers.

cancer is the beneficial 'side-effect' of contraception. For tamoxifen, a range of potential long-term risks and benefits have been identified. The most clearly identified risk is endometrial cancer for which a 2–3-fold excess has been consistently found. However, because endometrial cancer is much less common than breast cancer, and is more easily treated, a 40% reduction in breast cancer in the UK population eligible for this trial would lead to prevention of about 4 breast cancers for every endometrial cancer induced, and the estimate for fatal cancers is even more favourable (see Table 11.2). Beneficial 'side-effects' of tamoxifen in post-menopausal women have been observed for bone density, and a 15–20% reduction in low-density lipoprotein (LDL) cholesterol has also been consistently observed. An estimate of the magnitude of the *identified* potential risks and benefits for 10 000 50-year-old

women entering the UK-based trial is shown in Table 11.2. However, the greatest uncertainty is the possibility of late unforeseen side-effects. For tamoxifen, carcinogeneity must be a concern, in view of its established role as a liver carcinogen in the rat.[11] Apart from the increased risk of endometrial cancer, to date the data have been reassuring,[12,13] although one trial has suggested a possible increase in colorectal cancer.[14]

Long-term follow-up and high compliance

Prevention trials place heavy demands on the resources necessary to achieve high compliance and to maintain long-term follow-up. Treatments are likely to last for 5 years or more and require changes in daily habits.

Table 11.2 *Projected effects over 10 years of giving tamoxifen for 5 years to 10 000 women aged 50 years with a 2.5-fold relative risk of breast cancer*

	Benefits
Breast cancer (incidence down 40%)	↓ 200
Ischaemic heart disease (incidence down 20%)	
Incidence	↓ 90
Mortality	↓ 30
Spinal fractures (incidence down 33%)	↓ 50

	Risks
Endometrial cancer (incidence up 3-fold)	↑ 50
Thrombo-embolic disease	↑ 20
Serious eye problems (retinopathy)	↑ 1
Liver cancer	
Liver damage	↑ <1

Women who are participating in a prevention study do not have any symptom which is being alleviated, nor are there any really tangible signs that the treatment is 'doing anything'. The use of a placebo in double-blind studies makes it difficult to feed back any positive 'side-effects' such as a reduction in cholesterol levels, but does make it easier to deal with some side-effects, as they cannot be attributed so readily to active treatment, and it is easier to see whether they disappear by themselves over a few months. Before stopping treatment because of a side-effect, it can be useful to try a 3-month 'treatment holiday' and then restart treatment, to determine whether the side-effect is linked to the treatment.

In addition to achieving compliance with treatment over a protracted period, follow-up of participants needs to be sustained for even longer periods. A minimum of 10 years of follow-up is essential, and since entry is likely to be staggered over at least 3 years, a provision for keeping track of subjects for at least 15 years from the inception of the trial is required. For this reason, follow-up procedures need to be as simple as possible, especially after the treatment phase is over, and could be based on a passive system that simply records incident cancers and cause-specific mortality. However, extra visits may be considered necessary during the treatment period to maintain a high level of compliance. Of course, the controls must be followed by exactly the same procedure as those individuals who receive the active treatment.

Monitoring other trials

Prevention trials take a long time to complete, and are usually based on a substantial amount of information

from preliminary trials. In the case of tamoxifen, information on toxicity and long-term side-effects comes from the adjuvant use of this drug to treat women with breast cancer.

Even after commencement of a prevention trial, these trials will still provide a 10- to 15-year lead on long-term side-effects. Valuable as this information is, the adjuvant trials have not been designed to look specifically at long-term side-effects, and this information obtained can be incomplete and difficult to interpret. Mechanisms need to be in place for examining and interpreting the available data and deciding whether any changes are needed in the design or follow-up procedures for the prevention study.

DESIGN STRATEGY

The fundamental principles outlined above need to be translated into a specific evaluation strategy for any particular preventive measure. This task requires much careful thought and creative problem-solving, as prevention trials face very different problems to treatment trials and new design solutions are required. However, many of the basic tenets remain the same, particularly the need for randomized studies.

Need for randomization

The reason why randomization was introduced into clinical experimentation was to control for bias. When dealing with human populations, it is never possible to predict with great accuracy the natural history of a disease, although it is certainly possible to find important prognostic factors in many instances. Although prognostic factors should be actively sought and used to stratify results, rarely are they sufficiently informative to be able to use concurrent or historical controls as a reference group for evaluating the effects of a treatment for which moderate differences are expected. In this case, the only reliable method of evaluation is randomization, which guarantees an average distribution of both known and unknown prognostic factors. Some (usually slight) imbalances will occur by chance with randomization, and adjustment for known prognostic factors will help to re-establish balance. Adjustment for unknown prognostic factors is of course impossible, but the random fluctuation inherent in the distribution of any such factors is accommodated in the analysis.

The problems of bias are at least as great when evaluating preventive measures. This is primarily due to the fact that such studies can only be performed on volunteers, who will be self-selected to a greater or lesser extent. These self-selection biases can be large, and are not easily explained by known prognostic factors. A good example of this is the US Breast Cancer Detection

Demonstration Project in which participants had a substantially higher risk of breast cancer than the general population, and this could not be fully explained by their greater incidence of benign breast disease or a family history of breast cancer.[7] This has hampered evaluation of this very large project, and makes it impossible to use it to evaluate the impact of mammographic screening on breast cancer mortality. Randomization overcomes this problem and allows one to draw meaningful conclusions from studies of populations which may not be exactly representative of the general population. Questions of whether or not the results can be generalized to a larger population still need to be considered, but these are usually more quantitative questions relating to weighing up costs and benefits, rather than basic questions relating to the existence of an effect.

Placebos and blinding

The use of placebos and double-blind methods is essential for evaluating soft end-points, the occurrence of which is at least partially open to interpretation by the investigator or the subject. Studies on the side-effects or acceptability of a proposed intervention must employ these devices, as the side-effects attributable to placebo are not inconsequential when studying women near the age of menopause, as Powles *et al.*[10] and others have documented. However, a large multi-centre prevention study will have the occurrence of invasive breast cancer and death from breast cancer as its primary end-points, which are more objective. There is little difficulty in assessing the occurrence and date of death, but even the detection of invasive cancer can be influenced by the thoroughness of the investigation and even by the decision of the pathologist as to whether disease is invasive or *in situ*. Thus if double-blinding is not used, it is important that volunteers in both arms of the study are followed up by the same procedures, and that assessment of mammograms and biopsies is done blindly.

A case for *not* using placebos or blinding can be made in prevention studies. The argument centres primarily around the issue of compliance. This is the major problem for prevention studies. Use of a placebo requires that compliance be maintained in both arms of the trial. Moreover, the fact that the participating women do not know whether or not the pills they are taking contain an active ingredient can be an insidious influence which may undermine their willingness to continue with the treatment.

However, the use of placebo has counterbalancing effects which may improve recruitment and compliance. Use of placebo makes it easier for the physician to explain that a woman is at increased risk of breast cancer, because every woman has an equal chance of being on active treatment, and this continues to be the case even after randomization. Furthermore, it may be easier to restart patients who have stopped treatment because of some non-specific side-effect, as it could be argued that such an effect is less easily ascribed to the active treatment and is more easily related to factors which are unrelated to the trial.

Run-in period

Because of the importance of good compliance, every effort must be made to ensure that, once randomized, participants are likely to continue with their allocated treatment. Careful screening at the first appointment is probably the most important factor here, but another option is to provide a run-in period on active treatment *before* randomization. This is often for a period of around 3 months, and is primarily aimed at determining whether participants can maintain the habit of daily pill-taking. Randomization is not performed until after the run-in period, and thus the participants will have a better idea of what they are volunteering for. Two issues must be considered with regard to the utility of a run-in period. First, what proportion of non-compliance will be picked up by this measure? If non-compliance is primarily due to a slow but steady attrition rate, then it is unlikely to be helped by a run-in period, whereas if intolerance to a change in daily routine or specific side-effects are a primary concern, it can have a major benefit. Secondly, should active treatment or placebo be used during this run in period? Use of placebo is sufficient to determine whether a woman is prepared for and capable of developing the habit of daily pill-taking, and can weed out those who are not sufficiently motivated to do this. However, if lack of compliance is likely to be due to specific side-effects and intolerance, then the active treatment will have to be used during the run-in period. The possibility then exists that the short-term use of the agent in both arms of the trial will dilute the overall effect and, if this is to be done, the run-in period needs to be kept as strict as possible. A compromise is to mix the two and have, for example, a 3-month run-in period, of which only 1 month is on active treatment. That month could even be randomly allocated to look at specific side-effects.

Choice of end-point(s)

Several end-points are possible for prevention studies. The ultimate end-point is a reduction in breast cancer mortality. Very large numbers are needed to assess this reliably, and over 50 000 women at more than double the normal risk would be needed to detect reliably a one-third reduction in mortality. It is also the last end-point to become informative, so about 15 years of follow-up would be needed.

To obtain reliable information on this end-point it will be necessary to overview the three tamoxifen prevention trials. Breast cancer incidence is more easily evaluated, but of course less convincing, as tamoxifen could conceivably only prevent cancers with a good prognosis. Fewer participants are needed to evaluate this, and the results would become available about 5 years sooner. Each of the three trials is designed to detect reliably a one-third reduction in breast cancer incidence. With the publication of the early results on reduction of evidence in the NSABP P1 trial,[8] it seems less likely that a reliable overview of the mortality data from all three trials will be possible. However, the International Breast Cancer Intervention Study (IBIS) unlike the patients in a double-blind comparison although, like the participants in the US trial, all of them have been informed of the result. Fortunately, unlike the US women, the vast majority have agreed to continue with the blinded allocated treatment with IBIS.[15] Several other end-points are also important, including cardiovascular incidence and mortality, incidence and mortality from other cancers, and site-specific fracture rate, among others. In general, cause-specific and site-specific cancer rates should be compared between treated and control participants in a trial.

One of the major problems in prevention trials, is the long follow-up period required to accrue sufficient end-points. This is particularly acute for interventions and at initiating events, where 40 years of follow-up may be needed if breast cancer is the end-point. It is highly desirable to have some form of intermediate end-point or biomarker for such trials. Such end-points will never be entirely satisfactory, but they do provide an early indication as to whether the intervention is likely to be successful,[16] and this is clearly necessary if very many prevention trials are to be conducted. Intermediate end-points require validation against the final end-point (breast cancer incidence or death), so at least one long term is needed before they can be used. Another problem is that once an intermediate end-point is identified, intervention may be designed specifically against it, and then there is even less certainty about the validity of any result being translated to the final end-point. Spicer *et al.* have used mammographic dysplasia as an intermediate end-point in studies of oral contraceptives also designed to prevent breast cancer.[17] There is an urgent need to validate this as a useful intermediate end-point.

Number of participants

Three major factors determine the number of subjects needed for a trial, namely the absolute risk level of the participants, the size of the smallest reduction in risk that is thought to be worthwhile, and compliance rates. The first factor is related to the fact that trial size depends on the number of events which are observed, not on the total number of subjects entered. Thus, a trial in older women need not employ such a high relative risk as one in younger women. Both the American and UK-based tamoxifen trials employ stricter relative risk criteria in younger women in order to ensure that the absolute risk is always above a certain minimum value. Compliance

also strongly influences the required sample size. For example, compared to perfect compliance, twice as many participants are needed for 75% compliance and four times as many are required if only 50% compliance is achieved. In general, the question is more complex than this, as partial compliance is more likely to be the case, (e.g. stopping after 3 years of treatment, or missing treatment for some intermediate months, and this does not have such a severe effect on the sample size, but would only dilute, rather than abolish, any effect in partial non-compliers.

Factorial designs

In general, prevention trials need to be kept as simple as possible in order to achieve large numbers and good compliance. One circumstance in which a deviation from absolute simplicity can be contemplated is the possibility of using a factorial design to answer two (or more) questions in the same trial. The logistic complexity and cost of prevention trials means that it will not be possible to conduct very many of them, and as each treatment is likely to have at best a moderate chance of success, it would be useful to answer more than one question at a time. However, this should only be contemplated if the additional complexity is small and the added difficulties are not likely to affect compliance adversely. In particular, consideration must be given to the added difficulty of explaining a factorial experiment to the volunteers, and the possibility that one treatment might be considered unacceptable, thus leading to the loss of a participant for the other intervention.

Recruitment strategies

Some consideration also needs to be given as to how best to recruit patients. Ideally, what is needed is a source of a large number of high-risk women who will be easy to recruit and follow up, and who will show a high rate of compliance. The ideal sources are special clinics for women at increased risk of breast cancer, where counselling can also be offered. Where these clinics do not exist or do not cover the population fully, additional sources must be tapped. The most immediate sources are the symptomatic breast clinics, where women with high-risk benign disease can be invited. It is also possible to suggest that the sisters of women with early-onset breast cancer be approached. For women over the age of 50 years, routine mammographic screening centres are another source of volunteers. This source is particularly attractive if mammographic dysplasia is to be used as an entry criterion. An American study has shown that primary care physicians (PCPs) play an important role in influencing preventative health behaviour, specifically with regard to enrolment into a randomized breast cancer prevention trial. Efforts to increase recruitment to such a trial should include enlisting the support of PCPs.[18] Prevention trials will inevitably attract the attention of the general public and provision must be made for dealing with interest generated in this way. It is important to try to clarify the entry criteria and age groups when the trial is mentioned in the media, in order to reduce the number of ineligible women who express interest in joining the trial. It is difficult to maintain a balanced view of risks and benefits in the press, and much effort is needed to keep the press well informed.

REFERENCES

1 Tokunaga M, Norman JE Jr, Asano M *et al.* Malignant breast tumors among atomic bomb survivors, Hiroshima and Nagasaki, 1950–74. *J Natl Cancer Inst* 1979; **62**: 1347–59.

2 Boice JD Jr, Rosenstein M, Dale Trout E. Estimation of breast doses and breast cancer risk associated with repeated fluoroscopic chest examinations of women with tuberculosis. *Radiat Res* 1978; **73**: 373–90.

3 Modan B, Chetrit A, Alfandary E, Katz L. Increased risk of breast cancer after low-dose irradiation. *Lancet* 1989; 629–631.

4 Kelsey JL. A review of the epidemiology of human breast cancer. *Epidemiol Rev* 1979; **1**: 74–109.

5 Hsich C, Trichopoulos D, Katsouyanni K, Yuasa S. Age at menarche, age at menopause, height and obesity as risk factors for breast cancer: associations and interactions in an international case–control study. *Int J Cancer* 1990; **48**: 796–800.

6 Trichopoulos D, MacMahon B, Cole P. Menopause and breast cancer risk. *J Natl Cancer Inst* 1972; **48**: 605–13.

7 Brinton LA, Williams RR, Hoover RN *et al.* Breast cancer risk factors among screening program participants. *J Natl Cancer Inst* 1979; **62**: 37–44.

8 Fisher B, Constantino JP, Wickerham DC *et al.* Tamoxifen for the prevention of breast cancer. Report of the National Surgical Adjuvant Breast and Bowel Project P-1 Study. *J Natl Cancer Inst* 1998; **90**: 1371–88.

9 Powles T, Eales R, Ashley S *et al.* Interim analysis of the evidence of breast cancer in the Royal Marsden Hospital tamoxifen randomised chemoprevention trial. *Lancet* 1998; **352**: 98–101.

10 Powles TJ, Hardy JR, Ashley SE *et al.* The Royal Marsden Hospital pilot tamoxifen chemoprevention trial. *Breast Cancer Res Treat* 1994; **31**: 73–83.

11 Greaves P, Goonetilleke R, Nunn G *et al.* Ten-year carcinogenicity study of tamoxifen in Alderley park wistar-derived rats. *Cancer Res* 1993 **53**: 3919–24.

12 Muhlemann K, Cook LS, Weiss NS. The incidence of hepatocellular carcinoma in US white women with breast cancer after the introduction of tamoxifen in 1977. *Breast Cancer Res Treat* 1994; **30**: 201–4.

13 Fisher B, Costantino JP, Redmond CK *et al.* Endometrial cancer in tamoxifen-treated breast cancer patients: findings from the National Surgical Adjuvant Breast and Bowel Project NSABP; B-14. *J Natl Cancer Inst* 1994; **86**: 527–37.

14 Rutqvist LE, Mattson A. Cardiac and thromboembolic morbidity among postmenopausal women with early-stage breast cancer in a randomised trial of adjuvant tamoxifen. *J Natl Cancer Inst* 1993; **85**: 1398–1406.

15 Cuzick J. Centinals of the International Breast Cancer Intervention Study (IBIS). *Eur J Cancer Inst* 1998; **34**: 1647–8.

16 Boone CW, Kelloff GJ. Biomarker end-points in cancer chemoprevention trials. *IARC Sci Publ* 1997; **142**: 273–80.

17 Spicer DV, Ursin G, Pike MC *et al.* Changes in mammographic densities induced by hormonal contraceptive designed to reduce breast cancer risk. *J Natl Cancer Inst* 1994; **86**: 431–6.

18 Kinney AY, Richards C, Verne SW, Vogel VG. The effect of physical recommendation on enrolment in the Breast Cancer Prevention Trial. *Prev Med* 1998; **27**: 713–19.

12

Chemoprevention with tamoxifen: known benefits and toxicity

RICHARD R LOVE

Of the two broad approaches to breast cancer prevention – removal of identified risk factors and active intervention to reverse or stop the progression of preclinical disease – the active intervention approach, of which chemoprevention is the principal strategy, is significantly more complex and challenging. The reasons for this lie in our current understanding of the biology of breast cancer, and in the biology of current chemopreventive interventions, the prototype of which is tamoxifen. While the other chapters in this volume focus on aspects of the biology of breast cancer, on how tamoxifen works and on the important subject of the design of chemoprevention trials, some consideration of these topics is critical to addressing the subject to be covered here, namely chemoprevention with tamoxifen. This chapter will first place this strategy in its critical contexts and then offer a brief summary of the available data which have led to three large randomized trials. Finally, it will address the results of these trials and the challenging task of weighing the identified benefits and costs, and the implications of the data for public health.

CRITICAL BACKGROUND BIOLOGY OF BREAST CANCER AND TAMOXIFEN

Although much is known about the developmental biology of breast cancer, the available data currently leave us without complete, all-inclusive models for this disease process. Clearly, the implication of this situation is that perturbation of one part of the system may have consequences which are not well defined. This is easily said, but some further details make our ignorance clearer and its implications more important. Breast cancer is a disease with multiple causes, and recent interpretations suggest that certain causal complexes are associated with breast cancers having specific characteristics.[1] Generally, breast cancers are either hormonally dependent (at least at some periods in their development and natural history) or hormonally independent. Presumably these features, which appear to be quantitative for most individual cancers and not qualitative, are related to specific causes. This incompletely understood biology has significant implications for the application during development of an intervention which has hormonal manipulation as its major mode of action.

As a general rule, it appears that breast cancer probably develops through multiple stages of initiation, promotion (or regression) and progression. Based on data from radiation-caused cases, this process appears to occur over a period of many years (perhaps 10–20 years). As stated and currently understood, it is the protracted 'middle' stage, namely promotion, which appears to be a target for active prevention strategies.

These two general characteristics of breast cancer (i.e. that it is a multiple-cause disease with multiple developmental stages) present challenges when considering *which* individual patients (actually healthy subjects) should be targeted for a tamoxifen-preventive intervention, and *when* in their lives such an intervention might be applied. It would seem that our current understanding of the biology of breast cancer makes targeting a specific population impossible.[2] The processes, actions and reactions in biological systems suggest that a hormonal perturbation with tamoxifen will have undesirable consequences for breast and other tissues which we cannot currently predict.

The critical biology of tamoxifen also presents challenges in its potential role as a chemopreventive agent. Tamoxifen, as discussed in detail in Chapter 5, is a non-steroidal triphenylethylene derivative that acts like the steroid oestrogen, for which it is essentially a competitive antagonist. Like oestrogen, tamoxifen is pleomorphic in its effects in humans, and it is this characteristic which is central to its potential role as a chemopreventive drug. Although tamoxifen is non-specific or unselective with regard to the types of cells and tissues in which it produces some biological effects (it has documented effects in most human tissues), it is cell-specific and tissue-specific in its particular effects in different cells or tissues. Furthermore, these effects can be modulated significantly by the oestrogen levels that prevail. Tamoxifen's major effects are believed to result from interaction with oestrogen-receptor (binding) proteins in many types of human cells, with variable oestrogen agonist or antagonist effects. Other indirect hormonal effects occur with suppression of gonadotrophins in post-menopausal women, and with early follicular phase marked increases in circulating oestrogens in some premenopausal women.[3] Possibly non-hormonally mediated effects include modulation of stimulatory and inhibitory growth factors (TGF-α, TGF-294-β, EGF, IGF-1), inhibition of protein kinase C activity and polyamines, and interference with cytochrome P-450 activity.[4] One example of the cell-specific activity of tamoxifen is its apparent stimulation of breast cancer or breast stromal cells to produce the inhibitory growth factor TGF-β. The emergence of refractoriness to suppression of breast cancer growth with tamoxifen is postulated to be consequent to loss of this growth factor-influencing effect,[5] or to an alteration of the oestrogen receptor.[6] Further complicating predictions of tamoxifen's long-term tissue effects include observations that its metabolites are genotoxic and bind to DNA.

The above brief summary of tamoxifen's cellular action and pharmacology emphasizes that it does *not* have the characteristics of an ideal preventive intervention – that is, it does not have a single specific well-documented effect on only breast cells or malignant or premalignant breast cells. Instead, tamoxifen exerts effects in many tissues, and these effects are variable, tissue-specific and influenced by the existing hormonal milieu. In these circumstances, the potentially beneficial and harmful effects of tamoxifen, particularly in the long term, are understandably difficult to predict at tissue, whole body and treated population levels. The remainder of this chapter will attempt to summarize what is known about tamoxifen's organ and tissue effects, but this background should serve as a warning that our understanding is somewhat limited.

SOME CAVEATS ABOUT INTERPRETATION OF THE AVAILABLE INFORMATION ON TAMOXIFEN TOXICITY

The following discussion concerns target organ toxicities of tamoxifen. Two areas deserve attention to permit rational understanding and interpretation of the current data. First, based on the belief that tamoxifen acted primarily through combination with cellular oestrogen-receptor protein, whose presence was far more frequently detectable in the tumours of post-menopausal women, initial clinical studies and indeed the preponderance of mature studies have been conducted in post-menopausal hormone-receptor-positive tumour-bearing populations. These include both therapeutic and toxicological investigations. The 'side-effects' database in premenopausal women is remarkably small. As noted earlier, tamoxifen has been shown to cause hormonal perturbations with large increases in oestrogen levels in premenopausal women, and its tissue effects clearly appear to be modulated in at least two tissues, namely bone and vagina,[7-9] by the oestrogen milieu. Thus the tissue effects discussed below are primarily those observed in studies of post-menopausal women, and these may be very different to those eventually described in premenopausal subjects.

A second critical perspective that is needed here concerns the levels of reliability of clinical data from different sources. We can envisage a hierarchy of data sources according to reliability.[10] At the optimal end of such a hierarchy might be data from overviews or meta-analyses of all randomized trials *specifically designed to address particular questions*. Successively less reliable data might be from groups of trials, single trials, prospective and retrospective series studies, clinical observations and finally speculations based on some biological facts. The data from each of these types of study may be biased in critical ways which should prevent their generalization to larger populations. Three specific types of bias are of significance when interpreting the published tamoxifen data discussed below and also those under development.

The first type of bias is subject selection bias. Clinical studies have, through ethical necessity, investigated volunteers. Such populations differ from the population of individuals to whom we may ultimately wish to apply the intervention (or tamoxifen). Essentially all adjuvant studies of tamoxifen in breast cancer have been conducted in Caucasian populations whose dietary exposure and hormonal profiles might modulate the therapeutic and biological effects of the drug. The tamoxifen prevention trials currently in progress have recruited volunteers who are likely to be more healthy than their counterparts in the general population.

The second type of bias in interpreting data about side-effects or toxicities is early detection or surveillance bias. This is particularly important with regard to the evaluation of tamoxifen's effect on the uterine endometrium. The issue is that the process of screening or intense surveillance, particularly by laboratory or radiological technologies, leads to detection of 'disease' or 'side-effects' which might not otherwise be recognized or develop to a level of clinical significance.

The third source of bias concerns the methods used to detect particular effects or end-points, and when they are applied to the subjects being studied. This type of bias is very important in interpretation of the available data on the toxicities and effects of tamoxifen. Initially, adjuvant studies, which have been the main source of such data, were designed to ascertain major breast cancer-associated end-points. The collection of data on the side-effects of tamoxifen was often almost incidental, and the methods for this were imprecise. It is absolutely critical to appreciate this when interpreting other and more recent data about toxicities. The adjuvant studies were not designed to look at cardiovascular or osseous end-points. Quality-of-life data specifically focusing on gynaecological, central nervous system or ophthalmological consequences of tamoxifen treatment, particularly over the long term, were not sought, and thus the large adjuvant trial database cannot be used to provide reliable information about such side-effects. The often stated 'remarkable safety record' of tamoxifen must be understood in this light. Low-frequency consequences, consequences masked by variable background rates of events and therefore also the effects in disease-free, healthy populations cannot be estimated reliably on the basis of the treatment data available.

A further aspect of the interpretation of the available data about tamoxifen toxicity concerns other important numerical and statistical issues. The statistical strategies appropriate to analysis of the occurrence of certain toxicities (from tamoxifen in adjuvant trials), not defined a priori as of concern, must be carefully considered,[11] (see Chapter 11). Beyond these and the always pressing search for statistical significance, there is the challenge of paying adequate attention to biologically plausible serious low-frequency toxicities that have not yet been demonstrated to be reliably (or highly likely to be) consequent to tamoxifen. With tamoxifen, this type of challenge has arisen with regard to the question of proclivity to phlebitis, venous thrombosis and pulmonary thromboembolism. In individual studies (e.g. NSABP B-14),[12] the numbers of these events and study sizes have precluded a definitive statistical conclusion about cause, while multiple clinical studies and studies of coagulation-protection effects suggest that a real low frequency of this complication occurs consequent to tamoxifen. In studies of healthy populations, both the volunteers and public health advocates would argue that greater levels of prudence are warranted. Biological coherence of the available data may be more important than statistical proof of association.

HUMAN TISSUE AND ORGAN EFFECTS OF TAMOXIFEN AND THEIR POSSIBLE CLINICAL CONSEQUENCES

The myriad of effects of tamoxifen can be classified in several ways – for example, by the target organ affected at the cellular level, by the organ system affected as a consequence of cellular effects (in some cases the two are different), by risk factor or clinical effects, or by symptomatic or asymptomatic effects. In the following discussion, the target organ affected at cellular and tissue levels will be the organizational unit. After this discussion, a more specific consideration of the early results of three large chemoprevention trials will be presented.

Breast

The exploration of tamoxifen as a chemopreventive intervention stems naturally from its extensive use initially in metastatic breast cancer and more recently as adjuvant therapy of increasing duration in both pre- and post-menopausal women.[13] Although the known biology of tamoxifen provides many possible explanations for its clinically observed effects, the exact picture is far from clear. One of the unexplained issues is whether tamoxifen is essentially a cytostatic or both a cytostatic and a cytocidal agent. Initial adjuvant trials employed short therapy courses of 1–2 years, which were later anticipated to be less effective or only transiently effective in delaying the recurrence of disease, based on a presumed cytostatic mode of action. As these initial trials matured, it has become clear that a long-lasting impact of these brief courses is seen with persistent separation of disease-free and overall survival curves between treated and untreated groups.[13] This observation suggests a cytocidal effect in the clinic that is not predicted from the initial studies. The recent report of the NSABP P-1 trial is instructive and surprising (it will be discussed in detail later). While there was a slightly greater effect of tamoxifen in suppressing/preventing breast cancer in post-menopausal women, the difference between the two groups was not nearly as great as the adjuvant data suggested.[13,14] More recently, a report on the use of tamoxifen as an adjuvant to lumpectomy and radiotherapy in women with ductal carcinoma in situ found that the occurrence of invasive cancer in the affected breast was reduced by 45%.[15] These results have encouraging implications for interpretation of the early reports of a marked reduction in the incidence of breast cancer in the large American NSABP P-1 Breast Cancer Prevention Trial.[14] A modelling study by Trock has also suggested that the impact of tamoxifen on preclinical lesions might be prolonged, if not greater than expected.[16] On the other hand, as with the adjuvant populations, only long-term observation of treated and untreated women will clarify the actual consequences of tamoxifen treatment. Again, the initial report of the NSABP P-1 trial suggests that hormone-receptor-positive preclinical lesions are suppressed by tamoxifen, while oestrogen-receptor-negative lesions are unaffected.[14]

A second related issue concerns the efficacy of tamoxifen in hormone-receptor-positive and hormone-receptor-negative primary tumour-bearing patients. The implicit interpretation, based on clinical observations in adjuvant studies, is that tamoxifen is more effective in hormone-receptor-positive primary disease because the metastases that are suppressed are also hormone-receptor-positive. However, immunohistochemical studies of individual tumours suggest that most of them are admixtures of oestrogen or progesterone receptor protein 'positive' and negative cells, and that hormone-receptor positivity is a relative issue.

A third issue concerns the basis for the relative efficacy of adjuvant tamoxifen in pre- and post-menopausal groups. The general conclusion of the meta-analysis is that if one confines the analysis to the subgroups of pre-menopausal hormone-receptor-positive subjects, the favourable impact of tamoxifen is less than that in the comparable post-menopausal groups.[13]

These issues become germane when interpreting the available data on the reductions in the rates of contralateral breast cancer seen in women in adjuvant studies. For prevention studies, the questions raised concern what precisely we are treating, and what the guiding hypotheses in these efforts should be. For almost a decade, data have been available suggesting that reduced rates of contralateral breast cancers occur in adjuvantly treated women, and the updated meta-analysis reconfirms this conclusion, with a suggestion that longer adjuvant therapy is more effective in this regard (for women treated for 5 years, a proportional risk reduction of 47% was found; $P < 0.00001$).[13] The majority of the treated women in these adjuvant trials are likely to have had hormone-receptor-positive primary tumours, whose bearing on this observation of contralateral cancer suppression is uncertain. In addition, the majority of treated women were post-menopausal – a group which more often than not has hormone-receptor-positive primary tumours. The implicit argument in the prevention trials appears to be that in post-menopausal women, the preclinical 'disease' is likely to be hormone-receptor-positive and thus acted upon by tamoxifen. The argument in pre-menopausal women is less obvious. Of interest are the observations that in NSABP B-14, an adjuvant study of hormone-receptor-positive tumour-bearing patients, the rates of contralateral breast cancer were significantly lower in premenopausal women,[12] while in a Cancer Research Campaign (CRC) study which included unselected premenopausal women, no reductions were seen.[17] Why second tumours should have characteristics similar to those of the first is not obvious, but understandable. Presumably the causal complexes that are important in the first and second cancers are (with the exception of the role of tamoxifen) the same.[1] Furthermore, specific causal complexes might be expected to be associated with cancers that have specific biological characteristics. According to this argument, first-cancer oestrogen-receptor tumour-bearing women might be expected to have similar hormone-receptor positivity demonstrated in the second tumour. Specific data are not yet available on these issues. If the argument holds, then demonstrable breast cancer suppression by tamoxifen on *unselected* groups of premenopausal women (with less likelihood of hormone-receptor-positive tumours, and assuming tamoxifen action is related to the hormone-receptor status of the primary tumour) would not be expected (as was seen in the CRC study).[17]

Liver

Tamoxifen treatment results in a multitude of changes in liver tissues and their function which have consequences for several other organ systems. First, tamoxifen is metabolized by the liver and the cytochrome P-450 system. As a result, other xenobiotics (e.g. tricyclic antidepressants) metabolized by this system may be affected by tamoxifen consumption.[18] This complication merits more attention than it has received. It has also often been observed that tamoxifen is associated with increases in serum-assayed levels of hepatocellular enzymes. Cellular necrosis is occurring to some degree, which in extreme circumstances leads to fulminant hepatic failure (case reports) or cirrhosis.[19] Steatohepatitis, a process which can also lead to cirrhosis, has been reported. At present the frequency and modulators of these direct hepatocellular toxicities are not known.

The genotoxic effects of tamoxifen metabolites and the steroidal effect of tamoxifen as a hepatocellular tumour promoter have received considerable attention because of rodent experimental data which suggests significant levels of these processes.[20,21] Despite concern that new liver tumours in tamoxifen-treated women have been too readily assumed to be metastatic breast cancer and not of primary hepatocellular origin, the preponderance of clinical data strongly suggests that the development of primary liver cancers in humans is a negligible concern.[13,14] Dose, treatment duration and species differences in the animal experiments, as well as evidence that a threshold dose is not exceeded in humans, are important. Further reassurance comes from the human experience and laboratory studies of ethyl oestradiol. This compound appears to be the main steroid involved in the association of certain oral contraceptives with the very rare development of benign and malignant liver neoplasms. In liver tumour promoter potency studies, this hormone is perhaps 100-fold more powerful than tamoxifen.[21] One caveat is that tamoxifen-treated women who provide the reassuring database are selected with regard to their limited exposure to hepatic malignancy initiators such as hepatitis viruses and alcohol.

Tamoxifen has major effects on the production of several proteins and growth factors. Levels of the hormone transport proteins, sex hormone-binding globulin and thyroglobulin-binding protein are increased in serum, while levels of fibrinogen, antithrombin III, protein C, protein S and homocysteine are all lowered.[22–24] Low-density-lipoprotein (LDL) cholesterol levels are significantly decreased, possibly as a consequence of up-regulation of LDL receptors in the liver, as occurs with oestrogens or through other mechanisms,[25] while levels of lipoprotein(a), a very powerful atherogenic protein, are also decreased, probably as a result of a rate change in production.[26] Triglyceride levels generally and modestly increase,[22] and occasional patients appear to develop very serious hypertriglyceridaemia.[27] This effect was observed incidentally in several patients in one prevention trial, and led to termination of accrual.[28] Glucose metabolism appears to be unaffected, and the impact of tamoxifen on HDL cholesterol levels in one direction or the other must be modest, if it is significant at all.[26] Growth factor changes in thrombopoietin, IGF-I and other signal transducers may be liver mediated. Decreases in platelet counts of 7–9% are consistently seen, and more substantial decreases occasionally occur, although the consequences of these are unknown.[23] More frequent cholelithiasis would be predicted based on the cholesterol changes, but this has not been studied. Growth factor effects may be responsible for the suggested decreased mortality from cancers overall seen in the NSABP prevention trial.[14] The commonest clinical consequences of this array of risk factor alterations will be considered later in this chapter.

Most widely discussed have been the likely consequences of changes in cardiovascular risk factors. Although greater absolute and percentage LDL decreases with tamoxifen are seen with greater baseline levels of cholesterol, it is suggested that changes in HDL cholesterol levels are significantly more important in women.[29] While various data suggest that the decreases in fibrinogen and lipoprotein(a) levels that have been observed with tamoxifen should be associated with a decreased risk of coronary heart disease, again the general supportive data in women are sparse. Specific data on clinical outcomes in tamoxifen-treated women are of uncertain reliability. In a pair of randomized trials, reduced rates of myocardial infarction[30] and of hospitalization for heart disease[31] have been reported. The most recent adjuvant trial meta-analysis data demonstrate no impact of tamoxifen therapy on long-term non-breast-cancer mortality.[13] Perhaps this is to be expected, given that all of the risk factor effects might be expected to be demonstrable only during active tamoxifen treatment, which has until recently usually been of 2 years' duration or less. In addition, no favourable impact on cardiovascular end-points has been seen in the US prevention trial. This is perhaps also to be expected in view of the younger, healthy volunteer participant population.[14] However, an increased frequency of completed stroke (but not transient ischaemic attacks) was observed in tamoxifen-treated women in the NSABP P-1 trial,[14] when the decreased fibrinogen levels with tamoxifen would predict the opposite effects. The coagulation protein changes and clinical observations have long suggested that deep vein thrombosis and pulmonary embolism might be more frequent in tamoxifen recipients. Again, the NSABP P-1 data have now clarified that this is the case and provided some absolute risk estimates. These will be considered in the discussion below.

Uterine and other gynaecological tissues

The effects of tamoxifen on the uterine endometrium have been a focus of several studies in recent years, because of the suggestion that these effects are qualitatively similar to those of oestrogen, while being quantitatively less. A striking animal experiment reported in 1988, in which tamoxifen blocked the growth of breast carcinoma but facilitated the growth of a hormone-responsive endometrial carcinoma,[32] was followed in 1989 by a clinical report of an increased incidence of endometrial cancers in women adjuvantly treated with tamoxifen.[33] Subsequent reports support this general conclusion, although the magnitude of the increase in risk continues to remain in dispute.[34] The high prevalence of hysterectomy by the age of 60 years (approaching 40% in the USA) confounds interpretation of some of the available data. Increased surveillance using ultrasound to assess the thickness of the uterine endometrium and the practice of endometrial biopsies in asymptomatic women who are taking tamoxifen may also be responsible for uncovering endometrial lesions which may never have progressed clinically.[20] Nevertheless, the increased occurrence of endometrial carcinomas, hyperplasias, and endometrial and cervical polyps seems to be a clear consequence of tamoxifen treatment in postmenopausal women with an intact uterus. The cumulative dose is probably important, and the absolute risk with 5 years of therapy at 20 mg daily is approximately 1.5% for most menopausal women. After concern to the contrary raised by one report,[35] it now seems that the cancers which do develop in tamoxifen-treated women exhibit the same spectrum of histological features as are seen in patients without this therapy. The updated meta-analysis of adjuvant tamoxifen trials suggests a relative incidence risk of 3.7, a relationship between duration of therapy and cancer occurrence, and observes that unfortunately some of these iatrogenic cancers have been fatal.[13]

Other gynaecological tissue effects of tamoxifen have received less attention but deserve mention. Kedar et al. noted an increase in size of uterine fibroids with tamoxifen treatment, an observation consistent with growth factor changes measured serologically.[36] Gynaecological symptoms have often been more frequently reported in tamoxifen recipients, but the details have been poorly documented. Moderate or substantially increased vaginal discharge and associated genital pruritus occur in approximately 16% of tamoxifen-treated women.[37] We recently completed a longitudinal study of post-menopausal women which demonstrated that about 75% of subjects with oestrogen-deficient vaginal tissues prior to treatment will experience modest oestrogenic-maturational changes with tamoxifen associated with mild leucorrhoea and some genital pruritus. The remaining 25% of patients will experience modest vaginal tissue oestrogenic effects from endogenous oestrogen pretreatment, and no significant changes with tamoxifen therapy. Rarely, patients with significant oestrogen deficiency symptoms at baseline will show no changes with tamoxifen treatment.[9]

In post-menopausal women, tamoxifen may be associated with a decreased risk of ovarian cancer.[38] The mechanism by which this possible effect is mediated may be the decrease in gonadotrophins seen in this group of patients. In premenopausal women, the effects of tamoxifen on the ovary are clearly more frequent and adverse. Tamoxifen acts like clomiphene in these younger women, producing frequent ovulation, cysts, hormonal increases and occasional cystic necrosis.[39] Spicer et al. have suggested that if ovarian cancer is an epithelial disruption disease, then these more frequent events may be associated with increased risk of ovarian cancer.[39]

There are few data about the effect of tamoxifen on the fetus. As the half-life of this drug is long, by the time a woman who becomes pregnant can stop the agent, if the pregnancy continues the developing fetus will be exposed to tamoxifen or its metabolites for the entire first trimester. A recent report documented a case of Goldenhar's syndrome associated with tamoxifen treatment, and noted that 10 other cases of fetal/neonatal disorders have been reported to the American manufacturer.[40]

Central nervous system

Although for over a decade it has been known that anti-oestrogen binding sites are present in the brain in concentrations similar to those seen in the liver and uterus,[41] only recently have there been clinical studies of the central nervous system (CNS) in tamoxifen recipients. The first symptom to be noticed has been nausea, which occurs in tamoxifen recipients, often only during the first few weeks of therapy. Whether this is of CNS cause is uncertain. Several case reports have documented episodes of CNS dysfunction which have been very serious (encephalopathy in some circumstances). Sleep disturbance has been reported by patients for many years, but often the assumption has been that this is a consequence of vasomotor instability which is more evident at night. More detailed examinations of these symptoms have not been reported. In the same mechanistic mode, headaches, presumed to be vasomotor in aetiology, are less frequent in post-menopausal tamoxifen recipients.[37] The possibility that more profound, long-lasting and common CNS side-effects may be occurring has been signalled by a variety of observations. First, in one large adjuvant therapy trial, withdrawal for depression was noted in 1% of the subjects.[42] The total number of patients in this trial and the general setting (patients with life-threatening disease) contributed to the impression that this non-statistically significant observation was of no practical importance. The possibility that tamoxifen therapy might have major biological effects on the CNS has been suggested by clinical studies in patients with unresectable meningiomas[43] and malignant gliomas.[44] In the former, hormone receptors present in the tumour provided the rationale for this therapy. In the latter, the protein kinase-influencing effects of tamoxifen were considered to be an appropriate target, and tamoxifen was in fact localized to tumour tissue in one patient. What is remarkable is that objective tumour responses to tamoxifen were seen in both groups of patients.

This historical perspective of observations brings us to the last half decade, during which clinicians have increasingly acknowledged the occurrence of profound mood disturbance in some patients receiving tamoxifen. Exacerbation of diagnosed bipolar disorder and the development of profound clinical depression otherwise is regularly seen.[37] In 1993, in a study involving a concurrent historical control population, Cathcart et al. noted a significantly higher incidence of depression over time in tamoxifen recipients.[45] The relatively uncontrolled nature of the data reported has led to its being dismissed. However, a small and more detailed longitudinal study has supported the observation of depression,[46] and with increasing attention to the biology of oestrogen and the CNS, perhaps this relationship and the possible relationship of tamoxifen to degenerative brain disease will be rigorously studied. This mood area is one in which the methods used in studies are critical. We can gain little reassurance from the apparent absence of depression as a common side-effect of tamoxifen in adjuvant study reports, because those studies have not focused on this possible effect. Although the absolute excess fraction of women treated with tamoxifen who develop serious CNS side-effects may be small, in the context of chemoprevention, where the numbers of individual major *beneficial* events are small, this will be significant. Statisticians have belittled concern about this side-effect as speculative,[47] misinterpreting, in my estimation, the overall picture of the likelihood of this problem, and the absence of careful specific study. While the preliminary quality-of-life data from the NSABP P-1 trial did not suggest a general increase in depression in tamoxifen recipients, a detailed report which carefully considers missing data, and subjects dropping out for toxicity, may shed light on this depression-tamoxifen relationship.

Bone

Bone tissues have oestrogen receptors,[48] and animal studies have suggested bone density (and therefore strength and fracture risk) effects from tamoxifen treatment.[49] As women with lower peak bone mass age, gradual bone loss to critical threshold levels increases the risk of fracture. For post-menopausal women, bone fractures are a major cause of morbidity, and interventions that can be easily applied with major benefit have not been identified. The animal data have predicted with remarkable accuracy these more recently documented effects of tamoxifen on human bone density.[48] It is now clear that, in post-menopausal women, tamoxifen preserves bone mineral density with about one-third the favourable effect of oestrogen.[7,8] It is the trabecular bone, which provides structural integrity, which is maintained in these women, and thus over the long term an assessable reduction in fracture risks is predicted of perhaps one-quarter to one-third. The observed results in post-menopausal women are that, in contrast to untreated women who are losing bone mass and density, tamoxifen-treated subjects are not losing bone density and are perhaps actually increasing it during treatment.[50] The NSABP P-1 trial provided evidence that hip, spine and radial bone fracture rates, particularly in post-menopausal women, are indeed decreased by 20% with tamoxifen therapy.[14] In contrast, the situation in pre-menopausal women appears to be the reverse, namely that at different bone sites, premenopausal cycling women lose more bone mineral density with tamoxifen treatment than their placebo-treated controls.[8] Prediction of fracture risk based on these data is complex, primarily because of uncertainties about the effects during menopause should therapy be continued. Clearly more data are needed, but these findings reinforce the view that tamoxifen elicits remarkably different biological effects in different tissues and in different background hormonal milieus and that, in particular, premenopausal and post-menopausal recipients need to be considered separately.

Eye

Although the eye is often a target of animal toxicological investigations, the organization of investigations of systemic therapies such as tamoxifen has tended to ignore this organ. The pathophysiology through which tamoxifen-induced changes in structures of the eye might occur has been identified. The drug is an amphophilic compound which might be expected to bind with retinal proteins, binding to hormone receptors in any of the eye structures might occur, and chloride-channel blockage might contribute to corneal changes. On the basis of animal studies and case and small series reports, it has been suggested that corneal opacification, cataracts, macular oedema (usually reversible), a variety of retinal changes and optic neuritis may be related to tamoxifen.[38] Modest-sized studies, in which the frequencies of these and other ophthalmic complications were observed in tamoxifen-treated and control subjects, have suggested increases in intraretinal crystals and posterior subcapsular opacities.[51,52] The background rates of degenerative eye disorders of these types, and the likely low frequency of any of these specific complications consequent to tamoxifen appear to be responsible for these negative results. In the large NSABP P-1 trial, cataracts developed more frequently and were operated on in greater numbers of tamoxifen-treated (predominantly older) women.[14] The excess risk was low. The overall long-term additional benefits of requiring baseline ophthalmological evaluation for tamoxifen recipients are unclear.

Colon

Although the rates of colorectal malignancies have been approximately equivalent between the sexes, recent epidemiological studies have suggested a major protective effect of hormone replacement therapy against colon cancer,[53] and Scandinavian adjuvant studies with tamoxifen have suggested *increased* rates of this malignancy with this treatment.[54] Exposure to the genotoxic metabolites of tamoxifen may be the mechanism responsible for such serious consequences. In the updated meta-analysis of adjuvant trials, there appears to be no major difference in the numbers of colorectal cancers between tamoxifen-treated and control cases. Although the numbers of colon cancer cases in this analysis are greater for the tamoxifen-treated group, consequent to increased disease and overall survival, the tamoxifen-treated women are at risk for longer periods.[13] In the NSABP P-1 trial, 9 and 11 colon cancers were reported in the placebo and tamoxifen-treated women, respectively (non-significant difference).[14]

Skin

The most common toxicity from tamoxifen is increased vasomotor instability with hot flushes or flashes.[37] When carefully questioned, about half of post-menopausal women report significant increases in the number and intensity of these unpleasant episodes. Although various non-specific therapies have been proposed and evaluated, their ameliorating effects on these symptoms are only modest. On average, 20–25% of women who are treated with tamoxifen develop vasomotor symptoms that are sufficiently bothersome for them to want to stop treatment. In two recently reported randomized trials, 26% overall[28] and 24% of specifically tamoxifen-treated women[14] stopped therapy. From a variety of data it is clear that these vasomotor symptoms are the main reason for stopping treatment. One area of interest is the relationship between vasomotor instability symptoms and other toxicities, such as those of the CNS. In post-menopausal women, vasomotor symptoms diminish over time (measured over several months to 1–2 years). A maculopapular rash is occasionally seen with tamoxifen therapy.

Other important target organs

Changes in hormonal transport proteins have uncertain specific effects, but can confuse evaluations of endocrine organ function. Sex-hormone-binding and thyroid-binding globulin levels are increased, and T_4 levels are also increased, but euthyroidism is usually maintained.[55] Decreases in gonadotrophins are seen in post-menopausal women, which may be related to changes in libido. Modest hypercalcaemia of hyperparathyroidism, which is more common in women with breast cancer, appears to be controlled with tamoxifen. Fluid retention occurs in some tamoxifen-treated women, but over a 2-years period, weight gain and modest blood pressure changes are not seen.[26] Occasional joint or bursal inflammatory signs are observed in tamoxifen-treated subjects, and significant bronchospasm has been the subject of case reports. Neutropenia can occur and is sometimes fatal.

THE RESULTS OF CHEMOPREVENTION TRIALS WITH TAMOXIFEN

Three randomized trials of tamoxifen in healthy women have been reported by the National Surgical Adjuvant Breast Project (NSABP) (Trial NSABP P-1), the Royal Marsden Hospital and the European School of Oncology/Italian group.[14, 28, 56] These trials differ in size, subject years of follow-up, risk-factor characteristics of the studied women, and results (see Tables 12.1, 12.2 and 12.3). The NSABP trial is significantly larger, with many more subject-years of follow-up and higher numbers of breast cancers, while all three trials have 4–6 years of median follow-up (Table 12.2). Only the NSABP trial found a statistically significantly lower rate of breast cancer in the tamoxifen-treated group compared to the placebo group (Table 12.2).

The characteristics of the participants in these three trials appear to be different, although not clearly so in ways which might explain the tamoxifen benefit seen in the NSABP trial. Descriptions of the population characteristics in the three reports make it difficult to draw conclusions about differences and comparability (see Table 12.1). In general, the population enrolled in the Italian

Table 12.1 *Randomized trials of tamoxifen in healthy women: population characteristics*

Trial	Reference	Subjects with one first-degree relative with breast cancer	Subjects with one or more first-degree relative with breast cancer	Subjects <50	Subjects ≥ 60	Concurrent use of HRT	LCIS
NSABP P-1	14	57%	76%	39%	30%	0%	6.3%
Royal Marsden	56	96%	—	61%	—	23%	—
European Institute of Oncology/ Italian group	28	12%	15%	38%	12%	14%	—

Table 12.2 *Randomized trial results for tamoxifen treatment in healthy women*

Trial	Reference	Total number of subjects*	Subject-years of follow-up	Median follow-up (months)	Total number of breast cancers	Breast cancers/1000 subject-years					
						Placebo			Tamoxifen		
						All	Invasive	Non-invasive	All	Invasive	Non-invasive
NSABP P-1	14	13 175	52 401	54.6	368	6.8[a]	7.5[a]	2.1[b]	3.4[a]	3.8[a]	1.3[b]
Royal Marsden	56	2471	12 355	70	70	5.0[c]			4.7[c]		
European Institute of Oncology/ Italian group	28	5408	20 712	46	41	2.3[c]			2.1[c]		

* Subjects reported in analyses.
[a] $P < 0.00001$ for difference between placebo and tamoxifen groups.
[b] $P < 0.002$ for difference between placebo and tamoxifen groups.
[c] Non-significant difference between placebo and tamoxifen groups.

Table 12.3 *Risk reduction observed in patients with different characteristics in NSABP P-1 Trial*[14]*

Parameter	Risk reduction (%)
Overall risk reduction	49
Age (years)	
$\leqslant$ 49	44
50–59	51
$\geqslant$ 60	55
Lobular carcinoma *in situ*	56
Atypical hyperplasia	86
No first-degree relatives	54
Two first-degree relatives	45

* The reduction in risk was statistically significant in patient groups with each characteristic except for the group with lobular carcinoma *in situ*, in which the small numbers of cases yielded a result of borderline statistical significance.

trial was low risk, whereas the women in the NSABP and Royal Marsden trials were at much higher risk for breast cancer.[14,28,56] The Royal Marsden Trial recruited women specifically on the basis of a family history of breast cancer in first-degree relatives, and the report authors have suggested that a large fraction of participants are likely to be carriers of known genetic predisposing genes, based on family pedigree analysis.[56] The prevalence of such genetic mutations - BCRA1 and BCRA2 - among NSABP-participant women is the subject of current study.

Certainly the Royal Marsden population appears younger (Table 12.1) than those populations in the other two trials. The other possibly important difference concerns use of hormone replacement therapy (HRT). In the Royal Marsden Study, 42% of participants had used HRT before study entry, and 23% used HRT during study participation.[56] In contrast, 33% of NSABP P-1 participants had used HRT before participation, and none were reported to be using HRT during the study.[14] Untangling the possible consequences of these broadly described differences seems a daunting task, and while subset analyses of the relationship of these characteristics to effects of tamoxifen have been attempted, these can be criticized on several grounds.

There were statistically significant risk reductions for breast cancer observed in all usual risk and age groups in the NSABP P-1 Study (Table 12.3), and reductions in occurrence of both invasive and noninvasive tumours were observed (Table 12.2). A remarkable finding in the NSABP P-1 trial was that the incidence and numbers of oestrogen receptor-positive tumours were reduced, while those of oestrogen receptor-negative tumours were unchanged (Figure 12.1). The authors of the Royal Marsden report estimated that their study had 90% power to demonstrate a 50% reduction in risk (the level of reduction observed in the NSABP Study).

The results of the NSABP P-1 Study are consistent with those in adjuvant trials – both of adjuvant benefit

and of reductions in contralateral breast cancers,[13] and in an adjuvant breast conservation study looking at ipsilateral recurrence – NSABP B-24.[15] Additionally, the results are internally consistent (Table 12.3). What then do the broadly opposite conclusions from the Royal Marsden and Italian trials convey? First, the sizes of the trials are important. Power calculations are of *relative* power, and inconclusive results to date from the two smaller trials should not be surprising. Careful scrutiny of the wide variations in results of adjuvant therapy with tamoxifen in the EBCCTG tables reminds us of this reality.[13] Secondly, while the possible compliance differences among populations in these trials have been offered as an explanation for the differing results (in particular, dropout – mostly in the first year – of 26% of the participants in the Italian trial has been suggested as an explanation for the absence of a demonstrated benefit of tamoxifen in that trial), 23.7% of the subjects in the tamoxifen group in NSABP P-1 stopped therapy.[14,28] Again, untangling this issue in these trials will be daunting, but I suggest that in fact major differences in compliance do not explain the trial result differences. Thirdly, the possible 'genetic' risk-factor differences which are postulated to impact on the biological characteristics of clinical breast cancers have been invoked to explain the negative findings in the Royal Marsden trial.[56] Recent data have suggested that the main breast cancer genes are important in DNA repair.[57] If this is so, then they might be expected to play a role early in the development of breast cancers. How such observations can be consistent with differences in oestrogen/progesterone-receptor biology in clinical lesions diagnosed 10–20 years later is unclear. In summary, the broad conclusions of the NSABP trial seem highly likely to be correct, and the most obvious explanations for the inconclusive results of the Royal Marsden and Italian trials to date are statistical.

The trial results to date certainly do not answer several central questions about the use of tamoxifen in healthy women. It remains unclear whether this therapy has overall health benefits. The absence of mortality data and the long-term consequences of this hormonal therapy given for a fixed 5-year period are completely unknown. As will be discussed below, based on the data for breast cancer, endometrial cancer, stroke and pulmonary embolism from the NSABP P-1 trial, one could postulate a small mortality benefit in both pre- and post-menopausal women, but the cost-effectiveness of tamoxifen in high-risk women is likely to be low (see below). Furthermore, the groups of women who may benefit most from this intervention are not known. The benefit for a genetic family-history-positive, high-risk group, in particular, is in question. In addition, it must be noted that the NSABP trial was conducted almost exclusively in Caucasian women, and it must be considered uncertain whether the application of these results to other ethnic groups is appropriate.

New studies of tamoxifen vs. raloxifene (a less uterine oestrogenic selective oestrogen-receptor modulator

(SERM) (the STAR trial – NSABP P-2) in post-menopausal women in the USA, of idoxifene (another SERM) vs. placebo in Canada, an ongoing international trial of tamoxifen vs. no intervention as well as continuation and follow-up of the Royal Marsden and Italian study populations, will provide more data in the years to come. The NSABP trial population is not being followed further, and the circumstances and confounding factors in the Royal Marsden and Italian trials may significantly limit the amount of useful information that can be obtained from these trials.

A cost-effectiveness analysis of the use of tamoxifen in high-risk healthy women has been presented in a detailed poster.[58] Although the authors concluded that the cost-effectiveness of tamoxifen was within the range of commonly accepted therapies, detailed conclusions and aspects of the analysis are critical. First, and most importantly, the analyses assumed an *annual* breast cancer mortality range of 3.75–6% for years 1–8, when the actual annual mortality rate for *the invasive breast cancers prevented* (oestrogen-receptor-positive, likely lymph-node-negative) in a recently reported NSABP trial was less than 1%.[59] Based on the authors' own sensitivity analyses, this much lower rate would make the cost-effectiveness of tamoxifen comparable only to exorbitantly cost-ineffective therapy levels. Secondly, the benefit is greater in younger women or in post-menopausal women who have had a hysterectomy.

The tamoxifen prevention trial reports and the commentaries on these present information on relative risk, and the cost-effectiveness analysis data, while useful, are generally less clearly relevant to clinicians and individual women trying to make informed decisions about tamoxifen chemoprevention. However, the NSABP trial data in particular provide a partial picture of absolute risk and benefit data, as the numbers of prevented or excess events associated with tamoxifen treatment. Using the actual average *annual* rates in the NSABP report, and multiplying

these by 5 (except for the vasomotor and gynaecological symptom numbers), I have shown the data in Table 12.4.[60] The excess symptom data estimates are derived from the NSABP report and another publication of ours.[14,37]

> What this portrayal of absolute events shows is that, in high-risk cohorts under and over 50 years, the numbers of prevented breast cancers over 5 years are small; the number of prevented events in women under 50 markedly exceeds the number of unfavourable events (ignoring symptoms); the number of prevented events in women 50 and over is marginally more or less than the number of unfavourable events (without or with excess uterine cancer numbers); and that 15–25% (depending on how one looks at the symptom data) of all treated women will have what they view as significant toxicity.[59]

If some reasonable assumptions are made and additional data sources are drawn upon, projections about the approximate numbers of deaths over 10 years associated with tamoxifen therapy can be made. Taking the NSABP P-1 data on incident events (as outlined in Table 12.4), mortality data from NSABP P-1, the EBCCTG and NSABP B-20 (chemotherapy plus tamoxifen in oestrogen-receptor-positive, lymph-node-negative breast cancer), and assuming that such oestrogen-receptor-positive, lymph-node-negative cancers are the subtype prevented (NSABP P-1), and that disease-free survival at 5 years from NSABP B-20[60] predicts overall survival at 10 years (this has been true in EBCCTG data[13]), the projections show that for younger women, based on current data, the benefit is perhaps slightly greater. The results of this simple analysis are consistent with the much more detailed cost-effectiveness analyses discussed above – in critical age and hysterectomy variables. Most importantly, these analyses emphasize that possible benefits of tamoxifen are only likely to occur in healthy women who are at significantly increased risk for breast cancer.[61] In

Table 12.4 *Excess or prevented events if cohorts of 1000 high-risk healthy women aged < 50 years or aged ≥ 50 years with uteri are treated with tamoxifen for 5 years**

	Excess			Prevented	
	<50 years	≥50 years		<50 years	≥50 years
Stroke	—	4.7	Invasive breast cancer	14.7	18.0
Deep vein thrombosis	1.5	3.2	Non-invasive breast cancer	6.7	6.7
Deep vein thrombosis with pulmonary embolism	0.5	3.5	Fractures	—	7.6
Cataracts	—	15.5			
Uterine cancer	1.2	11.5	Subtotal	21.4	32.3
Subtotal	3.2	38.4			
Vasomotor symptoms†	170	170			
Gynaecological symptoms‡	160	160			

* Data from the NSABP trial were used.[14]
† Hot flashes ('bothersome, quite a bit, or extremely').
‡ Vaginal discharge ('moderately, quite a bit, or extremely').

healthy Western women, the overall occurrence and death from breast cancer are low-frequency events.[62]

APPLICATION OF CURRENT DATA ON TAMOXIFEN IN HEALTHY WOMEN IN CLINICAL PRACTICE

Although, whenever possible, women should be encouraged to be involved (or to continue to participate) in clinical trials of SERMs, other chemopreventive agents or other interventions targeting breast cancer, the possible use of tamoxifen in healthy women deserves consideration. The clinical decision-making about such treatment would seem initially to involve individual risk assessment. Although the published models are incomplete, they are none the less broadly useful.[14] Based on the above discussion, it is clear that only women who are found to be at increased risk (and the 1.66% risk over 5 years is an appropriate starting point)[14,61] should be further considered for tamoxifen treatment. Histories of proliferative uterine endometrial disease or polyps, deep venous thrombosis and/or pulmonary embolism or triglyceridaemia would appear to be significant contraindications. Note that the NSABP trial attempted to exclude women with some of these risk factors, and despite these efforts, thrombosis, embolism and uterine cancer rates were increased with tamoxifen treatment. Women who are receiving hormone replacement therapy (HRT) for vasomotor symptoms or who have significant levels of vasomotor symptoms are high-risk candidates for tamoxifen. Continuing HRT while on tamoxifen has uncertain consequences, while stopping HRT is likely to be associated with a recurrence of symptoms, and tamoxifen will exacerbate these. Women who experience symptoms before treatment are much more likely to find tamoxifen-exacerbated symptoms unbearable.

Reviewing with women the likely absolute numbers of excess and prevented events shown in Tables 12.4 and 12.5 is a logical next step. Finally, discussing the management of uterine cancer risk and vasomotor symptoms before beginning therapy is appropriate. The consensus in the American professional community is that education about the cardinal sign of endometrial cancer, namely

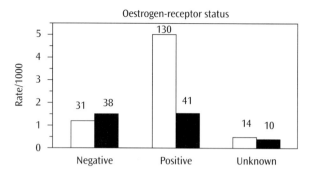

Figure 12.1 *Rates of invasive breast cancers in placebo and tamoxifen-treated groups in the NSABP P-1 trial. The lower rate of oestrogen-receptor-positive cases is highly statistically significant.*

vaginal bleeding, and annual bimanual gynaecological examination are appropriate in non-hysterectomized women.[63] Routine ultrasound or endometrial biopsy procedures are not recommended because of their non-specificity as tests for endometrial cancer. The figures shown in Tables 12.4 and 12.5 highlight the fact that, despite a major reduction in relative risk (of approximately 50%) in breast cancer in the NSABP trial (and accepting that result as 'truth'), the use of tamoxifen in selected healthy women at increased risk is a close call – that is, the benefits and risks are marginally different.

CONCLUSIONS

Although breast cancer is the most common majority malignancy in most populations of Western women, it is a low-frequency event.[62] A chemopreventive intervention such as tamoxifen, which now appears to be remarkably effective in reducing the incidence of breast cancer in high-risk women, also seems to be less than ideal for any healthy women, because it has adverse consequences which, even though they are also infrequent, manifest themselves in the large numbers of healthy treated women who are destined never to develop breast cancer. The trials reported to date have helped to clarify the importance of toxicity to populations of healthy women, have drawn attention to the

Table 12.5 *Excess or prevented deaths if 1000 high-risk healthy women aged < 50 years or aged ≥50 years with uteri are treated with tamoxifen for 5 years*

	Excess			**Prevented**	
	< 50 years	**≥ 50 years**		**< 50 years**	**≥ 50 years**
Stroke[14]	0	0.5	Breast cancer[13, 14]	1.5*	2.3†
Pulmonary embolism[14]	0	0.5			
Uterine cancer[14]	0	1			
Total	0	2.0			

* 10-year survival 90% based on Fisher *et al.*[59]

† 10-year survival 87% based on Fisher *et al.*[59]

challenges of evaluating interventions with multiple end-points and, in particular, their results have highlighted the need for long-term follow-up of treated women. An overall population-based strategy for breast cancer prevention has yet to be defined.

REFERENCES

1 Potter JD, Cerhan JR, Sellers TA *et al*. Progesterone and estrogen receptors and mammary neoplasia in the Iowa Women's Health Study: how many kinds of breast cancer are there? *Cancer Epidemiol Biomarkers Prev* 1995; **4**: 319–26.

2 Kiang K. Chemoprevention for breast cancer: are we ready? *J Natl Cancer Inst* 1991; **83**: 462–3.

3 Jordan VC, Fritz NF, Tormey DC. Endocrine effects of adjuvant chemotherapy and long-term tamoxifen administration in node-positive patients with breast cancer. *Cancer Res* 1987; **47**: 624–30.

4 Kelloff GJ, Crowell JA, Boone CW *et al*. Clinical development plan: tamoxifen. *J Cell Biochem* 1994; **20** (**Supplement**): 252–67.

5 Colletta AA, Wakefield LM, Howell FV *et al*. Anti-oestrogens induce the secretion of active transforming growth factor beta from human fetal fibroblasts. *Br J Cancer* 1990; **62**: 405–9.

6 Norris JD, Paige LA, Christensen DJ *et al*. Peptide antagonists of the human estrogen receptor. *Science* 1999; **285**: 744–6.

7 Love RR, Mazess RB, Barden HS *et al*. Effects of tamoxifen on bone mineral density in postmenopausal women with breast cancer. *N Engl J Med* 1992; **326**: 852–6.

8 Powles TJ, Hickish T, Kanis JA, Tidy A, Ashley S. Effect of tamoxifen on bone mineral density measured by dual-energy X-ray absorptiometry in healthy premenopausal and postmenopausal women. *J Clin Oncol* 1996; **14**: 78–84.

9 Love RR, Kurtycz DF, Dumesic DA, Laube DW, Yang FY. The effects of tamoxifen on the vaginal epithelium in postmenopausal women.

10 Coates A. Clinical trials. In: Love RR (ed.) *Manual of clinical oncology*. New York: Springer-Verlag, 1994: 224–32.

11 Simon R. Discovering the truth about tamoxifen: problems of multiplicity in statistical evaluation of biomedical data. *J Natl Cancer Inst* 1995; **87**: 627–9.

12 Fisher B, Costantino J, Redmond C *et al*. A randomized clinical trial evaluating tamoxifen in the treatment of patients with node-negative breast cancer who have estrogen-receptor-positive tumors. *N Engl J Med* 1989; **320**: 479–84.

13 Early Breast Cancer Trialists' Collaborative Group. Tamoxifen for early breast cancer: an overview of the randomised trials. *Lancet* 1998; **351**: 1451–67.

14 Fisher B, Costantino JP, Wickerham DL *et al*. Tamoxifen for prevention of breast cancer: report of the National Surgical Adjuvant Breast and Bowel Project P-1 Study. *J Natl Cancer Inst* 1998; **90**: 1371–88.

15 Fisher B, Dignam J, Wolmark N *et al*. Tamoxifen in treatment of intraductal breast cancer: National Surgical Adjuvant Breast and Bowel Project B-24 randomised controlled trial. *Lancet* 1999; **353**: 1993–2000.

16 Trock B. *Use of a carcinogenesis model to predict the effect of tamoxifen chemoprevention*. Unpublished report.

17 Houghton J, Riley D, Baum M. The Nolvadex Adjuvant Trial Organisation (NATO) and the Cancer Research Campaign (CRC) trials of adjuvant tamoxifen therapy. In: Jordan VC (ed.) *Long-term tamoxifen treatment for breast cancer*. Madison, WI: University of Wisconsin Press, 1994: 93–113.

18 Jefferson JW. Tamoxifen-associated reduction in tricyclic antidepressant levels in blood. *J Clin Psychopharmacol* 1995; **15**: 223–4.

19 Floren LC, Heberts MF, Venook AP, Jordan VC, Cisneros A, Somberg KA. Tamoxifen in liver disease – potential exacerbation of hepatic dysfunction. *Ann Oncol* 1998; **9**: 1123–6.

20 Jordan VC. Tamoxifen and tumorigenicity: a predictable concern (editorial). *J Natl Cancer Inst* 1995; **87**: 623–6.

21 Dragan YP, Xu Y, Pitot HC. Tumor promotion as a target for estrogen/antiestrogen effects in rat hepatocarcinogenesis. *Prev Med* 1991; **20**: 15–26.

22 Love RR, Newcomb PA, Wiebe DA *et al*. Effects of tamoxifen therapy on lipid and lipoprotein levels in postmenopausal patients with node-negative breast cancer. *J Natl Cancer Inst* 1990; **82**: 1327–32.

23 Love RR, Surawicz TS, Williams EC. Antithrombin III level, fibrinogen level, and platelet count changes with adjuvant tamoxifen therapy. *Arch Intern Med* 1992; **152**: 317–20.

24 Love RR, Anker G, Yang Y *et al*. Serum homocysteine levels in postmenopausal breast cancer patients treated with tamoxifen. *Cancer Lett* (in press).

25 Wasan KM, Ramaswamy M, Haley J, Dunn BP. Administration of long-term tamoxifen therapy modifies the plasma lipoprotein-lipid concentration and lipid transfer protein I activity in postmenopausal women with breast cancer. *J Pharm Sci* 1997; **86**: 876–9.

26 Love RR, Wiebe DA, Feyzi JM, Newcomb PA, Chappell RJ. Effects of tamoxifen on cardiovascular risk factors in postmenopausal women after 5 years of treatment. *J Natl Cancer Inst* 1994; **86**: 1534–9.

27 Hozumi Y, Kawano M, Miyata M. Severe hypertriglyceridemia caused by tamoxifen treatment after breast cancer surgery. *Endocr J* 1997; **44**: 745–59.

28 Veronesi U, Maisonneuve P, Costa A *et al*. Prevention of breast cancer with tamoxifen: preliminary findings from the Italian randomised trial among hysterectomised women. *Lancet* 1998; **352**: 93–7.

29 Bush T, Helzlsouer K. Tamoxifen for the primary prevention of breast cancer: a review and critique of the concept and trial. *Epidemiol Rev* 1993; **15**: 233–43.

30 McDonald CC, Stewart HJ. Fatal myocardial infarction in the Scottish adjuvant tamoxifen trial. *BMJ* 1991; **303**: 435–7.

31 Rutqvist LE, Mattsson A. Cardiac and thromboembolic morbidity among postmenopausal women with early-stage breast cancer in a randomized trial of adjuvant tamoxifen. The Stockholm Breast Cancer Study Group. *J Natl Cancer Inst* 1993; **85**: 1398–1406.

32 Gottardis MM, Robinson SP, Satyaswaropp PG, Jordan VC. Contrasting actions of tamoxifen on endometrial and breast tumor growth in the athymic mouse. *Cancer Res* 1988; **48**: 812–15.

33 Fornander T, Rutqvist LE, Cedermark B *et al*. Adjuvant tamoxifen in early breast cancer: occurrence of new primary cancer. *Lancet* 1989; **1**: 117–20.

34 Berliere M, Charles A, Galant C, Donnez J. Uterine side-effects of tamoxifen: a need for systematic pretreatment screening. *Obstet Gynecol* 1998; **91**: 40–4.

35 Magriples U, Naftolin F, Schwartz PE, Carcogiu ML. High-grade endometrial carcinoma in tamoxifen-treated breast cancer patients. *J Clin Oncol* 1993; **11**: 485–90.

36 Kedar RP, Bourne TH, Powles TJ *et al*. Effects of tamoxifen on uterus and ovaries of postmenopausal women in a randomised breast cancer prevention trial. *Lancet* 1994; **343**: 1318–21.

37 Love RR, Cameron L, Connell BL, Leventhal H. Symptoms associated with tamoxifen treatment in postmenopausal women. *Arch Intern Med* 1991; **151**: 1842–7.

38 Nayfield SG, Karp JE, Ford LG, Dorr FA, Kramer BS. Potential role of tamoxifen in prevention of breast cancer (review). *J Natl Cancer Inst* 1991; **83**: 1450–9.

39 Spicer DV, Pike MC, Henderson BE. Ovarian cancer and long-term tamoxifen in premenopausal women (letter). *Lancet* 1991; **337**: 1414.

40 Cullins SL, Pridjian G, Sutherland CM. Goldenhar's syndrome associated with tamoxifen given to the mother during gestation (letter). *J Am Med Assoc* 1994; **271**: 1905–6.

41 Sudo K, Monsm FJ, Katzenellenbogen BS. Antiestrogen binding sites distinct from the estrogen receptor: subcellular localization, ligand specificity, and distribution in tissues of the rat. *Endocrinology* 1983; **112**: 425–34.

42 Nolvadex Adjuvant Trial Organization. Controlled trial of tamoxifen as a single adjuvant agent in the management of early breast cancer. *Br J Cancer* 1988; **57**: 608–11.

43 Goodwin JW, Crowley J, Eyre HJ, Stafford B, Jaeckle KA, Townsend JJ. A phase II evaluation of tamoxifen in unresectable or refractory meningiomas: a South-West Oncology Group study. *J Neurooncol* 1993; **15**: 75–7.

44 Couldwell WT, Weiss MH, DeGiorgio CM *et al*. Clinical and radiographic response in a minority of patients with recurrent malignant gliomas treated with high-dose tamoxifen. *Neurosurgery* 1993; **32**: 485–90.

45 Cathcart CK, Jones SE, Pumroy CS, Peters GN, Knox SM, Cheek JH. Clinical recognition and management of depression in node-negative breast cancer patients treated with tamoxifen. *Breast Cancer Res Treat* 1993; **27**: 277–81.

46 Shariff S, Cumming CE, Lees A, Handman M, Cumming DC. Mood disorder in women with early breast cancer taking tamoxifen, an estradiol receptor antagonist. An expected or unexpected effect? *Ann N Y Acad Sci* 1995; **761**: 365–8.

47 Gray R. Response re: tamoxifen in healthy premenopausal and postmenopausal women: different risks and benefits (letter). *J Natl Cancer Inst* 1994; **86**: 63.

48 Bankson DD, Rifai N, Williams ME, Silverman LM, Gray TK. Biochemical effects of 17β-estradiol on UMR 106 cells. *Bone Miner* 1989; **6**: 55–63.

49 Kalu DN, Salerno E, Liu CC *et al*. A comparative study of the action of tamoxifen, estrogen and progesterone in the ovariectomized rat. *Bone Miner* 1991; **15**: 109–23.

50 Love RR, Barden HS, Mazess RB, Epstein S, Chappell RJ. Effect of tamoxifen on lumbar spine bone mineral density in postmenopausal women after 5 years. *Arch Intern Med* 1994; **154**: 2585–8.

51 Gorin MB, Day R, Costantino JP *et al*. Long-term tamoxifen citrate use and potential ocular toxicity. *Am J Ophthalmol* 1998; **125**: 493–501.

52 Longstaff S, Sigurdsson H, Keefe MO *et al*. A controlled study of the ocular effects of tamoxifen in conventional dosage in the treatment of breast carcinoma. *Eur J Cancer Clin Oncol* 1989; **25**: 1805–8.

53 Newcomb PA, Storer BE. Postmenopausal hormone use and risk of large-bowel cancer. *J Natl Cancer Inst* 1995; **87**: 1067–71.

54 Rutqvist LE, Johansson H, Signomklao T, Johansson U, Forander T, Wilking N. Adjuvant tamoxifen therapy for early-stage breast cancer and second primary malignancies. *J Natl Cancer Inst* 1995; **87**: 645–51.

55 Mamby CC, Love RR, Lee KE. Thyroid function test changes with adjuvant tamoxifen therapy in postmenopausal women with breast cancer. *J Clin Oncol* 1995; **13**: 854–7.

56 Powles T, Eeles R, Ashley S *et al*. Interim analysis of the incidence of breast cancer in the Royal Marsden Hospital tamoxifen randomised chemoprevention trial. *Lancet* 1998; **352**: 98–101.

57 Pfeiffer P. The mutagenic potential of DNA double-strand break repair. *Toxicol Lett* 1998; **96–7**: 119–29.

58 Noe LL, Becker RV III, Gradishar WJ, Gore M, Trotter JP. The cost-effectiveness of tamoxifen in reducing the incidence of breast cancer (Abstract No. 310). *Proc ASCO* 1999; **18**: 82a.

59 Fisher B, Dignam J, Wolmark N *et al*. Tamoxifen and chemotherapy for lymph node-negative, estrogen receptor-positive breast cancer. *J Natl Cancer Inst* 1997; **89**: 1673–82.

60 Love RR. Excess or prevented events in healthy women treated with tamoxifen. *J Natl Cancer Inst*.

61 Chlebowski R, Collyar DE, Somerfield MR, Pfister DG. American Society of Clinical Oncology technology assessment on breast cancer risk reduction strategies: tamoxifen and raloxifene. *J Clin Oncol* 1999; **17**: 1939–55.

62 Phillips KA, Glendon G, Knight JA. Putting the risk of breast cancer in perspective. *N Engl J Med* 1999; **340**: 141–4.

63 Barakat RR. Screening for endometrial cancer in the patient receiving tamoxifen for breast cancer. *J Clin Oncol* 1999; **17**: 1967–8.

13

Could cytotoxic chemotherapy have a future in the chemoprevention of breast cancer?

JEFFREY S TOBIAS AND JOAN HOUGHTON

Breast cancer has assumed an incidence and mortality of epidemic proportions among western women today. In the USA, for example, over 180 000 patients are diagnosed each year, with 100 deaths occurring daily from this disease – four deaths every hour round the clock. At least 1 in 10 of all women will develop breast cancer during their lifetime, and in some areas the figure is as high as 1 in 8. More than 70% of the patients have no known risk factors, and there have undoubtedly been rises in both incidence and mortality over the past 50 years, most probably as a result of delayed first pregnancy or nulliparity.[1,2]

THE CHALLENGE OF BREAST CANCER

Two crucial and unwelcome facts concerning the biology of breast cancer have gone largely unrecognized. First, despite many advances in both diagnosis and management, the disease is still usually fatal, not at the immediate point of diagnosis but at a later time, allowing both the medical profession and the public alike to sustain the present degree of complacency rather than sense the immediate danger of a more rapidly lethal diagnosis. Yet 75% of women diagnosed with breast cancer will be dead within 20 years.[3] With an ever increasing expected lifespan (e.g. almost 79 years in women in the UK), the average number of years of life lost by such patients is also increasing, and currently stands at almost 20 years per patient.[4] For young women (and it is no longer unusual to see patients aged 35 years or younger) the loss is greater still. Secondly, although the disease is diagnosed at a particular time-point during a woman's life, it must

be recognized that this most certainly does not coincide with the true biological appearance of the cancer. Breast cancer is quite different from acute infectious diseases, for example, in which an inflammatory change within the offending organ produces a rapid complex of symptoms which results in diagnosis within 1 or 2 weeks. Patients diagnosed as having breast cancer have merely been identified at a certain arbitrary time-point, well along the true path of the emerging illness, and with a latent period of many years between initiation of the malignant process and recognition of the disease. This general point remains equally true for patients diagnosed by screening rather than through symptomatic presentation. Our current concepts of genetic predetermination imply, of course, that at least for a proportion of patients, birth or even conception may rightly be regarded as 'time zero'.[5]

Despite our best attempts with patient education, mammography, ultrasound, tumour-marker analysis, and so on, there is no such thing as genuinely early diagnosis in breast cancer. The concept as understood at present is a fallacy. In biological terms, diagnosing an impalpable 0.5 cm tumour at mammography represents an insignificant shift to the left along the evolutionary pathway of breast cancer, compared to diagnosis at, say, 1.5 cm when the lump becomes palpable.[6] The difference between half a trillion or a trillion cells is truly trivial. What women (and doctors) want and need is diagnosis at a much earlier stage, say 10^2 or 10^3 cells, at a point where our weak but partly effective forms of systemic treatment might have a more valuable role. Sadly, our present approach, with its emphasis on radiological mammographic techniques, is not only ineffective in the younger age group, but possibly positively harmful in such patients,[7] to say nothing of the huge cost. Even in older women, screening on a national level has proved disappointing despite initial enthusiasm.[8]

In affluent western societies it seems probable that incidence rates of breast cancer will remain high for the foreseeable future, and may possibly even increase. Globally, the widespread 'Westernization' of traditional societies (there are many examples in Japan and the Pacific rim) will increase the world-wide epidemic still further. Increasing use of hormone replacement therapy (HRT) may possibly contribute, since the latter is thought to increase the risk of breast cancer by 2% per year of use,[9,10] with a cumulative increase, for example, of more than 20% over a 10-year exposure period. Furthermore, the increasing use of HRT is likely to make mammography even less reliable than at present because of the loss of radiological resolution engendered by these hormone combinations.[11–13]

In any highly lethal condition there can be no improvement in mortality figures without a lowering of the incidence rate, unless effective treatment is available. Since we cannot claim this at present, the question of what means of prevention are already available arises. Surgery (bilateral prophylactic mastectomy) is already in use, and tamoxifen is currently under clinical trial. For surgery, the concept and intent are clear, namely the removal of the sensitive end organ in patients at high risk, in order to eradicate the risk of malignant change altogether.[14,15] For women at high risk because of BRCA1 or 2 genetic mutation, both bilateral mastectomy and also prophylactic oophorectomy have been advocated or at least given serious consideration.[16,17] Yet we know that breast cancer is generally a systemic condition, and that distant metastases are presumably established before the surgical diagnosis is made, possibly augmented by the surgical shedding of malignant cells at biopsy and primary treatment.[18,19] This fact, coupled with the impossibility of providing an adequate and cosmetic total removal of all breast tissue, makes prophylactic mastectomy conceptually unappealing (to say nothing of the human concerns). Furthermore, the very long lead time of breast cancer development (years of carcinogenesis identified only at an arbitrary moment) clearly implies that the operation should be performed relatively early in a woman's life for optimum effect. None the less, surgical prophylaxis has found a foothold despite its aesthetic and other drawbacks, as many women at high risk fear the consequences of developing breast cancer more than they can bear, and feel that they are 'doing the best thing' by sacrificing their natural breasts. How terrible to undergo this mutilating procedure only to develop the disease at a later stage, as over 1% of high-risk women do.[20] Furthermore, in the Schrag analysis's of BRCA1 and 2 carriers, the median gain in an average 30-year-old woman was calculated to be only 3–5.3 years of life expectancy from prophylactic bilateral mastectomy, and from 0.3–1.7 years from prophylactic oophorectomy.

Gains in life expectancy decline with age at the time of prophylactic surgery and are minimal for 60-year-old women.[17]

Less dramatic and more widely accepted is the concept of tamoxifen chemoprophylaxis, now currently undergoing trial in Europe, Australia and the USA. However, the rationale is flawed by the reduced effectiveness of tamoxifen in oestrogen-receptor-negative tumours, particularly in younger patients, by the lengthy period for which it needs to be given and by the very small but real risk of carcinogenesis (endometrial cancer).[21–24] One recent study[25] of 2 years exposure confirmed that only 70% of women continue to take tamoxifen (or the placebo) for the whole trial period, despite their initial high motivation.

ADVANTAGES OF CYTOTOXIC CHEMOTHERAPY AS PROPHYLAXIS

Why might cytotoxic chemotherapy have advantages over surgery or tamoxifen? First, it is a systemic form of therapy that is known to be partially effective even in the most adverse group of patients with breast cancer, namely node-positive premenopausal women, with a therapeutic benefit at least as great as tamoxifen. Secondly, it also benefits the node-negative premenopausal group (with consistent improvement in disease-free survival), with increasing evidence that it has at least some effectiveness in the older age group. Thirdly, it does not appear to depend on oestrogen-receptor status for its effectiveness, certainly not to the same degree as tamoxifen.[26,27] Fourthly, it is genuinely cytotoxic rather than acting via a cytostatic pathway as tamoxifen probably does. One practical consequence of this is that effective doses can be given over a much shorter time period, arguably causing less disruption to the woman's life, at least from a temporal point of view. Randomized trials of peri-operative chemotherapy have taught us that even a single exposure to chemotherapy drugs can give long-lasting protection against the lethal effects of metastases apparently shed during the surgical procedure.[28–30] Furthermore, like tamoxifen but unlike surgery, chemotherapy is known to have a long-lasting benefit for at least 10 years, even though in most patients the chemotherapy will have been discontinued 9.5 years previously, with a statistically greater benefit at 10 years than at 5 years, and possibly even greater benefit at 15 years or beyond. Finally, data from the most recent (1998) global overview confirm that, like tamoxifen, adjuvant chemotherapy reduces the incidence of contralateral breast cancer, with a 20% reduction in the annual risk. This type of effect was one of the principal justifications for prevention trials using tamoxifen.

With regard to the number of courses needed for optimum effect, at least one study from Germany[30] has suggested that three courses of adjuvant combination chemotherapy (using CMF – cyclophosphamide, methotrexate and 5-fluorouracil – the best-researched type of chemotherapy) apparently have equivalent benefit to six courses. Although such practical concerns are not strictly the province of a hypothetical argument, it is of interest that CMF chemotherapy is inexpensive, easy to administer on an out-patient basis, and much more acceptable nowadays with the wide range of anti-emetic, counselling and other support measures available. One might envisage that further benefits could include protection against the emergence of other forms of chemosensitive malignancy, notably lymphoma, ovarian carcinoma and (possibly) colorectal and small-cell lung cancer. It is certainly not fanciful, from what we already know about the effectiveness of chemotherapy in early vs. late (bulky) tumours, to suggest that the currently available agents should be very much more effective with a small tumour bulk of, say, $10^2 - 10^5$ cells, than against the $10^8 - 10^9$ cells that most clinically apparent tumours contain.

PREVENTION RATHER THAN EARLY DETECTION

For a real reduction in mortality from breast cancer, it is clear that we cannot wait for the confirmed histological diagnosis which is at present regarded as the *sine qua non* before treatment can be considered. Indeed there is some evidence that surgery itself may be a major cause of shedding of malignant cells.[18,19] In our view, this probably applies just as much to a fine-needle aspiration as to a surgical operation. After all, from the point of view of a clump of cancer cells within the stroma of the breast, the arrival of a fine needle followed by high-pressure traumatic suction is likely to be just as disruptive, and therefore capable of distant cellular escape, as the more controlled and gentle surgical removal of the whole tumour with its margin of histologically normal tissue. Indeed, there is a growing body of opinion that even breast compression during mammography may be detrimental.[32,33] Thus both conceptually and from a practical point of view, an attempt at tumour control has to be made much earlier in the evolution of the cancer than is currently the case. The drawback, of course, is that one cannot identify the individual who is 'secretly' harbouring a lethal tumour, although clearly one can identify a *group* of individuals at high risk, in whom early diagnosis and treatment would be highly attractive if effective therapy were available.

Apart from the important conceptual difference between screening mammography (for early detection) and 'therapeutic' chemoprevention (for genuinely early 'treatment', albeit only for those who harbour an occult but developing malignancy), we know that the former

requires very wide uptake by the community, preferably on a national scale, for it to provide efficient use of resources.[34] However, with early chemotherapy, women who find the concept appealing and wish to participate could do so. Uptake on a national scale would not be required to make such a policy cost-effective. This applies to all chemopreventive agents, but apart from tamoxifen and fenretinide (4HPR), which are under trial, the only other group of substances that has been given serious consideration in this context is a modified version of the oral contraceptive pill[35] (and the retinoids and deltanoids, which have no track record whatever in the prevention of adenocarcinoma, despite their effectiveness in some studies in squamous-cell metaplasia.[36,37]). An alternative proposal, postulated from epidemiological studies, and now under trial, is to reduce fat intake. It is suggested that the mechanism may be related to a reduction in endogenous oestradiol levels, although for many women, chemical induction of an earlier menopause might have more appeal than the drastic dietary changes which would be essential over a protracted period of time.

If we are to make progress with the best possible use of currently available treatments, logic dictates the abandonment of the principle of 'healthy until diagnosed', with the inevitable complacency that this engenders. The alternative is to await newer and more effective treatments, which could be years or even decades away. In an epidemic in which over 10% of an apparently healthy female population will develop a disease which is usually fatal, we must start to think of 'illness' and 'health' in a new way. For breast cancer, the nature and size of the risk can be reasonably quantified for many women. Should we simply ignore this information, or can we make a really worthwhile paradigm shift (there were many references to this concept at the Brugge conference but, frankly, not many really new ideas) and use our new insights in a potentially valuable, protective manner? Although it is quite compatible to be both an individual and a point on a risk curve, we propose that it is probably more helpful, from the point of view of protection against breast cancer, to think of women in the latter way, in order to recognize where we might usefully intervene, prior to a diagnosis that comes too late. What use is a paradigm shift that does not lead to a testable hypothesis?

In fact, there are number of precedents already. For example, hypertension is not really a disease state itself, but is recognizably dangerous – to the point of requiring treatment in the majority of cases – because of the damage that can ensue. Hypertensive patients accept many years (and often decades) of continuous treatment because of the consequences of not doing so, although many are diagnosed at routine examinations when they are totally asymptomatic and, furthermore, antihypertensive drugs are certainly not without side-effects! In the field of oncology, every patient who accepts 'adjuvant' chemotherapy (now established in an increasing number of cancers, including osteosarcoma, breast, ovarian, colorectal and other cancers) is, consciously or not, recognizing the concept of risk as it applies to themselves as individuals. It is true that the typical premenopausal node-positive breast cancer patient undergoing six courses of chemotherapy has a vested interest, but it is equally true that at the time of treatment the assumed micrometastatic disease is entirely occult – the words 'secret' or 'invisible' would do equally well – making the treatment an act of faith rather than something that is deliberately given for a measurable, observable degree of residual disseminated disease. Even if we had reliable markers, as is the case with testicular cancers, the activity of currently available systemic treatments would be inadequate to cure the majority of patients (unlike the situation in testicular malignancy), even if treatment was provided at the earliest definable point of relapse because, at that point, the tumour burden, although not detectable at distant sites, is still too great.

CHEMOTHERAPY IS BOTH CYTOTOXIC AND ENDOCRINE ABLATIVE

According to cancer epidemiologists, the most effective way to lower the incidence (and therefore mortality) of breast cancer would be to reduce the mean age of menopause, a concept that is strongly supported both by epidemiological data[10,38] and by the known effectiveness of ovarian ablation as adjuvant therapy for early breast cancer. Both early menarche and late menopause, which are probably a result of high-level nutrition in the contemporary western world, increase the risk of breast cancer, particularly when augmented by late first pregnancy and only partial dependence on natural breastfeeding.[39] As chemotherapy clearly reduces ovarian function, one of its mechanisms of action should be to reduce the incidence of breast cancer via the ovarian–hypothalamic–pituitary axis. However, unlike tamoxifen or ovarian ablation, its benefits would not be limited to this single mechanism of action. Even when chemotherapy does not lead to immediate cessation of menses, earlier physiological menopause can be a consequence, and would probably be acceptable – and often even desirable – to the majority of women who have completed their families. Supplementary low doses of HRT could be offered to these women to prevent osteoporosis and other undesirable consequences of the menopause, as doses of circulating oestrogen metabolites would be far lower than with endogenous hormones, thus providing benefit without disadvantages.[40] Our experience with adjuvant tamoxifen and chemotherapy for established breast cancer would suggest that even a short-term switching off of ovarian function may be valuable, even if it is not complete or sustained in the long term.[41]

One hypothesis among several which could explain the current proven benefits of adjuvant systemic chemotherapy is that all patients may well benefit to an equal degree, a conclusion which is unjustifiable for tamoxifen, on the basis of the evidence currently available. We know that adjuvant systemic chemotherapy reduces recurrence events, even in node-negative patients with a relatively good prognosis. It is more difficult to demonstrate improved overall survival in this group, but this is likely to be nothing more than a statistical problem, namely the difficulty of demonstrating improved overall survival (OS) where short-term OS (up to 10 years) is already reasonably good. However, in terms of relative benefit, chemotherapy is equally effective in both node-positive and node-negative groups. For example, a single peri-operative course of adjuvant chemotherapy reduces the relapse rate even in node-negative patients to a dramatic extent.[30] These observations have considerable biological significance, lending support to the wider use of a treatment with important potential side-effects (such as systemic chemotherapy), as fewer patients with emerging breast cancer treated in this way would be undergoing a 'valueless' or 'unnecessary' treatment. Furthermore, the early treatment (with systemic chemotherapy) of impending relapse of breast cancer patients as defined by rising blood levels of CEA and CA 15-3 has already been shown to delay the onset of clinically identifiable metastatic disease, although not to the point of cure, in patients with established breast cancer.[42]

DISADVANTAGES OF USING CYTOTOXIC CHEMOPREVENTION

Previous studies using adjuvant chemotherapy to prevent relapse in established breast cancer have not only provided reliable data to show that this form of treatment is effective, but have also yielded estimates of the magnitude of improvement we might reasonably expect. It is possible that up until now we may have barely scratched the surface of what is achievable with currently available combinations of drugs. Use of chemotherapy much earlier in breast cancer seems logical in order to treat patients when the tumour burden is at its lowest, but we have to accept the fact that this inevitably means treatment at a time when there can be no certainty whatever that the 'subject' is truly a 'patient'. This drawback, coupled with the perceived toxicity of chemotherapy, will inevitably form the backbone of any rebuttal of our proposal, but it is worth reiterating that for the majority of patients, a diagnosis of breast cancer is tantamount to the identification of a fatal condition – one which will shorten the patient's life by, on average, 15–20 years – and for most, a diagnosis that is made too late. Inevitably a policy of early chemoprevention such as we are proposing would lead to 'over-treatment' in a substantial number of cases. In our view, however, this could be more than balanced by early destruction of occult breast cancers if the chemoprevention was successful. We should remember that, at present, despite all of our therapeutic attempts in established disease, we have no alternative but to 'under-treat' (i.e. treat unsuccessfully) the majority of patients. The disadvantage of unnecessary over-treatment that results from preventative therapy is inconvenience and physical upset for a few months, admittedly severe in a minority of patients but the penalty of our inadequate current treatment may be a 20-year loss of life. Short-term side-effects of chemotherapy such as partial and temporary hair loss, nausea and vomiting are upsetting for a few months, but are by no means inevitable, and the feasibility and acceptability of out-patient chemotherapy are improving all the time. For some women, surgical or radiation-induced ovarian ablation, a known method of adjuvant benefit for pre-menopausal patients,[43] carries its own disadvantages.

A further theoretical drawback relates to the possible ineffectiveness of chemotherapy during the early pre-malignant phase of carcinogenesis. Even if chemotherapy were to be effective in the manner we propose, might it be valueless during the lengthy period between the initial insult and the first genuinely 'malignant' cell divisions – that is, the very period we wish to exploit? In our view, the rate at which 'pre-malignant' and 'malignant' events succeed each other (presumably sequentially) remains poorly understood and, furthermore, pre-malignant or very early malignant changes could still, in any event, prove to be chemosensitive. A recent study of the natural history of breast cancer suggested that, for a typical post-menopausal patient, the initial malignant cell would generally have been present for approximately a decade, and sometimes longer.[44]

An increased incidence of chemotherapy-induced second malignancies is an even more important potential complication, but appears to be extremely rare for CMF-type regimens. Adjuvant trials of CMF vs. control have shown no increased risk of second malignancies in the treated patients over a 10-year period,[45] nor has a combined analysis of adjuvant trials using cyclophosphamide in a number of different centres.[46] In our view, these disadvantages, although theoretically important, might be regarded as acceptable compared to the high stakes of effective early control in a frequently fatal condition. Furthermore, in patients with a 'good' prognosis (i.e. only 1–3 positive axillary nodes or larger tumours with negative nodes), adjuvant chemotherapy with MF rather than CMF may provide equal benefit. This is an important point as cyclophosphamide is probably the most carcinogenic of the three agents.[47,48] At least it is now clear that there is no increased incidence of contralateral primary breast cancer following CMF chemotherapy. In fact, quite the reverse is true.[26]

The observation that tamoxifen markedly reduces this incidence (at least up to 3 years) has been the major stimulus for its use as a preventative agent. However, the use of contralateral disease as a model for primary breast cancer is open to debate. Data from the CRC Adjuvant Trial suggests that the process may represent a delay rather than a durable long-lasting prevention.[49] Further analysis at the next round of the Overview may show whether the difference demonstrated in the early years of trials, predominantly of 2 years of therapy, is maintained in the long term or diminished in size.

TRIAL OF CYTOTOXIC CHEMOPREVENTION

Our proposal, therefore, is that cytotoxic chemotherapy should seriously be considered as the best means of chemoprevention of breast cancer, that the most logical approach would be to use it in women aged 30–40 years who have completed their families, and that a randomized chemoprophylaxis study would be necessary to test this hypothesis, using *at least* three courses of (C)MF chemotherapy and with three possible end-points (the diagnosis of primary breast cancer, the diagnosis of malignant disease of all other types, and mortality). Clearly this would have to be a large national study, but judging by the enthusiasm of many women to enlist in the tamoxifen prevention programme, and their rapid and unprejudiced acceptance of promising new methods in breast cancer treatment, this should not prove overwhelmingly difficult.

The criteria for entry would be essentially similar to those for the trials of prevention with tamoxifen, but with further consideration as to the specific risk factors in pre-menopausal women. Genetic testing for breast cancer is likely to be available in the foreseeable future. Women with a high risk of developing the disease, although representing only about 5% of breast cancer cases, are likely to demand immediate therapy. It has been estimated that nearly 9 in 10 women who carry the BRCA1 gene will develop breast cancer by the age of 70 years,[50] and a recent population-based Icelandic study suggested a cumulative risk rate of 37% at age 70 years for BRCA2 carriers.[51] What do we have to offer them? For younger women, cytotoxic therapy over a few months may have more appeal and effectiveness than prolonged tamoxifen therapy.

In addition to women who are currently eligible for inclusion in tamoxifen chemoprevention studies, a further group of suitable subjects potentially includes those with a diagnosis of *in-situ* disease – a diagnosis of increasing numerical significance. Although surgical removal of the lesion is currently considered to be necessary (many of these patients are somewhat paradoxically now undergoing full mastectomy), could the time come when cytotoxic therapy is given and surgery is only instituted for disease that does not respond completely, as with neoadjuvant treatment for invasive disease? Once again, women may find this option less distressing than surgery followed by adjuvant therapy with tamoxifen and/or radiotherapy.

One final point should be made here. We know from recent studies that systemic chemotherapy confers some benefit, even to patients with established disease, for at least 10 years. We would therefore further propose that the use of 'early' chemotherapy, as we define it here (prior to the confirmed tissue diagnosis of breast cancer), might logically need to be repeated approximately every decade between the ages of, say, 30 and 70 years. Such preventative intervention may also be the best place to evaluate fully the role of biological response modifiers. Weisenthal et al.[52] have speculated that response to chemotherapy results in massive release and processing of tumour antigens, and that this response leads to a state in which the human immune system is primed ('vaccination in situ') to respond to exogenous macrophage-activation signals with potent and specific anti-tumour effects. This hypothesis needs further testing in animal models but, if true, may well add to the efficacy of 'early' treatment without contributing a great deal of toxicity. Or is this a paradigm shift too far?

We hope that the radical, even outrageous, nature of our proposal will be accepted in the spirit in which it is intended, in keeping with continued calls for fresh ideas in breast cancer research, and the stated aims of the US-based Breast Cancer Coalition of frustrated and angry women who are no longer prepared to accept that a mostly conservative medical establishment is genuinely giving of its best.

ACKNOWLEDGEMENTS

Joan Houghton is funded by the Cancer Research Campaign.

REFERENCES

1 MacMahon B, Cole P, Lin TM et al. Age at first birth and breast cancer risk. Bull WHO 1970; **43**: 209–21.

2 Ewertz M, Duffy SW, Adami H-O et al. Age at first birth, parity and risk of breast cancer: a meta-analysis of 8 studies from the Nordic countries. Int J Cancer 1990; **46**: 597–603.

3 Mueller CB, Ames F, Anderson GD. Breast cancer in 3558 women: age as a significant determinant in the rate of dying and causes of death. Surgery 1978; **83**: 123–32.

4 Rossof AH, Furner SE. Years of potential life lost from breast cancer: analysis of trends over time. Lancet Conference on the Challenge of Breast Cancer, Brugge, 1994: 80 (abstract).

5 Trichopoulos D. Hypothesis: does breast cancer originate in utero? Lancet 1990; **335**: 939–40.

6 Plotkin D, Blakenberg F. Breast cancer – biology and malpractice. Am J Clin Oncol 1991; **14**: 254–66.

7 Elwood JM, Cox B, Richardson AK. The effectiveness of breast cancer screening by mammography in younger women. Online J Curr Clin Trials 1993; **32**: 227.

8 Anon. Breast cancer: have we lost our way? Lancet 1993; **341**: 343–4.

9 Henderson BE, Ross RK, Pike MC. Hormonal chemoprevention of cancer in women. Science 1993; **259**: 633–8.

10 Grady D, Rubin SM, Petitti DB et al. Hormone therapy to prevent disease and prolong life in postmenopausal women. Ann Intern Med 1992; **117**: 1016–37.

11 Berkowitz JE, Gatewood OMB, Goldblum LE, Gayler BW. Hormonal replacement therapy – mammographic manifestations. Radiology 1990; **174**: 199–201.

12 Stomper PC, van Voorhis BJ, Ravnilar VA, Mayer JE. Mammographic changes associated with postmenopausal hormone replacement therapy: a longitudinal study. Radiology 1990; **174**: 487–90.

13 van de Mooren MJ, Marugg RC, Hendriks JHCL, Ruijs JHJ, Holland R. Effects of hormonal replacement therapy on mammographic breast cancer pattern in postmenopausal women. Lancet Conference on the Challenge of Breast Cancer, Brugge, 1994: 40 (abstract).

14 Hartmann LC, Schaid D, Woods JE et al. Efficacy of bilateral prophylactic mastectomy in women with a family history of breast cancer. N Engl J Med 1999; **340**: 77–84.

15 Eisen A, Weber BL. Prophylactic mastectomy – the price of fear. N Engl J Med 1999; **340**: 137–8.

16 Schrag D, Kuntz KM, Garber JE, Weeks JC. Decision analysis – effects of prophylactic mastectomy and oophorectomy on life expectancy among women with BRCA1 or BRCA2 mutations. N Engl J Med 1997; **336**: 1465–71.

17 Meijers-Heijboer EJ, Verhoog LC, Brekelmans CTM et al. Presymptomatic DNA testing and prophylactic surgery in families with BRCA1 or BRCA2 mutation. Lancet 2000; **355**: 2015–20.

18 Nissen-Meyer R. Chemotherapy and endocrine therapy of early breast cancer. Rev Endocr Related Cancer 1980; **Supplement 6**: 71–82.

19 Badwe RA, Baum M, Houghton J, Fentiman IS, Gregory WM. Does surgery perturb the natural history of breast cancer? Br J Cancer 1992; **66**: 9–12.

20 Eldar S, Meguid MM, Beatty JD. Cancer of the breast after prophylactic subcutaneous mastectomy. Am J Surg 1984; **148**: 692–3.

21 Andersson M, Storm HH, Mouridsen HT. Carcinogenic effects of adjuvant tamoxifen treatment and radiotherapy for early breast cancer. Acta Oncol 1992; **31**: 259–63.

22 Fornander T, Hellstrom A-C, Moberger B. Descriptive clinico-pathological study of 17 patients with endometrial cancer during or after adjuvant tamoxifen in early breast cancer. J Natl Cancer Inst 1993; **85**: 1850–85.

23 Fisher B, Costantino JP, Redmond CK et al. Endometrial carcinoma in tamoxifen-treated breast cancer patients: findings from the National Surgical Adjuvant Breast and Bowel Project (NSABP) B-14. J Natl Cancer Inst 1994; **86**: 527–37.

24 van Leeuwen FE, Benraadt J, Coebergh JWW et al. Risk of endometrial cancer after tamoxifen treatment of breast cancer. Lancet 1994; **343**: 448–52.

25 Powles TJ, Hardy JR, Ashley SE *et al*. A pilot trial to evaluate the acute toxicity and feasibility of tamoxifen for prevention of breast cancer. *Br J Cancer* 1989; **60**: 126–31.

26 Early Breast Cancer Trialists' Collaborative Group. Polychemotherapy for early breast cancer: an overview of the randomised trials. *Lancet* 1998; **352**: 930–42.

27 Zambetti M, Bonadonna G, Valagussa P *et al*. Adjuvant CMF for node-negative and estrogen-receptor-negative breast cancer patients. *J Natl Cancer Inst Monogr* 1992; **11**: 77–83.

28 Nissen-Meyer R, Kjellgren K, Malmio K *et al*. Surgical adjuvant chemotherapy. *Cancer* 1978; **41**: 2088–98.

29 Houghton J, Baum M, Nissen-Meyer R *et al*. Is there a role for peri-operative adjuvant cytotoxic therapy in the treatment of early breast cancer? In: Senn H, Goldhirsch A, Gelber RD, Osterwalder B (eds) *Recent results in cancer research – adjuvant therapy of primary breast cancer*. Berlin: Springer-Verlag, 1989: 54–61.

30 Goldhirsch A, Castiglione M and Gelber RD for the IBCSG. A single perioperative adjuvant chemotherapy course for node-negative breast cancer: five-year results of trial V. *J Natl Cancer Inst Monogr* 1992; **11**: 89–96.

31 Kaufmann M, Jonat W, Caffier H *et al*. Adjuvant cytotoxic chemotherapy. In: Salmon S (ed.) *Adjuvant therapy of cancer*. Orlando, FL: Grune and Stratton.

32 Watmough DJ, Quan KM. X-ray mammography and breast compression. *Lancet* 1992; **339**: 340–420.

33 van Netten JP, Mogentale T, Ashwood Smith MJ, Fletcher C, Coy P. Physical trauma and breast cancer. *Lancet* 1994; **343**: 979.

34 Patnick J, Austoker J. High compliance is essential in breast-screening programmes. *Br J Med* 1994; **308**: 65.

35 Spicer DV, Shoupe D, Pike MC *et al*. GnRH agonists as contraceptive agents: predicted significantly reduced risk of breast cancer. *Contraception* 1991; **44**: 289–310.

36 Sporn MB, Roberts AB, Anzano MA. New approaches to the prevention of breast cancer. *Lancet* Conference on the Challenge of Breast Cancer, Brugge, 1994: 14 (abstract).

37 Greenwald P, Kelloff G. The chemoprevention of cancer. In: Fortner J, Rhoads J (eds) *Accomplishments in cancer research 1992*. Philadelphia, PA: J B Lippincott Co., 1993.

38 Tricopoulos D, MacMahon B, Cole P. Menopause and breast cancer risk. *J Natl Cancer Inst* 1972; **48**: 604–13.

39 Chilvers CED, Pike MC, Hermon C, Crossley B. Breast cancer and breast-feeding. *Lancet* Conference on the Challenge of Breast Cancer, Brugge, 1994: 12 (abstract).

40 Pike MC, Berstein L, Spicer DV. In: Dekker NJE (ed.) *Current therapy in oncology*. St Louis, MO: Mosby-Year Book, 1993: 292–303.

41 Brincker H, Rose C, Rank F *et al*. Evidence of a castration-mediated effect of adjuvant cytotoxic chemotherapy in premenopausal breast cancer. *J Clin Oncol* 1987; **5**: 1771–8.

42 Jager W, Kramer S, Lang N. Disseminated breast cancer: does early treatment prolong survival without symptoms? *Lancet* Conference on the Challenge of Breast Cancer, Brugge, 1994: 54 (abstract).

43 Early Breast Cancer Trialists' Collaborative Group. Ovarian ablation in early breast cancer: overview of the randomised trials. *Lancet* 1996; **348**: 1189–96.

44 Semiglazov VF, Noiseyenko VK, Pozharisski KK, Chernomordikova NF. Natural history of breast cancer – new proposals to early detection. *Eur J Cancer* 1994; **30A**: 25 (abstract).

45 Valagussa P, Tancini G, Bonadonna G. Second malignancies after CMF for resectable breast cancer. *J Clin Oncol* 1987; **5**: 1138–42.

46 Holdener EE, Nissen-Myer R, Bonadonna G *et al*. Remaining problems of adjuvant chemotherapy in breast cancer. In: Senn H (ed.) *Recent results in cancer research. Adjuvant chemotherapy of breast cancer*. Heidelberg: Springer-Verlag, 1984: 188–96.

47 Curtis RE, Boice JD Jr, Moloney WC *et al*. Leukemia following chemotherapy for breast cancer. *Cancer Res* 1990, **50**. 2741–6.

48 Shapiro CL, Gelman R, Hayes DF *et al*. *J Natl Cancer Inst* 1993; **85**: 812–17.

49 Cancer Research Campaign Breast Cancer Trials Group. The effect of adjuvant tamoxifen: the latest results from the Cancer Research Campaign Adjuvant Breast Trial. *Eur J Cancer* 1992; **28A**: 904–7.

50 Ford D, Easton DF, Bishop DT, Norad SA, Goldgar DE. Risks of cancer in *BRCA*1-mutation carriers. *Lancet* 1994; **343**: 692–5.

51 Thorlacius S, Struewing JP, Hartge P *et al*. Population-based study of risk of breast cancer in carriers of *BRCA*2 mutation. *Lancet* 1998; **352**: 1337–9.

52 Weisenthal L, Dill PL, Pearson FC. Effect of prior cancer chemotherapy on human tumour-specific cytotoxicity *in vitro* in response to immunopotentiating biologic response modifiers. *J Natl Cancer Inst* 1991; **83**: 37–42.

Current and future management

14

To dissect or not – what is the role of axillary surgery in management and research?

TIM DAVIDSON

The question of axillary dissection remains one of the most controversial areas in the treatment of breast cancer. As a surgical procedure it has definite operative morbidity and in some patients long-term side-effects, yet its importance both for disease staging and for treatment has meant that it has been accepted as standard practice by many breast units. The place of axillary dissection has remained a matter of intense debate in the UK,[1–3] in Europe[4] and in the USA.[5]

In evaluating the role of axillary surgery in the management of breast cancer, a number of questions need to be addressed. These include operative treatment vs. radiotherapy to the axilla in the primary treatment of breast cancer, axillary node sampling vs. full axillary dissection, elective axillary dissection vs. 'wait-and-see' management of the axilla, and the place of sentinel-node biopsy.[6]

The arguments for and against axillary dissection can initially be considered in two main areas – first, those involving *staging* and prognosis, and secondly, those involving *treatment* for involved (or potentially involved) axillary lymph nodes. In this chapter we shall deal with the role of axillary surgery in relation to each of these areas, and also outline the current place of axillary surgery in research.

AXILLARY-NODE STAGING

The histological status of axillary nodes in early breast cancer remains the single best marker of disease behaviour and ultimate outcome.[7] Prognostic information from other parameters such as tumour size, histological grade, hormone-receptor status and the presence of vascular invasion can make a major contribution to assessing the prognosis in an individual patient, but is less accurate than formulae (such as the Nottingham prognostic index) which include axillary lymph-node status.

Clinical examination of the axilla is an important part of the initial staging evaluation, and the examination routinely evaluates the absence or presence of palpable nodes (N_0 vs. N_1), whether they are considered on the basis of size and consistency to be benign or to contain tumour (N_{1a} vs. N_{1b}), and whether they are mobile or fixed (N_1 vs. N_2). In addition, associated arm oedema or brachial plexus symptoms are possible indicators of locally advanced axillary disease.

However, in the majority of cases the accuracy of clinical examination is poor, with both false-positive and false-negative results in up to one-third of cases (Table 14.1). Clinical staging may be even more inaccurate if it is performed after a biopsy procedure on the breast, when reactive node enlargement may confound the issue.[8] Attempts to use immunoscintigraphy[9,10] and ultrasound[11] for non-invasive axillary staging have been disappointing. Magnetic resonance imaging (MRI) using a dedicated breast coil can identify enlarged involved axillary nodes, but is unable to evaluate the axilla in up to 25% of patients.[12]

The argument in favour of axillary dissection with respect to staging is that accurate prognostic information can be obtained upon which decisions about adjuvant treatment can rationally be made. The world overview on the management of breast cancer provided

Table 14.1 *Accuracy of physical examination in predicting histological involvement of axillary nodes in patients with operable breast cancer.*[2] *Reprinted by permission of Churchill Livingstone*

Series	Clinical assessment	
	False-positive (%)	False-negative (%)
Butcher *et al.* (1969)	25	32
Haagensen *et al.* (1971)	24	32
Bucalosi *et al.* (1971)	29	29
Schottenfeld *et al.* (1976)[17]	26	27
Danforth *et al.* (1986)[16]	11	38

robust evidence that systemic adjuvant therapy given to patients with involved axillary nodes decreases the odds of dying from breast cancer by up to 30%.[13] Although a reduction in the odds of dying is also observed in patients with node-negative breast cancer, the absolute benefit from adjuvant chemotherapy in these patients is proportionally less. In premenopausal early breast cancer, axillary-node staging has become the most important factor in determining whether adjuvant systemic chemotherapy is recommended.

In addition to establishing the tumour stage by nodal status, the prognosis in individual patients can be further stratified according to the total number of nodes involved as well as the anatomical level of involvement.[14,15] The axillary contents are divided anatomically into three levels (I, II and III) according to their relationship to the pectoralis minor muscle (Figure 14.1). The distribution of axillary lymph nodes (and axillary metastases) can be described according to the relationship to these three levels.

The number of nodes identified in an axillary dissection specimen will vary according to anatomical differences,

variations in the extent of surgical dissection and the expertise of the pathologist, together with the method of specimen analysis. In an analysis of 135 axillary dissection specimens Danforth *et al.* found that the number of lymph nodes ranged from 8 to 60, with a mean of 24 and a median of 23.[16] Most pathologists use either careful manual palpation of the unfixed axillary tissue for node identification, or serial sections, to locate lymph nodes.

From studies in which the axillary level was analysed individually, the node contents of levels I and II are comparable, together containing approximately 75% of the axillary nodes, with approximately 25% of nodes present at level III. This corresponds approximately to 9, 9 and 6 nodes for levels I, II and III, respectively.

It has been suggested that the *level* of axillary metastases correlates with prognosis. Data from the Memorial Sloan-Kettering study found that survival at 5 and 10 years was significantly poorer in patients with histologically positive nodes at levels II or III than in patients with negative nodes or positive nodes at only level 1.[17] Other series have argued that when patients are stratified by the *total number of positive nodes* (1–3 vs. 4) there were no differences in overall survival within these two groups.[5] It would therefore appear that once the total number of involved nodes is taken into consideration, the level of axillary involvement is probably not of independent prognostic significance. Prognosis and nodal involvement are correlated in Table 14.2.

Stratification according to risk of relapse is a major factor in the rationale of adjuvant chemotherapy, particularly with dose intensification and its attendant treatment morbidity and mortality, and the extent of axillary involvement allows such stratification. The Anglo-Celtic trial of high-dose chemotherapy with autologous stem-cell rescue requires four or more axillary nodes to be involved for trial

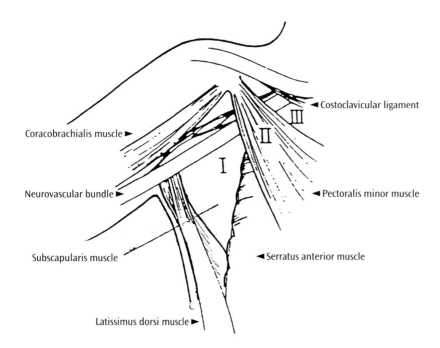

Figure 14.1 *Anatomical axillary levels. The axillary contents are divided into three levels (I, II and III) according to their relationship to the pectoralis minor muscle.*

Table 14.2 *Prognostic subsets in operable breast cancer.*[18] *Reproduced with permission from the BMJ Publishing Group*

Subset	Number of axillary nodes affected	Other discriminants*	Likelihood of being relapse free at 5 years (%)
1	None	Diameter < 1 cm	95
2	None	Diameter ≥ 1 cm Favourable histology or S-phase fraction < 10%	80
3	None	Diameter ≥ 1 cm Unfavourable histology or S-phase fraction ≥ 10%	50
4	1–3	Any histology	50
5	≥4	Favourable histology	50
6	≥4	Unfavourable histology	<25

* Favourable histology = ductal grade I, tubular, mucoid; unfavourable histology = ductal grades II and III, lobular, medullary.

entry. Where chemotherapy is considered inappropriate, information on axillary status is less important. In post-menopausal patients, the use of adjuvant tamoxifen for both node-positive and node-negative patients is now widely advocated because of the virtual absence of toxicity and the relatively low cost of this treatment. Staging information is clearly of less importance than in younger patients where different chemotherapy regimens might be advised on the basis of lymph-node status.

More exacting methods of histological analysis include processing to clear axillary fat from the specimen and serial micro-sectioning of lymph nodes.[19] The latter technique can identify occult metastases in up to 22% of cases initially thought to be node-negative, but the 5-year survival rate in such patients was not found to be significantly different to that for other lymph-node-negative patients, and the extra workload was not considered to be justified. However, a more recent study has found the disease-free and overall survival rates to be significantly worse, and is therefore at variance with previous studies.[20] Immuno-histochemical staining may offer an alternative and less time-consuming method of increasing sensitivity of node analysis and providing similar prognostic information.[21,22]

The argument against axillary clearance for *staging purposes alone* is based on a critical analysis of whether the overall management will be altered in an individual patient by knowledge of the lymph-node status. Any additional or more extensive surgical procedure for staging purposes, but which will not influence the progress of the disease either directly or indirectly by altering decisions about adjuvant treatment, may prove difficult to justify. Elsewhere in the field of surgical oncology (e.g. with mediastinoscopy for bronchial carcinoma, staging laparotomy for Hodgkin's disease, and second-look laparotomy for ovarian carcinoma), a reappraisal of these procedures has led to a more conservative approach in recent years.[23]

TECHNIQUE OF AXILLARY DISSECTION

The axilla is a potential pyramidal space consisting of four walls, an apex and a base. The anterior wall is formed by the pectoralis major and minor muscles, the posterior wall by the subscapularis and latissimus dorsi muscles, the medial wall by the serratus anterior muscle overlying the chest wall, and the lateral wall by the medial surface of the humerus and brachialis muscle. The base is formed by the axillary fascia deep to the skin of the axilla. The axilla contains the axillary artery and vein, brachial plexus, axillary lymph nodes, fat and connective tissue.

Axillary lymph-node dissection can be performed in conjunction with mastectomy, or separately as part of breast conservation surgery. During the axillary dissection, the pectoralis minor muscle may be removed or divided (to enhance the exposure of levels II and III), or it may be retracted medially to allow access to the apex of the axilla. All fatty and areolar lymph-node-bearing tissue inferior to the axillary vein is removed, beginning at the apex of the axilla and proceeding laterally along the vein to the point where is crosses the latissimus dorsi muscle. The long thoracic nerve to the serratus anterior and the thoracodorsal nerve to the latissimus dorsi are carefully identified and preserved. The intercostobrachial nerve is identified as it emerges from the chest wall and, if it is not involved with clinically positive nodes, many surgeons endeavour to preserve this sensory cutaneous nerve. The remaining attachment of the axillary contents to the tail of the breast is divided when performing breast conservation surgery, or removed *en bloc* with the mastectomy specimen. The skin incision is closed over a suction drain at the end of the procedure.

COMPLICATIONS OF AXILLARY DISSECTION

Dissection of the axilla is generally a well-tolerated operation. If the patient remains in hospital while the axillary drain is in place, a hospital stay of 5–7 days is generally required. The commonest post-operative problems, such as wound seroma and shoulder stiffness, are usually temporary in nature.[24]

The most common early complication of axillary dissection is seroma formation, which occurs at the rate of 40–50%.[25,26] Closed suction drainage is considered standard therapy following axillary dissection, and most surgeons leave the drain in place until drainage is less than 20–50 mL per day, which usually requires 4–6 days. Although some reports have suggested that restricting shoulder movements in the first 5 post-operative days reduces axillary drainage,[27] seroma formation remains a regular complication in all series, regardless of nodal status, both with shoulder immobilization and with early shoulder exercise,[28] and with both low-suction and high-suction drainage systems.[5] Seromas require needle aspiration in the clinic, but usually resolve after two or three aspirations with reducing volumes aspirated on each visit.

Shoulder stiffness following axillary dissection may result from oedema secondary to removal of axillary lymphatics, immobilization, post-operative pain that restricts shoulder movement, or muscle dysfunction due to injury to nerves such as the pectoral nerve. In many patients the functional range of movements is still restricted 1 month after surgery, but in almost all patients there is return of the full functional range of movements by 6 months.[29] This appears to be independent of whether early shoulder physiotherapy is practised or whether the arm is immobilized for 5 days.[30,31] Most surgeons recommend a programme of early graduated shoulder mobilization within the patient's tolerance of pain, starting on the first post-operative day.

Nerve injuries may occur during axillary dissection involving the nerves to the serratus anterior, latissimus dorsi and pectoral muscles,[32] the brachial plexus and the intercostobrachial nerve. The most frequent nerve injury results from sacrifice of the intercostobrachial nerve during axillary dissection,[33] and the degree of disability can vary from a small area of anaesthesia in the armpit to troublesome paraesthesia and dysaesthesia along the medial aspect of the upper arm.[34] In a minority of patients, troublesome paraesthesias can be permanent, and a randomized trial of nerve preservation where the intercostobrachial nerve was not macroscopically involved by tumour at the time of axillary dissection[35] suggests that these symptoms can be avoided in some but not all patients if the nerve is preserved.

Lymphoedema is a rare but potentially significant complication of axillary dissection. After axillary dissection alone, the incidence of arm oedema is in the range 2–4%, although in some series it is much lower.[36] Two important factors that significantly increase the risk of this complication are infection and radiotherapy.[37,38] Axillary infection may compromise the remaining lymphatic channels from the arm,[39] and patients who have undergone axillary dissection are advised to seek immediate treatment for any cellulitis or inflammation of the affected arm or the area draining to the axilla. Adequate physiotherapy[40] and attendance at a specialist lymphoedema clinic are vital in order to avoid the development of chronic oedema in such patients.

It is now well recognized that the combination of axillary dissection and axillary radiotherapy can result in arm oedema in up to 40% of patients.[41,42] Consequently, following axillary dissection, the axilla is always excluded from the radiotherapy field when post-operative radiation is delivered to the breast following breast conservation surgery (or, more rarely, to the chest wall following mastectomy).

Because the incidence of regional tumour recurrence following full axillary dissection is low (Table 14.3), recurrent tumour is a rare cause of lymphoedema, but must nevertheless be considered when arm oedema arises as a late complication following adequate surgery.

Table 14.3 *Axillary recurrence in 10 years after level III axillary clearance, radiotherapy or watch policy[43]*

	Clearance	Radiotherapy	Watch policy
Axillary relapse (%)	3	8	21
Uncontrolled axillary relapse (%)	1	3	12

AXILLARY CLEARANCE VS. SAMPLING

Less extensive procedures than full axillary clearance have been advocated on the basis that they can provide adequate staging information while not incurring the same morbidity as axillary clearance. Unguided biopsy of a single axillary node has been shown to be inaccurate,[8] although recent attempts to use lymphatic mapping to identify a sentinel node for biopsy have achieved far greater accuracy,[44,45] and this technique is rapidly gaining acceptance in breast units where nuclear medicine facilities are available. To date, the most commonly practised surgical alternative to axillary dissection has been axillary sampling.

Axillary sampling involves resection of the axillary tail and tissue adjacent to it containing the central lymph-node group. Critics of axillary sampling stress the imprecision of the sampling procedure in its variation and extent,[46] ranging from a virtual level I axillary clearance to retrieval of a small amount of axillary fat containing a small number of nodes. In up to 18% of axillary sampling specimens no nodes are retrieved.[47] However, in centres where the sampling technique is well defined, the procedure has been shown consistently to yield at least four lymph nodes with identical node positivity rates in patients randomized to sampling or clearance.[48]

A further criticism of axillary sampling is the incomplete information available if patients are to be offered high-dose adjuvant therapy on the basis of the extent of nodal involvement. It is evident that only with a full axillary clearance can the group of patients be most accurately stratified according to risk of relapse.

The problem posed by lesser axillary procedures than full clearance is how to treat the remaining nodes.[49–51]

Clinical assessment of axillary-node involvement is unreliable for determining initially which patients should undergo sampling and which should undergo full dissection. In patients where axillary sampling shows the absence of lymph-node involvement by tumour, the incidence of 'skip metastases' (node metastases in level II or III in the absence of level I involvement) is undoubtedly low, and probably no more than 5%.[52] However, when level I nodes are found to be positive, at least 44% of patients will have involvement of higher levels in the axilla as well.[53] Leaving the axillary tumour untreated, particularly near the apex of the axilla where disease progression may be difficult to detect clinically, runs the risk of brachial plexus and subclavian vessel involvement, and the often insurmountable problem of uncontrolled axillary disease.

Patients with involved nodes found on axillary sampling are therefore generally advised either to undergo a second operation to complete the axillary dissection, or to include the axilla in the radiotherapy field. This latter option raises the question of lymphoedema of the arm as one of the sequelae of combined treatment of the axilla. The risk of lymphoedema following either axillary clearance or axillary irradiation alone is of the order of 2–6%,[41,54] but is significantly increased to almost 40% if a combination of both procedures is used. Bearing this in mind, the surgeon who has performed the axillary sampling must be aware that if initial surgery has been more extensive than planned, it may with subsequent radiotherapy to the axilla contribute to serious long-term morbidity in the arm.

The axillary recurrence rate among patients with clinically negative nodes who do not undergo axillary surgery is in the region of 20%.[5] This recurrence rate is considerable in terms of the need for further hospital admission and surgery, even if all of these patients are resectable at the time of recurrence.[55] If progressive axillary disease is not detected early enough, perhaps as a result of difficulties with regular and experienced follow-up, axillary nodal disease may prove to be inoperable.[56] For these reasons, it is argued that patients with clinically positive axillary nodes, and those in whom axillary sampling has shown the presence of nodal involvement, are best served by treatment with full axillary clearance. This offers the greatest likelihood of controlling local disease and eliminating the need to treat the partially dissected axilla with post-operative radiotherapy.

The sentinel-node biopsy technique, now extensively validated in patients with stage I melanoma, has recently been introduced in breast surgery in the hope of avoiding axillary dissection in node-negative patients. The optimal techniques and protocols, involving both radio-labelled colloidal albumin for radiolocalization and Patent Blue dye for visual localization, are currently being evaluated.[44,45] Sentinel-node biopsy would appear to be a promising and feasible procedure in about 75% of patients with clinically T1–2 N0–1 breast cancer.[57] The technical equipment, particularly the gamma-probe, is relatively expensive, and close collaboration between surgical and nuclear medicine departments is required, but sentinel lymphadenectomy holds promise for allowing accurate selection of those patients in whom axillary surgery can safely be avoided.

TREATMENT OF THE AXILLA – SURGERY OR RADIOTHERAPY?

The axillary nodes receive about 75% of the total lymph drainage of the breast (Figure 14.2), and the most common initial site of spread of breast cancer is the axilla. The incidence of axillary metastases correlates with several characteristics of the primary tumour, including the size of the primary tumour (Table 14.4) and its location within the breast. Lesions located in the upper outer quadrant of the breast have the highest incidence of axillary-node metastases, although it is unclear whether this relates to the proximity of these lesions to the axilla or drainage patterns of breast lymphatics. Among all patients with symptomatic outer quadrant primary tumours (irrespective of size), 40–51% will have axillary metastases.[5]

The argument in favour of surgical clearance for treating the axilla in patients with operable breast cancer is that it achieves excellent tumour control, with axillary recurrence rates of 2% or less.[53,54] A number of randomized trials have addressed the question of axillary-node treatment, either by surgery or by radiotherapy.[60,61] Neither trial showed any difference in terms of overall survival rates, and axillary recurrence after surgical clearance and after axillary irradiation alone were 1% and 3%, respectively.[60] The axillary recurrence rate if the axilla is untreated is significantly higher, with about 20% of patients requiring subsequent axillary dissection for disease progression. The strenuous desire to avoid the consequences of uncontrolled axillary recurrence remains the primary reason for treating the axilla.

The impact of axillary treatment on *survival* remains a controversial issue.[62,63] Two large randomized trials (the NSABP B-04 and CRC trials) suggest that delayed treatment of involved axillary nodes is not associated with a worse outcome, these nodes being a marker and not a determinant of a poor prognosis. If there is a survival benefit, it would seem likely that this is in a subgroup of patients with one to three axillary nodes involved.[64,65] The demonstration of a survival advantage in patients randomized to axillary dissection must be interpreted with caution if adjuvant chemotherapy or hormone therapy is given more frequently to patients who are demonstrated on node dissection to have nodal involvement.[4]

Axillary irradiation represents an alternative and effective means of treating the axilla, with local control rates equivalent to that of axillary clearance.[54,66] To achieve this effect, radiotherapy must be given to a total

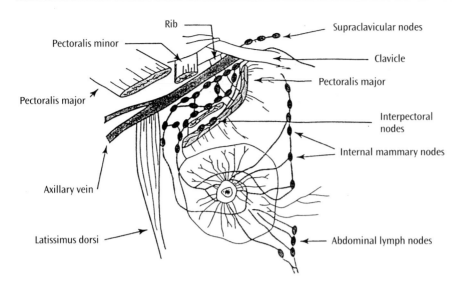

Figure 14.2 *Lymph drainage of the breast.*

dose of at least 45–50 Gy. Lower doses, such as those used in the Guy's Hospital trial,[67] are associated with an unacceptably high local recurrence rate. From the point of view of treatment alone (although not with regard to staging information), radical axillary irradiation is therefore an acceptable alternative to axillary dissection.

Although many of the complications of axillary dissection are short term,[68] major long-term complications may arise from axillary radiotherapy, albeit rarely. Radiation-induced brachial plexus neuropathy can vary in severity, and in occasional cases can lead to disabling pain and progressive loss of function of the limb. The risks of neuropathy are undoubtedly related to radiotherapy technique, particularly fraction size, and can be minimized by careful attention to avoiding overlapping fields and to radiation dosimetry.[69] Radiation-induced sarcoma is also an extremely rare long-term complication of radiotherapy, and may of course arise whether the breast alone or the breast and axilla are included in the radiotherapy field. The risk of radiation-induced sarcoma is in the region of 21 cases per 100 000 patient-years in patients surviving more than 5 years,[70] but when

such sarcomas arise they carry a formidable mortality, and at this site may require forequarter amputation for local control.[71,72]

PATIENTS IN WHOM AXILLARY TREATMENT IS UNNECESSARY

An alternative approach to management of the axilla in patients with early breast cancer is that of a simple 'watch policy' for patients with clinically uninvolved nodes. Although about 20% of patients will undergo subsequent axillary dissection because of disease progression in the axilla, the corollary – that 80% of patients avoid axillary surgery or axillary radiotherapy – is evident. A deleterious effect on survival of delaying axillary treatment has not been proven, and indeed the absence of a major survival difference despite a significant axillary recurrence rate suggests that untreated nodes do not serve as a reservoir for further systemic metastases, and that they represent a marker rather than a source of disease progression. However, such a watch policy requires rigorous and regular patient follow-up if the distressing sequelae of uncontrolled axillary disease are to be avoided.

Over one-third of all breast cancers occur in women over 70 years of age, and following trials to evaluate whether tamoxifen alone represents an effective treatment in these patients, there is now consensus that many of these patients require surgery for local control at the primary site.[73] In many patients, wide local excision of the tumour together with tamoxifen treatment achieves adequate control of the tumour for their remaining lifespan. In these patients, staging information is not relevant, and most clinicians would agree that axillary dissection represents over-treatment in such patients when the axillary nodes are not clinically involved by tumour. The post-operative problem of shoulder stiffness is often compounded in elderly patients with a degree of underlying arthritis, and many clinicians agree that a watch

Table 14.4 *Incidence of axillary metastases according to primary tumour size: Haagensen's personal series*[58]

Primary Tumour Size (cm)	Number of patients	Incidence of axillary metastases (%)
No palpable tumour	26	19.2
<1	22	22.7
1.0–1.9	119	24.2
2.0–2.9	223	30.5
3.0–3.9	180	46.7
4.0–4.9	147	46.3
5.0–5.9	101	60.4
6.0–6.9	77	51.9
≥ 8.0	27	51.9
Total	922	40.6

policy is appropriate management for the axilla in the frail patient over 70 years of age.

In post-menopausal patients under 70 years of age, chemotherapy is increasingly being offered in addition to tamoxifen as adjuvant treatment for node-positive breast cancer. This has followed the demonstration that poly-chemotherapy is well tolerated and may contribute an additional survival benefit in this group of patients.[74] It would therefore appear to be a logical argument for treating fit post-menopausal patients under 70 years in the same way as pre-menopausal patients, and offering them the staging and treatment benefits of axillary dissection.

The role of axillary dissection in patients with *locally advanced disease* (e.g. T4 or 'inflammatory' breast cancer) is less well defined than in early breast cancer. With surgery alone these patients are considered to be inoperable because of very high local recurrence rates. With neoadjuvant chemotherapy, many such patients become 'operable' and mastectomy with post-operative radiotherapy is recommended. In such cases, or in the presence of distant metastases, palliative local surgery may be confined to the breast in the form of a simple 'salvage' mastectomy and the axilla included in the irradiation fields. Alternatively, if palpable axillary nodes remain, the axilla is cleared at the same time and post-operative radiotherapy is confined to the chest wall.[75]

With the advent of national breast screening programmes and the detection of an increasing number of small (< 1 cm diameter), good-prognosis tumours, it is evident that axillary dissection may represent over-treatment in this subgroup of screen-detected tumours where the risk of nodal metastases is under 10%. This is true for well-differentiated tumours less than 1 cm in diameter, and for those of special histological type such as tubular or medullary patterns. The prognosis of these tumours appears to be so good that the role of axillary clearance (as well as that of post-operative radiotherapy to the breast) has been questioned, and the long-term outcome in this group of patients is in many ways similar to that for ductal carcinoma *in situ* (DCIS). Sentinel-node biopsy for these clinically early tumours offers the prospect of identifying those patients with axillary-node involvement, while at the same time allowing axillary clearance to be be avoided in the majority of cases.

DCIS now accounts for up to 20% of screen-detected breast lesions. Where DCIS is detected in the absence of invasive tumour, there is no indication for axillary dissection (or indeed any axillary treatment). In a very small percentage of cases, axillary dissection performed in patients with completely excised DCIS may show evidence of lymph-node involvement (thus implicating an area of micro-invasion that was missed on histological sectioning), but the incidence is too low to justify the morbidity of axillary surgery. Similarly, in patients undergoing prophylactic surgery either because of genetic predisposition or a strong family history, or

because of biopsies showing proliferative lesions with atypia, axillary clearance is not included in the procedure of prophylactic simple mastectomy and reconstruction.[76]

AXILLARY DISSECTION, SENTINEL-NODE BIOPSY AND FUTURE RESEARCH

Although axillary-node status remains the single most important prognostic marker currently available in assessment of early breast cancer, efforts are continuing to identify possible non-invasive alternative methods of staging. Conventional ultrasound examination of the axillary node has not proved accurate, and has the same pitfalls as clinical examination because of the poor correlation in many cases between node enlargement and node involvement by tumour.[77] More recently, high-resolution colour doppler ultrasound has attempted to increase the accuracy of this investigation by assessing vascularity in conjunction with lymph-node size and volume.

In other clinical settings, magnetic resonance imaging (MRI) has the ability to differentiate between malignant and benign tissue densities more readily than conventional radiology. MRI of the axilla is able to detect large axillary nodes with obvious tumour involvement, but has poor specificity and is unlikely to identify microscopic tumour burden in axillary lymph nodes.[12] Positron emission tomography (PET) scanning is also currently under assessment as a non-invasive staging modality which can distinguish between malignant and benign breast lesions in certain patients.[78,79]

Preliminary results are encouraging. For example, in the study by Smith *et al.* from Aberdeen,[79] overall sensitivity was 90% and specificity was 97% (50 patients), which is a very much better result than that achieved by clinical examination alone. The use of monoclonal antibodies raised against breast cancer cell lines is a further area of investigation. Gamma-camera scanning of the axilla following administration of radiolabelled monoclonal antibody has confirmed the presence of tumour deposits in the axilla in patients subsequently undergoing axillary dissection, but the ability of this imaging technique to provide reliable staging information remains unproven, and it is unlikely to achieve sufficient resolution to record the numbers of nodes involved.

Although alternatives to axillary clearance continue to be sought and new imaging modalities refined, full axillary dissection needs to be performed in these patients under investigation so that novel techniques can be compared to 'gold-standard' histological findings. The introduction of sentinel-node biopsy offers the possibility of more accurate selection of patients with involved nodes for axillary surgery, with conservative management of the sentinel-node-negative axilla. However, the reliability of this procedure in everyday clinical practice has yet to be proven in multicentre trials. At present, following the first use of this staging technique by Giuliano et al.,[80] it seems clear that sentinel-node biopsy using radionuclide localization can accurately predict the probability of axillary lymph-node metastases. A negative sentinel-node biopsy 'has a 95–100% likelihood of representing a clear axillary nodal basin'.[81] Similar results have been reported from elsewhere,[82] and a large-scale multicentre study recently reported from the USA provided further details of both the sensitivity and the specificity of the sentinel-node technique.[83] A total of 443 patients were included (enrolled between May 1995 and September 1997), all of whom had clinically negative axillary nodes, but with a treatment plan which included axillary lymphadenectomy. The overall rate of identification of 'hot spots' following injection of technetium[99m] sulphur colloid was 93%, and the accuracy of these sentinel nodes with regard to the confirmed status of the axillary nodes was 97% (392 of 405 cases), with a specificity of 100%. Overall, despite these high figures, the authors considered that the use of sentinel-node biopsy 'can be technically challenging, and the success rate varies according to the surgeon and the characteristics of the patient'.

In an accompanying editorial, McMasters and colleagues noted that, despite the potential benefits of avoiding formal axillary-node dissection, and the considerable promise of the sentinel-node biopsy technique, at present it is still clearly premature to regard sentinel-node biopsy as an adequate substitute for axillary dissection, since the frequency of false-negative rates remains uncertain.[84] Recent work from The Netherlands suggests that the sentinel-node biopsy technique (using radiocolloid combined with Patent Blue dye injected peritumorally) may even be valuable in patients who have undergone previous excisional biopsy.[85]

REFERENCES

1 Boote DJ, Stockdale AD, Phillips RH. Axillary dissection in breast cancer. Lancet 1991; 337: 486.
2 Sacks NPM, Barr LC, Allan SM, Baum M. The role of axillary dissection in operable breast cancer. Breast 1992; 1: 41–9.
3 Greenall MJ, Davidson T. How should the axilla be treated in breast cancer? Eur J Surg Oncol 1995; 21: 2–7.
4 Cabanes PA, Salmon RJ, Vilcoq JR et al. Value of axillary dissection in addition to lumpectomy and radiotherapy in early breast cancer. Lancet 1992; 339: 1245–8.
5 Danforth DN. The role of axillary lymph node dissection in the management of breast cancer. Princip Pract Oncol 1992; 6: 1–16.
6 Veronesi U, Paganelli G, Galimberti V et al. Sentinel node biopsy to avoid axillary dissection in breast cancer with clinically negative lymph nodes. Lancet 1997; 349: 1864–7.
7 Fentiman IS, Mansel RE. The axilla; not a no-go zone. Lancet 1991; 337: 221–3.
8 Davies GC, Millis RR, Hayward JL. Assessment of axillary node status. Am Surg 1980; 192: 148–51.
9 Thompson CH, Stacker SA, Salehi N et al. Immunoscintigraphy for the detection of lymph node metastases from breast cancer. Lancet 1984; 11: 1245–7.
10 McLean RG, Ege GN. Prognostic value of axillary lymphoscintography in breast carcinoma patients. J Nucl Med 1986; 27: 1116–24.
11 Bruneton JN, Caramella E, Hery M et al. Axillary lymph node metastases in breast cancer: preoperative detection with ultrasound. Radiology 1986; 158: 325–6.
12 Davidson T, Mumtaz H, Hall-Craggs MA et al. The impact of magnetic resonance imaging in determining surgical management in breast cancer. Breast 1997; 6: 177–82.
13 Early Breast Cancer Trialists' Collaborative Group. Systemic treatment of early breast cancer by hormonal, cytotoxic or immune therapy. Lancet 1992; 339: 1–15, 71–85.
14 Fisher B, Bauer M, Wickerham DL, Redmonds CK, Fisher ER. Relation of the number of positive axillary nodes to the prognosis of patients with primary breast cancer. Cancer 1983; 52: 1551–7.
15 Veronesi U, Rilke F, Luimi A et al. Distribution of axillary node metastases by level of invasion. An analysis of 539 cases. Cancer 1987; 59: 682–7.
16 Danforth DN Jr, Findlay PA, McDonald HD et al. Complete axillary lymph node dissection for stage 1–11 carcinoma of the breast. J Clin Oncol 1986; 4: 655.
17 Schottenfeld D, Nash AG, Robbins GF et al. Ten-year results of the treatment of primary operable breast carcinoma: a summary of 304 patients evaluated by the TNM system. Cancer 1976; 38: 1001.
18 Rubens RD. Management of early breast cancer. BMJ 1992; 304: 1361–4.
19 Friedman S, Bertin H, Mouriesse H et al. Importance of tumour cells in axillary node sinus margins discovered by serial sectioning in operable breast carcinoma. Acta Oncol 1988; 27: 483–7.
20 International (Ludwig) Breast Cancer Study Group. Prognostic importance of occult axillary lymph-node micrometastases from breast cancers. Lancet 1990; 335: 156–8.
21 Wells CA, Heryet A, Brochner J, Gatter KC, Mason DY. The immunocytochemical detection of axillary micrometastases in breast cancer. Br J Cancer 1984; 50: 193–7.
22 Berry N, Jones DB, Marshall R, Smallwood J, Taylor I. Increased detection of axillary lymph node metastases from primary breast cancer by immunohistochemical staining with monoclonal antibodies. Br J Surg 1985; 72: 10–35.
23 Davidson T, Sacks N. The management of women with a high risk of breast cancer: the controversy of prophylactic mastectomy. In: Eeles RA, Ponder BAJ, Easton DF, Horwich A (eds) Genetic predisposition to cancer. London: Chapman & Hall, 1996: 273–81.
24 Budd DC, Cochran RC, Sturtz DL, Fouty WJ. Surgical morbidity after mastectomy operations. Am J Surg 1978; 135: 218.

25 Cameron AEP, Ebbs SR, Wylie F, Baum M. Suction drainage of the axilla: a prospective randomized trial. *Br J Surg* 1988; **75**: 1211.

26 Bryant M, Baum M. Postoperative seroma following mastectomy and axillary dissection. *Br J Surg* 1987; **74**: 1187.

27 Flew TJ. Wound drainage following radical mastectomy: the effect of restriction of shoulder movement. *Br J Surg* 1979; **66**: 302.

28 Dawson I, Stam L, Heslinga JM. Effect of shoulder immobilization on wound seroma and shoulder dysfunction following modified radical mastectomy: a randomized prospective clinical trial. *Br J Surg* 1989; **76**: 311.

29 Lotze MT, Duncan MA, Gerber LH et al. Early versus delayed shoulder following axillary dissection. *Ann Surg* 1981; **193**: 228.

30 Pollard R, Callum KG, Alman DG, Bates T. Shoulder movement following mastectomy. *Clin Oncol* 1976; **2**: 343.

31 Jansen RFM, van Geel AN, de Groot HG et al. Immediate versus delayed shoulder exercises after axillary lymph node dissection. *Am Surg* 1990; **160**: 481.

32 Scanlon EF. The importance of the anterior thoracic nerves in modified radical mastectomy. *Surg Gynecol Obstet* 1981; **152**: 789.

33 Vecht CJ, Van de Branch HJ, Wajer OJM. Post-axillary dissection pain in breast cancer due to a lesion of the intercostobrachial nerve. *Pain* 1989; **38**: 171.

34 Paredes JP, Puente JL, Potel J. Variations in sensitivity after sectioning the intercostobrachial nerve. *Am J Surg* 1990; **160**: 525.

35 Bundred NJ et al. Randomised trial of preservation of intercostobrachial nerve in axillary dissection. *Eur J Surg Oncol* 1998.

36 Hoe AL, Ivens D, Royle GT, Taylor I. Incidence of arm swelling following axillary clearance for breast cancer. *Br J Surg* 1992; **79**: 261–2.

37 Swedborg I, Wallgren A. The effect of pre and postmastectomy radiotherapy on the degree of edema shoulder-joint mobility and gripping force. *Cancer* 1981; **47**: 877.

38 Aitken RJ, Gaze MN, Rodger A, Chetty U, Forrest APM. Arm morbidity within a trial of mastectomy and either nodal sample with selective radiotherapy or axillary clearance. *Br J Surg* 1989; **76**: 568–71.

39 Britton RC, Nelson PA. Causes and treatment of postmastectomy lymphedema of the arm: report of 114 cases. *J Am Med Assoc* 1962; **180**: 95.

40 Rodier JF, Gaddoneix P, Dauplat J et al. Influence of the timing of physiotherapy upon the lymphatic complications of axillary dissection for breast cancer. *Int Surg* 1987; **72**: 166.

41 Kissin MW, Querci della Rovere G, Easton D, Westbury G. Risk of lymphoedema following the treatment of breast cancer. *Br J Surg* 1986; **73**: 580–4.

42 Larson D, Weinstein M, Goldberg I et al. Edema of the arm as a function of the extent of axillary surgery in patients with stage 1–11 carcinoma of the breast treated with primary radiotherapy. *Int J Radiat Oncol Biol Phys* 1986; **12**: 1575.

43 Bundred NJ et al. Management of regional nodes in breast cancer. In: Dixon JM (ed.) *ABC of breast diseases*. London: BMA Press, 1994.

44 Krag DN, Weaver DL, Alex JC, Fairbank JT. Surgical resection and radiolocalization of the sentinel lymph node in breast cancer using a gamma probe. *Surg Oncol* 1997; **2**: 335–40.

45 Guiliano AE, Dale PS, Turner RR et al. Improved axillary staging of breast cancer with sentinel lymphadenectomy. *Ann Surg* 1995; **222**: 394–401.

46 Kissin MW, Thompson EM, Price AM et al. The inadequacy of axillary sampling in breast cancer. *Lancet* 1982; **1**: 1210–12.

47 Forrest APM, Stewart HJ, Roberts MM, Steele RJC. Simple mastectomy and axillary node sampling in the management of primary breast cancer. *Am J Surg* 1982; **196**: 371–8.

48 Steele RJC, Forrest APM, Gibson T et al. The efficacy of lower axillary sampling in obtaining lymph node status in breast cancer: a controlled randomised trial. *Br J Surg* 1985; **72**: 368–9.

49 Kjaergaard J, Blichert-Toft M, Anderson JA et al. Probability of false-negative nodal staging in conjunction with partial axillary dissection in breast cancer. *Br J Surg* 1985; **72**: 365–7.

50 Locker AP, Ellis IO, Morgan DAL et al. Factors influencing local recurrence after excision and radiotherapy for primary breast cancer. *Br J Surg* 1989; **76**: 890–4.

51 O'Dwyer PJ. Axillary dissection in primary breast cancer. *BMJ* 1991; **302**: 36–61.

52 Rosen PP, Groshen S. Factors influencing survival and prognosis in early breast carcinoma (TINOMO-TINIMO). Assessment of 644 patients with median follow-up of 18 years. *Surg Clin North Am* 1990; **70**: 937–62.

53 Veronesi U, Luini A, Galimberti V et al. Extent of metastatic axillary involvement in 1446 cases of breast cancer. *Eur J Surg Oncol* 1990; **16**: 127–33.

54 Mazeron JJ, Otmezguine Y, Huart J, Pierquin B. Conservative treatment of breast cancer: results of management of axillary lymph node area in 3353 patients (letter). *Lancet* 1985; **1**: 1387.

55 Baum M, Coyle PJ. Simple mastectomy for early breast cancer and the behaviour of the untreated axillary nodes. *Bull Cancer (Paris)* 1977; **64**: 603.

56 Helman P, Bennett MB, Louw JH et al. Interim report on trial of treatment for operable cancer. *South Afr Med J* 1972; **46**: 1374.

57 Roumen RMH, Valkenberg JGM, Geuskens LM. Lymphoscintigraphy and feasibility of sentinel node biopsy in 83 patients with primary breast cancer. *Eur J Surg Oncol* 1997; **23**: 495–502.

58 Haagensen CD. *Diseases of the breast*. Philadelphia, PA: WB Saunders, 1971.

59 Graverson HP, Blichert Toff M, Anderson JA et al. Breast cancer: risk of axillary recurrence in node-negative

patients following partial dissection of the axilla. *Eur J Surg Oncol* 1988; **14**: 407–12.

60 Fisher B, Redmond C, Fisher ER. Ten-year results of a randomised clinical trial comparing radical mastectomy and total mastectomy with or without radiation. *N Engl J Med* 1985; **312**: 674–81.

61 Cancer Research Campaign Working Party. CRC (Kings/Cambridge) trial for early breast cancer. A detailed update at the tenth year. *Lancet* 1980; **11**: 55–60.

62 Harris JR, Osteen RT. Patients with early breast cancer benefit from axillary treatment. *Breast Cancer Res Treat* 1985; **5**: 17–21.

63 Stotter A, Atkinson EN, Fairston BA. Survival following locoregional recurrence after breast conservation therapy for cancer. *Ann Surg* 1990; **212**: 166–72.

64 Haagensen CD, Bjodian C. A personal experience with Halsted's radical mastectomy. *Ann Surg* 1984; **199**: 443–50.

65 Cascinelli N, Greco M, Bufalino R *et al*. Prognosis of breast cancer with axillary node metastases after surgical treatment only. *Eur J Cancer Clin Oncol* 1987; **23**: 795–9.

66 Amalric R, Santamaria F, Robert F *et al*. Radiation therapy with or without primary limited surgery for operable breast cancer. *Cancer* 1982; **49**: 30–4.

67 Hayward JL. The Guy's trial of treatments of 'early' breast cancer. *World J Surg* 1977; **1**(3): 314–16.

68 Clarke D, Martinez A, Cox R *et al*. Breast edema following staging axillary node dissection in patients with breast carcinoma treated by radical radiotherapy. *Cancer* 1982; **49**: 2295.

69 Yarnold JR. Early-stage breast cancer; treatment options and results. *Br Med Bull* 1991; **47**: 372–87.

70 Kurtz JM, Amalric R, Brandone H, Ayme Y, Spitalier JM. Contralateral breast cancer and other second malignancies in patients treated by breast-conserving therapy with radiation. *Int J Radiat Oncol Biol Phys* 1988; **15**: 277–84.

71 Davidson T, Westbury G, Harmer CL. Radiation-induced soft tissue sarcoma *Br J Surg* 1986; **73**: 308.

72 Pitcher ME, Davidson TI, Fisher C, Thomas JM. Post-irradiation sarcoma of soft tissue and bone. *Eur J Surg Oncol* 1994; **20**: 53–6.

73 Dixon JM. Management of breast cancer. *BMJ* 1992; **305**: 114.

74 DeVita VT. Breast cancer therapy; exercising all our options. *N Engl J Med* 1989; **320**: 527–9.

75 Pierce L, Bader J, Cowan K *et al*. The effect of systemic therapy upon local-regional control in locally advanced breast cancer. *Int J Radiat Oncol Biol Phys* 1991; **21** (**Supplement 1**): 155.

76 Davidson T, Sacks N. Principles of surgical oncology. In: Horwich A (ed.) *Oncology: a multidisciplinary textbook*. London: Chapman & Hall Medical, 1995: 101–15.

77 Tate J, Lewis V, Archer T, Guyer PG, Royle GT, Taylor I. Ultrasound detection of axillary lymph node metastases in breast cancer. *Eur J Surg Oncol* 1989; **15**: 139–42.

78 Crowe JP, Lee MD, Adler MD *et al*. Positron emission tomography and breast masses: comparison with clinical, mammographic and pathological findings. *Ann Surg Oncol* 1994; **1**: 132–40.

79 Smith IC, Ogston KN, Whitford P *et al*. Staging of the axilla in breast cancer: accurate *in vivo* assessment using positron emission tomography with 2-(fluorine-18)-fluoro-2-deoxy-ᴅ-glucose. *Ann Surg* 1998; **228**: 220–7.

80 Giuliano AE, Kirgan DN, Guenther JM, Morton DL. Lymphatic mapping and sentinel lymphadenectomy for breast cancer. *Ann Surg* 1994; **220**: 391–401.

81 Querci della Rovere G, Bird PA. Sentinel-lymph-node biopsy in breast cancer. *Lancet* 1998; **352**: 421–2.

82 O'Hea BJ, Hill ADK, El-Shirburny AM *et al*. Sentinel lymph node in breast cancer: initial experience at Memorial Sloan-Kettering Cancer Center. *J Am Coll Surg* 1998; **186**: 423–7.

83 Krag D, Weaver D, Ashikaga T *et al*. The sentinel node in breast cancer – a multicenter validation study. *N Engl J Med* 1998; **339**: 941–6.

84 McMasters KM, Giuliano AE, Ross MI *et al*. Sentinel-lymph-node biopsy for breast cancer – not yet the standard of care. *N Engl J Med* 1998; **339**: 990–4.

85 van der Ent FWC, Kengen RAM, van der Pol HAG, Hoofwijk AGM. Sentinel node biopsy in 70 unexpected patients with breast cancer: increased feasibility by using 10 mCi radiocolloid in combination with a blue dye tracer. *Eur J Surg Oncol* 1999; **25**: 24–9.

15

Neoadjuvant systemic primary therapy – is surgery the true adjuvant?

RICHARD G MARGOLESE

The use of chemotherapy as an adjunct to breast cancer surgery became a clinical reality in the mid-1970s. Following the initial reports of improved disease-free survival (DFS) with adjuvant therapy, there was great initial optimism that evaluation of better drugs, better schedules or better combinations of drugs would continue to increase long-term cure rates in a steady fashion. Two decades later it is surprising and disappointing that forward momentum has been so slow. The difficulties of improving upon the significant initial results are causing clinical investigators to widen the search for better avenues to progress. An important issue in this context is the timing of chemotherapy with respect to surgery. Since surgery was standard therapy and adjuvant chemotherapy was the experimental innovation, it logically followed that chemotherapy would be given after surgery. This probably corresponds to the placement of the automobile engine at the front of the car simply because that is where the horse was and no one thought to consider the matter much further. A better understanding of cancer growth and spread has resulted in a reconsideration of these temporal relationships.

BIOLOGICAL BACKGROUND

Kinetics

The basis for adjuvant therapy was laid by the research of Skipper et al.,[1] who reported that small tumours might be more sensitive to chemotherapy than established tumours because they were more likely to be in the exponential growth phase. Therefore, early distant metastases may exhibit a better response to chemotherapy than the older primary tumour. In itself this view does not suggest that timing of chemotherapy is important, but rather that micrometastases are more sensitive than the clinically apparent tumour. If removal of the primary tumour and the decrease in total tumour cell burden alters the growth characteristics of residual metastases, the timing of the treatments may be important.

Experiments to document this have been conducted by Gunduz and Fisher et al.,[2] who demonstrated in a rodent model that there is an increase in labelling index (LI) of metastases following amputation of a transplanted primary tumour. This results in a faster tumour doubling time and a measurable increase in size of the metastases compared to non-amputated animals. Radiation of the primary tumour sufficient to retard growth had similar results.

In a second set of experiments,[3] they speculated that accelerated tumour growth was caused by recruitment of non-cycling cells from G_0 into the proliferative phase. If so, this would make them more vulnerable to chemotherapy. Subsequent investigations revealed that cyclophosphamide or tamoxifen given prior to operation resulted in prevention of LI increase, suppression of tumour growth, and prolonged survival of the animal. Early post-operative chemotherapy treatment of the animals provided a mild improvement in outcomes compared to later chemotherapy, but pre-operative therapy provided the greatest benefit.

The stimulation of metastatic growth may possibly be due to a serum growth factor. Serum derived from mice following primary tumour removal was injected into tumour-bearing recipients and produced changes in the pulmonary metastases similar to those in animals whose primary tumour was removed.[3]

Resistant cells

Clinicians and researchers alike have long been frustrated by the frequency with which cancer cells display resistance to cytotoxic agents. The Goldie–Coldman[4] thesis attributes this to spontaneous mutations which will obviously occur more frequently as cell populations increase. Not only does the absolute number of resistant cells increase, but also the percentage of resistant cells in the total cell population increases as new mutations occur. If metastatic cells proliferate faster following primary tumour removal, the number of resistant phenotypes may also increase. It follows that early treatment, when the lowest numbers of tumour cells are present, will encounter the smallest number of resistant cells and thus be potentially more effective.

It is not clear whether a few weeks' or even a few months' lead time in chemotherapy treatment makes a difference against the background of many years for which tumours are likely to be present, but there is some mathematical and experimental evidence to support this theory, and clinical testing is warranted.

CLINICAL STUDIES

There has been extensive experience with pre-operative chemotherapy where the aim was organ or structure preservation. Osteosarcoma,[5] head and neck tumours,[6] bladder[7] and oesophageal cancers[8] have all been studied, as has locally advanced (stage III) breast cancer.[9–11] None of these reports come from randomized prospective trials. All of them are aimed at improved local control or downstaging essentially inoperable malignancies to allow surgery. Most of them present their results in comparison with historical controls or in terms of responders vs. non-responders. Although this approach may help to generate information for use in designing a prospective trial, none of these reports provides the kind of conclusive evidence that is necessary to change current practices.

Of particular interest is the suggestion that, in all of these tumours, primary chemotherapy achieves objective response rates that are much better than those obtained when treating clinical metastases that appear during post-surgical follow-up. It is unclear whether or not this differential represents increased drug resistance in metastases compared to primary tumours. It is speculated that metastases have different genetic mutations to the primary tumours, and this set of changes may be what enables the cell to metastasize in the first place. These differences may also reflect increased drug resistance.

On the other hand, treatment before the perturbations of surgery may indeed be more effective at the level of both the primary tumour and the metastases for the reasons discussed earlier. If so, there is the potential for better response and increased disease-free survival (DFS) and survival (S), but an appropriately designed prospective randomized trial will be necessary to demonstrate this.

Breast trials: history

In the National Surgical Adjuvant Breast Project (NSABP) Protocol B-01, thiotepa was administered at the time of surgery and repeated on the following 2 days. The timing of this treatment had nothing to do with the topic of this chapter. Rather, it was a primitive attempt at adjuvant therapy and started with the idea that metastases may result from manipulation of the primary tumour during surgery. The chemotherapy was therefore timed to coincide with surgery in an attempt to eliminate any such dislodged cells. One subset of treated patients showed a long-lasting improvement in DFS and S, and established the first evidence for the benefit of adjuvant chemotherapy.[12] This trial led to many others using drug schedules which evolved into the more traditional approach for adjuvant therapy, 2–5 weeks after surgery, but the question has remained whether or not the timing of the thiotepa treatment had anything to do with the favourable outcome for some patients.

A second trial of historic interest is the Scandinavian trial led by Nissen-Meyer.[13] Cyclophosphamide was administered for 6 consecutive days starting on the day of operation, and the patients were compared to a group that received no chemotherapy. All of the patients received post-operative radiation. Later, these findings were compared with another group that received radiation therapy and was then similarly randomized to adjuvant chemotherapy or control. Because these patients received radiation therapy first, their chemotherapy was started an average of 3 weeks after mastectomy. These patients failed to demonstrate any benefit from the therapy, whereas those treated with immediate chemotherapy showed a benefit attributable to the treatment. If the delay of 3 weeks was responsible for the lack of benefit in the second group, it would support the rationale for pre-operative chemotherapy, even though more modern clinical trials do show a benefit even when treatment is initiated several weeks after surgery.

Breast trials: early reports of primary chemotherapy

The idea of pre-operative chemotherapy in breast cancer has been extensively clinically tested, but not in the same setting as routine adjuvant chemotherapy. Initial studies were in locally advanced and essentially inoperable breast cancer, or in operable cases with large tumours where there would be a reluctance to attempt breast-conserving surgery (BCS). Primary chemotherapy was first given in the hope of downsizing the primary to enable surgical control with mastectomy. With some initial success, the aim of later protocols was changed to make BCS more achievable and more likely to succeed in locally advanced cases. The idea that pre-operative chemotherapy could result in improved DFS or S was not a primary objective of these early studies.

All of these studies can thus be analysed in three groups, namely locally advanced cases where the objective is better local control, operable cases in non-randomized studies where the aim is downsizing and increased use of BCS and, later, randomized trials aimed primarily at downsizing the primary and secondarily at increasing DFS and S.

LOCALLY ADVANCED TUMOURS

There has been extensive experience of the treatment of stage III disease by initial chemotherapy. Lipmann et al.[9] used a special strategy to recruit cells into division with a combination of tamoxifen and oestrogen, followed by combination chemotherapy. They reported a 90% response rate, with a 20% complete clinical response rate. Chevalier et al.[10] treated 45 women with inflammatory breast cancer using intensive primary chemotherapy followed by surgery or radiation therapy, with a good response in 91% of the patients. There was a 30% complete clinical response rate and 66% partial response rate. A total of 39 patients underwent modified radical mastectomy, and 10 of these specimens showed no residual invasive tumour. These response rates are typical of other reports, but in none of these is it clear whether long-term survival was improved, and the effect of factors such as patient selection cannot be determined from this type of design. However, these studies do confirm that high objective response rates are obtained with initial chemotherapy, and led to further research on the possible uses of primary chemotherapy.

NON-RANDOMIZED STUDIES

Jacquillat et al.[14] administered combination chemotherapy to 250 patients with T_1 to T_4 tumours, but there was no control group. These 250 patients were derived from 270 patients referred to their treatment centre. A total of 20 patients were excluded because of previous excisional biopsy or patient choice of primary surgery. Patients received primary chemotherapy and consolidation therapy with vinblastine, thiotepa, methotrexate and 5-fluorouracil (5FU) with or without adriamycin. These authors believed that the main advantage of primary chemotherapy is the availability of an indicator of effectiveness, namely the complete remission rate. A second objective is tumour downsizing to permit the choice of breast-conserving treatment. To maximize this, they chose radiation therapy as the exclusive local-

regional treatment. Tamoxifen was given to 195 patients; 24 of the 55 patients who did not receive tamoxifen were premenopausal, and 66 of the 195 patients who were treated with tamoxifen were premenopausal.

The response as demonstrated by shrinkage of the tumour was rapid. In total, 75% (178 of 250) of the patients showed a tumour volume reduction of more than 50% after a median of 3 doses. In 74 patients (30%) there was no clinical tumour detectable at the end of primary chemotherapy. None of the 250 patients showed progression during chemotherapy. The actuarial rate of local-regional recurrence was 13% for small tumours, 19% for large tumours and 18% for tumours of intermediate size. These were usually treated by local resection. The rate of breast preservation was 94% at 5 years, with cosmetic results rated as good or excellent for most patients.

The better clinical responses occurred in patients with smaller tumours and less differentiated tumours. Tumour regression was also better in patients who were receiving tamoxifen. In 160 of the 176 patients with clinically persistent tumour, complete remission was achieved after external irradiation. In the remaining 16 patients, the tumours disappeared after an interstitial boost. None of the patients required mastectomy, which was indicated only for cases with failure of complete local control. The 5-year disease-free survival and overall survival rates corresponded to clinical staging. The 5-year DFS rate was 100% for stage I, 82% for stage IIA, 61% for stage IIB and 46% for stage III.

Bonadonna et al.[15] studied 165 women with tumours larger than 3 cm in diameter. Initial chemotherapy was administered in the hope of increasing BCS in this group of larger tumours. Five different treatment regimens were used to compare several 3-drug combinations of cyclophosphamide, methotrexate, 5FU and adriamycin. Patients who were node-positive or oestrogen-receptor-negative also received post-operative chemotherapy. Those patients who responded received two or three courses of the same combination post-operatively. For those who did not respond, a non-cross-resistant combination was used (doxorubicin for those who did not respond to CMF, and mitomycin and vinblastine for those who did not respond to anthracyclines). All but four of the 161 assessable patients showed measurable tumour shrinkage, and 127 patients (81%) achieved shrinkage to < 3 cm in diameter, allowing a breast-conserving procedure to replace a modified mastectomy.[15]

Seven patients achieved complete histopathological remission, and 27 patients showed a complete clinical response. There was no discernible difference in response or progress of disease with respect to any of the treatment regimens chosen, nor was there any detectable difference in response related to menopausal status, age or DNA content. The response was inversely proportional to initial tumour size. The frequency of response was higher in receptor-negative tumours. However, tissue samples for receptor determinations were infrequently obtained at initial biopsy, and correlations with response cannot be made with confidence. Although the follow-up time is short (median 18 months), only 1 of 201 women treated by BCS has shown an ipsilateral tumour recurrence.[16]

This was neither a prospective nor a comparative study, so no conclusions can be drawn about the long term prognosis. However, it is clear that for any of the drug combinations, the delivery of 3 treatment cycles is sufficient to effect a meaningful clinical response in the local tumour. It is not clear whether tumour response will be an indicator of the overall usefulness of the pre-operative drug regimen.

This study demonstrates a significant decrease in primary tumour size, allowing 81% of patients to be converted from intended mastectomy to breast-conserving surgery. However, this benefit may be less real than it appears, as defining a diameter of 3 cm as the limiting feature is somewhat arbitrary.

The National Surgical Adjuvant Breast and Bowel Project (NSABP) has always accepted larger tumours for primary surgery. The difference is mainly one of perspective, and depends on expectations for local control. If large tumours are considered to be unsuitable for BCS, then downsizing is important, but this would be less of a problem if some or all of the large tumours were in fact suitable for BCS initially. In the early lumpectomy trials, the NSABP accepted patients with tumour sizes of 4 cm or less.[17] The Milan QUART study[18] was originally conducted on patients with tumours of diameter 2 cm or less, although in later studies this was increased to a 2.5 cm limit. In subsequent protocols, NSABP surgeons accepted tumours of diameter 5 cm or less for lumpectomy. Long-term local results with radiation therapy and post-operative adjuvant therapy as routinely practised have demonstrated very high levels of local control. In protocol B-06, patients treated by lumpectomy and post-operative radiation had a local recurrence rate of 10% over 12 years.[19] The figure was lower for node-positive patients (who received adjuvant chemotherapy) than for node-negative patients (who did not), suggesting a role for chemotherapy in promoting local control by a possible synergy with radiotherapy, as lumpectomy patients who received chemotherapy but not radiotherapy did not benefit to the same extent.

Local recurrence rates in node-negative patients also appear to be improved when adjuvant therapies[20–23] are used. This is confirmed in protocol B-13 (a trial of chemotherapy vs. observation in oestrogen-receptor-negative patients), where the average annual local failure rate is 0.57%.[24] In B-14 (a comparison of placebo vs. tamoxifen in oestrogen-receptor-positive patients), the rate is 0.5% per year. The rates in control patients were 2.78% and 1.24%, respectively, i.e. the same as in the B-06 population[24] (see Table 15.1).

Table 15.1 *Local recurrence rates in B-06 compared to later protocols where systemic adjuvant therapy was added to radiation therapy, resulting in lower rates of tumour recurrence in the breast*

Trial number	Number of patients	Number of events	Average annual failure rate (%)
B-06	558	47	1.38
B-14			
Surgery only	121	9	2.78
MTX + 5FU	117	2	0.57
B-14			
Placebo	537	19	1.24
Tamoxifen	537	8	0.50

MTX + 5FU, methotrexate and fluorouracil.

Thus it is unclear whether in the population of patients typified by the Milan study[15] primary chemotherapy is warranted, as the goal of BCS could have been achieved with good local control rates by the standard approaches of lumpectomy, radiation and routine post-operative adjuvant therapy according to NSABP selection standards, in the 79% of patients whose tumours were up to 5 cm in diameter. For larger tumours, a significant clinical response is less frequent with pre-operative therapy, so this approach may be less useful at this end of the spectrum of tumour size.

While downstaging for breast preservation may be important in some cases, if pre-operative chemotherapy only succeeded in downsizing the tumours and had no effect on long-term outcomes, it is doubtful that this would become a widely accepted technique when all of the negative features (e.g. lack of prognostic information) are considered. On the other hand, if there is an improvement in disease-free survival or survival, the negative features would be of much less importance and its usefulness would be enormous. Furthermore, if response to primary therapy corresponded to improved disease-free survival, we would have a useful tool for selecting individual treatment regimens, or choosing which patients should or should not receive adjuvant chemotherapy. For this reason, the most valuable studies would be the prospective randomized comparisons of pre-operative chemotherapy compared to standard post-operative chemotherapy.

Randomized studies

Mauriac *et al.*[25] reported in 1991 on one of the first studies aimed at improving survival. A total of 272 women with operable breast carcinomas larger than 3 cm in diameter were randomized to receive standard post-operative adjuvant chemotherapy or initial chemotherapy followed by surgery in order to determine whether induction chemotherapy could reduce the number of mastectomies which would otherwise be necessary. A secondary end-point was disease-free survival and survival. In the initial chemotherapy group, 84 patients received BCS and 44 patients received radiation therapy above. The initial chemotherapy group showed a better overall survival (P=0.04). However, all of the patients in this group received chemotherapy. In the post-operative group, 32 patients who were found at initial surgery to be node-negative and oestrogen-receptor-positive received no adjuvant chemotherapy. It has subsequently been demonstrated that node-negative patients benefit from adjuvant tamoxifen therapy or chemotherapy. As the pre-operative group included some node-negative patients, all of whom received therapy, a treatment bias exists, and these results must be treated with caution. An update of this trial, published recently,[26] reported no overall survival advantage. However, more than 50% of the patients in the pre-operative group survived with conserved breasts, although the local recurrence rate was 'non-negligible'.

Scholl et al.[27] randomized 196 patients with an operable tumour (T2–3) at the Institute Curie. Group I received two monthly cycles of doxorubicin, cyclophosphamide and 5FU followed by local therapy and four chemotherapy cycles post-operatively. Group II received local therapy followed by six monthly cycles of chemotherapy. Some node-negative patients received incomplete initial chemotherapy, and none of them received adjuvant post-operative chemotherapy. Furthermore, because of the inclusion of pre- and post-menopausal patients and different clinical treatment decisions, it was necessary to analyse the patients in four different groups. Local therapy for all patients consisted of radiation either as primary treatment in the adjuvant group or between cycles two and three in the primary chemotherapy group. Surgery was limited to those patients who had a persisting mass after completion of radiation and was intended to be as conservative as possible.

Significant downstaging of tumour size was achieved. The best responses were obtained in patients who received the largest fraction of the planned chemotherapy dose. When all of the patients were analysed, no difference was found in disease-free survival or survival. In the subgroup of patients whose treatment did not deviate from the planned protocol, the survival curve showed a non-significant trend (P=0.3) in favour of the primary chemotherapy group. In those patients who achieved a greater than 50% reduction in tumour size from primary chemotherapy there were fewer metastases (P=0.1) and an improved disease-free survival (P=0.05) compared to those with little or no objective tumour shrinkage, but again this advantage disappeared when all of the patients were included. Only 72% of the randomized patients actually received the therapy as assigned, and some post-menopausal patients received hormone treatment. As only two courses of primary chemotherapy were given, a clear evaluation of that modality may not have been achieved. The observation of a better response in patients who received more than 75% of the planned dose suggests that many of the patients may not have been adequately treated. In a later report, four cycles of pre-operative FAC were compared to conventional adjuvant FAC. Local recurrence and breast conservation rates were similar, and no survival difference was reported.[28]

An early report (median follow-up 28 months) of a UK trial which randomized 212 patients with primary operable breast cancer demonstrated a significant reduction in the need for mastectomy among patients who were treated with neoadjuvant therapy.[29] The follow-up period is obviously too short, and the trial had insufficient power to allow reliable evaluation of the relapse rate or survival duration.

In addition to the three European trials mentioned above, a randomized prospective trial of pre-operative chemotherapy has been carried out by the National Surgical Adjuvant Breast Project (NSABP).[30] The clinical rationale for this study also derives from the excellent response rates previously reported where treating patients with locally advanced breast cancer, and the evidence that a reduction in primary tumour size could allow an increased number of breast-preserving operations, but the primary objective was now improved DFS and S.

Patients with clinically palpable tumours had their diagnosis established by fine-needle aspiration cytology or core-needle biopsy. Consenting patients were then randomized to receive four cycles of adriamycin (60 mg/m²) and cyclophosphamide (600 mg/m²) at 3-week intervals. Group I received this treatment prior to surgery. Group II underwent standard surgery and then received chemotherapy. All of the lumpectomy patients received 5000 Gy of radiation therapy without a boost. All patients aged 50 years or older received tamoxifen regardless of oestrogen-receptor status. Patients were assessed with tumour measurements prior to each chemotherapy cycle. A declaration by the treating surgeon was made at the time of diagnosis as to whether or not that patient was suitable for lumpectomy at the time.

Although differences in disease-free survival and survival were not demonstrated through 5 years of follow-up,[31] it is clear that a significant reduction in tumour size occurred with initial chemotherapy. The complete response (CR) rate was highest in tumours of diameter ≤ 2 cm (Table 15.2). BCS was achieved in 67% of pre-operative chemotherapy patients and 57% of post-operative patients. Among the patients who showed a complete response, lumpectomy was achieved in 81% of cases, and among patients with a partial response, 62% had a lumpectomy.

Pathological lymph-node status was also downstaged by pre-operative chemotherapy. In the pre-operative group, 59% of patients had negative nodes, compared to 42% of the post-operative group. There was a correlation between tumour response and pathological nodal status. Among patients who showed a complete response, 73%

Table 15.2 *Initial pre-operative chemotherapy with adriamycin and cyclophosphamide × 4 doses showing the response of the primary tumour according to the initial pretreatment tumour size*

Response	%	Tumour diameter (cm)		
		≤ 2 (%)	2.1–4.0 (%)	≥ 4.1 (%)
Complete (CR)	37	50	38	18
Partial (PR)	43	29	45	55
Stable disease (SD)	17	15	14	25
Progressive disease (PD)	4	6	4	2

had negative nodes, compared to 55% of those who showed a partial response (see Table 15.3). Thus in a randomized trial, pre-operative chemotherapy with AC results in an 80% primary tumour response, a 17% incidence of axillary-node downstaging, and modestly increased rates of breast conservation (63% vs. 57%). The latter indicates NSABP surgeons' confidence in lumpectomy, even without downstaging.

This trial addresses one of the disquieting aspects of many of the other reports in which all patients in the pre-operative treatment group receive chemotherapy, but those with initial surgery who are found to have negative lymph nodes often do not receive the scheduled post-operative therapy. In the NSABP trial, all patients received identical therapy, enabling a more realistic evaluation of the importance of downstaging. The real question is whether downstaging is correlated with improved DFS and S, or whether this treatment effect simply identifies the longer survivors by the 'market' of response. It is encouraging that axillary-node status correlates with primary tumour response, but objective outcome data are still needed. An important corollary question will concern the future evaluation of combined pre- and post-operative therapy compared to either one alone.

These studies have shown that chemotherapy is safe and that it provides high rates of primary tumour response, enabling increased rates of breast preservation. Even if pre-operative chemotherapy does not result in achievement of the primary goal, namely better DFS and S, it may be preferable in some cases because it increases breast preservation (although it may not always be necessary). Against this must be weighed the disadvantages with regard to loss of prognostic factors and the need to treat patients who would turn out to have very favourable tumours with less need for chemotherapy, but who would have already received initial chemotherapy. This problem is balanced somewhat by the finding that smaller tumours have the highest response rates. This provides a good rationale for treating patients with T_1 lesions, at least during the research phase.

One specific concern with regard to the possible treatment of patients who might have a very good prognosis is the possibility that they will receive initial chemotherapy with more toxic agents, such as anthracyclines or taxanes. Should initial chemotherapy become standard, this situation could be offset by the development of reliable prognostic features which would enable better selection of patients. These could include S-phase determination or other prognostic markers which may be evaluated by needle aspiration cytology in a pre-operative setting (see below).

We must also consider our biased view that chemotherapy is more important in patients with bad tumours. In fact, common sense would indicate that chemotherapy is more important in patients who demonstrate a good response and show increased DFS and S. If it should turn out that some good-prognosis patients do even better when they are treated by primary chemotherapy, this would change our perspective on who should receive treatment and who should not do so.

The French reports[14,25] suggest that surgery may not be necessary in all cases. Although these results are impressive, a prospective clinical trial is still necessary to confirm these preliminary findings and allow comparisons of local, regional and distant recurrence rates over a longer period. The avoidance of surgery is a logical outcome of the series of trials that have accompanied the challenge to the Halsted hypothesis since the 1960s. In the coming years we shall probably continue the trend

Table 15.3 *Incidence of negative nodes, positive nodes and number of positive nodes for patients who received post-operative adriamycin and cyclophosphamide compared to those who received pre-operative adriamycin and cyclophosphamide at the same dosages*

Treatment Group	Nodal status at operation				
	Negative	Positive	Number of positive nodes		
	(%)	(%)	1–3 (%)	4–9 (%)	≥10 (%)
Post-operative	42	58	31	17	9
Pre-operative	59	41	25	12	4
CR	71	29	20	7	1
PR	53	47	29	14	4
SD	52	48	27	15	6
PD	38	62	38	13	13

towards diagnosis of earlier and smaller tumours, and this category will dominate the spectrum of clinical presentations. If we are to make an impact on long-term cure rates, it will be in this category of patient, so it is important to treat patients with small tumours in current trials to determine whether this will become an important strategy for widespread clinical use.

TECHNICAL PROBLEMS

It is clear from preliminary studies that meaningful shrinkage of primary tumours can be achieved. Whether or not this results in an improvement in long-term survival has yet to be ascertained, but the management of patients in whom the primary tumour has diminished significantly poses some new technical challenges.

Several of these relate to departures from routine adjuvant therapy, but a number of surgical issues also arise.

Surgical problems

SUB-CLINICAL TUMOURS

With high rates of complete response, the problem of identifying the lesion at the time of surgery can present difficulties. NSABP investigators have held workshops on this subject, and have devised a simple method of mapping or marking the tumour using visible skin naevi or blemishes as landmarks, or making a small tattoo, as is often done by radiation oncologists when delineating their fields. Some of these tumours may remain visible on mammography and can therefore be localized with standard pre-operative wire techniques. Serial mammograms of the treated breast can be worthwhile in rapidly responding patients in order to track the lesion for identification even as a small architectural distortion. The simplest technique is the use of a transparent grid which is laid over the patient's breast at the time of diagnosis (see Figure 15.1). The patient is placed in the same position as she will be in the operating room, the tumour is indicated with an ink mark on the skin, and the grid is placed over this with the centre point over the nipple and a fixed mark for orientation made at the medial end of the clavicle. With the co-ordinates noted, the tumour can then be relocated at the time of surgery and the incision planned even if there is a complete response.

THE COMPLETE RESPONSE AND SURGICAL MARGINS

It appears that tumours do not necessarily shrink in a uniform fashion similar to a melting ice cube, but they may regress irregularly leaving pockets of tumour cells near the periphery of the original tumour (see Figure

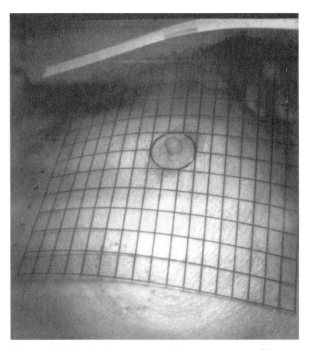

Figure 15.1 *Simple 1 cm-square grid on a transparent film with a circle cut out at the centre. This is placed over the treated breast and the coordinates are noted for the future location of responding tumours.*

15.2). Therefore, when performing a lumpectomy on a patient who has had significant reduction in the size of the tumour, the original tumour boundaries should be excised (see Figure 15.3). Sometimes pre-operative mammography will show that the true dimensions are larger than the new clinical size, but occasionally even mammographic signs of malignancy may disappear, making the mapping technique very important.

The technique of lumpectomy is the same as for a palpable tumour even if there is no palpable mass. The incision is placed according to previously determined measurements, and a tissue mass corresponding to the original tumour dimensions is removed. This enables the pathologist to evaluate and report on the margins. In most cases, pathological evidence of tumour remains even though it is not clinically palpable. The most important technical point is to make the incision directly over the presumed site of the original tumour. Cosmetic periareolar incisions with tunnelling are not suitable because they increase the likelihood of incomplete excision.

Radiation therapy after lumpectomy

In retrospective studies, Bucholz et al.[32] found that delaying radiation therapy for 6 months to allow for chemotherapy administration resulted in a higher local failure rate, which was itself associated with an increased rate of distant metastases and a decreased overall survival rate. We do not know what factors led to the delay in these patients (did more worrying tumours receive more

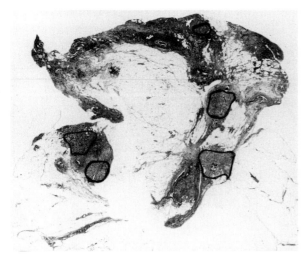

Figure 15.2 *Photomicrograph of tumour excised after complete clinical response, showing islands of remaining tumour.*

chemotherapy?). Recht *et al.* also found that patients with more than a 16-week delay before beginning radiation therapy had a significantly higher local failure rate 4 years later.[33] However, in a similar review, Buzdar *et al.* found no such association.[34] Their patients had a minimum of 20 weeks' delay of radiotherapy, but the incidence of local failure was not influenced by this, or by the order in which chemotherapy and radiotherapy were administered.

These reports concern treatments given after routine surgical treatment. With pre-operative chemotherapy, the issue of radiation therapy presents no additional problems. When traditional surgery is followed by adjuvant chemotherapy, radiation therapy is often given after the completion of chemotherapy, especially in situations where anthracyclines are used. Surgery took place very soon after diagnosis, and the issue of delay relates to the interval between diagnosis and initiation of radiotherapy. The same time-frame exists here; it is only the

surgery that has changed. With primary chemotherapy, diagnosis and surgery may be separated by an interval of several weeks while chemotherapy is given, but the overall timing from diagnosis to radiotherapy is virtually the same regardless of when the surgery is performed. Although this question is not answered by these conflicting reports, it appears that the timing of surgery with respect to chemotherapy will have little impact on the issue of timing of radiotherapy.

Oestrogen-receptor values

These were the main criteria used to select patients for adjuvant hormone therapy with or without chemotherapy. Quantitative cytosol determinations have been the accepted technique, and also more recently immunocytochemical analysis (ERICA). Even more recently, other prognostic indicators such as DNA content have entered clinical use. Their determination in pre-operative settings is also being explored, but as yet no reliable treatment guidelines exist, and their clinical usefulness has not been determined.

Remvikos *et al.* evaluated S-phase fractions (SPF) with flow cytometry on pre-operative cytological samples.[35] Patients were entered in the Institute Curie trial comparing primary and post-operative adjuvant chemotherapy. A high SPF was associated with relapse ($P<0.0008$) and local regional recurrence ($P<0.02$). However, when this analysis was combined with the type of treatment, SPF was not useful for predicting outcome in the primary chemotherapy group ($P=0.06$). The rate of tumour response to initial chemotherapy was lower for tumours with low SPF. Thus SPF was only highly predictive in non-responding patients. Although the feasibility of the technique for cytological samples is established, it is not clear how useful the values will be in selecting patients for therapy.

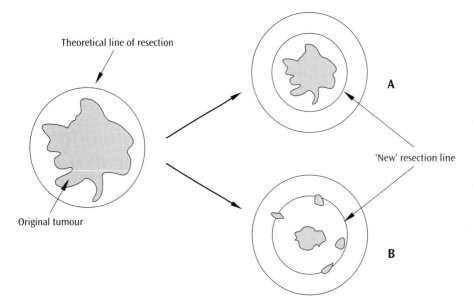

Figure 15.3 *A hypothetical tumour shrinks to 50% of its former size with pre-operative chemotherapy. Panel A suggests (incorrectly) that the tumour shrinks in a homogenous fashion allowing for a smaller line of resection. Panel B shows a more realistic outcome, where pockets of tumour cells may remain even at the periphery of the old tumour. Adequate resection may require wider resection margins.*

Lymph nodes status

This has always been the main criterion for selecting patients for post-operative adjuvant therapy. With the demonstration that node-negative patients also benefit from adjuvant therapy,[36] we can combine patients with different nodal status into a more unified group which facilitates the pre-operative approach to treatment. However, there are still unanswered questions about whether node-negative patients should receive the same chemotherapy as node-positive patients, and whether some node-negative patients should only receive tamoxifen instead of chemotherapy or both.

NSABP protocols B-09[37] and B-16[38] indicate that chemotherapy and tamoxifen combinations are superior to either treatment alone in node-positive women. Similarly, recent studies have provided data on node-negative patients. In Protocol B-20, tamoxifen and chemotherapy provided better DFS at 5 years than tamoxifen alone, generating greater confidence that a unified approach, necessary for pre-operative chemotherapy, is appropriate.[39] The old divisions of nodal status and oestrogen receptors, while useful for exploring early adjuvant therapies, may turn out to be less important than was originally thought for clinical use. In fact, we may be able to devise a better delineation of low-and high-risk groups using clinical and cytological indicators.

Fine-needle aspiration cytology

This is not reliable for differentiating ductal carcinoma *in situ* (DCIS) from invasive carcinoma. Although it can be argued that some T_1 tumours are suitable for pre-operative treatment because they are most responsive, it is nevertheless concerning that some patients with DCIS may inadvertently be treated with chemotherapy, and possibly even with such toxic drugs as anthracyclines and taxanes. More frequent use of core-needle biopsies and careful patient selection may minimize these concerns. It would be most useful to have markers to select the invasive cancers such as cadherins or extracellular matrix regulators, but these are not currently available for clinical use.

Powles *et al.*[40] evaluated the accuracy of fine-needle aspiration cytology with regard to predicting treatment with cytotoxic drugs. In a total of 868 women who were seen in their breast clinic, clinical examination together with fine-needle aspiration cytology detected over 99% of cancers, with a 12% false-positive rate. The cytological diagnosis of definite carcinoma was obtained in 69% of women with breast cancer, with no false-positive results.

It is understood that a small number of false-positive results will occur. Cytologists can have considerable difficulty in distinguishing some fibroadenomas from carcinomas. One way of minimizing these problems is to require clear cytological signs of malignancy and to require core biopsy for any borderline changes of the type

often reported as 'suspicious for carcinoma'. In the long term, if primary chemotherapy is established as useful, these problems will have to be seen in perspective. We now give post-operative adjuvant therapy to many patients who do not need it (not all untreated patients develop recurrences). The usefulness of primary chemotherapy will have to be established in the same way (are the benefits of treatment worth the risk, even of unnecessary treatment?). Before this conclusion can be reached, more research is needed to establish risk–benefit ratios and to examine the methods of patient selection.

CONCLUSION

After nearly a century of dominance of breast cancer therapy by radical surgery, we have moved to a situation that is best described as less surgery accompanied by increasing reliance on adjuvant chemotherapy. Having reached the point where many regard surgery as the adjuvant therapy of cancer, we are now entering a phase where the very usefulness of surgery is being questioned. Two French studies have evaluated primary chemotherapy and radiation therapy without surgery in selected cases, and have demonstrated the feasibility of this approach. The issue is now complicated by the advent of newer therapies that are grouped together under the common heading of 'biologics'. These include many different kinds of agents whose only common feature is that they are not the typical cytotoxic chemotherapies we have been studying for 20 years. There is a reasonably strong possibility that these will provide new ways of controlling or reversing the growth of tumours. This will have an important impact on the role of surgery in the treatment of breast cancer. As we move from an approach that seeks to kill cancer cells to one which seeks to control or change the growth of cancer cells, we shall be faced with the challenge and opportunity of further integrating yet another therapeutic approach into the established practices of surgery, chemotherapy and radiotherapy. The timing and sequencing of these may be important, and rigorous prospective clinical trials will clearly be necessary in order to guide us.

REFERENCES

1 Skipper HE. Kinetics of mammary tumor cell growth and implications for therapy. *Cancer* 1971; **28**: 1479.

2 Gunduz N, Fisher B, Saffer EA. Effect of surgical removal on the growth and kinetics of residual tumor. *Cancer Res* 1979; **39**: 3861–5.

3 Fisher B, Gunduz N, Saffer EA. Influence of the interval between primary tumor removal and chemotherapy on kinetics and growth of metastases. *Cancer Res* 1983; **43**: 1488–92.

4 Goldie JH. Arguments supporting the concept of non-cross-resistant combinations of chemotherapy. *Cancer Invest* 1994; **12**: 324–8.

5 Rosen G. Preoperative chemotherapy for osteogenic sarcoma. *Cancer* 1982; **49**: 1221.

6 Schuller DE. Preoperative reductive chemotherapy for locally advanced carcinoma of the oral cavity, oropharynx and hypopharynx. *Cancer* 1983; **51**: 15.

7 Schultz PK, Herr HW, Zhang ZF *et al*. Neoadjuvant chemotherapy for invasive bladder cancer: prognostic factors for survival of patients treated with M-VAC with 5-year follow-up. *J Clin Oncol* 1994; **12**: 1394–401.

8 Leichman L, Steiger Z, Seydel HG *et al*. Preoperative chemotherapy and radiation therapy for patients with cancer of the esophagus: a potentially curative approach. *J Clin Oncol* 1984; **2**: 75–9.

9 Sorace RA, Bagley CS, Lichter AS *et al*. The management of non-metastatic locally advanced breast cancer using primary induction chemotherapy with hormonal synchronization followed by radiation therapy with or without debulking surgery. *World J Surg* 1985; **9**: 775–85.

10 Chevallier B, Bastit P, Graic Y *et al*. Becquerel studies in inflammatory non-metastatic breast cancer. Combined modality approach in 178 patients. *Br J Cancer* 1993; **67**: 594–601.

11 Perloff M, Lesnick J. Chemotherapy before and after mastectomy in stage III breast cancer. *Arch Surg* 1982; **117**: 879–81.

12 Fisher B, Ravdin RG, Ausman RK, Slack NH, Moore GE, ana Noer RJ. Surgical adjuvant chemotherapy in cancer of the breast: results of a decade of co-operative investigation. *Ann Surg* 1968; **168**: 337.

13 Nissen-Meyer R, Kjellgren K, Malmio K, Mansson B, Norin T. Surgical adjuvant chemotherapy: results with one short course with cyclophosphamide after mastectomy for breast cancer. *Cancer* 1978; **41**: 2088–98.

14 Jacquillat C, Weil M, Baillet F *et al*. Results of neoadjuvant chemotherapy and radiation therapy in the breast-conserving treatment of 250 patients with all stages of infiltrative breast cancer. *Cancer* 1990; **66**: 119–29.

15 Bonadonna G, Veronese U, Brambilla C *et al*. Primary chemotherapy to avoid mastectomy in tumors with diameters of three centimeters or more. *J Natl Cancer Inst* 1990; **82**: 1539–45.

16 Bonadonna G, Valagussa P, Brambilla C, Moliterni A, Zambetti M, Ferrari L. Adjuvant and neoadjuvant treatment of breast cancer with chemotherapy and/or endocrine therapy. *Semin Oncol* 1991; **18**: 515–24.

17 Fisher B, Bauer M, Margolese R *et al*. Five-year results of a randomized clinical trial comparing total mastectomy and segmental mastectomy with or without radiation in the treatment of breast cancer. *New Engl J Med* 1985; **312**: 665–73.

18 Veronesi U, Salvadori B, Lun A *et al*. Conservative treatment of early breast cancer (long-term results of 1232 cases treated with quadrantectomy, axillary dissection and radiotherapy). *Ann Surg* 1990; **211**: 250–9.

19 Fisher B, Anderson S, Redmond CK, Wolmark N, Wickerham DL, Cronin WM. Re-analysis and results after 12 years of follow-up in a randomized clinical trial comparing total mastectomy with lumpectomy with or without irradiation in the treatment of breast cancer. *N Engl J Med* 1995; **333**: 1456–61.

20 Fisher B, Redmond C, Dimitrov N *et al*. A randomized clinical trial evaluating sequential methotrexate and fluorouracil in the treatment of patients with node-negative breast cancer who have estrogen-receptor-negative tumors. *N Engl J Med* 1989; **320**: 473–8.

21 Fisher B, Constantino J, Redmond C *et al*. A randomized clinical trial evaluating tamoxifen in the treatment of patients with node-negative breast cancer who have estrogen-receptor-positive tumors. *N Engl J Med* 1989; **320**: 479–84.

22 Mansour EG, Gray R, Shatila AH *et al*. Efficacy of adjuvant chemotherapy in high-risk node-negative breast cancer. An inter-group study. *N Engl J Med* 1989; **320**: 485–90.

23 The Ludwig Breast Cancer Study Group. Prolonged disease-free survival after one course of peri-operative adjuvant chemotherapy for node-negative breast cancer. *N Engl J Med* 1989; **320**: 491–6.

24 Margolese R. Surgical considerations in selecting local therapy. *J Natl Cancer Inst Monogr* 1992; **11**: 41–8.

25 Mauriac L, Durand M, Avril A, Dilhuydy JM. Effects of primary chemotherapy in conservative treatment of breast cancer patients with operable tumors larger than 3 cm. *Ann Oncol* 1991; **2**: 347–54.

26 Mauriac L, MacGrogan G, Avril A *et al*. Neoadjuvant chemotherapy for operable breast carcinoma larger than 3 cm: a unicentre randomized trial with a 124-month median follow-up. Institut Bergonie Bordeaux Groupe Sein (IBBGS). *Ann Oncol* 1999; **10**: 47–52.

27 Scholl SM, Asselain B, Palangie T *et al*. Neoadjuvant chemotherapy in operable breast cancer. *Eur J Cancer* 1991; **27**: 1668–71.

28 Scholl SM, Asselain B, Beuzeboc P *et al*. Neoadjuvant versus adjuvant chemotherapy in premenopausal patients with tumours considered too large for breast-conserving surgery. An update. *Proc Am Soc Clin Oncol* 1995; **14**: 125.

29 Powles TJ, Hickish TF, Makris A *et al*. Randomized trial of chemoendocrine therapy started before or after surgery for treatment of primary breast cancer. *J Clin Oncol* 1995; **13**: 547–52.

30 Fisher B, Rockette H, Robidoux A *et al*. Effect of pre-operative therapy for breast cancer (BC) on local-regional disease: first report of NSABP B-18. *Proc ASCO* 1994; **13**: 64.

31 Fisher B, Brown A, Mamounas E *et al*. Effect of preoperative chemotherapy on local-regional disease in women with operable breast cancer: findings from National Surgical Adjuvant Breast and Bowel Project B-18. *J Clin Oncol* 1997; **15**: 2483–93.

32 Bucholz AT, Austin-Seymour M, Moe RE *et al*. Effect of delay in radiation in the combined modality treatment of breast cancer. *Int J Radiat Oncol Biol Phys* 1993; **26**: 23–35.

33 Recht A, Come SE, Gelman RS *et al*. Integration of conservative surgery, radiotherapy, and chemotherapy for the treatment of early-stage, node-positive breast cancer: sequencing, timing, and outcome. *J Clin Oncol* 1991; **9**: 1662–7.

34 Buzdar AU, Shu Wan Kau RN, Terry L *et al*. The order of administration of chemotherapy and radiation and its effect on the local control of operable breast cancer. *Cancer* 1993; **71**: 3680–4.

35 Remvikos Y, Jouve M, Beuzeboc P, Viehl P, Magdelenat H, Pouillart P. Cell cycle modifications of breast cancers during neoadjuvant chemotherapy: a flow cytometry study on fine-needle aspirates. *Eur J Cancer* 1993; **29A**: 1843–8.

36 Fisher B, Dignam J, Mamounas EP *et al*. Sequential methotrexate and fluorouracil for the treatment of node-negative breast cancer patients with estrogen-receptor-negative tumors: eight-year results from National Surgical Adjuvant Breast and Bowel Project (NSABP) B-13 and first report of findings from NSABP B-19 comparing methotrexate and fluorouracil with conventional cyclophosphamide, methotrexate, and fluorouracil. *J Clin Oncol* 1996; **14**: 1982–92.

37 Fisher B, Redmond C, Brown A *et al*. Adjuvant chemotherapy with and without tamoxifen in the treatment of primary breast cancer; five-year results from the National Surgical Adjuvant Breast and Bowel Project trial. *J Clin Oncol* 1986; **4**: 459–71.

38 Fisher B, Redmond C, Legault-Poisson S *et al*. Postoperative chemotherapy and tamoxifen compared with tamoxifen alone in the treatment of positive-node breast cancer patients aged 50 years and older with tumours responsive to tamoxifen: results from the National Surgical Adjuvant Breast and Bowel Project B-16. *J Clin Oncol* 1990; **8**: 1005–18.

39 Fisher B, Dignam J, Wolmark N *et al*. Tamoxifen and chemotherapy for lymph-node-negative, estrogen-receptor-positive breast cancer. *J Natl Cancer Inst* 1997; **89**: 1673–82.

40 Powles TJ, Trott PA, Cherryman G *et al*. Fine-needle aspiration cytodiagnosis as a prerequisite for primary medical treatment for breast cancer. *Cytopathology* 1991; **2**: 7–12.

16

Adjuvant radiotherapy in the management of early breast cancer

JOAN HOUGHTON AND JEFFREY S TOBIAS

INTRODUCTION

Radiotherapy has been used to manage breast cancer patients since the 1940s.[1] The major objective of post-mastectomy irradiation has been to reduce the risk of local relapse, and that this is clearly achieved is now well documented by a number of large trials both following mastectomy and more recently also following breast-conserving surgery (see Table 16.1). Moreover, several meta-analyses of the early trials have been conducted to review the evidence relating to mortality.[2–5] However, it is still unclear from these analyses to what extent survival is modified. In the last two decades the use of breast conservation surgery has become widespread, mainly for patients with good-prognosis disease. The early trials of breast conservation included radiation therapy as part of the 'treatment package', although two trials did also evaluate breast conservation without radiation therapy,[6,7] and concluded that the local relapse rates were unacceptably high even though distant metastatic spread and survival do not appear to have been compromised.

A number of questions still need to be addressed in evaluating the place of radiotherapy in the current management of early breast cancer.

- Is it possible to define subgroups of patients who do or do not need radiation treatment?
- Do patients who are to receive adjuvant systemic therapy also need to receive local prophylactic radiotherapy and, if so, in what sequence should these treatments be employed?

- Is the likelihood of survival modified for patients given prophylactic radiotherapy?
- From the patient's perspective, what are the risks and benefits of treatments?

This chapter will address these issues, relying mainly on the data generated within randomized clinical trials, especially the two large trials organized by the CRC Breast Cancer Trials Group, and will also highlight research questions that need to be addressed or which are currently receiving attention.

IS IT POSSIBLE TO DEFINE SUBGROUPS OF PATIENTS WHO DO OR DO NOT NEED TO BE TREATED?

For mastectomy patients it has been well documented that, in the absence of prophylactic radiotherapy, there is a substantial risk of local relapse. To date, none of the published overviews of breast cancer have addressed this question, but the latest overview by the Early Breast Cancer Trialists' Collaborative Group (EBCTCG) will do so.[5] However, review of the individual trials gives a clear indication that local recurrence is reduced (relatively) by about 60% at 10 years. This will translate into an approximate absolute reduction in incidence of 15–20%. The extent to which an individual patient will benefit obviously depends on a number of factors, such as the size of the tumour and nodal status at presentation, which determine the likelihood of relapse. Therefore, even

Table 16.1 *Randomised trials of radiotherapy versus the same management without radiotherapy*

Type of surgery and study name	Year Started	Total patient numbers	Breast/chest wall (BW) irradiation	Axilla & fossa (AF) irradiation	Internal mammary chain irradiation	Systemic chemo or endocrine therapy
Mastectomy only						
Manchester Trial	1970	714	37–45Gy (I5f/21d) o	As BW	As BW	OvAbl
CRC (Kings/Cambridge)	1970	2800	Various	Various	Various	None
NSABP B-04	1971	770	50Gy (25f/35d) m	As BW (60–70Gy if NI b)	As BW	None
Scottish D	*1978*	*93*	*37–45Gy (10–20f/19–30d) om*	*As BW*	*None*	*± Tam*
CRC	*1986*	*59*	*4–45 Gy (20f/28d)*	*As BW for about half*	*Generally none*	*Endocrine*
Mastectomy with axillary sampling						
Wessex	*1973*	*151*	*46Gy (20f/28d) m*	*55Gy (22f/30d) m*	*As BW*	*None*
Edinburgh 1	1974	348	43Gy (I Of128d) m	As BW	None	None
Danish BCG 82b pre	1982	1832	50Gy (25f/35d) om	As BW	As BW	CMF
Danish BCG 82c post	1982	1481	50Gy (25f/35d) om	As BW	As BW	Tam
Nottingham	1985	77	45Gy (I 5f/?d)	As BW	As BW	Various
Mastectomy with axillary clearance						
Berlin-Buch ABC**	1962	255	55Gy (?f/40d) m	As BW	As BW	None
Oslo X-ray	1964	552	25-3 1 Gy (?f/28d(o	36–52Gy (?f/28d) o	As BW	OvIrr
Oslo Co-60	1964	563	None	50Gy (20f/28d) m	As AF	OvIrr
Heidelberg XRT*	1969	143	None	65Gy (24–30f/42d) m	As AF	None
Stockholm A**	1971	960	45Gy (25f/35d) m	As BW	As BW	None
SASIB	1971	377	34–60Gy (10–24f/24–42d) m	44–60Gy (as BW)	40–56Gy (as BW)	None
Mayo Clinic	1973	241	50Gy (24f/52d) m	As BW	As BW	± CFP
INT Milan 1	1973	56	None	45Gy (20f/28d) m	As AF	None
DFCI Boston	1974	218	45Gy (20f/35d) m	As BW	None	ACvCMFvMF
Piedmont OA (1)	1975	280	45–50Gy (30fl142d) m	As BW	As BW	Mel v CMF
(2) [NI –3 or T <3]			None	45Gy (I6f/28d) m	None	Mel v CMF
SECSG 1	1976	257	50Gy (?f/35d) m	As BW	As BW	CMF
Glasgow	1976	219	3 8Gy (1 5f/2 1 d) o	As BW	As BW	CMF
Cologne(X)		No data	50Gy (?f/35d) m	As BW	Not known	AC
MD Ander, 7730B*	1977	97	45–50Gy (25–27f/32–35d) m	As BW	ASBW	FAC
S Swedish BCG (1)	1978	7668	35Gy (20f/48d) m	48Gy (20f/48d) m	As AF	C or Tam
(2) [perigiand+1			35Gy (20f/48d) m	60Gy (25f/55d) m	ASAF	C or Tam
Toronto-Edmont.	1978	50	40Gy (I 4f/I 6d) m	As BW	None	OvIrr + CMFP
BCCA Vancouver	1978	318	40Gy (I6f/21d)	3 8Gy (1 6f/21 d)	ASAF	CMF ± Ov1rr
Dusseldorf U.	1978	88	40Gy (20f/28d) m	As BW	None	LMF
Coimbra	1979	124	36Gy (I2f/28d) om	39–45Gy (I2f.28d) m	ASAF	AC
Metaxas Athens	1979	71	50–60Gy (25–30fl35–42d) om	50Gy (25f/35d) om	ASAF	Various
Helsinki	1980	99	45Gy (I 5f/?d) m	As BW	30Gy (I0f/?d) m	CAFT
NSABC Israel	1980	112	46–50Gy (23–25f/28–35d) m	As BW	40Gy (20fl28d) m	CMF
ECOG EST3181	1962	332	46Gy (23f/3 Id) m	As BW	As BW	CAFH + Tam
BMFT 03 Germany	1984	199	50Gy (25f/35–42d) m	As BW	44Gy (as BW)	CMF
Conservative surgery with axillary clearance						
NSABP B-06	1976	1449	50GY (25f/35df) m	None	None	N+ FMel
Uppsala-Orebro	1981	381	54Gy (27f/38d) m	None	None	None
St George's	1982	400	54Gy (27f/39d)	50Gy (25f/25d) m if N+	None	ER+/– Tam/CM
Ontario COG	1984	837	53Gy (21f/28d) m	None	None	None
Scottish	1985	589	40–50Gy (20–25f/28–35d) m	As BW	None	Er+/– Tam/CM
West Midlands(X)		No data	40–50Gy (1 5–25f/?d)	As BW	As BW	Tam
CRC, UK*	1986	486	40–45Gy (20f/28d)	As BW for about half	Generally none	Endocrine
Uppsala-Orebro(X)		No data	54Gy (27f/35d) m	None	None	ER+ Tam
Milan 111(X)		No data	50Gy(25f/35d) m	None	None	CMF/tam
NSABP B-21 (X)		No data	50Gy (25f/35–43d) om	None	None	± Tam

No local recurrence data; **: preoperative radiotherapy; (X): no data; pre/post: pre/post-menopausal.' N: nodes; T: tumour (cm); o/m: ortho/mega-voltage; Gy: Gray; F.. fractions; d: days; A: adriamycin; C: cyclophosphamide; F: 5-fluorouracil; Ft: Futrafur.' H: halotestin; L: chlorambucil; M: methotrexate; Mel: melphalan; OvAbl/Ovirr: ovarian ablation/irradiation; P: prednisone; Tam: Tamoxifen; v: vs.

though the relative risk reduction may be similar, the absolute reduction in different prognostic subgroups can be very different. The early trials in which patients were randomized following mastectomy provide only limited information on the effects of treatment in prognostic groups that are used clinically today,[8] but more information will be available from the more recent trials following breast conservation therapy. Table 16.2 compares the data from the two CRC trials of radiotherapy, the more recent of which included patients who were also receiving adjuvant hormonal therapy. As the relative reduction in prognostic groups is similar, it becomes a matter of judgement whether the underlying risk is high enough to warrant the treatment.

Table 16.2 *Prognostic factors for local relapse and effect of radiation therapy*

Parametre	DXT Number of events	DXT Number of patients	WP Number of events	WP Number of patients	Relative risk*
Pathologic grade					
DCIS	3	21	3	20	0.93 (0.19–4.68)
Grade 1	15	106	29	124	0.63 (0.35–1.15)
Grade 2	104	559	225	564	0.43 (0.35–0.54)
Grade 3	54	291	163	317	0.35 (0.26–0.45)
Pathologic size					
<2 cm	47	266	90	255	0.48 (0.35–0.88)
≥2 cm	119	651	312	717	0.41 (0.33–0.49)
Nodes involved[†]					
Node negative	22	137	38	150	0.61 (0.37–1.02)
Node positive	23	174	78	162	0.27 (0.18–0.40)
All patients with pathologic audit[‡]	176	977	420	1025	0.41 (0.35–0.49)

DCIS: ductal carcinoma in situ.

*The 95% confidence intervals are shown in parentheses
[†]The test for interaction between treatment in the node negative and node positive was significant ($\chi^2 = 6.40$; p = 0.01)
[‡]Material was not available for the assessment of all factors in all patients in whom the full pathologic audit was undertaken. There was no difference in outcome for those patients in whom the audit was undertaken, as shown by comparing the overall relative risk in this table with that for all patients (0.44 (0.39 – 0.51)

In the largest trial of post-mastectomy radiation (the CRC King's/Cambridge Trial),[9] local relapse was defined as confirmed disease on the chest wall or in the ipsilateral axilla, supraclavicular area, or internal mammary nodes. In all analyses of local recurrence, the event was included only if it was the first report of treatment failure, regardless of whether distant disease was diagnosed at the same time. The radiotherapy (DXT) group had a significantly reduced risk of local failure (RR = 0.44, 95% confidence interval (CI) 0.39–0.51). Interestingly, the reduction in risk continued, although to a lesser degree, even after 10 years (see Table 16.3).

The distribution of recurrences at the various sites is shown in Table 16.4. The previously demonstrated risk factors for local disease[8] continue to provide a definition

Table 16.3 *Local recurrence by length of follow-up*

Follow-up interval (years)	Number	Relative risk*	Logrank p value
0–4.99	2800	0.40 (0.34–0.46)	< 0.001
5–9.99	1699	0.67 (0.51–0.88)	0.004
10–14.99	1152	0.61 (0.37–1.01)	0.06
15+	602	0.22 (0.06–0.82)	0.02
10+	1152	0.54 (0.34–0.87)	0.01
All	2800	0.44 (0.39–0.51)	< 0.001

*The 95% confidence intervals are shown in parentheses

of patients at higher risk of developing local relapse. The prognosis of patients developing local recurrence is poor, with less than one-third surviving for 5 years. Patients in the DXT group have a poorer survival after the diagnosis of local relapse than those who did not receive prophylactic irradiation (RR = 1.42, 95% CI 1.20–1.68). Detection of supraclavicular nodes as the first site of treatment failure is indicative of a particularly poor prognosis (see Table 16.4).

Table 16.4 *Sites of first local relapse*

Site	DXT	WP	Relative risk*	Logrank p value
Chest wall	69	135	0.50 (0.38–0.66)	<0.001
Axilla	79	277	0.31 (0.25–0.38)	<0.001
Supraclavicular nodes	28	31	0.85 (0.51–1.42)	0.54
Internal mammary nodes	1	3	[†]	
Multiple sites[‡]	53	96	0.53 (0.38–0.73)	<0.001
All sites[§]	230	542	0.42 (0.36–0.48)	<0.001

*the 95% confidence intervals are shown in parentheses
[†]too few events have occurred to allow accurate estimation
[‡]Patients having recurrence simultaneously at more than one local site are included only in this category
[§]not all patients had detailed site information available and have therefore been excluded from this table (DXT group = 30; WP group = 26)

The protocol of this trial did not stipulate the management of local recurrence, and therefore patients received a variety of treatments. Most of those in the watch policy group had the recurrence surgically excised and received delayed radiotherapy, whereas patients in the DXT group had the recurrence removed surgically and were then treated with hormones. Even more distressing for the patient than the development of local disease is its persistence on the chest wall or in the axilla. Therefore major outcome in trials of local therapy is not just the development of local recurrence, but also the ultimate incidence of uncontrolled disease in patients who die of breast cancer. To gain an idea of the persistence of local disease, we looked at the individual sites of disease at first relapse and assessed whether recurrence was still present at the same site at the time of death. The results of these analyses are shown in Tables 16.5 and 16.6.

Table 16.5 *Survival after development of local relapse*

Site of recurrence	5-Year survival (% ± SE)		Median survival (years)		Logrank p value
	DXT	WP	DXT	WP	
Chest wall	34.8 ± 11.4	36.5 ± 8.2	2.91	2.39	0.09
Axilla	26.2 ± 9.9	38.3 ± 5.9	2.06	3.18	0.01
Supraclavicular nodes	10.7 ± 11.7	21.1 ± 15.4	0.69	1.37	0.21
Multiple sites*	17.0 ± 10.3	17.2 ± 7.8	1.25	1.70	0.81
All sites*	23.9 ± 5.3	32.2 ± 3.9	1.35	2.68	< 0.001

Patients with first relapse only in the internal mammary nodes have been excluded from this table because the numbers were small

*The same definitions for 'multiple' and 'all' sites have been used as for Table 16.4

Table 16.6 *Persistent local disease at death*

Site	Initial local relapse (number of patients)		Number of subsequent deaths		Number of patients with relapse at same site at death	
	DXT	WP	DXT	WP	DXT	WP
Chest wall	69	135	62	113	30 (48%)	54 (48%)
Axilla	79	277	69	221	36 (52%)	89 (40%)

Returning to the subject of local relapse, it is necessary to determine whether a reduction in this alone is sufficient for recommending treatment in specified prognostic groups. Various suggestions have been made for determining the underlying risk, and the Nottingham Prognostic Index (NPI)[9] is one of the simplest and most commonly used in the UK. The higher the NPI, the more likely it is that the patient is at increased risk of relapse, and therefore the greater the rationale for employing post-operative radiotherapy.

However, in coming to this conclusion the significance of local relapse must be considered. In a study conducted by the National Surgical Adjuvant Breast and Bowel Project (NSABP) on data from Protocol B-06, the question of the relevance of ipsilateral breast tumour recurrence (IBTR) on the subsequent development of distant disease was addressed.[10] Using a multivariate model in which local relapse was considered as a time-dependant variable they showed that IBTR is a powerful independent predictor of distant disease, with a three-fold increase in risk for patients in whom IBTR developed. However, it was concluded that there was no causal relationship between IBTR and subsequent distant metastatic spread.

In other words, data from both the old CRC mastectomy trial and the NSABP lumpectomy trial indicate that IBTR is a marker of poor prognosis and not a cause of metastatic spread.

How do these studies influence our current management of breast cancer? Before answering this question,

we should first look at the evidence from trials that have addressed the question in the presence of adjuvant systemic therapy.

IS PROPHYLACTIC RADIOTHERAPY ESSENTIAL WHEN THE PATIENT IS ALSO TO RECEIVE SYSTEMIC ADJUVANT TREATMENT?

The first reliable evidence of the effectiveness of adjuvant systemic therapy came from the 1985 Breast Cancer Trials Overview.[11] Although individual trials had previously reported advantages, mainly in disease-free survival, the evidence up to that time had been unreliable. The trials included in that overview evaluated the role of tamoxifen and systemic chemotherapy in women who had previously received appropriate local therapy (as defined in each trial protocol), and were typically recruiting patients in the late 1970s and early 1980s.

In contrast, the trials of post-mastectomy radiation were mainly initiated before 1975 when patients were not offered adjuvant systemic treatment. Some of the trials that evaluated local excision rather than mastectomy had allowed the administration of other adjuvant therapies, but the availability of agents in the early 1980s was limited and the evidence for the benefit of these treatments had not accumulated. However, the question has been addressed in a number of trials which have been reported recently. The largest of those trials were from the Danish Breast Cancer Group, which conducted two trials. A total of 1708 premenopausal patients were randomized to receive or not to receive irradiation of the chest wall and regional lymph nodes. All patients were prescribed CMF (eight courses for those also allocated to radiotherapy, and nine to the rest). There was not only a significant reduction in local control but also an improvement in survival for patients allocated to radiotherapy.[12] A similar trial among postmenopausal patients (n = 1375) who were allocated tamoxifen rather than CMF as adjuvant therapy showed very similar results, with a survival rate at a median follow-up of 123 months of 45% in the radiotherapy patients compared to 36% in the control group (P=0.03).[13] The authors concluded that the trials not only demonstrated a decrease in the risk of locoregional recurrence, but were also associated with improved survival in high-risk patients following mastectomy and limited axillary dissection.

A smaller trial performed in Canada in premenopausal mastectomy patients with node-positive breast cancer demonstrated a 33% reduction in risk of recurrence and a 29% reduction in mortality after 15 years of follow-up for those patients who received radiotherapy and chemotherapy, compared to those who received chemotherapy alone.[14]

IS THE CHANCE OF SURVIVAL MODIFIED IN PATIENTS WHO ARE GIVEN PROPHYLACTIC RADIATION THERAPY?

The positive effect of radiotherapy on the survival of patients following surgery for breast cancer has already been mentioned. The results of the two Danish studies clearly allow this possibility.[11,12] However, this is only the latest evidence in an area which has been debated since the 1970s.[15] Publication of an overview (meta-analysis) of trials of simple or radical mastectomy with randomization to either radical radiotherapy or a watch policy demonstrated a small excess in mortality among irradiated patients after 10 years or more.[2]

This finding led the Cancer Research Campaign (CRC) Breast Cancer Trials Group (BCTG) to undertake an in-depth analysis of late mortality among the survivors of the original 2800 randomized patients,[16] which showed a small excess late mortality from non-breast cancers and cardiac disease. The CRC (King's/ Cambridge) Trial for Early Breast Cancer was set up in 1970 to determine 'whether treatment of the regional lymph nodes in patients with clinically early carcinoma of the breast affects the survival of patients, the site or time of recurrence of the tumour, and the morbidity of patients'.[17] These objectives were set as a contentious debate raged among oncologists concerning the mechanism of spread of the disease from the local area. The traditional view that breast cancer cells spread in continuity along lymphatic channels and were temporarily checked in the lymph nodes before spreading to the next group of nodes had been challenged by animal experiments,[18,19] as these suggested that cancer cells could gain direct access to the vital organs at an early stage via the bloodstream. Thus lymph nodes, rather than determining outcome, were but markers of poor prognosis – hence the desire to determine whether sterilization of the lymphatic regions around the breast tumour affected outcome. In retrospect, the policy of non-surgical interference with the axilla has limited the conclusions that can be drawn from this trial, as axillary histology was available only as an incidental finding in 623 of the 2002 patients who had completed the pathological audit.

A total of 2800 patients were randomized to simple mastectomy and radiotherapy (DXT) or simple mastectomy and careful observation (watch policy) between June 1970 and April 1975. Patients under 70 years of age with no previous history of malignancy and with stage I or II disease were eligible. Some surgeons elected not to randomize patients with palpable nodes in the axilla, which resulted in a preponderance of clinically stage I patients (2104 of 2800 patients). The two treatment groups were comparable with regard to major prognostic and pathological factors.[8,9] The protocol suggested that a dosage in the range 1320–1510 rets was used to deliver treatment to the chest wall, axilla and supraclavicular and internal mammary areas by either ortho- or super-voltage, as available at the local centre.

During a prolonged follow-up period, there was no difference in survival between the two groups, with a relative risk (RR) of 1.01 (95% CI 0.92–1.11). There was a slight increase in the risk of death beyond 5 years, but it was non-significant, and the difference appears to diminish after 10 years, although this may be due to lack of power. There were 1978 patients still alive at 5 years (watch policy = 995; DXT = 983), but this number decreased to 1011 at 15 years (watch policy = 517; DXT = 494). More detailed analysis of the cause-specific mortality demonstrates that an increased risk to the irradiated patients of dying of causes other than breast cancer was present (RR = 1.49, 95% CI 1.18–1.89).

Patients with primary cancer in the left breast who were irradiated had an increased mortality risk after 5 years. A test for interaction between tumours of the left and right breasts was just significant ($P=0.04$). As the excess of deaths among patients with left-sided disease could be due to irradiation of the heart or major vessels, we examined cause-specific mortality in more detail in the two treatment groups. The excess mortality among the irradiated patients is still apparent when deaths due to cardiac disease alone are considered, and the interaction between left- and right-sided tumours is significant ($P=0.02$). Because irradiation of the cardiac region appears to influence survival, we also looked at the type of radiation given. Trial patients were treated with whatever equipment was available locally. This practice resulted in some patients having supervoltage only, some having orthovoltage only, and others receiving both.

Stratified analyses were performed of patients who were treated at centres where supervoltage only was used compared to those treated at centres where orthovoltage was used either alone or in combination with supervoltage. Orthovoltage, which has greater lateral scatter and delivers a higher radiation dose to the heart, would therefore be expected to increase the risk of cardiac death. Analyses comparing quality of radiation and side of the primary tumour in the various cause-specific categories showed that, overall, patients who received supervoltage only ($n = 264$) did not appear to be at reduced risk of late cardiac mortality compared to those who received some orthovoltage ($n = 719$; RR = 0.88, 95% CI 0.49–1.57; $P = 0.66$). These findings must be viewed with some caution because the comparisons are non-randomized subsets.

There is now little doubt that the radiotherapy techniques used during trials of simple or radical mastectomy with and without radical radiotherapy have increased the risk of irradiated patients dying from a late excess of cardiac disease. This fact has been demonstrated in other individual trials,[20–22] by a review of registry data[23] and in the overview of trials.[3] The significance of these results for modern management of early breast cancer is unclear. Overall, there is a 7% reduction in breast cancer deaths in the CRC trial for patients who received radiotherapy, though it fails to reach the level of statistical significance.

Nevertheless, the latest overview does suggest that it may be a real finding, particularly in the more recent trials, which employed simple mastectomy.

However, a comparison of reconstructed orthovoltage dosage given to irradiated patients in the CRC trial with modern radiotherapy techniques following breast conservation[24] demonstrates that, although the dose to the myocardium is reduced by modern techniques, the left anterior descending artery still receives a high dose of radiation. The clinical relevance of this observation is not yet clear, but should highlight the need for caution in the use of prophylactic therapy for those at low risk of local relapse. Fortunately, the patients at increased risk of cardiac disease following irradiation are those who are long-term survivors of breast cancer, and are therefore the very individuals who are least likely to require irradiation for control of local disease.

FROM A PATIENT'S PERSPECTIVE, WHAT ARE THE RISKS AND BENEFITS OF TREATMENTS?

For patients, the decision as to whether to opt for immediate radiotherapy or take a chance and delay treatment until and if a recurrence develops is a difficult one. We know that the pathological factors which influence the development of local relapse are the size of the tumour, its histological grade and the nodal status. Patients in the highest risk groups for these prognostic factors should certainly be considered for prophylactic radiotherapy, particularly as they are less likely to live long enough for the late toxic side-effects to become manifest. For other patients, the risk–benefit equation is still unclear. About 50% of the patients who develop local recurrence in the chest wall or axilla will die with disease present at the same site. Prophylactic irradiation reduces by about 50% the number of patients who suffer this distressing sequela, but the actual numbers are relatively small because only about 10% of patients (143 of 1424 subjects) in the trial developed persistent disease following mastectomy in the absence of radiotherapy.

The costs involved in treating all patients undergoing conservation therapy for early breast cancer, particularly those with small tumours found on screening mammography, place enormous burdens on health resources. It is therefore essential to refine the role of radiotherapy in such patients. Trials for good-prognosis patients are now being reported, and the need for large numbers of patients is obvious. We therefore await with interest the results of the latest overview and the findings from individual large trials.

REFERENCES

1 Harris JR. Postmastectomy radiotherapy. In: Harris JR, Hellman S, Henderson IC, Kinne DW (Eds) *Breast diseases 1987*. Philadelphia, PA: JB Lippincott.

2 Cuzick J, Stewart H, Peto R *et al*. Overview of randomized trials of post-operative adjuvant radiotherapy in breast cancer. *Cancer Treat Rep* 1987; **71**: 15.

3 Cuzick J, Stewart H, Rutqvlst L *et al*. Cause-specific mortality in long-term survivors of breast cancer who participated in trials of radiotherapy. *J Clin Oncol* 1994; **12**: 447–53.

4 Early Breast Cancer Trialists' Collaborative Group. Effects of radiotherapy and surgery in early breast cancer. *N Engl J Med* 1995; **333**: 1444–55.

5 Early Breast Cancer Trialists' Collaborative Group. Favourable and unfavourable effects on long-term survival of radiotherapy for early breast cancer: an overview of randomised clinical trials. *Lancet* 2000; **355**; 1737–70.

6 Fisher B, Anderson S, Redmond CK, Wolmark N, Cronin WM. Re-analysis and results after 12 years of follow-up in a randomised clinical trial comparing total mastectomy with or without irradiation in the treatment of breast cancer. *N Engl J Med* 1995; **333**: 1456–61.

7 Veronesi U, Banfi A, Del Vecchio M *et al*. Comparison of Halsted mastectomy with quadrantectomy, axillary dissection and radiotherapy in early breast cancer: long-term results. *Eur J Cancer Clin Oncol* 1996; **22**: 1085–9.

8 Elston CW, Gresham GA, Rao GS *et al*. The Cancer Research Campaign (King's/Cambridge) trial for early breast cancer: clinico-pathological aspects. *Br J Cancer* 1982; **45**: 655.

9 Cancer Research Campaign Working Party. Cancer Research Campaign (King's/Cambridge) Trial for Early Breast Cancer. *Lancet* 1980; **2**: 55.

10 Fisher B, Anderson S, Fisher ER *et al*. Significance of ipsilateral breast tumour recurrence after lumpectomy. *Lancet* 1991; **338**: 327–31.

11 Early Breast Cancer Trialists' Collaborative Group. *Treatment of early breast cancer: worldwide evidence 1985–1990. Vol. 1*. Oxford: Oxford University Press, 1990.

12 Overgaard M, Hansen PS, Overgaard J *et al*. Post-operative radiotherapy in high-risk premenopausal women with breast cancer who receive adjuvant chemotherapy. *N Engl J Med* 1997; **15**: 3192–200.

13 Overgaard M, Jensen MB, Overgaard J *et al*. Post-operative radiotherapy in high-risk post-menopausal breast cancer patients given adjuvant tamoxifen: Danish Breast Cancer Cooperative Group DBCG 82c randomised trial. *Lancet* 1999; **353**: 1641–8.

14 Ragaz J, Jackson SM, Le N *et al*. Adjuvant radiotherapy and chemotherapy in node-positive premenopausal women with breast cancer. *N Engl J Med* 1997; **337**: 956–62.

15 Stjernsward J. Decreased survival related to irradiation post-operatively in early operable breast cancer. *Lancet* 1974; **2**: 1285–6.

16 Haybittle JL, Brinkley D, Houghton J, A'Hem RPA, Baum M. Postoperative radiotherapy and late mortality: evidence from the Cancer Research Campaign trial for early breast cancer. *BMJ* 1989; **298**: 1611.

17 CRC Breast Cancer Trials Group. *Breast trial protocol*. 1970.

18 Crile G Jr. The effect on metastasis of removing or irradiating regional nodes of mice. *Surg Gynecol Obstet* 1968; **126**: 1270.

19 Fisher B, Fisher ER. Studies concerning the regional lymph nodes in cancer. 1. Initiation of immunity. *Cancer* 1971; **27**: 1001.

20 Jones JM, Riberio GG. Mortality patterns over 34 years of breast cancer patients in a clinical trial of postoperative radiotherapy. *Clin Radiol* 1989; **40**: 204.

21 Host H, Brennhovd MD, Loeb M. Postoperative radiotherapy in breast cancer – long-term results from the Oslo study. *Int J Radiat Oncol Biol Phys* 1986; **12**: 727.

22 Rutqvist LE, Lax I, Fornander T, Johansson H. Cardiovascular mortality in a randomised trial of adjuvant radiation therapy versus surgery alone in primary breast cancer. *J Radiat Oncol Biol Phys* 1992; **22**: 887.

23 Rutqvist LE, Johansson H. Mortality by laterality of the primary tumour among 55 000 breast cancer patients from the Swedish Cancer Registry. *Br J Cancer* 1990; **61**; 866.

24 Fuller SA, Haybittle JL, Smith REA, Dobbs HJ. Cardiac doses in postoperative breast irradiation. *Radiother Oncol* 1992; **25**: 19.

FURTHER READING

Kurtz JM. Radiotherapy for early breast cancer: was a comprehensive overview of trials needed? *Lancet* 2000; 1739–40.

Whelan TJ, Julian J, Wright J *et al*. Does locoregional radiation therapy improve survival in breast cancer? A meta-analysis. *J Clin Oncol* 2000; **18**; 1220–9.

17

'Moving the goalposts' – a review of clinical trial strategies in early breast cancer

JEFFREY S TOBIAS, JOAN HOUGHTON AND DIANNE L RILEY

INTRODUCTION

The last two decades have seen important changes, both local and systemic, in the treatment of early breast cancer. This progress has been largely attributable to the careful testing of newer therapies in large randomized trials, which have not only allowed significance testing of the benefits but also, with the development of meta-analysis, provided reliable estimates of the size of the benefits. The Cancer Research Campaign (UK) Breast Cancer Trials Group has been a major contributor in this area of research, and the purpose of this paper is to review some of the studies and achievements of the group, and to set these within the context of our understanding of the biology and treatment of this disorder.

Twenty years ago, most patients with 'early' (stage I and stage II) cancer were treated by mastectomy, with post-operative radiotherapy offered for node-positive cases. Little else was possible, although a few rebellious spirits claimed that local excision with post-operative radiotherapy and preservation of the breast was as effective.[1] This form of treatment has now become commonplace.

Remarkable as this rejection of a long-held surgical cornerstone has been, the rapid introduction of systemic agents (hormone therapy and chemotherapy) for breast cancer has been even more dramatic and, unlike the welcome change in local treatment of the primary, has resulted in statistically significant and worthwhile survival benefits.[2] Simple and safe treatment with tamoxifen or combination chemotherapy has become rapidly accepted not only because we now regard breast cancer as essentially a systemic illness in virtually all patients,[3] but also because the scientific medical community has for the most part been convinced by the strength of the data now available, and also by the pressure which our increasingly well-informed patients are applying.

THE CONTRIBUTION OF RANDOMIZED CLINICAL TRIALS TO BREAST CANCER RESEARCH

For the Breast Cancer Trials Group of the Cancer Research Campaign (CRC), the design and implementation of large-scale studies – simple in objective and permissive and pragmatic in approach – was an early goal[4] (see Table 17.1). Our philosophy has always been to make studies as appealing as possible, recognizing that surgeons, radiation and medical oncologists in the UK see large numbers of patients and have no time to spare for unnecessarily detailed documentation. Our studies have been carefully researched prior to launch, usually by means of a questionnaire, to assess whether participating colleagues regarded a particular question as being of sufficient importance to warrant a prospective study and to justify the expense, energy and time involved. In the 1970s, the most important question was to establish whether or not tamoxifen, with its proven efficacy in advanced disease and an excellent record of tolerance and safety, should be recommended as standard treatment for all patients with 'early' post-menopausal breast cancer. The studies (see Table 17.2) performed by the CRC and

Table 17.1 *Chronological representation of the trials undertaken by the CRC Breast Cancer Trials Group*

				Under-Fifties Trial	Mx or LE ± XRT Tamoxifen and Zoladex 920 in 2×2 design
				Over-Fifties Trial	Mx or LE ±XRT 3220 Tamoxifen 2 vs. 5 years
			CRC Adjuvant Trial	Mx or LE ±XRT Tamoxifen and cyclophosphamide 2230 in 2×2 design	
		NATO	Mx ± XRT 1131 Tamoxifen vs. none		
	King's Adjuvant Trial	Mx ± XRT 535 Chemotherapy (MM)			
CRC (King's/ Cambridge) Trial	Mx 2800 Watch policy vs. XRT				
1970	1975	1980	1985	1990	1995

Key	Indicates period of accrual	Primary therapy Randomized therapy	Number of patients randomized		Period of follow-up

the Nolvadex Adjuvant Trial Organisation (NATO) group provided data from thousands of patients which substantially predicted the results obtained from the large world-wide overview published in 1992.[2] Furthermore, data from the CRC studies were among the earliest to suggest that the benefits might apply not only to post-menopausal patients, but also to the important group of younger women, who represent approximately 25% of all breast cancer patients, and furthermore, to a proportion of those of all ages with oestrogen-receptor-negative disease.

An important principle that we learned was to conduct the study before assuming the answer – in the case of tamoxifen, for example, to use a relatively safe and inexpensive compound which might have effects mediated via its hormonal characteristics in all patients whether oestrogen-receptor positive or negative, without assuming that, because of theoretical objections, it was unlikely to be effective in the oestrogen-receptor-negative group. Equally, for premenopausal patients, one of the consequences of our early tamoxifen studies has been the development of trials addressing its possible role in

adjuvant therapy based on what might best be described as 'straws in the wind' from the earlier CRC data in relatively small numbers of younger patients.

The development of a multicentre group (see Figure 17.1) such as the CRC Breast Cancer Trials Group requires commitment and enthusiasm. We have often wondered what participants might gain from their involvement, given the extra work and documentation required, coupled with the complete lack of personal or financial reward. Apart from the natural desire to become involved in important research, many participants feel that the *esprit de corps*, the access to recent and unpublished group data, and the stimulation of Working Party and Group meetings is adequate reward, although all trial organizers realize that these benefits are often fragile in the face of a mounting workload, and should not be taken for granted.

Some important studies that were judged to be of high priority at the time, have proved in practice to be less appealing than had been anticipated, or too complicated, impractical or ethically contentious to complete. One example was our failed attempt to perform a randomized

Table 17.2 *Brief description of the CRC Breast Cancer Trials Group protocols*

Trial	Randomized arms	Primary treatment	Eligible patients	Number of patients	Result summary
NATO	No adjuvant therapy Tamoxifen 10 mg bd for 2 years	Mastectomy ± RT	Premenopausal node-positive Post-menopausal node-positive or negative	1131	Significantly increased time to relapse and increased survival
CRC Adjuvant Trial	2×2 design No adjuvant therapy Tamoxifen 20 mg daily for 2 years Cyclophosphamide (peri-operatively) Tamoxifen and cyclophosphamide	Mastectomy ± RT Local excision + RT	All patients with operable, non-metastatic breast cancer	2230	As for the NATO trial
Over-Fifties Trial	Tamoxifen for 2 years Tamoxifen for 5 years	Mastectomy ± RT Local excision + RT Elective chemotherapy may be given	All patients over the age of 50 but under 75 years with operable, non-metastatic breast cancer	3220	5 yr significantly better than 2 yr in relapse-free survival
Under-Fifties Trial	2×2 design No adjuvant hormone therapy Tamoxifen for 2 years Zoladex for 2 years Tamoxifen and Zoladex	Mastectomy ± RT Local excision + RT Elective chemotherapy may be given	All patients under the age of 50 years with operable, non-metastatic breast cancer	920	Zoladex adds significant advantage in relapse-free survival

RT, radiotherapy.

Group structure

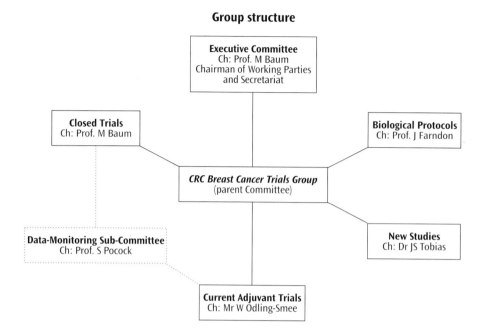

Figure 17.1 *The committee structure of the Cancer Research Campaign Breast Cancer Trials Group.*

comparison of local excision (in patients with operable, 'early' breast cancer) vs. mastectomy,[5] despite (or perhaps in part because of) the success of the Milan[6] and National Surgical Adjuvant Breast and Bowel Project (NSABP)[7] studies addressing similar questions. At the time this was widely described as 'the study everybody needs but nobody wants,'[8] and so it proved. Our study closed after 18 months, during which time only 145 patients were recruited – nowhere near the number required to give a reliable answer.

Although there was a useful fall-out in our understanding of the psychology of breast cancer and its treatment,[9] the more important lesson we learned was that informed consent, now regarded as an essential prerequisite in any prospectively randomized study, and especially so in this trial,[10] could greatly inhibit clinicians, as many found the necessary discussions of the treatment options too arduous or upsetting, both for themselves and for their patients.[11] Increasingly, CRC Working Parties have focused on the issue of informed consent as it relates to clinical trial participation, since it has become such a barrier.[12,13] Our system, which required the approval of all research studies by local ethics committees, bent over backwards to preserve the fundamental rights and autonomy of individual patients, but in doing so delays were inevitable, and the ethical absurdity of an identical study being judged acceptable in one health district but unacceptable in a geographically adjacent one was a constant reality. The recent introduction of multicentre research ethics committees should ease this process, but we are too low down on the learning curve to comment further at present. To those of us who recognize that advances in cancer management come far more often from unsteady infantile steps than from giant strides, these obstacles to patient participation have become extremely frustrating.

Recent studies closely reflect these constraints. In the majority of patients with 'early' breast cancer (i.e. the post-menopausal group), our own studies,[14,15] and also those from colleagues in the Scottish Breast Cancer Group,[16] showed clearly that cohorts of patients given either 2 years of adjuvant tamoxifen treatment (CRC) or 5 years of such treatment (Scottish study) survived longer than controls who received no tamoxifen or delayed tamoxifen, yet the important issue of optimization of treatment duration had not been resolved. What could be more dull than a 2-year vs. 5-year tamoxifen study? Yet this important question is one which the CRC Breast Cancer Trials Group viewed as being of high enough priority in 1985 for them to launch a major large-scale prospectively randomized trial, even though many individual non-trialist surgeons throughout Europe and the USA had already decided, without any supportive data, that if tamoxifen for 2 years was good, then it followed that it must be better still if given for ever. This feeling, too, coloured the view of patients in the study, as more have refused randomization at the 2-year point out of fear of discontinuation than for any other reason (see Figure 17.2). This example illustrates well the relatively small window of time during which a study can be performed, as more and more patients, impressed by media coverage and friendly advice relating to the benefits of tamoxifen, wish to continue with it and refuse randomization. However, later in the study the pendulum swung again, as fear about the real but small risk of tamoxifen-induced endometrial cancer once more put this question firmly centre stage.

In younger women, in whom adjuvant chemotherapy is clearly of overall survival benefit, the most important issues for major study groups probably relate to the characterization of patient subgroups which would be likely to benefit – a more important issue than with tamoxifen,

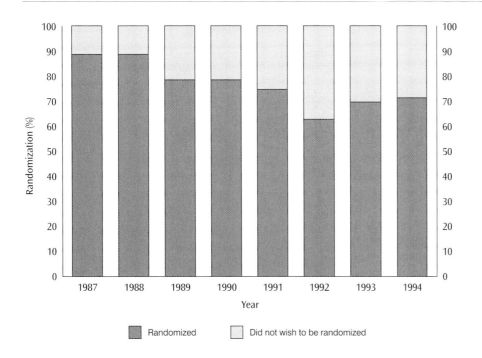

Figure 17.2 *Patients registered into the trial of tamoxifen (over-fifties trial) at the time of diagnosis but who subsequently refused the offer of randomization after having been on therapy for 2 years.*

as chemotherapy is more unpleasant, intensive of professional labour, and hazardous. Based on the present data, probably less than 50% of patients who receive such therapy are likely to benefit significantly from it (about 25% of the patients will not recur and have been cured by their initial surgery, whilst the other 25% will die of their disease even though they have been receiving adjuvant therapy). An alternative hypothesis is that all patients who are treated with chemotherapy may derive some advantage from it, including those whose lives cannot be saved but who at least can be given a degree of extension of life as a result of the adjuvant treatment. Although the first generation of adjuvant chemotherapy studies were mostly based on year-long treatment (12 courses), 6 months of chemotherapy appears to be as good, raising the question that the duration of such treatment might perhaps be safely reduced still further (e.g. to a total of only 3 months). Yet the CRC Breast Cancer Trials Group chose essentially to address a different 'unknown', namely the potential value of intensification of adjuvant hormone therapy by offering either tamoxifen or goserelin (or both, or neither, in a 2×2 factorial study design) (see Figure 17.3). This study was designed in 1987, following the first analysis of the World Overview which suggested that, in premenopausal women, hormone manipulation by ovarian ablation may be extremely powerful, and possibly even as valuable as chemotherapy,[2] although with less morbidity and lower cost. The choice of goserelin was itself determined by changing social patterns as much as by the availability of this and allied agents, which for the first time have offered a reversible form of ovarian suppression. Significant numbers of premenopausal breast cancer patients now wish both to have 'adequate' systemic treatment and to preserve their fertility. Even here, within the short space of 5 years, the goalposts have

moved rapidly enough to require a response from the study group, since the publication of the World Overview in 1992 persuaded many participants that the 'control' arm was no longer tenable, so the study has in effect now become a simpler two-arm randomization either to tamoxifen alone or to tamoxifen plus goserelin (Zoladex). This represents a welcome return to simplicity, as many participants found the lengthy discussion of four possible treatment options too confusing for the patients to grasp and accept with proper understanding. Once again we have been reminded that simplicity is a key element of success in large-scale multicentre studies.

A new and successful initiative is a joint collaboration with the pharmaceutical industry in an adjuvant trial of anastrazole, one of the new generation of aromatase inhibitors, in post-menopausal women, the so-called ATAC study. In determining the design of the trial we consulted a number of ethics committees for their opinion. Initially we thought that it would not be possible to run a trial in this group in which tamoxifen, now accepted as 'standard treatment', was deliberately not administered within one of the study groups. The design would therefore have to compare the new drug in combination with tamoxifen against tamoxifen alone. However, the view of the ethics committees was that, provided there was evidence of activity for anastrazole similar to that for tamoxifen, it was acceptable to invite patients to join with their informed consent. Similar advice was given by the Consumers Advisory Group for Clinical Trials, consisting mainly of lay women with experience of breast cancer who are willing to review trial protocols and comment on their likely acceptability to future patients. We were therefore able to design a three-arm trial to test for equivalence between the two single agents or for superiority of the combination. Another new feature for our collaborative

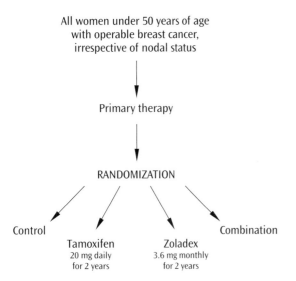

All women under 50 years of age
with operable breast cancer,
irrespective of nodal status

↓

Primary therapy

↓

RANDOMIZATION

Control

Tamoxifen
20 mg daily
for 2 years

Zoladex
3.6 mg monthly
for 2 years

Combination

Randomization options

Option A
• Control
• Tamoxifen
• Zoladex
• Tamoxifen and Zoladex

Option B
• Tamoxifen
• Tamoxifen and Zoladex

Option C
• Control
• Zoladex

Figure 17.3 *Design of the under-fifties trial showing the randomized options available to participating clinicians.*

group was the use of double-dummy placebos to ensure that both doctors and patients were blind to the treatment being given. This delivers another benefit in terms of trial methodology – if a patient suffers recurrence whilst on treatment, which lasts for 5 years, in order to have the trial treatment unblinded, the trial office has to be contacted. This allows rapid and accurate recording of the primary end-point for the trial.

The collaboration between industry and academic collaborative groups has been a learning process for all involved. To meld the requirements for registration for the industry and to run a pragmatic simple trial as has been our past practice has been extremely challenging. Being able to use an exciting new drug in the adjuvant situation soon after benefit was demonstrated in advanced disease was attractive to breast cancer doctors and patients alike. The advantages for rapid evaluation by a single large trial (over 9000 patients are included in the internationally-collaborative ATAC study, and recruitment has now been completed) provides the possibility of early outcome data and a single toxicity database. Less attractive to our collaborating clinicians has been learning to run a trial to the requirements of Good Clinical (Research) Practice (GCP). The additional paperwork and the detail which has to be recorded are irksome, but are to some extent offset by being provided with the finance to resource the work, and by the regular visits of trial monitors – who soon let you know if your record-keeping is not up to scratch! All in all this has been a rewarding experience, and we eagerly await the first release of data.

LESSONS FOR THE FUTURE

Quite apart from the specific knowledge we have gained in studying over 10 000 patients with 'early' breast cancer over a 15-year period (see Figure 17.4), we have learned

enough about clinical trial methodology to try to apply certain rules to every clinical study.

1 The trial design must be flexible and sufficiently pragmatic to accommodate real variations in the clinical approaches of the many participants. Doctors are by nature individualists – even those who are prepared to submit to the discipline of clinical trials.

2 It is important to recognize the nature of the disease itself, and if it has a lengthy natural history and an inevitable protracted period of recruitment (in order to achieve large numbers) we may well be overtaken by new understanding or discoveries from other groups, and must then react accordingly. The resolve should always be towards simplification of a study (see above), rather than towards adding complexity.

3 As generations of trials develop, so does the complexity of the questions being addressed, which in turn results in increasing difficulties in achieving the initial aims. This might be, for example, because patient groups have to be subdivided and therefore become smaller; or because clinicians find it increasingly difficult to discuss the large number of options with their patients; or because patients themselves become confused by the uncertainty and, wishing for more direction from their medical adviser, feel unable to submit to the apparently brutal and insensitive randomized decision-making process. In designing third- or fourth-generation trials, all the basic issues should be reconsidered in depth, and may need to be readdressed. For example, do we really need to subgroup the population for this trial? Is this practicable within our collaborators' preferred approaches for management of this disease? And the list goes on.

4 All good studies lead to further questions – indeed, the paradox of increased complexity is a common phenomenon after completion of a large-scale study. Large groups such as ours frequently have to choose

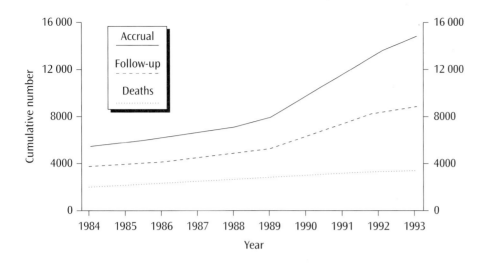

Figure 17.4 *Cumulative numbers of patients entered, number of deaths and number of patients under follow-up by the CRC Breast Cancer Trials Group.*

between several further questions which need to be addressed, making prioritization between competing questions an increasingly common (and important) part of our work.

THE ROLE OF LARGE COLLABORATIVE GROUPS WITHIN THE CONTEXT OF META-ANALYSIS

Over the past 5 years the most important new departure in medical trial technology has been the rapid acceptance of meta-analysis as a highly effective means of increasing the power of similar studies. Although independently designed and performed, often in distant parts of the globe, these trials have essentially asked the same question and can therefore be analysed together with respect to the main question(s) addressed by the randomization. As pointed out in a *New England Journal of Medicine* editorial:

> among the methods that can be used to compare new treatments with existing ones, the gold standard is the randomised controlled trial.... Meta-analyses are studies of studies; they are attempts to synthesise the results of many trials. In the 10 or so years since meta-analysis began to have an impact on the medical literature, dramatic progress has been made in the use of this technique.[17]

Within the context of breast cancer, the highly influential meta-analysis report on systemic treatments for early breast cancer[2] rests largely, of course, on the large numbers accrued by well-organized multicentre groups such as the CRC Breast Cancer Trials Group within the UK. As recently pointed out by Lau *et al.*,[18] the use of accumulative meta-analysis of therapeutic trials may, through sequential addition of new results of studies as they are published, provide additional useful information on a novel therapeutic question well before the completion and publication of a Worldwide Overview, thus greatly reducing the time required for the results to achieve general attention and impact within wider medical circles. For instance, Lau *et al.* point to the 33 trials of thrombolytic therapy for acute myocardial infarction (1959–1988), stressing that the important positive conclusion was achieved after only 8 trials had been completed (in 1973). The 25 subsequent trials, involving an additional 34 500 patients, had little or no effect on the overall findings, although they clearly added statistical power. In these circumstances, a tightly knit and committed study group such as ours may assume greater responsibility, as we have been able to provide relatively early data on the important issues of the day, by designing studies quickly and efficiently and implementing them without unnecessary delay. The lesser bureaucratic requirements of many UK-based study groups, compared to their counterparts in the USA, should also allow us a continued prominent role in the future.

Although techniques of meta-analysis have become rapidly accepted as a highly efficient means of providing powerful statistical evidence to support or refute a novel treatment policy, the success of meta-analysis depends, of course, on the commitment of contributing groups, and the proper design and implementation of the studies that they carry out. Recent overviews in breast cancer have been successful because many large groups, including our own, decided at much the same time that the important questions to be asked were similar. This permitted the rapid analysis and publication of a relatively straightforward (and, as it turned out, highly influential) overview, since so many of the studies were strikingly similar in both intent and design. The success of and publicity about meta-analysis techniques has further stimulated interest in clinical trials, even though single studies are inevitably numerically small, compared to the numbers of patients contributing to the overview. Physicians and surgeons who are disinclined to enter their patients into randomized studies can no longer state, as they often did in the past, that 'no one ever learned anything from a randomized trial', as important results were held to be self-evident. By contrast, in our view one of the most important effects of meta-analysis for single and multi-centre study groups has been the *highlighting of the individual clinician's contribution*. This improves the overall sense of achievement when an important discovery, such as the quantitative assessment of benefit for tamoxifen or combination chemotherapy, has been made as a result of (often international) collaboration.

Increasingly, emphasis has been placed on the methods by which patients can more easily be entered into randomized clinical trials, together with a reassessment of the ethics of clinicians who choose *not* to enter their patients into such studies. In view of the pressures which are often brought to bear upon those who wish to participate in clinical studies, it seems to us entirely appropriate to question the ethics of those who are *unwilling* to contribute, even though so many important questions have yet to be answered. The proportion of patients who are entered into such studies remains discouragingly low, the CRC Breast Cancer Trials Group still only managing to recruit about 7% of the available patient population, despite its ethos for simple studies and extremely practical questions with major clinical implications.

CONCLUSION

In conclusion, the many questions addressed by a major multicentre breast cancer study group alter as the results of previous studies become available. We have seen this over the last 25 years or so with the rapid emergence of both tamoxifen and combination chemotherapy as valuable additions to treatment, and the subsequent and essential refinement of treatments that then become necessary. At the same time, studies have inevitably become more complex. For example, with regard to the important question of adjuvant hormone therapy in premenopausal patients, there are many (mainly the node-positive and younger group) in whom adjuvant chemotherapy must also be given in order to satisfy the requirements of 'best possible care'. Provided that individual treatment centres establish their choices for additional treatment of this kind, this need not become a barrier to continuing with the initial randomized study (in this case of adjuvant hormone therapy). Since the statistical power of a large study is adequate provided that no systematic bias enters – as would be the case if the investigator was also free to choose at will which patients should have chemotherapy – the goalposts will have moved, even during a single study, because of a single important publication which could not possibly be ignored.

Study groups have to maintain the commitment and enthusiasm of their participants, satisfy local and central ethics committees, devise scientific studies of real interest, promote rapid recruitment and achieve success in the difficult area of competitive assessment for trial funding. In our view, these tasks are more likely to be achieved by collaboration within a group with a proven track record, the ability to recruit large numbers of patients into a study, and a continuing interest in addressing the important questions that have already started to reduce the death rate from this all too common and fatal disorder.

REFERENCES

1 Pierquin B, Owen R, Maylin C *et al*. Radical radiation therapy of breast cancer. *Int J Radiat Oncol Biol Phys* 1980; **6**: 17–24.

2 Early Breast Cancer Trialists' Collaborative Group. Systemic treatment of early breast cancer by hormonal, cytotoxic, or immune therapy: 133 randomised trials involving 31 000 recurrences and 24 000 deaths among 75 000 women. *Lancet* 1992; **339**: 1–15, 71–85.

3 Fisher B. The evolution of paradigms for the management of breast cancer: a personal perspective. *Cancer Res* 1992; **52**: 2371–83.

4 Cancer Research Campaign Working Party. Trials and tribulations: thoughts on the organisation of multicentre clinical studies. *BMJ* 1980; **280**: 918–20.

5 Riley D, Baum M, Houghton J. Current management questionnaires and protocol design. *Eur Surg Res* 1984; **16**: 88.

6 Veronesi U, Banfi A, Salvadori B *et al*. Breast conservation is the treatment of choice in small breast cancer: long-term results of a randomized trial. *Eur J Cancer* 1990; **26**: 668–70.

7 Fisher B, Redmond C *et al*. for the National Surgical Adjuvant Breast and Bowel Project. Lumpectomy for breast cancer: an update of the NSABP experience. *J Natl Cancer Inst Monogr* 1992; **11**: 7–13.

8 Lefanu J. The breast cancer trial that nobody wants but everybody needs. *Med News* 1983.

9 Fallowfield LJ, Baum M, Maguire GP. Effects of breast conservation on psychological morbidity associated with diagnosis and treatment of early breast cancer. *BMJ* 1986; **293**: 1331–4.

10 Cancer Research Campaign Working Party on Breast Conservation. Informed consent: ethical, legal and medical implications for doctors and patients who participate in randomized clinical trials. *BMJ* 1983; **286**: 1117–21.

11 Tobias JS, Souhami RL. Fully informed consent can be needlessly cruel. *BMJ* 1993; **307**: 1199–201.

12 Baum M, Zilkha K, Houghton J. Ethics of clinical research: lessons for the future. *BMJ* 1989; **299**: 251–3.

13 Tobias JS, Houghton J. Is informed consent essential for all chemotherapy studies? *Eur J Cancer* 1994; **30A**: 897–9.

14 Baum M, Houghton J, Riley D on behalf of the Cancer Research Campaign Breast Cancer Trials Group. Results of the Cancer Research Campaign Adjuvant Trial for perioperative cyclophosphamide and long-term tamoxifen in early breast cancer reported at the tenth year of follow-up. *Acta Oncol* 1992; **31**: 251–7.

15 Houghton J, Riley D, Baumm. The Nolvadex Adjuvant Trial Organisation (NATO) and the Cancer Research Campaign (CRC) trials of adjuvant tamoxifen therapy on behalf of the CRC Breast Cancer Trials Group. In: Jordan VC (ed.) *Long-term tamoxifen treatment for breast cancer*. WI: University of Wisconsin Press, 1994: 93–112.

16 Scottish Cancer Trials Office. Adjuvant tamoxifen in the management of operable breast cancer: the Scottish trial. *Lancet* 1987; **ii**: 171–5.

17 Kassirer JP. Clinical trials and meta-analysis. *N Engl J Med* 1992; **327**: 273–4.

18 Lau J, Antman EM, Jimenez-Silva J *et al.* Cumulative meta-analysis of therapeutic trials for myocardial infarction. *N Engl J Med* 1992; **327**: 248–54.

18

Chemotherapy for post-menopausal patients with primary breast cancer

PETER M RAVDIN AND CK OSBORNE

INTRODUCTION

A discussion of chemotherapy for post-menopausal women with breast cancer involves an overview of what has been achieved by clinical research, what the current standards seem to be, and finally what new directions are being pursued. These areas can be most succinctly reviewed by firstly a discussion of the results of the Early Breast Cancer Trialists' Collaborative Group (EBCTCG) meta-analysis of randomized adjuvant chemotherapy and endocrine therapy clinical trials (see Table 18.1),[1–3] secondly a discussion of various 'standard of care' recommendations from different sources (see Table 18.3), and thirdly a discussion of the currently pursued clinical research questions as reflected in ongoing trials (see Table 18.4).

WHY DISCUSS CHEMOTHERAPY OF PREMENOPAUSAL AND POST-MENOPAUSAL WOMEN SEPARATELY?

There are three issues that may result in somewhat different treatment strategies being selected in premenopausal women and post-menopausal women. First, the options and relative efficacies of endocrine therapies may differ in the two groups. Secondly, the average biological characteristics of the disease itself may differ in the two groups. Thirdly, the ability of women in the two groups to tolerate the toxicity and to derive benefit from given therapies may differ.

Differences in hormonal therapy options

Breast cancer is the only major malignancy in which it has been useful to dichotomize patients by menopausal status. Menopausal status rather than simply age is a useful parameter when discussing breast cancer because the underlying hormonal milieu of the patient has a direct impact on the treatment options that are appropriate. Ovarian ablative therapies are only of value in premenopausal patients, while tamoxifen and aromatase inhibitors are perhaps more effective in post-menopausal patients. Thus the relative effectiveness of the appropriate endocrine therapy vs. chemotherapy may well differ. A general statement about adjuvant therapy, reinforced by the Early Breast Cancer Trialists' Collaborative Group (EBCTCG)[4] meta-analysis (but certainly a broad simplification), is that adjuvant chemotherapy is superior to adjuvant endocrine therapy for premenopausal patients, while the reverse is true for post-menopausal patients. However, the latest meta-analysis of trials of tamoxifen does not use age as a major stratification variable, since with the larger number of patients and the longer duration of treatment it is clear that tamoxifen has a substantial benefit with regard to recurrence and survival not only in older women but also in those under the age of 50 years. The age-related trend for benefit from chemotherapy clearly remains.

Basic biological differences?

Is there evidence that breast cancer is biologically different in pre- and post-menopausal women? Most studies have shown that post-menopausal women have, on average, biologically less aggressive tumours than those of younger women. Comparisons of histological features,[5] steroid-hormone receptors, and proliferative rates based on S-phase measurements[6] are all consistent with this conclusion. The differences are most apparent when the comparisons are made with younger samples of premenopausal women.

Age and menopausal status are not themselves strong *independent* predictors of outcome. When age and menopausal status are included in multivariate analyses with other prognostic variables as predictors of disease-free survival or overall survival, they are not usually independently predictive, or they have only a minor impact on outcome. Population registry-based studies which appear to suggest that older post-menopausal patients have poorer outcomes than younger patients are flawed by a lack of documentation that the older patients received equally definitive primary or subsequent therapy.[7,8] Our current theoretical understanding of the basic biology of tumours of pre- and post-menopausal women would not dictate any major differences in therapy between the two groups, except for considering oestrogen-receptor and progesterone-receptor status. Based on a higher frequency of oestrogen-receptor and progesterone-receptor positivity in post-menopausal women compared to premenopausal women, one would predict a greater efficacy of hormonal therapy in post-menopausal women on average.

Differences in toxicity and risk/benefit ratios in post-menopausal women

The question of whether chemotherapy is as well tolerated and can be given at the same dose intensities in pre- and post-menopausal women has been examined, as the pharmacology of some drugs is affected by age,[9] and older patients may be more susceptible to haematological toxicity.[10] An analysis of outcomes of patients by age in the Eastern Cooperative Oncology Group studies found that, for patients with metastatic breast cancer, there was a trend with increasing age towards increased haematological toxicity, but this did not reach the level of statistical significance. This conclusion was based on a comparison of toxicity in women under 60 years of age with women aged 60–65 years.[11] Another study of toxicity of chemotherapy regimens for metastatic breast cancer, which included a substantial number of patients aged ≥ 70 years, also showed no significant differences in the ability of older and younger women to tolerate chemotherapy overall, but

did report more myelosuppression in older patients.[12] The overall conclusion of these studies has been that the increase with age in risk of toxicity due to chemotherapy is modest. Therefore, at the present time American national co-operative breast cancer protocols do not exclude women because of advanced age, except in the case of some protocols involving intensive therapy that requires stem-cell support. In general, attenuation of doses or denial of the option of adjuvant therapy solely on the basis of age may not be appropriate.

However, one cannot totally deny the importance of age, because as women grow older the frequency of existing comorbidities and the risk of developing new ones increases. Thus the average number of remaining expected years of life decreases, and the gain after successful therapy is less for older women than for younger women. Markov analyses of this problem show that the absolute benefit for women receiving adjuvant chemotherapy, in terms of months of survival gained, decreases by 50% between the ages of 60 and 75 years because of this effect.[13] This suggests that the criteria for a prognostic group (in terms of tumour size, nodal status and other prognostic parameters) that might experience a certain net gain in life expectancy depends to some extent on the woman's age, particularly in women aged ≥ 75 years. For older women, where the gains produced by therapy are decreased by this simple effect, the net benefit becomes less. The net impact of adjuvant therapies on quality of life, in terms of the balance between time lost to toxicity but later regained in terms of longer symptom-free periods before relapse and longer survival, is of particular interest in older women.[14,15]

Figures 18.1 and 18.2 illustrate the issues that may be considered in adjuvant therapy decision-making in younger vs. older post-menopausal women. Figures 18.1 and 18.2 were prepared on the assumptions firstly that natural mortality (i.e. non-breast-cancer related) is similar in breast cancer patients to that in women in the general population, secondly, breast cancer-related mortality in the general population is similar to that reported from a large American patient series,[16] and thirdly, adjuvant therapy has the same efficacy (a 20% proportional reduction in mortality) in women aged 50 years as in those aged 70 years. Figure 18.1 shows how small a net benefit is projected to be due to adjuvant therapy for patients with low-risk tumours, and also how at the age of 70 years natural mortality dominates rather than breast cancer-related mortality. Figure 18.2 shows that even for patients with TI tumours and 1–3 positive nodes where breast cancer-related mortality is around 20% at 10 years, the overall improvement in prognosis afforded by adjuvant therapy is modest. Again, in older patients, natural mortality dominates the outcome.

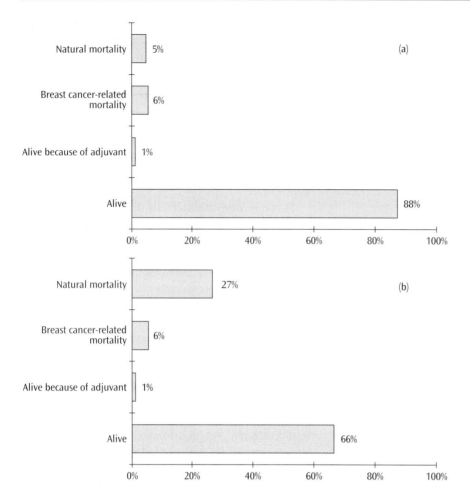

Figure 18.1 *Projections of survival at 10 years with relative contributions of natural and breast cancer-related mortality and impact of adjuvant therapy. (a) For a 50-year-old woman with a T (0–1.0 cm in diameter) and no involved nodes. (b) For a 70-year-old woman with a T (0–1.0 cm in diameter) and no involved nodes.*

OVERVIEW OF ADJUVANT CHEMOTHERAPY IN POST-MENOPAUSAL PATIENTS – INFORMATION FROM THE EBCTCG META-ANALYSIS OF ADJUVANT THERAPY TRIALS

The completed clinical studies of adjuvant therapy are the foundation of current treatment standards and of ongoing and future clinical trials.[17] The most influential papers in the discussion of adjuvant therapy planning have been those detailing the results of the EBCTCG meta-analyses of randomized adjuvant chemotherapy trials. The earlier overview papers[1,2] included subset analyses based not on menopausal status but rather on age (< 50 vs. ≥ 50 years), because in many of the trials age rather than menopausal status was used as an entry criterion, and/or menopausal status of the patients was unknown or uncertain. None the less, age < 50 vs. ≥ 50 years is a useful substitute for menopausal status. For the patients included in the EBCTCG analysis, > 90% of those who were < 50 years of age were premenopausal, while > 90% of the patients aged ≥ 50 years were post-menopausal. This is not surprising given that 50 years is the approximate median age at menopause.

The results of the EBCTCG meta-analyses are summarized in Table 18.1, which can be viewed as supporting

three basic tenets relating to post-menopausal patients, even though all of these tenets have been challenged as over-simplifications or as incorrect, or have been accepted only with important qualifications.

Tenet 1

Post-menopausal patients receiving adjuvant chemotherapy experience net benefit in terms of both disease-free survival and overall survival.

The first meta-analysis of adjuvant polychemotherapy trials found that premenopausal patients derived benefit from adjuvant chemotherapy, but failed to demonstrate a clear benefit in post-menopausal patients.[1] Thus adjuvant chemotherapy became a widely accepted standard for premenopausal patients, while its value in post-menopausal patients remained suspect. However, the second EBCTCG analysis[2] included additional trials and an additional 5 years of follow-up, and it did show that the benefits of adjuvant chemotherapy were not restricted to premenopausal women, but occurred in post-menopausal women as well (see Table 18.1). The latest meta-analysis[3] showed that with longer follow-up the advantage remains, although with slightly lower magnitude; for women over 50 years of age the proportional

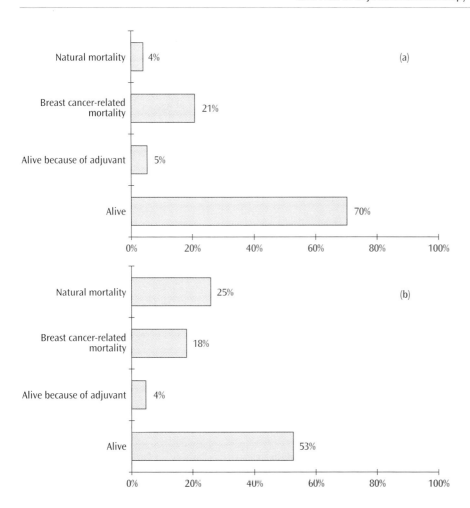

Figure 18.2 *Projections of survival at 10 years with relative contributions of natural and breast cancer-related mortality and impact of adjuvant therapy (a) For a 50-year-old woman with a T (0–2.0 cm in diameter) and 1–3 nodes. (b) For a 70-year-old woman with a T1 (0–2.0 cm in diameter) and 1–3 involved nodes.*

reduction in annual hazard for relapse was 19±3%, and for death was 11±3%. This benefit was modest but statistically significant.

For example, suppose a 60-year-old woman with an oestrogen-receptor-negative tumour with a 30% risk of relapse and a 25% risk of breast cancer-related death at 10 years follow-up was to receive adjuvant chemotherapy. This woman might be expected to have a *proportional* (note not *absolute*) risk reduction for relapse of 19%. There would be a 30% risk of relapse or a 6% absolute reduction in risk, and a *proportional* risk reduction for mortality of 11% of the 25% risk of mortality, i.e. only about 3%.

However, this modestly encouraging result must be viewed with some important cautions.

First, in the previous meta-analysis[2] this benefit was clearly demonstrated in the node-positive subset of patients, but did not reach the level of statistical significance in node-negative patients. However, in the latest analysis[3] the result is significant in both nodal groups. The lack of significance in node-negative patients in the earlier meta-analysis was possibly an artefact due to the lower relapse and death rates, making statistically significant differences more difficult to demonstrate. The early results of the recent NSABP[18] and Intergroup[19] trials in node-negative patients suggest that current chemothera-

peutic regimens do offer significant benefit in this population. In NSABP trial B-13, post-menopausal node-negative patients receiving 6 cycles of methotrexate and 5-fluorouracil had a greater than 30% reduction in the proportional risk of relapse, which was statistically significant (P < 0.01). Intergroup Trial 1180, in which post-menopausal node-negative patients received 6 cycles of cyclophosphamide, methotrexate, 4-fluorouracil and prednisone (CMFP), also showed a more than 50% reduction in the risk of relapse. Thus individual clinical trial results show a beneficial effect of chemotherapy in post-menopausal node-positive patients, and an uncertain but probable benefit in high-risk node-negative patients.

Secondly, the benefit was demonstrated by the EBCTCG analysis in post-menopausal subsets of women between 50 and 69 years of age in terms of a reduction in the risk of relapse. So few women under 70 years of age were included in the analysis that it was impossible to draw meaningful conclusions about the benefit of adjuvant chemotherapy for these older women. The meta-analysis also suggested a trend towards less benefit for post-menopausal women with increasing age. Reductions in the risk of relapse were 22%, 18% and then non-demonstrable for post-menopausal women aged 50–59, 60–69 and ≥ 70 years, respectively. Reductions in the risk

Table 18.1 *EBCTG meta-analyses – benefits of adjuvant therapy in pre- and post-menopausal patients expressed as percentage proportion risk reduction of relapse or death ± SD*

		Risk of relapse		Risk of death	
		Premenopausal < 50 years of age	Post-menopausal ≥ 50 years of age	Premenopausal < 50 years of age	Post-menopausal ≥ 50 years of age
C vs. no C*					
	Overall	35 ± 4	20 ± 3	27 ± 5	11 ± 3
	Node-negative	31 ± 6	23 ± 7	20 ± 8	20 ± 7
	Node-positive	39 ± 5	20 ± 3	30 ± 5	10 ± 3
	OR < 10	40 ± 7	30 ± 5	35 ± 9	17 ± 6
	OR ≥ 10	33 ± 8	18 ± 4	20 ± 10	9 ± 5
T vs. no T (treatment for about 5 years)†	Overall	45 ± 8	47 ± 4	32 ± 10	26 ± 4
	Node-negative		49 ± 4		25 ± 5
	Node-positive		43 ± 5		28 ± 6
	OR < 10		6 ± 11		−3 ± 11
	OR ≥ 10		43 ± 3		23 ± 4
T + C vs. T*					
	Overall	21 ± 13	19 ± 3	25 ± 14	11 ± 4
C + T vs. C† (T for 5 years)	Overall		52 ± 8		47 ± 9

C, chemotherapy; T, tamoxifen; OR, oestrogen receptor.

* Data from the chemotherapy meta-analysis.[3]

† Data taken from the tamoxifen meta-analysis.[2] Apart from the overall results which are based on all trials of tamoxifen, the other results are from OR-positive or OR-unknown patients.

of death were 14%, 8% and then non-demonstrable in women aged 50–59, 60–69 and ≥ 70 years, respectively. Whether this apparent decrease in efficacy was due to less intense therapy in the trials including many of the older post-menopausal patients, or whether it reflects a true difference in efficacy, was not addressed in the meta-analysis. Although it seems possible that women over 70 years of age would experience the same reduction in relapse and mortality that is seen in younger post-menopausal women, based on their similar response rates to chemotherapy for metastatic disease, the benefits of adjuvant chemotherapy in women over 70 years of age remain largely unexplored and have not yet been confirmed, and so are thus uncertain.

Thirdly, the net benefit of adjuvant chemotherapy in post-menopausal patients may or may not be obtained in women who are receiving concurrent endocrine therapy. There may be subsets of post-menopausal women who obtain a substantial risk reduction from the tamoxifen alone, and who would derive no additional benefit from chemotherapy. Thus, for these women, chemotherapy would not be worthwhile. This will be discussed in more detail below.

Fourthly, although analyses such as the meta-analysis suggest that there was a net benefit for post-menopausal patients who received adjuvant chemotherapy, this simple statement obscures the enormous differences between dif-

ferent chemotherapeutic regimens. Chemotherapeutic regimens can differ in the drugs included, their doses, their sequencing, how many cycles were delivered, how the doses were modified, and what supportive care was given for possible toxicity. There is no accepted standard adjuvant chemotherapy for post-menopausal women. Some general principles have emerged, but are not beyond debate. The earlier meta-analysis showed that, in general, polychemotherapy was more effective than monodrug therapy. In addition, shorter-duration therapies (4–6 cycles) were as effective as longer-duration regimens.

Another important question is whether doxorubicin-containing regimens offer an advantage, and whether the benefit differs according to menopausal status. The meta-analysis gave the results of 11 trials making direct comparisons between anthracycline-containing regimens and CMF in about 7000 women. There was an advantage of 12±4% in terms of recurrence and 11±5% for survival in proportional terms, which translates into an absolute advantage of just over 3% for recurrence and a little less than this for death. Most of these trials began in the early 1980s, and so the follow-up is still short.

These results of course reflect only the data from the few trials that have been published. Preliminary results of a Southeast Cancer Study Group (SEG) study comparing the two regimens showed a non-statistically significant trend in overall survival in favour of CAF.[20] Preliminary results of a European study comparing CMF with epirubicin-based CEF also showed a trend favouring the anthracycline-based regimen, but again it did not reach the level of statistical significance.[21] Neither of these studies was designed to answer the question of the relative efficacy and safety of anthracycline-based regimens in post-menopausal patients. A trial relevant to this discussion is the Oncofrance trial in node-positive patients reported at 10 years of follow-up. This trial demonstrated a significant DFS and S advantage for CAF compared to CMF, but this benefit was restricted to premenopausal patients, and was not seen in post-menopausal patients.[22] The question of which is superior, CMF or CAF, may be addressed in a subset analysis of the recently completed very large Intergroup trial 0102 in high-risk, node-negative patients, but data for this are not yet available.

A large study was reported by the NSABP,[23] comparing 4 cycles (about 3 months) of AC (doxorubicin plus cyclophosphamide) with 6 cycles (about 6 months) of standard CMF. After 3 years of follow-up, no difference between the arms was apparent. If the efficacy is similar, then which regimen is preferred? The AC regimen was completed in less than half the time of the CMF regimen, it was associated with one-third the number of physician visits and fewer treatment days and, although alopecia was worse, there were fewer days of nausea with AC. Cardiac toxicity was not a major problem. The investigators concluded that AC is arguably the optimal regimen. However, approximately 75% of the patients in this study were premenopausal, and because the study was not analysed by menopausal status, its relevance to these issues in the post-menopausal population is unclear. Thus basic questions about which widely used adjuvant chemotherapies would be most effective for post-menopausal women remain unanswered.

Tenet 2

Post-menopausal patients benefit more from adjuvant endocrine therapy than from adjuvant chemotherapy.
The meta-analyses appear to show that endocrine therapy is more effective than adjuvant chemotherapy (with a more than twofold reduction in risk for both relapse and death when given for 5 years) to post-menopausal patients.[2,3]

However, when discussing the potential advantages of either of these therapies, it is essential to take into account the value of oestrogen and progesterone receptors in directing therapy. In the oestrogen-receptor-positive subset of post-menopausal patients, tamoxifen does appear to be much more efficacious than chemotherapy (see Table 18.1). However, it is uncertain whether this is the case for adjuvant therapy of oestrogen-receptor-negative patients, in whom tamoxifen is clearly less effective. The chemotherapy meta-analysis showed that, for post-menopausal patients, the proportional reduction in recurrence appeared to be nearly twice as large in women with

oestrogen-receptor-negative disease ($30\pm5\%$) as in those with oestrogen-receptor-positive disease ($18\pm4\%$). The difference between these effects was statistically significant. This is in contrast to the results obtained in the premenopausal group, where there was no evidence of different outcomes according to oestrogen-receptor status.

The meta-analysis showed that the benefit in terms of relapse among oestrogen-receptor-negative patients receiving tamoxifen for any duration (not just 5 years as in Table 18.1), although statistically significant, was small ($10\pm4\%$, with the lower confidence limit close to zero). There was no significant advantage in terms of mortality. This analysis was not stratified by the age (or menopausal status) of the patients. It should be emphasized that the oestrogen-receptor-negative category in the meta-analysis is a mixture of true oestrogen-receptor-negative tumours in which oestrogen-receptor was not detectable in the assay, and low oestrogen-receptor-positive tumours with oestrogen-receptor levels of < 10 fmol/mg protein. These low oestrogen-receptor-positive tumours have previously been shown to respond well to endocrine therapy for advanced disease, and might be expected to benefit from adjuvant tamoxifen. Whether tumours in which oestrogen-receptor is undetectable also derive benefit from adjuvant tamoxifen is not known, but it seems unlikely given the paucity of responses in patients with metastatic disease with no detectable oestrogen receptor. Thus it would seem reasonable to some to consider treating oestrogen-receptor-negative post-menopausal patients with tamoxifen rather than chemotherapy as adjuvant therapy, particularly in view of the low efficacy of some standard chemotherapy regimens in this population, and the low toxicity of tamoxifen, but the benefit – particularly for these patients – is in any case small.

This view has not been accepted uncritically. Individual chemotherapy trials including oestrogen-receptor-negative post-menopausal patients do report levels of benefit for adjuvant chemotherapy beyond those expected for tamoxifen alone in this population.[17] Whether the apparent tamoxifen benefit for oestrogen-receptor-negative patients remains with a more stringent oestrogen-receptor cut-off of < 3 fmol/mg protein, or in oestrogen-receptor-negative/progesterone-receptor-negative populations, and when the oestrogen-receptor and progesterone-receptor determinations are performed with high levels of quality control, remains an open question.

Tenet 3

Combined therapy with endocrine therapy and chemotherapy is often better than either alone.

TAMOXIFEN PLUS CHEMOTHERAPY VS. TAMOXIFEN ALONE

Based on the earlier meta-analysis results which suggested that adjuvant tamoxifen would be superior to adjuvant chemotherapy in most post-menopausal women, tamoxifen has been accepted as the standard of care for many of these women, particularly those at moderate risk for recurrence who are oestrogen-receptor or progesterone-receptor positive. This standard is not altogether satisfactory, however, given that tamoxifen is only modestly active as an adjuvant. Thus an obvious question is whether combined therapy with both tamoxifen and endocrine therapy would be better than tamoxifen alone. The latest EBCTCG analyses show that, when comparing the effects of tamoxifen alone with those of tamoxifen plus chemotherapy, there was a highly significant $19\pm3\%$ reduction in the annual odds of relapse and a $10\pm4\%$ reduction in the annual odds of death in the group that received combined therapy. It could be argued that the prolongation of disease-free and overall survival that results from the addition of chemotherapy to tamoxifen would make combined therapy the preferred treatment, but the added toxicity and cost must also be considered. This remains the subject of controversy, and a focus of ongoing clinical research for the following reasons.

First, patient selection may be crucial in determining whether combined chemoendocrine therapy is superior to endocrine therapy alone. There are several trials that suggest no additional benefit beyond that of tamoxifen alone by the addition of chemotherapy (see Table 18.2). On examination of the 9 major trials of combined therapy vs. tamoxifen alone, 6 of the 8 trials suggest that combined therapy is better. The 3 trials which show no additive effect were all restricted to patients who were oestrogen-receptor- and/or progesterone-receptor-positive. This raises the important possibility of whether the inclusion of oestrogen-receptor-negative patients in the other trials explains the apparent benefit from chemotherapy. Thus it is still open to question whether oestrogen-receptor-positive post-menopausal patients should receive combined therapy.

Secondly, it is also possible that the duration and timing of tamoxifen therapy or the type of chemotherapy may be important parameters. Perhaps some of the trials showed a benefit for combined therapy because the duration of tamoxifen was not optimal (i.e. it was too short). It is also possible that in some circumstances the addition of tamoxifen concurrently with a chemotherapy regimen might decrease the efficacy of the chemotherapy, as has been suggested by the results of NSABP B-09.[22] In addition, trials that used particularly efficacious chemotherapy regimens might be more likely to show a benefit for combined therapy.

Thirdly, the EBCTCG meta-analysis suggests that the addition of chemotherapy to tamoxifen reduces the risk of relapse mortality, but only 2 of the 9 studies in Table 18.2 show a significant improvement in survival in the combined therapy arm. We need to wait for the data from these and other trials to mature before drawing firm conclusions.

CHEMOTHERAPY PLUS TAMOXIFEN VS. CHEMOTHERAPY ALONE

A second question is whether, for patients who are selected to receive chemotherapy, the addition of tamoxifen is worthwhile. Reviews of this topic in general suggest that the addition of tamoxifen is indeed worthwhile, with the EBCTCG meta-analysis showing that combined therapy reduced the annual odds of relapse by $52\pm8\%$ and those of death by $47\pm9\%$ compared to chemotherapy alone.

First, the major caveat with this interpretation is whether the oestrogen-receptor status makes a difference (i.e. could similar results have been achieved in certain subsets with tamoxifen alone?). Many of the trials upon which the meta-analysis was based excluded oestrogen-receptor-negative patients,[31] or did not require oestrogen-receptor status. One large trial (NSABP B-09)[32] that did include a large number of post-menopausal patients with either oestrogen-receptor-positive or oestrogen-receptor-negative status, randomizing them to either melphalan and 5-fluorouracil (PF) or PF plus tamoxifen found the

Table 18.2 *Studies of polychemotherapy plus tamoxifen in combination vs. tamoxifen alone in post-menopausal women*

Study	Chemotherapy	Duration of tamoxifen (years)	Subset	n	FU (years)	DFS benefit?	OS benefit?
Ludwig 3[23]	CMFPT	1	N+	463	7	Yes $P=0.01$	Trend $P=0.08$
Danish BCG[24]	CMF	1	Any N	1350	4	Yes $P=0.03$	No
Case Western[25]	CMFVP	2	N+,OR+	94	4.5	Yes $P=0.04$	Trend $P=0.1$
SWOG 7827[19]	CMFVP	1	N+,OR+	966	6.5	No	No
NCI Canada[26]	CMF	2	N+,OR+ or PgR+	705	?	No $P>0.5$	No
Lyon[27]	FEC	2	N+	739	3.1	Yes? $\pm$ trend	Trend
NSABP B-16[28]	AC	5	N+	1170	3.0	Yes $P<0.001$	Yes $P<0.04$
	PAF					Yes $P<0.001$	No
GROCTA[29]	CMF,E	5	N+,OR+	233	3.3	No	No
Nomura et al.[30]	MMC	2	OR+	1579	8.2	Yes $P=0.04$	Yes $P=0.02$

N+, node-positive; OR+, oestrogen-receptor-positive; PgR+, progesterone-receptor-positive.

advantage of combined therapy only in the post-menopausal oestrogen-receptor-positive patients and not in the post-menopausal oestrogen-receptor-negative patients. The Eastern Cooperative Oncology Group reported just the opposite from a smaller trial including only 170 post-menopausal patients (about 33% oestrogen-receptor-negative) with CMFVP as the chemotherapy. They found that the benefit of combined therapy was restricted to relapse (with no effect on survival), and was present in both the oestrogen-receptor-positive and oestrogen-receptor-negative subsets, but was only statistically significant in the oestrogen-receptor-negative group. Thus although combined therapy might be preferable to chemotherapy alone, it is still debated whether the combination is useful in both oestrogen-receptor-positive and oestrogen-receptor-negative subsets of patients, and whether its desirability is dependent on the type of chemotherapy and the timing and duration of the tamoxifen given.

PRESENT STANDARDS OF CARE

With the EBCTCG meta-analysis of clinical trials as a driving force, several sets of basic guidelines for adjuvant therapy have been drafted, based on the 1992 publication. These guidelines are similar, but they do differ in significant details as the authors weigh individual trials and regimens somewhat differently (see Table 18.3).

All of the guidelines are in basic agreement that, for patients with node-negative breast cancers ≤ 1 cm in diameter, no adjuvant therapy is the standard of care because these patients have such a low-risk of recurrence.[36] These patients have only a 10% or less risk of mortality at 10 years, so treatment of this low-risk population would require 100 patients to be treated (with an attendant therapy-related cost, and morbidity and mortality) to prevent at most two breast cancer-related deaths. Details of the discussions for these guidelines show that treatment recommendations were affected by

the prognostic evaluation of the patient, with patients perceived at being at highest risk for recurrence and death within any given category considered to be the best candidates for the most aggressive treatment options, because they have the most to gain.

All guidelines favour tamoxifen as part of the adjuvant programme for oestrogen-receptor-positive post-menopausal patients. The guidelines differ on whether to recommend addition of chemotherapy in oestrogen-receptor-positive patients, with no guideline mandating it. In one set of guidelines, chemotherapy combined with tamoxifen is considered to be an additional option for all moderate-risk patients, and at the other end of the spectrum one set of guidelines recommends tamoxifen alone, with chemotherapy not included as an option.

The guidelines diverge most in the treatment recommendations for oestrogen-receptor-negative post-menopausal patients. The most aggressive guidelines recommend that both node-positive and node-negative patients who are oestrogen-receptor-negative receive some form of adjuvant chemotherapy. The other sets of guidelines suggest a list of options including chemotherapy, hormonal therapy with tamoxifen, or observation, with the least aggressive set of guidelines not including chemotherapy at all as a standard option for oestrogen-receptor-negative node-negative post-menopausal women. For many clinicians, consideration of the patient's age, the presence of other illnesses, and tumour-related factors (such as S-phase, histological grade, etc.) may influence decisions about adjuvant therapy in this group of patients.

The inclusion of tamoxifen as an option for oestrogen-receptor-negative post-menopausal women is interesting and reflects the observation from the meta-analysis that even post-menopausal women with low oestrogen-receptor levels (< 10 fmol/mg protein) did appear to benefit from tamoxifen, with a relative risk reduction for relapse or death similar to that seen for chemotherapy in post-menopausal patients (both oestrogen-receptor-positive and oestrogen-receptor-negative patients). This may need

Table 18.3 *Recommendations for conventional therapy from three different recent sources**

Source		Premenopausal		Post-menopausal	
		OR+	OR–	OR+	OR–
St Gallen[33]	N–†	C ± tamoxifen	C	Tamoxifen or Tamoxifen ± C	C ± tamoxifen
	N+	C ± tamoxifen	C	Tamoxifen ± C	C ± tamoxifen
Osborne et al.[34]	N–†	C or tamoxifen	C	Tamoxifen	C or tamoxifen or observation
	N+	C	C	Tamoxifen ± C	C or tamoxifen
Henderson[35]	N–†	Tamoxifen or observation	C or observation	Tamoxifen	Tamoxifen or observation
	N+	C	C	Tamoxifen	Observation or tamoxifen or C

N–, node-negative; N+, node-positive; OR+, oestrogen-receptor-positive; OR–, oestrogen-receptor-negative; C, chemotherapy.
* These guidelines were written as recommendations for conventional therapy, and were not intended to preclude investigational clinical trial therapy outside these limits.
† For patients with tumours ≤ 1 cm in diameter and axillary node negative, guidelines indicate that observation only is the preferred course except in the context of a clinical trial.

to be reassessed in the light of the latest tamoxifen meta-analysis although this does not include an analysis by age and oestrogen-receptor status.

These recommendations are for standard therapy. However, standard therapy is in fact not very satisfactory, with the majority of women who would have relapsed and died without adjuvant therapy still destined to relapse and die of breast cancer even if they receive adjuvant therapy. This unsatisfactory situation is being addressed by an active programme of clinical trials, which deserve vigorous support and in which all women with breast cancer should be invited to participate.

NEW HORIZONS AND FUTURE DIRECTIONS IN ADJUVANT THERAPY FOR POST-MENOPAUSAL WOMEN

The immediate goals for the improvement of adjuvant therapy in post-menopausal women are reflected in ongoing clinical trials. To illustrate the major issues now being addressed, we can review some of these ongoing trials. For the sake of simplicity, this chapter will only review the current American studies being performed by the Intergroup committee and the NSABP. An overview of these trials is presented in Tables 18.4 and 18.5.

Studies involving combined chemoendocrine therapy

Intergroup trial 0100 is addressing whether the combination of tamoxifen and chemotherapy (CAF) is superior to tamoxifen alone in node-positive, oestrogen-receptor- or progesterone-receptor-positive, post-menopausal women. The three arms compare tamoxifen for 5 years alone vs. CAF chemotherapy followed by tamoxifen for 5 years vs. concurrent CAF and tamoxifen with tamoxifen continued for 5 years. The most important question to be answered in this study is whether CAF chemotherapy gives additional benefit in post-menopausal receptor-positive women taking adjuvant tamoxifen. This is the only trial that has addressed this issue in women who receive an extended course of tamoxifen and who are given a conventional CAF regimen. This trial may thus in part help to confirm or reject the results of NSABP B-16 in which tamoxifen was compared with tamoxifen plus AC, which suggested that combined therapy was superior to tamoxifen alone.[27] It is interesting to note that all other ongoing Intergroup studies give tamoxifen to receptor-positive patients after completion of chemotherapy. This widely used practice is supported by the results of the meta-analysis, which suggested that the addition of tamoxifen to chemotherapy improved DFS.

This question may be definitively answered by one ongoing and one recently completed trial with modern adjuvant chemotherapeutic regimens (and biological correlative studies) for post-menopausal, node-negative patients. The ongoing NSABP B-23 trial randomizes patients between CMF and AC, with a secondary randomization to tamoxifen or observation. The recently completed, but as yet unanalysed Intergroup trial 0102, which randomized node-negative patients after a conventional CMF or CAF adjuvant regimen to either

Table 18.4 *Ongoing clinical trials of the North American Intergroup Group Committee and the NSABP*

	Premenopausal		Post-menopausal	
	OR+	**OR−**	**OR+**	**OR−**
N−*	I 0137	I 0137	I 0137	I 0137
	C1 vs. C2	C1 vs. C2	C1 vs. C2	C1 vs. C2
	I 0142	NSABP B-23		NSABP B-23
	T vs. T + Ooph	(C1 vs. C2) ± T		(C1 vs. C2) ± T
N+			I 0100	
			T vs. T + C1	
	I 0137†	I 0137	I 0137†	I 0137
	C1 vs. C2	C1 vs. C2	C1 vs. C2	C1 vs. C2
	I 0148†	I 0148	I 0148†	I 0148
	C1 vs. C2 vs. C3	C1 vs. C2 vs. C3	C1 vs. C2 vs. C3	C1 vs. C2 vs. C3
	I 0121†	I 0121	I 0121†	I 0121
	C1 vs. C1 + BMT	C1 vs. C1 + BMT	C1 vs. C1 + BMT	C1 vs. C1 + BMT
	CALGB 9082†	CALGB 9082	CALGB 9082†	CALGB 9082
	C1 + C2 vs. C1 + BMT	C1 + C2 vs. C1 + BMT	C1 + C2 vs. C1 + BMT	C1 + C2 vs. C1 + BMT

N−, node-negative; N+, node-positive; OR+, oestrogen-receptor-positive; OR−, oestrogen-receptor-negative; T, tamoxifen; Ooph, oophorectomy; C1, chemotherapy of one type; C2, chemotherapy of another type; BMT, bone-marrow transplantation.
* In all node-negative protocols patients with tumours ≤ 1 cm in diameter were excluded.
† In Intergroup trials I 0137, I 0148 and I 0121, and CALGB 9082, tamoxifen is started by all oestrogen-receptor-positive patients after the completion of therapy.

NSABP B-27	NSABP B-30	I 0151
C1 vs. C2 vs. C3	C1 vs. C2 vs. C3	T vs. T + F

tamoxifen or observation, also asks a similar question about combined therapy.

It seems unlikely that this question will be studied further because of the relatively low cost and toxicity of tamoxifen, particularly if the recently completed Intergroup trial 0102 and the ongoing NSABP B-23 trial confirm the benefit of the addition of tamoxifen after completion of chemotherapy.

Table 18.5 *Current (1995) Intergroup and NSABP Adjuvant Trials*

Intergroup Trial 0137
    Cycles of AC (combined) vs.
        A as single agent followed by C as a single agent

Intergroup Trial 0142
    Tamoxifen vs.
        tamoxifen plus oophorectomy

NSABP Trial B-23
    AC vs.
        CMF

Intergroup Trial 0100
    Tamoxifen vs.
        CAF then tamoxifen vs.
        CAF with tamoxifen and then tamoxifen

Intergroup Trial 0148
    First randomization
        CA with A at standard dose vs.
        CA with A at intermediate dose vs.
        CA with A at high dose
    Then second randomization
        Taxol vs.
            observation

Intergroup Trial 0121
    CAF vs.
        CAF followed by high-dose therapy with stem-cell support

CALGB Trial 9082
    CAF followed by randomization to:
        high-dose therapy with stem-cell support vs.
        standard-dose therapy with no stem-cell support

Intergroup Trial I 0151
    Tamoxifen vs.
        tamoxifen + fenretinide

NSABP Trial B-37
    Pre-operative AC vs.
        pre-operative AC followed by Docetaxel vs.
        pre-operative AC + post-operative Docetaxel

NSABP B-30
    Adjuvant AC followed by Docetaxel vs.
        A + Docetaxel vs.
        AC + Docetaxel

Studies evaluating the importance of chemotherapy dose intensity

The work of Hryniuk and Levine, suggested that the higher the dose intensity of chemotherapy, the greater the effectiveness of adjuvant chemotherapy regimens for breast cancer.[37] While this view is almost certainly true for very-low-dose regimens, it is still debated whether efficacy keeps increasing with high-dose intensities. It is clear that for adjuvant regimens, lowering doses below standard regimens can result in decreased effectiveness. Thus it might be inferred that reducing the dose of therapy in standard regimens when treating older post-menopausal women would result in reduced effectiveness, and is therefore to be discouraged.[38]

The relationship between dose intensity and efficacy of a conventional cyclophosphamide/doxorubicin (CA) regimen is being investigated by Intergroup trial 0148. This study addresses whether increasing the dose of doxorubicin causes increased efficacy.

The second approach is a less conventional one illustrated by Intergroup trial 0121. These studies are examining whether dose intensification beyond that of standard regimens to levels that require autologous stem-cell reinfusion improves outcome. In these protocols, patients with more than 10 positive nodes receive several cycles of a conventional CAF regimen and are then randomized either to receive or not to receive a single cycle of high-dose therapy that requires autologous stem-cell support. There have been promising pilot trials of such regimens,[39] but with no completed phase III comparisons to conventional therapy, adjuvant regimens requiring stem-cell support must be considered investigational at this stage. These trials do include both premenopausal and post-menopausal women, but because the high-intensity drug regimens can cause severe morbidity, and may be more poorly tolerated by older women, women over 60 years of age have generally been excluded.

Studies of combination vs. sequential polychemotherapy

The meta-analysis included 13 studies of prolonged combination chemotherapy compared to prolonged single-agent therapy. Polychemotherapy appeared to be more efficacious in 10 of these studies, and produced a reduction of $13\pm5\%$ and $17\pm5\%$ in the annual odds of recurrence or death in comparison to monotherapy, respectively. Thus the cumulative data suggest that combination drug therapy is better than single-agent therapy in both DFS and S. However, it should be emphasized that none of these studies used the single agent optimally with regard to dose, and thus it is possible that sequential single agents given at maximum tolerable dose intensity might be more effective than combination chemotherapy regimens. An obvious potential problem with combination drug regimens is that doses of each of the agents in the combination must often be reduced because of overlapping toxicity. Thus it is quite plausible that a single agent or series of single agents given at their optimal dose and schedule would be equivalent or even superior to combination therapy. Certainly such sequential monotherapy regimens would be easier to introduce, as phase I and phase II studies of drug combinations would not be necessary. Intergroup trial 0137 is designed to test the efficacy of adjuvant doxorubicin and cyclophosphamide given either as combined therapy or as two sequential monotherapy programmes, with the patient first receiving several cycles of single-agent doxorubicin and then several cycles of single-agent cyclophosphamide. The doses were selected so as to deliver an identical total dose of the chemotherapeutic agents in both arms.

Studies of new agents in adjuvant therapy

A number of new cytotoxic agents have recently become available and have been studied in phase I and phase II clinical trials in patients with breast cancer.[40,41] Three of the more promising agents have been navelbine, paclitaxel (Taxol) and docetaxel (Taxotere).

Agents such as the taxanes attract particular interest because of their novel mechanism of action (stabilization of abnormal microtubule assembly), and because of clinical trial evidence of non-cross-resistance with doxorubicin. As an example of a study in which the possible role of one of the new agents in adjuvant regimens is being tested, Intergroup trial 0148 randomizes patients who have received adjuvant CA regimens to either observation or several cycles of adjuvant Taxol.

AREAS OF ONGOING OR IMPORTANT NEW RESEARCH FOR POST-MENOPAUSAL WOMEN

Approximately 20 years ago the exciting new agents for the adjuvant treatment of breast cancer were tamoxifen and the exciting new concept was the use of multiple agents in adjuvant programmes. Most of the research over the last 20 years has explored the opportunities raised by the availability of these agents and this concept. At the present time we are on a second threshold of applying new information derived from basic research, and a deeper understanding of the clinical problems that must be addressed to produce therapies of high efficacy.

The fundamental problems are therapeutic index (how to treat neoplastic tissue without causing unacceptable toxicity to normal tissue), and tumour heterogeneity (the fact that cells within a tumour express different phenotypes, and subpopulations with resistance to any given treatment strategy exist or occur

during therapy). These problems may be more successfully addressed as we understand on a more fundamental level the processes that are important to the growth of neoplastic tissue. The agents that we regard as chemotherapeutic drugs are molecules that interact with important macromolecules in tissue. For example, recent research has shown that anthracyclines are not merely mechanical intercalators in DNA, but are specific agents that inhibit with high affinity topoisomerase H, an enzyme that is critical for DNA replication.[42] Such knowledge can be used to screen more rapidly for interesting new agents, and may find application in the understanding and interference with intrinsic or acquired resistance to chemotherapeutic agents. At the intracellular level, a more profound understanding may be obtained of the control of the cell cycle, cell differentiation, and programmed cell death.[43] At the intercellular level, an understanding of autocrine and paracrine interactions, angiogenesis[44] or immune targeting may be exploited.

Today, our only well-validated strategies for prediction of the response to therapy in breast cancer patients are oestrogen-receptor and progesterone-receptor determinations used to predict responsiveness to endocrine therapy. Ultimately, tumours will be analysed for characteristics that would predict responsiveness to specific therapies. For example, tumours that greatly over-express hormone receptors such as the Her2/neu gene product or the epidermal growth factor receptor can be targeted by immunoglobin–toxin complexes, or by molecules designed to elicit immune responses,[45] and such research is in the phase I and phase II levels of clinical development today. These possibilities as well as others hold substantial promise for greatly improving therapy for breast cancer.

SUMMARY

Standard adjuvant therapy for node-positive, oestrogen-receptor-positive post-menopausal women includes tamoxifen. Combined tamoxifen and chemotherapy may be even more effective in some patients, but questions remain about the optimal chemo-endocrine regimen and the patient population that is most likely to benefit. For oestrogen-receptor-negative patients, standard adjuvant regimens are less well defined. For all post-menopausal patients treatment recommendations must take into consideration the degree of risk of relapse and death due to breast cancer. The existence or probability of developing other comorbidities, as well as overall quality-of-life issues, should also play a role in adjuvant therapy decision-making. Clinical research has played a major role in improving outcome for post-menopausal women, and continued patient participation in clinical trials should remain a top priority.

REFERENCES

1 Early Breast Cancer Trialists' Collaborative Group. Effects of adjuvant tamoxifen and of cytotoxic therapy on mortality in early breast cancer: an overview of 61 randomized trials among 28 896 women. *N Engl J Med* 1988; **319**: 1681–92.

2 Early Breast Cancer Trialists' Group. Tamoxifen for early breast cancer; an overview of the randomised trials. *Lancet* 1998; **351**: 1451–67.

3 Early Breast Cancer Trialists' Group. Polychemotherapy for early breast cancer; an overview of the randomised trials. *Lancet* 1998; **352**: 930–42.

4 Early Breast Cancer Trialists' Collaborative Group. Systemic treatment of early breast cancer by hormonal, cytotoxic, or immune therapy. *Lancet* 1992; **339**: 1–15, 71–85.

5 Nixon AJ, Neuberg D, Hayes DF *et al.* Relationship of patient age to pathologic features of the tumor and prognosis for patients with stage I or II breast cancer. *J Clin Oncol* 1994; **12**: 888–94.

6 Wenger CR, Beardsley S, Owens MA. DNA ploidy, S-phase, and steroid receptors in more than 127 000 breast cancer patients. *Breast Cancer Res Treat* 1993; **28**: 9–20.

7 Host H, Lund E. Age as a prognostic factor in breast cancer. *Cancer* 1986; **57**: 2217–21.

8 Adami H-O, Malker B, Holmberg L, Persson I, Stone B. The relationship between survival and age at diagnosis in breast cancer. *N Engl J Med* 1986; **315**: 559–63.

9 Balducci L, Parker M, Sexton W, Tantranond P. Pharmacology of antineoplastic agents in the elderly patient. *Semin Oncol* 1989; **16**: 76–84.

10 Begg CB, Elson PJ, Carbone PP. A study of excess hematologic toxicity in elderly patients on chemotherapy protocols. In: *Cancer in the elderly: approaches to early detection and management*. New York: 1989.

11 Begg CB, Cohen JL, Ellerton J. Are the elderly predisposed to toxicity from cancer chemotherapy? An investigation using data from the Eastern Cooperative Oncology Group. *Cancer Clin Trials* 1980; **3**: 369–74.

12 Christman K, Muss HB, Case LD, Stanley V. Chemotherapy of metastatic breast cancer in the elderly. *J Am Med Assoc* 1992; **268**: 57–62.

13 Desch CE, Hillner BE, Smith TJ, Retchin SM. Should the elderly receive chemotherapy for node-negative breast cancer? A cost-effectiveness analysis examining total and active life-expectancy outcomes. *J Clin Oncol* 1993; **11**: 777–82.

14 Gelber RD, Goldhirsch A, Cavalli F, for the International Breast Cancer Study Group. Quality-of-life-adjusted evaluation of adjuvant therapies for operable breast cancer. *Ann Intern Med* 1991; **114**: 621–8.

15 Goldhirsch A, Gelber RD, Simes RJ, Glasziou P, Coates AS. Costs and benefits of adjuvant therapy in breast cancer: a quality-adjusted survival analysis. *J Clin Oncol* 1989; **7**: 36–44.

16 Rosen PP, Groshen S, Saigo PE *et al.* A long-term follow-up study of survival in stage I (T1N1M0) and stage II (T1N1M0) breast carcinoma. *J Clin Oncol* 1989; **7**: 355–66.

17 Henderson IC. Chemotherapy for metastatic disease. In: Harris JR, Hellman S, Henderson IC, Kinne DW (eds) *Breast diseases*. Philadelphia, PA: JB Lippincott, 1991: 604–55.

18 Fisher B, Redmond C, Dimitrov NV *et al.* A randomized clinical trial evaluating sequential methotrexate and fluorouracil in the treatment of patients with node-negative breast cancer who have estrogen-receptor-negative tumors. *N Engl J Med* 1989; **320**: 473–8.

19 Mansour EG, Gray R, Shatilia AH *et al.* Survival advantage of adjuvant chemotherapy in high-risk node-negative breast cancer: ten-year analysis – an intergroup study. *J Clin Oncol* 1998; **16**: 3486–92.

20 Carpenter JT, Velez-Garcia E, Aron BS *et al.* Five-year results of a randomized comparison of cyclophosphamide, doxorubicin (adriamcyin) and fluorouracil (CAF) vs. cyclophosphamide, methotrexate and fluorouracil (CMF) for node-positive breast cancer: a Southeastern Cancer Study Group study. *Proc Am Soc Clin Oncol* 1994; **13**: 66 (A 68).

21 Coombes RC, Bliss JM, Marty M *et al.* for the International Collaborative Cancer Group (IOCG). A randomized trial comparing adjuvant FEC with CMF in premenopausal patients with node-positive resectable breast cancer. *Proc Am Soc Clin Oncol* 1991; **10**: 41 (A 37).

22 Misset JL, Gil-Dalgado M, Chollet Ph, Belpomme D, Fargeot P, Fumeleau P. Ten-years results of the French trial comparing adriamycin, vincristine, 5-fluorouracil and cyclophosphamide to standard CMF as adjuvant therapy for node-positive breast cancer. *Proc Am Soc Clin Oncol* 1992; **11**: 54 (A 41).

23 Goldhirsch A, Gelber RD. Adjuvant chemo-endocrine therapy or endocrine therapy alone for postmenopausal patients: Ludwig Studies III and IV. In: Senn H, Goldhirsch A, Gelber RD, Osterwalder B (eds) *Results in cancer research – adjuvant therapy of primary breast cancer*. Berlin: Springer-Verlag, 1989: 153–62.

24 Mouridsen HT, Rose C, Overgaard M *et al.* Adjuvant treatment of post-menopausal patients with high-risk primary breast cancer. *Acta Oncol* 1988; **27**: 699–705.

25 Pearson OH, Hubay CA, Gordon NH *et al.* Endocrine versus endocrine plus five-drug chemotherapy in postmenopausal women with stage II estrogen-receptor-positive breast cancer. *Cancer* 1989; **64**: 1819–23.

26 Pritchard KI, Paterson AH, Fine S *et al.* Randomised trial of cyclophosphamide, methotrexate, and fluorouracil chemotherapy added to tamoxifen as adjuvant therapy in postmenopausal women with node-positive estrogen and/or progesterone receptor-positive breast cancer: a report of the National Cancer Institute of Canada Clinical Trials Group. *J Clin Oncol* 1997; **15**: 2302–11.

27 Gerard JP, Hery M, Gedouin D *et al.* Postmenopausal patients with node-positive resectable breast cancer. Tamoxifen vs FEC (6 cycles) vs. FEC 50 (6 cycles) plus tamoxifen vs. control – preliminary results of a 4-arm randomized trial. The French Adjuvant Study Group. *Drugs* 1993; **45**: 60–7.

28 Fisher B, Wolmark N, Wickerham DL, Redmond CK. Current NSABP trials of adjuvant therapy for breast cancer. In: Salmon SE (ed) *Adjuvant therapy of cancer. VI.* Orlando, FL: Grune & Stratton, 1990: 275–85.

29 Boccardo F, Rubagotti A, Bruzzi P *et al.* for the Breast Cancer Adjuvant Chemo-Hormone Therapy Cooperative Group. Chemotherapy versus tamoxifen versus chemotherapy plus tamoxifen in node-positive, estrogen receptor-positive breast cancer patients: results of a multicentric Italian study. *J Clin Oncol* 1990; **8**: 1310–20.

30 Nomura Y, Shirouz M, Takayama T. Direct comparisons of adjuvant endocrine therapy, chemotherapy and chemoendocrine therapy for operable breast cancer patients stratified by estrogen receptor and menopausal status. *Breast Cancer Res Treat* 1998; **49**: 51–60.

31 Rivkin SE, Green S, Metch B *et al.* Adjuvant CMFVP versus tamoxifen versus concurrent CMFVP and tamoxifen for postmenopausal, node-positive and estrogen receptor-positive breast cancer patients: a Southwest Oncology Group Study. *J Clin Oncol* 1994; **12**: 2078–85.

32 Fisher B, Redmond C, Brown A *et al.* Adjuvant chemotherapy with and without tamoxifen in the treatment of primary breast cancer: 5-year results from the National Surgical Adjuvant Breast and Bowel Project Trial. *J Clin Oncol* 1986; **4**: 459–71.

33 Glick JH, Gelber RD, Goldhirsch A, Senn H-J. Meeting highlights: adjuvant therapy for primary breast cancer. *J Natl Cancer Inst* 1992; **84**.

34 Osborne CK, Clark GM, Ravdin PM. Adjuvant systemic therapy of primary breast cancer. In: Harris JR, Lippman ME, Morrow MS, Henderson IC, Kinne DW (eds) *Diseases of the breast.* Philadelphia, PA: JB Lippincott, 1995.

35 Henderson IC. Adjuvant systemic therapy for early breast cancer. *Cancer* 1994; **74**: 401–9.

36 National Institutes of Health Consensus Development Panel. Consensus statement: treatment of early-stage breast cancer. *J Natl Cancer Inst Mongr* 1992; **11**: 1–5.

37 Hryniuk W, Levine MN. Analysis of dose intensity for adjuvant chemotherapy trials in stage II breast cancer. *J Clin Oncol* 1986; **4**: 1162–70.

38 Muss HB. The role of chemotherapy and adjuvant therapy in the management of breast cancer in older women. *Cancer* 1994; **74**: 2165–71.

39 Peters WP, Ross M, Vrendenburgh JJ *et al.* High-dose chemotherapy and autologous bone-marrow support as consolidation after standard-dose adjuvant therapy for high-risk primary breast cancer. *J Clin Oncol* 1993; **11**: 1132–43.

40 Hortobagyi GN. Overview of new treatments for breast cancer. *Breast Cancer Res Treat* 1992; **21**: 3–13.

41 Rowinsky EK. Update on the antitumor activity of paclitaxel in clinical trials. *Ann Pharmacother* 1994; **28 (Supplement 5)**: S18–22.

42 Loflin PT, Zwelling LA. Topoisomerase II and the path to apoptosis. *Contemp Oncol* 1994; **11**: 46–57.

43 Fisher DF. Apoptosis in cancer therapy: crossing the threshold. *Cell* 1994; **78**: 539–44.

44 Hayes DF. Angiogenesis and breast cancer. *Hematol Oncol Clin North Am* 1994; **8**: 51–71.

45 Valone FH, Kaufman PA, Fanger MW, Guyre PM, Memoli V. Phase Ia/Ib trial of bispecific monoclonal antibody (BSAb) therapy (anti-Her-2/neu x nati-CD64) (MDX-210) for breast or ovarian cancers that over express Her-2/neu. *Proc Am Assoc Cancer Res* 1994; **35**: A1311.

19

New concepts in the treatment of breast cancer using high-dose chemotherapy

WILLIAM P PETERS AND ROGER DANSEY

INTRODUCTION

During the past 10 years, there has been increasing interest in the use of high-dose chemotherapy with autologous bone-marrow support in the treatment of metastatic and primary breast cancer. Analysis of data submitted to the North American Bone Marrow Transplant Registry indicates that breast cancer is now the most common diagnosis for which a transplant is performed in the USA. In fact, there are more transplants performed for breast cancer than the combined numbers of allogeneic bone-marrow transplants for acute and chronic myeloid leukaemia. There are even more autologous transplants performed for breast cancer than for non-Hodgkin's or Hodgkin's disease. Yet despite this enthusiastic adoption of the use of high-dose therapy, it is only recently that prospective randomized trials have been completed that support the value of high-dose therapy in metastatic breast cancer.[1] Furthermore, the results of prospective, multicentre trials in high-risk primary breast cancer are still years away.

This rapid adoption of high-dose therapy reflects general dissatisfaction with the treatment results of conventional-dose therapy and the uniform treatment results from high-dose efforts, reported from numerous centres in phase I and II trials, which demonstrate an increased objective response rate and provide suggestive evidence of a higher frequency of durable complete remissions compared to the general experience with conventional-dose therapy. Most reports of high-dose therapy have

indicated a complete response frequency of between 45% and 70% in patients with hormone-insensitive metastatic breast cancer, with overall complete and partial response rates in excess of 85%.[2–4] For young women with metastatic breast cancer, these rates appear particularly attractive when coupled with the data from several series which indicate that between 15% and 25% of poor-prognosis patients remain progression-free more than 3 to 5 years after treatment.

Phase II studies in high-risk primary breast cancer involving 10 or more axillary lymph nodes were undertaken because the relapse rates associated with the use of conventional-dose therapy were consistently above 60% at 5 years, and because of the premise that the higher objective response rates observed in high-dose therapy might translate to significant improvements in disease-free survival in the adjuvant setting where the tumour volume was lower. These studies have found that the use of high-dose combination alkylating agent therapy as consolidation after conventional-dose therapy has resulted in unexpectedly high disease-free and overall survival. With follow-up in excess of a median of 7 years and a minimum of 5 years, 64% of patients with a median of 14 involved lymph nodes at diagnosis have remained alive and disease-free after 5 years.[1] These data have prompted two multicentre trials of high-dose consolidation in this patient population. The results of these trials will undoubtedly be very influential in determining the ultimate role of high-dose therapy in the treatment of breast cancer. Data from other trials are not necessarily supportive of the experience from our own research group.[5,6]

UNDERLYING CONCEPTS OF HIGH-DOSE THERAPY

The use of high-dose therapy is derived from laboratory and clinical observations about tumour cell growth properties and the ability of chemotherapy to affect the growth of both quiescent and replicating tumour populations. The fundamental concepts were to a large extent derived by Howard Skipper and Frank Schabel from murine models exploring dose, dose intensity, schedule and class of chemotherapy.[7–9] Many of these observations were provided through a series of 'Booklets' published by the Southern Research Institute and circulated in limited numbers to investigators involved in chemotherapy programme design and testing.

This review will concentrate on three of Skipper's rules and their application to high-dose therapy as well as their interpretation in the light of two new sets of prospective randomized trial data using high-dose therapy conducted by the authors.

Skipper Rule 1 – the total tumour cell kill hypothesis

'In order to achieve cure, it is necessary to eradicate the tumour stem cells (both T/O and T/R cell in both the primary and metastatic sites) using tolerated local and/or systemic treatment.'

While at first glance this hypothesis may seem obvious, there are several important implications of the rule which merit consideration in the development and interpretation of high-dose studies. It is perhaps fundamental to the concept of high-dose therapy that eradication of the tumour stem-cell burden is the therapeutic aim. The total body tumour stem-cell burden represents one of the major barriers to the cure of metastatic cancer. It has thus become a principle of contemporary oncology that efforts targeted at smaller tumour burdens are more likely to be successful. The objective of all therapeutic strategies aimed at cure has to be total eradication of all tumour stem cells. The mechanism by which these tumour cells are eradicated is to a large extent irrelevant. Surgery has the capability of rapidly reducing the body tumour burden of localized tumours. Similarly, radiation therapy can effectively sterilize limited tumour burdens. Systemic cancer dissemination implies the necessity of systemic treatment – chemotherapy, immunotherapy or other molecular therapeutic approaches. Clinical experience has demonstrated that *localized* tumours can be eradicated by either local or systemic treatment, but not by the same mechanisms. Metastatic tumours are more likely to be cured by a combination of both local *and* systemic treatment.

Derivative from this rule is the fact that, as tumour stem-cell burden increases, the potential for multiple drug resistance limiting the efficacy of the therapeutic regimen increases as well. Skipper constrains the rule by noting the necessity for eradicating both sensitive and resistant cell populations from both primary and metastatic sites. The implication is that, if a few or potentially even one tumour stem cell remains at the end of treatment, it may successfully proliferate to kill the host. This observation has been consistently observed in animal models and is likely to be true for humans. Immune responses, either natural or induced, and capable of dealing with small tumour burdens, may be able to modify this limitation, but they do not fundamentally alter the underlying principle.

The biological tendency of tumours to spontaneous drug resistance mutation is generally accepted as a major reason for the inherent chemoresistance of large tumours. Goldie and Coldman mathematically modelled this drug resistance and have postulated that the transition from sensitive to resistant tumour populations can occur over as few as six tumour-cell-doubling periods.[10]

For high-dose studies, these observations have implications both for the selection of the disease setting to be studied and for the selection of multiple drugs and modalities of therapy for combination in the high-dose setting. Observations in the metastatic disease setting have relied on a combination of conventional-dose chemotherapy programmes consolidated with high-dose chemotherapy. Furthermore, many studies have demonstrated that bulky tumours at pretreatment sites of disease are frequently the sole sites of recurrence and this has resulted in the combined use of surgery and radiation therapy to sites of pretreatment bulk disease.

The selection of earlier disease settings, such as the adjuvant treatment of breast cancer, would also be expected to improve the results obtained with high-dose therapy due to a shorter natural history (and consequently less opportunity for the development of multiple drug resistance) and because of the smaller total body tumour stem-cell burden. Other considerations, such as the kinetic properties of smaller tumours, probably also play a role, but will not be discussed further here.

Skipper Rule 2 – the dose–response rule and first-order kinetic rule

'There is an invariable direct relationship between the single dose of a given chemotherapy agent and the number of drug-sensitive tumour stem cells killed. In a given cancer, the same dose of a given drug will kill the same fraction or percentage (but not the same number) of widely different tumour burdens of drug-sensitive cancer stem cells. It follows that *in vivo* dose–response curves or *in vitro* concentration–response curves should be (and are) exponential for homogeneous drug-sensitive tumour stem-cell populations.'

The fractional kill doctrine – that is, that in a given cancer the same dose of a drug will kill the same fraction of drug-sensitive cancer stem cells – implies that the total body burden of cancer will quickly become limiting to any given dose of chemotherapy. One potential way to overcome this limitation is to escalate the dose of chemotherapy substantially. For certain classes of drugs, especially the alkylating agents, the dose–response relationship is log-linear within the clinically relevant dose range. This means that doubling the dose of chemotherapy will result – even in resistant tumour types – in a log or greater increase in tumour cell kill. Thus for the more resistant epithelial phenotypes, the use of dose-intensified therapy offers the potential to magnify the tumour stem-cell kill sufficiently to eradicate the body burden of cancer cells.

Of course, the limitation on the use of dose intensification is the damage to normal cell populations for which the dose–response relationship also holds. Among the alkylating agents, the common dose-limiting side-effect is myelosuppression. This can be avoided by the use of autologous bone marrow or, more recently, by the use of peripheral blood progenitor cells (commonly called stem cells) which can repopulate the marrow after an otherwise lethal dose of combination chemotherapy. Limiting toxicity to dose escalation is then relegated to the next major toxicity – generally a visceral organ toxicity. Among the alkylating agents, the non-myelosuppressive toxicities differ widely. For example, cyclophosphamide is limited by cardiotoxicity, cisplatin is limited by nephrotoxicity and carmustine is limited by pulmonary or hepatic toxicity. Although these toxicities represent substantial and formidable challenges, the fact that they differ offers the potential to combine several agents in high-dose autologous stem-cell-supported regimens with non-overlapping toxicities. These predictions from animal and phase I clinical trials have been largely supported by subsequent clinical observations.

Over the last 5 years, rapid developments in the supportive care of patients have markedly changed the tolerability of high-dose regimens.[11] The treatment-related mortality associated with high-dose chemotherapy has fallen rapidly from over 20% to between 2% and 5% in most experienced centres. To a large extent this has been a result of the use of peripheral blood progenitor cells and haematopoietic growth factors which have resulted in shorter periods of myelosuppression and improvement of patient tolerance of the high-dose programme.

The dose escalation that has generally been achievable in these settings is in the range of 2- to 10-fold, although in selected cases even higher dose increases have been possible. Such dose escalations, particularly for the more sensitive epithelial tumours, would reasonably be expected to improve tumour stem-cell kill. The consistent clinical observation of frequent complete remissions is consistent with this hypothesis. Furthermore, the fraction of patients with metastatic breast cancer who show durable progression-free responses is consistent with the potential of high-dose therapy to eradicate the tumour stem-cell burden. My group has reported that a single treatment with high-dose cyclophosphamide, cisplatin and carmustine with autologous bone-marrow support has resulted in 14% of patients (3 of 22) with measurable, hormone-insensitive metastatic breast cancer achieving a complete remission and remaining continuously disease-free for in excess of 10 years.[2,3,12] In this trial, the therapeutic result can only be attributed to the high-dose treatment, as no other intervention – surgery, radiation therapy, induction chemotherapy or hormonal therapy – was utilized. Although the series is small, the demonstration that a single high-dose treatment can result in the eradication of a metastatic malignancy is supportive of Skipper's Rule 2.

From this rule is derived the *dose-intensity rule* which states that 'the dose intensity (dose per unit time) of anticancer drugs is the dominant treatment design variable with respect to the degree of therapeutic response (cure or nearness to cure at the nadir). However, duration of treatment and total dose often correlate most strongly with the duration of response in treatment failures.' The implication of this rule is that comparisons between various high-dose regimens are most appropriately made by examining the long-term progression-free fractions, and *not* the median duration of response. The latter will be more indicative of the ability of treatment to modify the growth characteristics of cellular populations that remain after chemotherapy.

Skipper Rule 3 – the inverse rule

'There is an invariable inverse relation between the cancer stem-cell burden and curability by chemotherapy used alone or in an adjuvant setting.'

This rule has at the same time both an obvious and an obscure relationship to the total tumour cell kill hypothesis discussed above. There is the obvious relationship that, as the tumour volume becomes larger, the required tumour stem-cell kill necessary for cure is increased. Given the inherent limitations on tumour cell kill imposed by the dose–response rule, large tumour burdens will be less effectively killed than small tumours. Less obvious is the relationship of this rule to the development of spontaneous drug resistance by mutation as espoused by Goldie and Coldman.[11] This interpretation of Rule 3 takes the form of an invariable *direct* relationship between the tumour stem-cell burden and the presence of specific resistant cells. In other words, the longer or larger a tumour has grown, the greater the probability that the development of drug resistance will be manifested and result in reduced curability.

The two interpretations of this rule are operative at the same time, and reflect different populations within a tumour. The first interpretation relates to the effect of total tumour burden on the effectiveness of a given chemotherapy programme on chemotherapy-sensitive populations. The second interpretation relates to the effect of total tumour burden on the development of drug-resistant populations. The operative effect of both of these interpretations is that increasing tumour burden rapidly alters the curability of tumours by chemotherapy, for reasons related to both chemotherapy effectiveness and intrinsic drug resistance.

RANDOMIZED TRIALS OF HIGH-DOSE THERAPY IN METASTATIC BREAST CANCER

Recently, randomized trials using high-dose therapy have been reported in the treatment of metastatic breast cancer although the study from South Africa has been withdrawn.

The AFM randomized trial evaluated a high-dose chemotherapy strategy in 425 patients with hormone-insensitive metastatic breast cancer.[13] Patients were treated with up to four cycles of doxorubicin, 5-fluorouracil and methotrexate (AFM), and if a complete remission was achieved they were randomized to either immediate consolidation with high-dose combination alkylating agents (cyclophosphamide, cisplatin and carmustine; CPB + ABMS), or to observation with the use of the high-dose CPB if the cancer recurred. The trial demonstrated that the use of induction AFM followed by immediate high-dose CPB resulted in a significantly improved disease-free survival compared to that obtained with the induction AFM alone, but that the *strategy* of AFM induction, namely observation, and CPB + ABMS at recurrence resulted in a better overall survival. Indeed, in this group the overall survival at 5 years was in excess of 40%, compared to 22% in the patients treated with immediate high-dose consolidation. This result, which at first appears counterintuitive, can possibly be interpreted in the context of the Skipper rules described above. Conventional chemotherapy, when applied in metastatic disease, appears to be incapable of efficiently eradicating the total tumour stem-cell burden.

At first glance, the AFM randomized trial would appear to be a violation of the inverse rule. As the patients on the observation arm are subsequently treated with high-dose therapy at the time of recurrence from a complete remission, by definition the tumour burden of these patients is greater than that of those who are treated with immediate high-dose therapy in complete remission. The observation that overall survival was superior in this patient population would appear to argue that, for these patients, either the inverse rule was not operative, the dose–response rule was not operative, or other factors intervened to negate the effect of the rules.

The reconciliation begins with a consideration of the dose–response rule as described above. This rule states that, for a given tumour and drug, the same dose of drug will kill the same fraction of *drug-sensitive* cells. In this regard, the results of the AFM randomized trial are consistent with fractional kill which is greater than that obtained with conventional-dose therapy. The disease-

free survival is significantly prolonged, possibly indicating that there was a greater effect of the high-dose therapy in the *failing* population. The interpretation of overall survival is more complicated in the AFM randomized trial, because *both* arms received the high-dose therapy, but on a different schedule, or more precisely at a strategically different time.

The key to interpreting the findings of these studies is a consideration of the Skipper rules *as modified by drug resistance in the inverse rule*. Fundamental to the interpretation of the inverse rule is the hypothesis that the presence of drug-resistant populations is directly related to the tumour stem-cell burden. Thus at the time of the application of high-dose therapy in either study at either time, there is a probability of the presence of drug-resistant populations (T/R in Skipper terminology) which will not be sensitive to even high-dose therapy. This T/R population limits the effectiveness of the treatment, which is reflective not of the effectiveness of the high-dose regimen on the sensitive population (the first interpretation of the inverse rule above) but rather of the limit on effectiveness resulting from the development of intrinsic resistance. Within the difference in tumour burden which occurs between complete and partial responses, the approach to eradication of the total tumour cell burden is limited not by the magnitude of the cell kill, but by the development of intrinsic resistance.

What might be the explanation for the longer overall survival in the patients who are treated with the strategy of induction therapy, observation and transplant at recurrence? Here the explanation is most easily understood by adding the time of observation to the effect of tumour cell kill. If the limitation to cure is the presence of resistant cells, the median duration of the survival curve will reflect the growth characteristics of the surviving population (presumably T/R). As shown in Figure 19.1, the regrowth characteristics of tumour stem-cell populations from a 'floor' of a T/R population would be expected to be similar and would therefore add to the overall survival by the amount of time added by the total cell kill of T/0 cells at whatever time it is applied.

In reality, the data suggest tumour growth characteristics that are consistent with a fraction of the patients (approximately 20%) who have not, at the time of high-dose treatment, developed a cell population resistant to the high-dose regimen. It also implies that the relative short interval between randomization to observation and recurrence (approximately 4 months) is not sufficient to change the total number of T/R cells in the host substantially. Of course, the *fraction* of T/R cells present will differ substantially between the arms, as the high-dose therapy will be expected to have killed a much larger fraction of the T/0 cells.

The above analysis is based on the number of T/R cells that remain essentially unchanged after induction therapy until the use of high-dose therapy on either arm. This could, of course, be incorrect, and the number of T/R cells might either increase or decrease. Assuming that the T/R

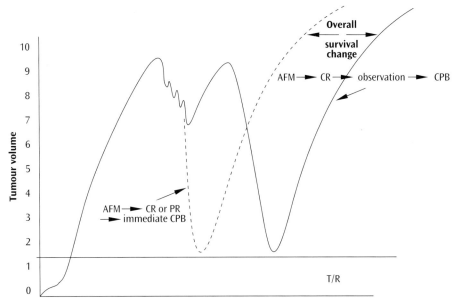

Figure 19.1 *Regrowth of tumour stem-cell populations after high-dose therapy administered at different times during the AFM Randomized Trial. Because of the limitation of total tumour cell kill by the presence of T/R cells, the regrowth of tumour populations from their minimal level after high-dose therapy is able to explain the difference in overall survival data. The results observed with the regrowth from the minimal level reached when patients with CR or a PR are transplanted are consistent with the data for overall survival. The longer overall survival after recurrence from observation is the result of the additional time that the patient has on observation. Other hypotheses to explain these observations are discussed in the text.*

cells are entirely unaffected by the induction therapy, they would continue to grow and perhaps develop additional resistance through spontaneous mutation. The longer the interval between induction therapy and the use of high-dose therapy, the greater the likelihood that this might occur. On the other hand, it is possible that the resistance characteristics of the tumour might favourably change due to reversal of the resistant phenotype. The basis for this hypothesis is that, although alkylating agents are effective anti-cancer agents in G_0 cells, they are more effective when the cells are cycling. It would not be unreasonable to expect that T/R cells might not be killed by induction therapy, but that their kinetic activity would be significantly affected due to sublethal drug injury. At this point these cells would be less sensitive to high-dose therapy if it was administered immediately. On the other hand, if there is a delay in administering high-dose therapy such that tumour cell repair occurs, followed by an increase in the kinetic activity of the tumour, the effectiveness of the same high-dose therapy would be improved because of the greater effectiveness of the alkylating agents in this tumour with a high growth fraction.

IMPLICATIONS FOR FUTURE TRIALS

These data raise important questions and suggest potentially significant opportunities in the application of high-dose therapy to breast cancer. The testing of high-dose therapy earlier in the natural history of breast cancer, such as the high-risk setting, is important, and considerations derived from the inverse rule and the dose–response relationship both indicate that this would be a better setting for improving the efficacy of the treatment. On the other hand, these studies and their interpretations raise questions about the appropriate timing of the high-dose therapy, and whether there is any role for the use of induction chemotherapy to affect the plateau seen after high-dose therapy. It is conceivable that the early and single use of high-dose therapy would allow maximization of the tumour cell kill and obviate any additive advantage of combination with conventional-dose therapy. The data do indicate that there will be a need for additional therapy to attempt to eliminate the residual tumour cell populations after high-dose therapy. Combining this approach with alternative strategies which utilize different mechanisms of tumour cell kill may prove to be very important.

ACKNOWLEDGEMENTS

The authors would like to acknowledge that the clinical study data from which these observations are derived were performed chiefly by colleagues at the Duke University Medical Center. The continuous support of our teams of nurses, support staff and physicians at our current transplant unit and in our previous centres is very much appreciated. We would also like to thank both

Howard Skipper and Larry Norton for their valuable discussions and creative ideas concerning high-dose therapy over the last 15 years.

REFERENCES

1 Peters W, Rosner G, Vredenburgh J *et al*. A prospective, randomized comparison of two doses of combination alkyating agents (AA) as consolidation after CAF in high-risk primary breast cancer involving ten or more axillary lymph nodes (LN): preliminary results of CALGB 9082/SWOG 9114/NCIC MA-13. *Proc ASCO* 1999; **18**.

2 Peters WP, Shpall EJ, Jones RB *et al*. High-dose combination alkylating agents with bone marrow support as initial treatment for metastatic breast cancer. *J Clin Oncol* 1988; **6**: 1368–76.

3 Peters WP, Ross M, Vredenburgh JJ *et al*. High-dose chemotherapy and autologous bone marrow support as consolidation after standard-dose adjuvant therapy for high-risk primary breast cancer. *J Clin Oncol* 1993; **11**: 1132–43.

4 Bezwoda WR, Seymour L, Dansey RD. High-dose chemotherapy with hematopoietic rescue as primary treatment for metastatic breast cancer: a randomized trial. *J Clin Oncol* 1995; **13**: 2483–9.

5 The Scandinavian Breast Cancer Study Group 9401. Results from a randomized adjuvant breast cancer study with high dose chemotherapy with CTC$_6$ supported by autologous bone marrow stem cells versus dose escalated and tailored FEC therapy. *Proc ASCO* 1999; **18**.

6 Stadtmaner EA, O'Neill A, Goldstein LJ *et al*. Phase III randomized trial of high-dose chemotherapy (HDC) and stem cell support (SCT) shows no difference in overall survival or severe toxicity compared to maintenance chemotherapy with cyclophosphamide, methotrexate and 5-fluorouracil (CMF) for women with metastatic breast cancer who are responding to conventional induction chemotherapy: the 'Philadelphia' Intergroup Study (PSI-1). *Proc ASCO* 1999; **18**.

7 Skipper HE. Adjuvant chemotherapy. *Cancer* 1978; **41**: 936–40.

8 Skipper HE, Schabel FM, Jay R, Wilcox WS. Experimental evaluation of antitumor agents: on the criteria and kinetics associated with curability of experimental leukemia. *Cancer Chemother Rep* 1964; **35**: 1–11.

9 Skipper HE, Schabel FM, Wilcox WS. Experimental evaluation of potential anticancer agents. XXI. Scheduling of arabinosyl cytosine to take advantage of its S-phase specificity against leukemic cells. *Cancer Chemother Rep* 1976; **51**: 125–32.

10 Goldie JH, Coldman J. Application of theoretical models to chemotherapy protocol design. *Cancer Treat Rep* 1966; **70**: 127–36.

11 Anderson KC. Hematologic complications and blood-bank support. In: Holland JF, Frei III E, Bast Jr RC *et al*. (eds) *Cancer medicine*, 4th edn. Baltimore, MD: Williams and Wilkins, 1997; 3155–78.

12 Hurd DD, Peters WP. Randomized, comparative study of high-dose (with autologous bone marrow support) versus low-dose cyclophosphamide, cisplatin, and carmustine as consolidation to adjuvant cyclophosphamide, doxorubicin, and fluorouracil for patients with operable stage II or III breast cancer involving 10 or more axillary lymph nodes (CALGB Protocol 9082). Cancer and Leukemia Group B. *J Natl Cancer Inst Monogr* 1995; 41–4.

13 Carter *et al*. *The Royal Society Medicine* 1999.

20

Adjuvant systemic chemotherapy – where do we go from here?

GIANNI BONADONNA AND PINUCCIA VALAGUSSA

INTRODUCTION

Breast cancer is a substantial public health problem throughout the Western industrialized world. Because of its high incidence, even small improvements in the efficacy of the treatment applied may represent tens of thousands of lives saved.

Up to approximately 30 years ago, treatment philosophy was dominated by the anatomical and mechanistic dogma of tumour cell dissemination first by direct extension into contiguous tissue and then, by an orderly progression through the lymphatic circulation, to the rest of the body.[1] It was only towards the end of the 1960s that a few clinical and laboratory findings challenged the Halstedian hypothesis, revealing that regional lymph nodes were of biological rather than anatomical importance.[2] It also became apparent that extensive local-regional treatment could possibly only achieve cure in a minority of patients, i.e. in women who were not harbouring micrometastases that already existed at the time of diagnosis in many breast cancer patients.

More important information was derived from the seminal studies conducted in experimental animal systems.[3,4] These studies highlighted the importance of drug dose and tumour cell burden, and suggested that micrometastatic foci could be more vulnerable to the effects of cell-cycle-specific agents.[5]

The golden age of adjuvant chemotherapy began in the early 1970s. The above-mentioned hypotheses were first tested through randomized clinical trials by the National Surgical Adjuvant Breast and Bowel Project (NSABP) and the Milan Cancer Institute. The NSABP study utilized single-agent chemotherapy with melphalan delivered for 2 years,[6] while the Milan study employed a multiple-drug regimen known as CMF (cyclophosphamide, methotrexate and fluorouracil) for 12 monthly cycles.[7] The early results of both trials, activated in patients with node-positive breast cancer, raised both hopes and innumerable controversies. Furthermore, they stimulated many research physicians to set up further prospective trials to confirm or rule out the validity of the multidisciplinary approach. It would serve no useful purpose here to summarize the many individual trials and their results. Rather, this chapter will attempt to describe how the strategic approach has been progressively changing over the years. Building on prior experience is important in the effort to improve further the control of high-risk breast cancer.

THE CMF LESSON

Long-term results

The recently published 20-year results of the first CMF adjuvant programme confirmed that the scientific principles underlying the clinical strategy were correct.[8] The positive effects of adjuvant chemotherapy in reducing the risk of disease relapse, which were mainly achieved during the first 3 years after surgery, were maintained throughout the subsequent years. In contrast to relapse-free survival, the total survival difference between CMF-treated and control patients progressively increased from the seventh year after surgery, and this beneficial effect persisted over the years. Overall, the benefit translated into a 34% reduction in the relative risk of relapse and a 26% reduction in the relative risk of death.

The results of the CMF programme confirmed the importance of nodal extent, for there was a consistent inverse relationship between the number of involved lymph nodes and treatment outcome (see Table 20.1). In this trial, the significant achievements in premenopausal women were not duplicated in postmenopausal patients. Many oncologists interpreted these results as meaning that the predominant effect of chemotherapy was due to an ovarian suppression-mediated mechanism, as many premenopausal women became amenorrhoeic (either temporarily or permanently) while on drug treatment. However, it is unlikely that all of the benefit obtained by chemotherapy in premenopausal patients is achieved through a hormonal mechanism in patients who have positive oestrogen or progesterone receptors. The Milan findings have always confirmed the lack of difference in treatment outcome between women with drug-induced amenorrhoea and those without it.[8] The recent international overview has also demonstrated a significant, albeit smaller, benefit of polychemotherapy in post-menopausal women.[9] Furthermore, the positive effects of CMF in node-negative and oestrogen-receptor-negative tumours further help to dispel the hypothesis that polychemotherapy and ablative endocrine therapy work through exactly the same mechanisms.

When the results of the first CMF study were analysed according to age groups (see Table 20.2) rather than menopausal status, it became evident that only women over 60 years of age failed to benefit from adjuvant CMF. In this latter subgroup, by trial design or protocol deviation, CMF included initial low doses and was often arbitrarily reduced during most cycles.[11] This important pharmacological aspect will be discussed later.

As mentioned previously, many similar studies with CMF-based regimens were activated in different countries during the late 1970s and, as also reported in the international overview,[9] they were able to achieve results comparable to those summarized above.

Table 20.2 Main therapeutic results from the first CMF adjuvant programme relative to age groups: data at 20 years

Age group	Relapse-free survival		Overall survival	
	Control group (%)	CMF group (%)	Control group (%)	CMF group (%)
< 40 years	14	30	14	39
40–49 years	24	31	28	45
50–59 years	23	38	30	39
≥60 years	24	22	17	20

Duration of adjuvant CMF

In June 1973, when the first CMF programme was initiated, we decided empirically to deliver this drug regimen for 12 monthly cycles, i.e. for 1 year. Although fairly well tolerated, this regimen was not devoid of side-effects, and a few of our patients refused to complete the planned programme. Consequently, in September 1975 we started a new prospective study with the aim of evaluating the possibility of reducing the treatment duration without compromising the therapeutic effects. The available 18-year results (see Figures 20.1 and 20.2) confirm both our initial observations[12] that 6 cycles of adjuvant CMF are as effective as the same regimen delivered for a longer time, as well as the reproducibility of treatment outcome in patients entered into two successive trials and who received 12 cycles of adjuvant CMF. Comparable findings have been reported by other investigators testing shorter vs. longer duration of CMF- or adriamycin-based combinations.[13–17] By contrast, one cycle of peri-operative chemotherapy (i.e. chemotherapy delivered soon after surgery) is definitely inferior to 6 cycles of post-operative chemotherapy.[18]

All of the above-reported findings allow speculation about drug resistance at a clinical level. Most probably a few cycles of effective combination chemotherapy delivered at full or near full doses are sufficient to kill most

Table 20.1 Main therapeutic results from the first CMF adjuvant programme: data at 20 years

	Relapse-free survival				Overall survival			
	Control group		CMF group		Control group		CMF group	
	%	Median (months)	%	Median (months)	%	Median (months)	%	Median (months)
Total*	25	40	32	83	23	104	34	137
Number of involved nodes								
1–3	29	63	37	144	24	131	38	174
>3	16	20	22	44	21	77	25	82
Menopausal status								
Premenopausal	26	32	37	141	24	96	37	180
Post-menopausal	24	59	26	64	22	128	22	113

* Adjusted relative risk: for relapse-free survival 0.65 (95% confidence intervals 0.51–0.83), P<0.001; for overall survival 0.76 (95% confidence intervals 0.60–0.97), P = 0.03.

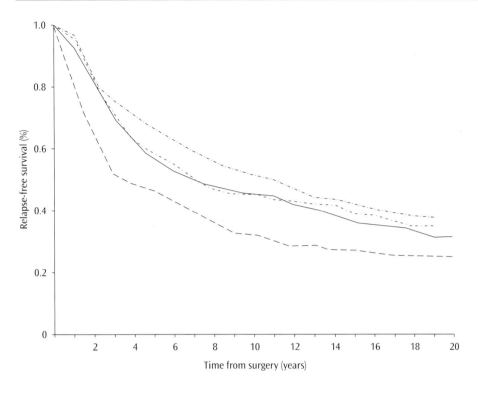

Figure 20.1 *Milan experience with CMF in two successive randomized studies comparing control (– – –) vs. standard CMF for 12 cycles (—) and standard CMF for 12 (— - - —) vs. 6 cycles (— -): relapse-free survival.*

(and sometimes all) drug-sensitive tumour cells, while early and late metastases are due to the overgrowth of primary resistant neoplastic cells. These considerations were instrumental in the design of subsequent trials. Practically, prolonged treatments (i.e. more than 4–6 cycles of the same regimen) are unable to achieve an additional effect, and are associated with an increased acute (and probably delayed) toxicity and increased financial costs.

Trials in node-negative tumours and the role of cyclophosphamide in the combination

The favourable effects of CMF-based adjuvant regimens were also confirmed in trials conducted in node-negative patients who had oestrogen-receptor-negative tumours.[10,19,20] The 12-year analysis of the study performed at the Milan Cancer Institute[10] reported that 71%

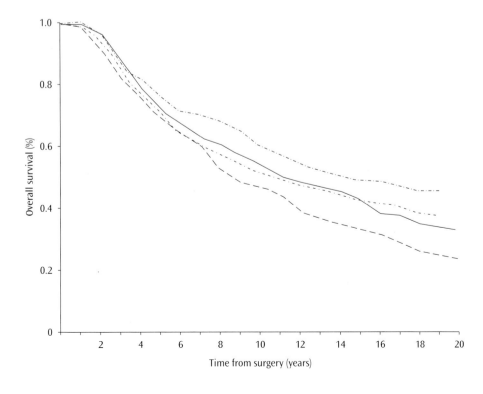

Figure 20.2 *Milan experience with CMF in two successive randomized studies comparing control (– – –) vs. standard CMF for 12 cycles (—) and standard CMF for 12 (— - - —) vs. 6 cycles (— -): overall survival.*

of patients given adjuvant CMF remained disease-free, compared to 48% of women in the control group (P=0.008). Similar results were obtained for total survival, and treatment outcome after CMF was unrelated to tumour size, grade and proliferative activity, or to menopausal status.

The first NSABP trial[19] delivered a sequential methotrexate and fluorouracil regimen (MF) instead of the CMF combination, on the assumption that this so-called 'high-risk' subgroup of patients should not be exposed to the risk of haematological malignancies that could result from the use of alkylating agents.[21] Initial findings indicated a significant improvement in disease-free survival for women treated with MF compared to those who received no systemic therapy. In October 1988, the NSABP implemented a new protocol to compare the merits of MF vs. conventional CMF. The recently published results,[22] while confirming on a longer follow-up the efficacy of MF compared to local-regional therapy alone, also reported that conventional CMF provided a significantly better (33%, P<0.001) overall disease-free survival over 5 years of follow-up than that observed after MF, and an overall survival advantage of borderline significance (20%, P=0.06). Despite a subgroup analysis which revealed that the absolute 5-year difference favouring CMF was higher in younger (84% vs. 72%, P<0.001) than in older women (80% vs. 74%, P=0.13), these results show that the addition of cyclophosphamide to MF is justifiable at the cost of a modest increase in acute toxicity.

The role of dose rate or dose intensity

The concept that dose is a critical factor in achieving higher cell kill by chemotherapy has long been recognized in animal models,[23] in which a small increase in drug dose results in a disproportionately large increase in tumour cell kill. Clinically, the interaction between tumour and drug(s) is much more complex. Dose response is in fact a property of tumour size, type, proliferative rate and genetic resistance, as well as the differential sensitivity of the normal and tumour cells to the effect of the drug(s). Therefore, in humans, attempts to define the optimal treatment have resulted in a plethora of schedules, combinations and schemes to reduce doses and delay treatments.

With regard to the adjuvant chemotherapy of breast cancer, only following the retrospective analysis of received doses of CMF conducted at the Milan Cancer Institute[11] was there an increasingly widespread interest in the subject of dose rate and intensity. Despite the limitations intrinsic to retrospective evaluations, it is worth mentioning that the 20-year analysis also confirmed the prognostic importance of received dose rate. Regardless of nodal extent and menopausal status, women receiving full or near full doses of the planned treatment fared sig-

nificantly better during the entire period of follow-up than patients receiving low-dose chemotherapy.[8] In this latter subgroup, the treatment effect was only transient compared to that for women in the control group. It is noteworthy that, despite reduced doses, these patients were not spared the acute toxicities associated with the administration of chemotherapy.

Dose intensity is a mathematical concept that was developed by Hryniuk and Levine[24] a few years after the Milan data were first published. It consists of the amount of drug delivered per unit time, and for a single-drug regimen it may be expressed simply as mg/m^2 of body surface per week, regardless of the schedule used. These authors reported that retrospective analysis of published data showed a highly significant relationship between projected dose intensity and 3-year relapse-free survival. Their results raised many controversies,[25] but although conclusions from data-derived results may be biased, it was evident that the findings of trials refuting the dose-intensity hypothesis included most of the case series given single-agent or low-dose combination chemotherapy.

Recently, a few prospective randomized studies of this subject have been undertaken. One CMF study, in which all three drugs were delivered intravenously every 3 weeks, was activated in advanced breast cancer. By halving the normally recommended doses for intravenous administration, Tannock et al. showed that the lower doses were unable to produce worthwhile therapeutic results in terms of objective remission rate.[26]

The other available data are derived from studies of adjuvant chemotherapy using anthracycline-containing regimens. The French Adjuvant Study Group has recently reported in abstract form the results from two consecutive prospective studies employing the fluorouracil, epirubicin and cyclophosphamide (FEC) regimen. In the first trial,[27] node-positive premenopausal women were allocated to receive the classical doses of the three drugs, with epirubicin at 50 mg/m^2, either for 6 or 3 cycles, whereas in the third arm 3 cycles of the combination were delivered, but the epirubicin dose was 75 mg/m^2. In the second trial,[28] the classical 6-cycle regimen was compared with a 3-cycle regimen where the dose of epirubicin was increased to 100 mg/m^2. The univariate analysis of the first trial failed to reveal any significant differences, but a multivariate analysis demonstrated a difference (P=0.031) favouring the classical 6-cycle regimen. By contrast, the 3-year analysis of the second trial showed that the 3-cycle arm with the increased dose of epirubicin gave an improved relapse-free survival (P=0.02) compared to the classical regimen.

The NSABP has conducted a prospective trial in which 2092 node-positive breast cancer patients were randomly assigned to receive a combination of adriamycin and cyclophosphamide (AC) with three different dose levels of the alkylating agent. Adriamycin was always administered at a dose of 60 mg/m^2 for 4 cycles, while the doses of cyclophosphamide were 600 mg/m^2 for 4 cycles vs. 1200 mg/m^2 for 2 cycles vs. 1200 mg/m^2 for 4 cycles, respectively. The 3-year analysis, reported in abstract form,[29] failed to detect a benefit from the higher doses of the alkylating agent.

In 1994, the Cancer and Leukemia Group B published the therapeutic results of a prospective study in which 1572 women were randomly allocated to receive three different dose levels for each of the three drugs (cyclophosphamide, adriamycin and fluorouracil) of the CAF regimen.[30] The low-dose arm represented half as much drug treatment as the high-dose arm, both schedules being delivered over a period of 4 months. The inter-mediate-dose arm delivered a reduced dose of the three drugs for each cycle, but for a 6-month period, and therefore the total amount of chemotherapy was the same as in the high-dose schedule. At 5 years, the low-dose arm yielded a significantly worse treatment outcome, in terms of both relapse-free and overall survival, than the other two arms. No statistically significant difference was found between the high- and intermediate-dose arm, but there was a trend favouring the high-dose arm.

Despite some inconsistencies in the above findings, overall the data suggest the possibility of a dose-intensity or dose-threshold effect for the drugs or drug regimens used. They confirm once again that clinical trials involve more complexity (i.e. features of patient eligibility criteria, drugs used and routes of administration and patient compliance) than any mathematical model may encompass and probably tolerate. The important lesson to be learned from these studies is that the doses of the drugs combined in an effective regimen should not be arbitrarily reduced. Not only does lowering the doses not prevent side-effects, but also, most importantly, final treatment outcomes are adversely affected.

Patterns of relapse after adjuvant chemotherapy

Whether the main effect of adjuvant chemotherapy consists of the reduction of new disease manifestations in either local-regional or distant sites, or in both, is still a matter of controversy. Despite a description of the sites of first disease relapse, summarized in some published reports, evaluations using appropriate methods and showing relapse site-specific incidence over time are still scarce. Indeed, these informative analyses can be instrumental in the design of new and more effective adjuvant regimens.

The 20-year analysis of the first CMF programme revealed that there were no important differences between the two treatment groups in the incidence of local-regional relapses.[8] Although only moderate, the main therapeutic effect of adjuvant CMF was to suppress distant micrometastases, regardless of their anatomical sites. The results reported by the International (Ludwig)

Breast Cancer Study Group (IBCSG) are quite dissimilar.[31] These investigators grouped together the findings from different prospective studies and subdivided their regimens into two categories, namely more vs. less effective systemic treatment. The more effective treatment consisted of prolonged CMF-based regimens or tamoxifen for 1 year, while the less effective treatment included patients given one cycle of peri-operative CMF or no adjuvant systemic therapy. In contrast to the Milan findings, the IBCSG experience failed to detect any effect in bone and visceral dominant sites of disease recurrence, and the efficacy of the more effective treatment was apparently limited to a dramatic reduction of soft tissue relapses (from 36% to 18%).

These findings merit a number of comments. First, the more effective IBCSG regimen included tamoxifen therapy for many patients, and it is well known that this anti-oestrogen can significantly decrease the incidence of both local-regional recurrences and contralateral breast cancers.[32] Secondly, the incidence of soft tissue relapses as first and isolated manifestation of disease relapse is strikingly high in the less effective treatment (36% at 10 years), and is double that for the same type of relapses detected in the control group of the Milan Cancer Institute (18% at 10 years). Another issue of concern in the experience of the IBCSG is the high incidence of bone metastases in patients treated with CMF plus low-dose prednisone (17%), compared to patients in whom the latter drug was not administered (8%, $P=0.004$). As chronic treatment with prednisone is known to enhance bone absorption and to interfere with bone repair, the authors proposed a theoretical mechanism for the enhancement of tumour growth in the bone possibly caused by the steroid.[33] Whatever the mechanism underlying this effect, this information about a higher risk of osseous metastases in CMF-treated patients warrants careful consideration because bone is a not infrequent site of disease relapse in breast cancer patients.

NEWER STRATEGIES

Once it became evident that adjuvant CMF, or its variants, significantly affected treatment outcome compared to local-regional therapy alone, many research centres designed new prospective randomized studies in an attempt to improve therapeutic results further. Other classes of putatively more effective growth-inhibiting compounds were introduced into the adjuvant regimens. Alternatively, adjuvant chemotherapy and hormonal therapy were delivered simultaneously.

Anthracycline-containing combinations

Anthracyclines (i.e. adriamycin and epirubicin) are among the most effective agents for the treatment of metastatic breast cancer.[34] Adriamycin was first introduced in the adjuvant setting in 1973 when the MD Anderson Institute in Houston activated a prospective non-randomized study in node-positive patients.[35] In addition to its high efficacy, the inclusion of this antibiotic was justified by the limited incidence of congestive heart failure when cumulative doses were less than 400 mg/m^2 of body surface. Several prospective trials were then activated comparing anthracycline-containing and non-anthracycline-containing regimens. As is shown in Table 20.3, consistent evidence for the superiority of the anthracycline combinations was not obtained.

There are several possible explanations for the inconsistencies in treatment outcome. The majority of the studies integrated the anthracycline into a classical combination regimen in which all of the drugs are usually given simultaneously and recycled over time to allow haematological recovery. To avoid overlapping toxicity from the different drugs used in a combination, a compromise in the dose of each single agent is necessary, thus resulting in a dose level that is lower than its permissible single-agent dose. Both retrospective[24] and prospective[30] evaluations have demonstrated that adriamycin is capable of exhibiting a rising dose–response relationship within the usual dose range. It is plausible that the lack of a clear advantage for the anthracycline regimens may, at least in a few studies, be ascribed to the suboptimal dose of these agents when integrated in a combination of drugs.

Two of the studies reported in Table 20.3 deserve extra mention. One of the largest modern studies conducted by the NSABP group in node-positive patients compared adriamycin and cyclophosphamide (AC) for 4 cycles with standard CMF for 6 monthly cycles.[40] The two regimens had a similar treatment outcome, but the AC regimen was preferred by patients and nurses alike because of its shorter duration and a reported better tolerance, even if total alopecia was more frequent with adriamycin than with CMF. Another recent study compared dose-intensive cyclophosphamide, epirubicin and fluorouracil (CEF) with CMF in premenopausal women with node-positive breast cancer.[41] After a median follow-up of 37 months, an improved relapse-free survival was reported for CEF-treated patients (71% vs. 62%, $P=0.05$), while survival rates were superimposable in both treatment arms. A troublesome finding in this study was the occurrence of 4 cases of secondary leukaemia, all documented in the epirubicin group and within a median period of 18 months after entry to the study. The fact that alkylating agents can induce acute leukaemia, especially when combined with radiation therapy, has long been recognized.[21] More recently, topoisomerase II inhibitors have also been reported to potentially induce secondary leukaemia, usually with a typical 11q23 translocation.

Simultaneous administration of chemotherapy and hormone therapy

About half of the individual trials which compared the combined administration of both modalities with the delivery of either modality alone have shown an added benefit in relapse-free survival with the use of combined treatment, but a significant benefit in overall survival was only observed in a few trials.

The international overview suggested that the addition of tamoxifen to standard chemotherapy provided an increased benefit for patients aged 50 years and older.[9]

Table 20.3 *Representative randomized studies comparing anthracycline-containing vs. non-anthracycline-containing regimens in the adjuvant therapy of breast cancer*

First author of study	Systemic treatments	Total number of patients	Follow-up period (months)	Comments
Misset[36]	AVCF vs. CMF	249	120	AVCF significantly superior for both relapse-free and overall survival
Fisher[37]	PAF ± T vs. PF ± T	1790	88	PAF significantly superior to PF in terms of relapse-free survival. No significant difference between PAFT and PFT
Carpenter[38]	CAF vs. CMF	528	60	No difference in treatment outcome
Marty[39]	FEC vs. CMF	716	54	Two different schedules of both regimens. No difference in treatment outcome
Fisher[40]	AC vs. CMF	1473	44	No difference in treatment outcome, but AC preferred for its shorter duration
Levine[41]	Intensive CEF vs. CMF	710	37	CEF significantly superior in terms of relapse-free survival. Four cases of leukaemia detected in the CEF regimen

A, adriamycin; V, vincristine; C, cyclophosphamide; F, fluorouracil; M, methotrexate; P, melphalan; T, tamoxifen; E, epirubicin.

Similar comparisons for younger women have failed in the past to demonstrate any significant improvement when the endocrine treatment was represented by tamoxifen. When the hormonal manipulation consisted of ovarian ablation, an added benefit was observed, but the standard deviation associated with the reported results was relatively high, and thus no firm conclusions could be drawn. It is worth mentioning that the overview findings were derived from indirect comparisons, and the weight that can be given to such comparisons is a matter of controversy.

The NSABP has recently published the results of a trial which compared tamoxifen alone with tamoxifen plus CMF or MF chemotherapy in patients with axillary lymph-node-negative and oestrogen-receptor-positive primary breast cancer.[42] Through 5 years of follow-up, chemotherapy plus tamoxifen results in significantly better disease-free survival than tamoxifen alone (P=0.002). There was a 35% reduction in the event rate for women who received CMF plus tamoxifen, and a 28% reduction for women who were given MF plus tamoxifen. A similar benefit was observed in both distant disease-free survival and total survival. The risk of treatment failure was reduced regardless of tumour size, tumour oestrogen or progesterone receptor level, or patient age. However, the reduction was greatest in patients aged 49 years or less.

In view of the heterogeneity of steroid receptors, the combined treatment with hormone manipulations and cytotoxic drugs seems rational. However, the concomitant administration of both modalities may indeed result in an antagonistic effect due to their specific mode of action.[43] One reasonable basis for this antagonism is that anti-oestrogens are probably cytostatic for cancer cells, whereas certain chemotherapy agents are cell-cycle active and thus require DNA synthesis to exert their maximum effect. It is possible that a definite improvement in treatment outcome may be achieved by delivering the two modalities sequentially rather than concurrently. Therefore adjuvant treatment should start with chemotherapy, which would affect fast-growing receptor-poor cells, and should be followed by prolonged administration of endocrine therapy (e.g. tamoxifen), to keep in check the relatively slower-growing receptor-rich cells.

Sequential non-cross-resistant chemotherapy

In an attempt to circumvent, at least in part, the phenomenon of primary drug resistance, an alternative to the simultaneous administration of various agents in a single combination is to deliver them in sequences of drug regimens.

Two adjuvant trials were designed in the early 1980s at the Milan Cancer Institute. Due to the clinical non-cross-resistance of CMF and adriamycin (ADM), the

sequential administration of these two regimens was tested in two different patient subsets. To avoid non-compliance with oral cyclophosphamide,[11] all of the three drugs in the CMF regimen were administered intravenously and recycled every 21 days, whereas ADM, when included, was always given intravenously as a single agent at a dose of 75 mg/m² every 21 days and for four administrations.[44,45]

In women with 1 to 3 positive nodes, the aim of the study was to assess whether ADM was able to overcome drug resistance possibly induced by a 6-month treatment with CMF.[12] Therefore, we elected to deliver 12 courses of the intravenous 3-weekly CMF regimen, i.e. to deliver a total amount of the three drugs comparable to that administered with standard CMF over 6 months, and to compare it with 8 courses of the same combination followed by 4 courses of adriamycin. The 10-year analysis (see Table 20.4) confirmed our previous finding of the inability of adriamycin, delivered after CMF, to improve treatment outcome.[44] It is worth noting that the adequate delivery of full or near full doses of chemotherapy regardless of patient age, failed to affect treatment outcome between pre- and post-menopausal women.

In patients with more than 3 positive nodes, we elected to test randomly the sequential delivery of adriamycin given before CMF (ADM→CMF) vs. its administration alternated after every two courses of CMF (CMF/ADM). Table 20.4 also summarizes the most relevant results of this trial, which confirmed the superiority of the sequential ADM→CMF regimen compared to the alternating CMF/ADM regimen (relapse-free survival, P=0.002; overall survival, P=0.002), and to the administration of standard CMF.[45] With the only variation being the sequence of drug delivery, the median duration of relapse-free survival was almost doubled after sequential ADM→CMF (86 months) compared to CMF/ADM (47 months).

The contrasting results achieved in the two different trials when both ADM and CMF were delivered merit a

Table 20.4 *Main therapeutic results in two different studies exploring the role of non-cross-resistant regimens and comparison with the first CMF programme; data at 10 years*

	Relapse-free survival (%)	Overall survival (%)
Nodes 1 to 3		
Control vs.	38	52
CMF × 12	53	62
CMF iv vs.	59	75
CMF → ADM	57	75
Nodes > 3		
Control vs.	18	32
CMF × 12	29	43
ADM → CMF vs.	42	58
CMF/ADM	28	44

number of comments. Overall, treatment duration, total drug dose and total received dose intensity were superimposable in the three regimens. The total treatment duration required was 33 weeks. However, in one regimen the four cycles of anthracycline were administered after 24 weeks of CMF, in the alternating plan they were spread over 27 weeks, and in the remaining regimen the four cycles were administered within the first 9 weeks of treatment. Thus in the sequential ADM→CMF regimen the dose intensity of the anthracycline administration, i.e. its administration at full dose and on time at the start of the regimen, was significantly increased and by itself could account for the superiority of the treatment outcome. These observations confirm that the type of drug sequence is important, and further studies on this topic could provide more biological insights into the design of optimal regimens in the adjuvant treatment of breast cancer.

Use of haematopoietic growth factors in conventional chemotherapy

As mentioned previously, both prospective trials[30] and retrospective analyses[11, 24] have confirmed that dose is an important variable in treatment outcome.

In conventional regimens, myelosuppression is the most important factor limiting either the delivery of higher doses of some drugs or the possibility of shortening the intervals between treatment cycles. The recent introduction into clinical practice of some haematopoietic colony-stimulating growth factors (CSFs) has been shown to be able to reduce the haematological toxicity of some of the standard drug regimens. Consequently, CSFs have been used in pilot studies of conventional adjuvant chemotherapy to test the feasibility of higher-dose-intensity regimens. The majority of these trials, most of which have only been published in abstract form, reported that these dose-intense regimens were feasible and devoid of major toxicities. However, no therapeutic results are yet available which demonstrate that these dose-intense regimens can indeed improve treatment outcome over full-dose standard polychemotherapy. Of note, the results obtained with non-cross-resistant regimens have shown that the complexities inherent to the delivery of chemotherapy are not simply related to the total amount of drugs or to their intensity per week of treatment. Consequently, in current clinical practice CSFs must be delivered only following the recommendations of the American Society of Clinical Oncology.[46]

High-dose chemotherapy

A substantial increase in chemotherapy dose clearly requires more supportive care than only the administration of CSFs. Early experience with high-dose chemotherapy and autologous bone-marrow transplantation has raised the hope that this treatment modality could improve treatment outcome over standard conventional chemotherapy. Recently, the introduction of CSFs to harvest circulating haematopoietic stem cells for auto-transplantation has greatly increased the feasibility of high-dose therapy and reduced the risk involved.[47]

A number of relatively small non-randomized trials have been published which suggest that high-dose therapy with bone-marrow support may be superior to conventional treatment. The topic of high-dose chemotherapy has been extensively discussed in the preceding chapter by Peters and Dansey. We therefore only wish to summarize briefly two of the non-randomized studies. The largest and most publicized one is the study by Peters et al.[48] In patients presenting with 10 or more positive axillary nodes, four cycles of the classical CAF regimen were delivered as initial treatment. Subsequently, 85 women who were in clinical complete remission received one cycle of high-dose CPB (cyclophosphamide, cisplatin and BCNU) with autologous bone-marrow support. After a median follow-up of 2.5 years, the event-free survival rate was 72%, significantly superior to that of a matched control group (43%). The toxicity was substantial, with a fairly high rate of toxic deaths (12%).

A different strategy was adopted by Gianni et al. in the treatment of a similar patient subset.[49] A total of 67 women under the age of 56 years were entered into a protocol which utilized high-dose cyclophosphamide, vincristine with high-dose methotrexate, cisplatin and high-dose melphalan. The treatment programme was initiated within 4 weeks after surgery, and all of the drugs were administered sequentially within a period of 8 weeks. Circulating progenitor cells, which were harvested following the delivery of high-dose chemotherapy and GM-CSF, were reinfused at the end of the chemotherapy programme. At 5 years after surgery, the relapse-free and overall survival rates were 57% and 70%, respectively, and both rates were superior to those observed in a similar patient subgroup, i.e. with ≥ 10 positive nodes and aged < 56 years, treated with the sequential ADM→CMF regimen (40% and 60%, respectively) in a previous prospective randomized study.[45]

Some investigators have argued that the favourable results obtained so far with high-dose chemotherapy can be largely ascribed to the selection criteria[50] and additional staging tests, such as bone-marrow examinations and CT scan of brain and liver, currently in use in many high-dose protocols, and which led to exclusion of 25% of otherwise eligible patients.[51] Although this cannot be denied altogether, it is worth mentioning that this was not the case for the study conducted at the Milan Cancer Institute, where both the patients entered into the high-dose protocol[49] and those entered into the conventional regimen[45] underwent the same staging tests. Clearly, the issue of the value of the high-dose regimens can only be answered by the results of the prospective randomized studies that are currently ongoing in a number of different countries.

SEQUENCES OF LOCAL-REGIONAL AND SYSTEMIC THERAPY

Sequencing of radiation therapy and chemotherapy

Data from animal models suggest that early initiation of adjuvant chemotherapy is important in order to achieve optimal therapeutic results. In the majority of clinical trials, adjuvant chemotherapy was planned to start within 4 to 6 weeks after surgery. One large prospective trial was designed by the IBCSG investigators to assess whether the earlier initiation of adjuvant CMF could improve treatment outcome.[18] Patients were randomly allocated to receive either one cycle of intravenous CMF immediately after operation (peri-operative chemotherapy), or no immediate adjuvant systemic therapy. On confirmation of pathological involvement of the axillary nodes, patients were allocated to either a single cycle of chemotherapy (already applied), or conventionally timed cycles of standard CMF, or to both peri-operative and conventionally timed chemotherapy. Although limiting the administration of chemotherapy to a single cycle resulted in a significantly inferior treatment outcome, no advantage of the earlier initiation of adjuvant CMF over conventionally timed chemotherapy with the same regimen was detected.

Very little information is currently available about the efficacy of adjuvant chemotherapy when started beyond the conventional 6 weeks after surgery. This is an important issue in view of the fact that many more patients are now being treated with conserving surgery and post-operative irradiation. Should patients who are candidates for adjuvant chemotherapy be treated concurrently with post-operative irradiation, or should chemotherapy be delivered before or after irradiation? This issue is of considerable importance, as local-regional radiotherapy delivered concurrently with or before chemotherapy can adversely affect the administration of optimal doses of growth-inhibiting compounds and consequently reduce the beneficial effects of drug treatment against distant micrometastases.

Conflicting results were reported by different investigators who retrospectively reviewed their experiences with regard to the appropriate timing of adjuvant chemotherapy and irradiation. Recently, Recht et al. reported the results of a 5-year analysis of a prospective trial in 244 women at substantial risk of distant micrometastases.[52] Following breast-conserving surgery, patients were randomly assigned to receive a 12-week course of chemotherapy either before or after radiation therapy. Overall, treatment outcome did not differ significantly between the two treatment groups. A higher risk of local recurrence was detected in the chemotherapy-first group (14% vs. 5%), whereas a higher risk of distant metastases was documented in the radiotherapy-first group (32% vs. 20%), the difference in the pattern of first site of disease relapse being of borderline statistical significance (P=0.07). Of note, overall survival favoured the chemotherapy-first group (81% vs. 73%, P=0.11). Another important finding of this prospective trial was a significant difference (P<0.01) in the median dose of chemotherapy delivered, which was lower in the radiotherapy-first group.

The results of this study cannot be extrapolated to other regimens, especially those requiring 6 months or longer to complete the chemotherapy programme. Furthermore, a cause for concern in the appropriate sequence of chemotherapy and radiotherapy is the growing use, in an adjuvant setting, of full doses of powerful drugs, such as adriamycin and paclitaxel, which could have an undesirable toxic effect when delivered concomitantly with or immediately after irradiation.

Two recently published trials merit some comments on the role of post-operative irradiation as an adjuvant to chemotherapy. These studies concluded that adjuvant radiotherapy and chemotherapy given to high-risk pre-menopausal women who had undergone mastectomy significantly decrease the rate of disease relapse,[53] and also reduce mortality compared to adjuvant chemotherapy alone.[54] However, it is worth emphasizing that the adjuvant regimen delivered (i.e. intravenous CMF for eight courses every 4 or 3 weeks) is associated with a low dose intensity. In fact, in our experience, when CMF was administered with a higher cumulative dose of the three drugs in two different programmes,[8,55] results similar to those obtained with the addition of classical post-operative irradiation were achieved with chemotherapy alone (see Table 20.5). In addition, after radical mastectomy plus full axillary dissection, the rate of loco-regional recurrences was only 12% in the Milan study,[8] compared to rates of 26% and 25% reported in the Danish[53] and Canadian[54] trials, respectively, where axillary dissection was limited to one or more level I and II lymph nodes. Once more, the optimal delivery of adjuvant chemotherapy associated with optimal removal of involved nodes was able to influence treatment outcome favourably.

Sequencing of surgery and chemotherapy

The possibility that in high-risk subsets surgery may not be the correct form of primary therapy stimulated a few medical oncologists to initiate treatment with drugs rather than with a local-regional modality. The first attempts with primary (neoadjuvant, pre-operative, pre-irradiation) chemotherapy arose from the need to achieve, in locally advanced breast cancer, prompt tumour response using only a few chemotherapy cycles to facilitate the delivery of either mastectomy or radiotherapy, or both modalities.[56,57] Following the initially promising results, the concept of primary chemotherapy

Table 20.5 *Ten-year results with adjuvant CMF in four different series of high-risk premenopausal patients*

First author of study	Schedule	Relapse-free survival (%)		Overall survival (%)	
		CMF	CMF+RT	CMF	CMF+RT
All patients					
Bonadonna[8]	Classical 12-monthly cycles	51	—	60	—
Overgaard[53]	IV q 4 weeks for 8 courses	34	48	45	54
Ragaz[54]	IV q 3 weeks for 8 courses	41	56	54	64
Nodes 1 to 3					
Bonadonna[55]	IV q 3 weeks for 12 courses	60	—	75	—
Overgaard[53]	IV q 4 weeks for 8 courses	39	54	54	62

RT, classical post-operative radiotherapy to all lymph-node-bearing areas.

was introduced in the treatment of large but resectable breast cancers.

The use of chemotherapy before surgery is supported by important laboratory observations which show that, in many animal models, the presence of a primary malignancy inhibits metastatic cell proliferation, while removal of the primary neoplasm accelerates metastatic cell proliferation. Non-curative surgical cytoreduction is combined with increased proliferation of the remaining tumour cells.[58] Briefly, the consequences of non-curative tumour removal are a measurable increase in the proliferation of the remaining malignant cells. It should be noted that pre-operative chemotherapy prevents this increase. The formal identification of the biological and biochemical mechanisms underlying these observations has not yet been clarified.

Recent studies on angiogenesis and its regulation have implicated the control of neovascularization as a major determinant of tumour cell apoptosis and consequently of tumour growth.[59] In particular, it has been proposed that the disappearance of circulating angiogenesis inhibitors, as a result of primary tumour removal, could account for metastatic development. These observations call for a profound reconsideration of the basic strategy of combined-modality treatment of breast cancer. The most important aspect is the definition of the 'optimal' timing of surgery and other local-regional forms of therapy in relation to the long-term goal of improving treatment outcome. The early and non-curative removal of primary tumour as performed in adjuvant chemotherapy programmes could be somewhat detrimental to curability. Chemotherapy before surgery should then be aimed at attempting to eradicate micrometastases while decreasing and eventually eliminating the primary tumour burden.

Two recent review articles have summarized the most pertinent data obtained by several research groups with various primary drug regimens.[56,57] Briefly, despite the heterogeneity of patient selection and evaluation, as well as the type of drugs and doses utilized, the findings of a few prospective randomized studies showed that the relapse-free and overall survival rates were similar, if not superior, to those achieved after conventional post-operative chemotherapy. Another positive effect of primary chemotherapy was its ability to achieve breast conservation rates in the range 62–87%. The data from the two large studies initiated at the Milan Cancer Institute clearly indicated that various drug regimens, given at full dose, could induce prompt tumour shrinkage which allowed limited breast surgery such as quadrantectomy plus complete axillary dissection.[60] In addition, and more importantly, prognosis was related to the degree of tumour response, and 86% of the patients who achieved pathological complete remission remained alive and disease-free at the 8-year analysis, compared to a lower relapse-free survival rate in women who showed only a partial or no objective response after primary chemotherapy ($P=0.034$). Similar results have also been obtained in the large NSABP study in which patients were randomized to receive 4 cycles of adriamycin plus cyclophosphamide either before or after surgery.[61] The lesson is clear – primary chemotherapy should include a full-dose regimen of the most effective drugs in order to facilitate the achievement of pathological complete remission which appears to represent a marker of treatment outcome.

WHERE DO WE GO FROM HERE?

The clinical experience amassed over the past quarter of a century (i.e. after the beginning of modern trials with systemic adjuvant therapy) has been considerable and fruitful. In recent years, new cytotoxic drugs, namely taxanes (paclitaxel and docetaxel) and vinorelbine, have proved to be very effective in overt metastatic disease, even when patients have been previously treated with anthracyclines.[62–64]

Paclitaxel has been tested by numerous institutions world-wide, and as a single agent it can induce objective responses in approximately 40% of patients who are refractory to the anthracyclines. The most impressive results have been achieved when paclitaxel was combined with adriamycin in previously untreated patients. In a recent study at the Milan Cancer Institute,[65] the combination of these two agents has achieved a rate of partial and complete responses (94% overall and 41% complete rate) that ranks this combination in the same range of anti-tumour activity that is observed with high-dose or high-intensity chemotherapy regimens for metastatic breast cancer. The combination entails an increased risk of cardiac toxicity when the cumulative dose of adriamycin approximates 480 mg/m^2. However, no instances of congestive heart failure were observed when the cumulative dose of anthracycline was limited to 300 mg/m^2.

Docetaxel appears to be as effective as paclitaxel. However, further studies are mandatory to assess objectively the cost–benefit ratio of this drug, which is often associated with skin toxicity and fluid retention.[63] Vinorelbine appears to be as effective as both taxanes, but its minimal non-haematological toxicity probably makes this drug easier to administer.[64]

One of the priorities in the next few years should therefore involve the incorporation of these new drugs into innovative combination regimens. The association of the 'best' drugs can yield exciting new results which may greatly exceed the potential risk of acute and delayed iatrogenic morbidities. Indeed, major research centres (e.g. Intergroup, NSABP and the Milan Cancer Institute) have already activated co-operative randomized studies including taxanes.[55] In fact, building on treatment efficacy appears to be a more fruitful strategy than wasting years (as in the past for adriamycin) dissecting side-effects.

Another future possibility is the use of factors that are predictive of treatment response. Retrospective analyses have reported that c-erbB-2 expression can predict response to specific types of drugs, such as methotrexate,[66] adriamycin[67] and paclitaxel.[68,69] Investigators from the IBCSG have observed that methotrexate-containing adjuvant chemotherapy was more effective in patients with c-erbB-2-negative tumours than in women whose tumours over-expressed this oncogene.[66] By contrast, investigators from the Cancer and Leukemia Group B found that higher doses of an adriamycin-containing regimen were more effective than lower doses in c-erbB-2-positive tumours, but no effect of the dose intensity was apparent in tumours that did not express this oncogene.[67] In a series of 49 patients with advanced breast cancer who were treated with different doses and schedules of paclitaxel by 3-hr infusion and doxorubicin, a significantly higher rate of complete responses was documented in c-erbB-2-positive tumours (50%) than in negative tumours (17%, $P = 0.014$), and this was irrespective of other prognostic factors such as visceral metastases and the number of lesions.[69] Although intriguing, the above-mentioned findings, as well as preliminary reports on the potential ability of p-53 and other molecular factors to predict responsiveness to treatment, still require confirmation and validation

through well-designed prospective studies. No less important, for the majority of these variables standardization of laboratory techniques and appropriate definition of cut-off values are mandatory if the results are to be reproducible among different case series. Should these caveats be overcome and well-designed and large prospective studies confirm the results of retrospective analyses, then we shall be able to offer a type of 'individualized' treatment to patients who are candidates for adjuvant or primary chemotherapy.

At present, novel therapies involving the use of growth factors, monoclonal antibodies and angiogenetic inhibitors are still in their infancy, and require accurate testing in rigorous clinical trials in patients with advanced breast cancer.

It is quite possible that high-dose chemotherapy with haematopoietic support may prove to be superior to current conventional adjuvant chemotherapy. Optimization of the dose–response effect, the use of sequential non-cross-resistant agents, a shortened duration of treatment (approximately 8 weeks), the possibility of administering most of the treatment phases in an out-patient clinic, as well as the dramatic reduction in the previously reported incidence of iatrogenic fatalities (now in the range 0–2%), all represent important aspects. Should treatments utilizing high-dose sequential chemotherapy emerge as a superior adjuvant modality in the ongoing randomized trials, the findings will disclose an entirely new avenue of clinical research.

The topic of primary chemotherapy also merits more attention. As preliminary findings have revealed that the degree of primary tumour response is most probably a simple and useful marker of outcome,[60,61] future innovative studies should be aimed at increasing the rate of pathological complete (or near-complete) remission through well-designed and well-executed effective drug regimens similar to those mentioned earlier for the classical post-operative treatment. In women who achieve complete or almost complete tumour disappearance at radiological examinations and/or fine-needle aspiration, appropriate controlled studies should subsequently define whether breast surgery could be replaced by breast irradiation. In the remaining patients who show substantial tumour shrinkage on completion of the chemotherapy programme, breast-conserving surgery will probably remain a necessary procedure.

In conclusion, clinical research in this area remains fruitful and interesting, and in the years to come we shall learn how to better integrate and use the various treatment modalities (surgery, irradiation, chemotherapy and endocrine treatment) in an attempt to further decrease tumour mortality in operable breast cancer.

In the early 1970s, treatment of patients who were free of clinically detectable metastase with adjuvant systemic chemotherapy, because some of them might develop distant disease in the future, was a revolutionary departure from the previous treatment strategy. Both laboratory and clinical results provided biological and therapeutic models that became very helpful in developing contemporary multidisciplinary strategy and more effective poly-drug regimens. It is now time to conceive a more radical departure from the old dogma that resectable tumours must always be excised as the first therapeutic approach. As a result of the availability of better tools and properly conducted trials, medical treatment has assumed a more central role in the treatment of breast cancer. Innovative strategies aimed at increasing the cell kill of distant micrometastases should help further crossing of the boundaries of medical compartments so that local-regional therapy can aid systemic treatment in achieving curability.

REFERENCES

1 Fisher B. Personal contributions to progress in breast cancer research and treatment. *Seminars in Oncology* 1996; **23**: 414–27.

2 Fisher B, Fisher ER. The interrelationship of hematogenous and lymphatic tumor cell dissemination. *Surgery, Gynecology and Obstetrics* 1966; **122**: 791–8.

3 Martin DS, Fugman RA, Stolfi RL, Hayworth PE. Solid tumor animal model therapeutically predictive for human breast cancer. *Cancer Chemotherapy Reports* 1975; **5**: 89–109.

4 Skipper HE, Schabel FM Jr. Tumor stem cell heterogeneity: implication with respect to the classification of cancers by chemotherapeutic effect. *Cancer Treatment Reports* 1984; **68**: 43–61.

5 Schabel FM, Griswold DP, Corbett TH *et al.* Increasing the therapeutic response rates to anticancer drugs by applying the basic principles of pharmacology. *Cancer* 1984; **54**: 1160–7.

6 Fisher B, Carbone P, Economou SG *et al.* L–Phenylalanine mustard (L-PAM) in the management of primary breast cancer: a report of early findings. *New England Journal of Medicine* 1975; **292**: 117–22.

7 Bonadonna G, Brusamolino E, Valagussa P *et al.* Combination chemotherapy as an adjuvant treatment in operable breast cancer. *New England Journal of Medicine* 1976; **294**: 405–10.

8 Bonadonna G, Valagussa P, Moliterni A *et al.* Adjuvant cyclophosphamide, methotrexate, and fluorouracil in node-positive breast cancer. The results of 20 years of follow-up. *New England Journal of Medicine* 1995; **332**: 901–6.

9 Early Breast Cancer Trialists' Collaborative Group. Systemic treatment of early breast cancer by hormonal, cytotoxic, or immune therapy. 133 randomised trials involving 31 000 recurrences and 24 000 deaths among 75 000 women. *Lancet* 1992; **339**: 1–15, 71–85.

10 Zambetti M, Valagussa P, Bonadonna G. Adjuvant cyclophosphamide, methotrexate and fluorouracil in node-negative and estrogen-receptor-negative breast cancer. Updated results. *Annals of Oncology* 1996; **7**: 481–5.

11 Bonadonna G, Valagussa P. Dose–response effect of adjuvant chemotherapy in breast cancer. *New England Journal of Medicine* 1981; **304**: 10–15.

12 Tancini G, Bonadonna G, Valagussa P *et al.* Adjuvant CMF in breast cancer: comparative 5-year results of 12 versus 6 cycles. *Journal of Clinical Oncology* 1983; **1**: 2–10.

13 Velez-Garcia E, Moore M, Vogel CL *et al.* Postmastectomy adjuvant chemotherapy with or without radiation therapy in women with operable breast cancer and positive axillary lymph nodes. The Southeastern Cancer Study Group experience. *Breast Cancer Research and Treatment* 1983; **3 (Supplement 1)**: 49–60.

14 Jungi WF, Alberto P, Brunner KW *et al.* Short- or long-term chemotherapy for node-positive breast cancer. LMF 6 versus 18 cycles: SAKK study 27/76. *Recent Results in Cancer Research* 1984; **96**: 175–7.

15 Henderson IC, Gelman RS, Harris JR, Canellos GP. Duration of therapy in adjuvant chemotherapy trial. *National Cancer Institute Monograph* 1986; **1**: 95–8.

16 Falkson HC, Gray R, Wolberg WH *et al.* Adjuvant trial of 12 cycles of CMFPT followed by observation or continuous tamoxifen versus four cycles of CMFPT in postmenopausal women with breast cancer. An Eastern Cooperative Oncology Group phase III study. *Journal of Clinical Oncology* 1990; **8**: 599–607.

17 Rivkin SE, Green S, Metch B *et al.* One versus 2 years of CMFVP adjuvant chemotherapy in axillary node-positive and estrogen-receptor-negative patients. A Southwest Oncology Group study. *Journal of Clinical Oncology* 1993; **11**; 1710–16.

18 The Ludwig Breast Cancer Study Group. Combination adjuvant chemotherapy for node-positive breast cancer: inadequacy of a single perioperative cycle. *New England Journal of Medicine* 1988; **319**: 677–83.

19 Fisher B, Redmond C, Dimitrov NV *et al.* A randomized clinical trial evaluating sequential methotrexate and fluorouracil in the treatment of patients with node-negative breast cancer who have estrogen-receptor-negative tumors. *New England Journal of Medicine* 1989; **320**: 473–8.

20 Mansour EG, Gray R, Shatila AH *et al.* Efficacy of adjuvant chemotherapy in high-risk node-negative breast cancer. An Intergroup study. *New England Journal of Medicine* 1989; **320**: 485–90.

21 Valagussa P, Bonadonna G. Carcinogenic effects of cancer treatment. In: Peckam M, Pinedo H, Veronesi V (eds) *Oxford textbook of oncology*. Oxford: Oxford University Press, 1995: 2348–58.

22 Fisher B, Dignam J, Mamounas EP *et al.* Sequential methotrexate and fluorouracil for the treatment of node-negative breast cancer patients with estrogen-receptor-negative tumors: eight-year results from National Surgical Adjuvant Breast and Bowel Project (NSABP) B-13 and first report of findings from NSABP B-19 comparing

methotrexate and fluorouracil with conventional cyclophosphamide, methotrexate and fluorouracil. *Journal of Clinical Oncology* 1996; **14**: 1982–92.

23 Skipper HE, Laboratory models: the historical perspectives. *Cancer Treatment Reports* 1986; **76**: 3–7.

24 Hryniuk W, Levine MN. Analysis of dose intensity for adjuvant chemotherapy trials in stage II breast cancer. *Journal of Clinical Oncology* 1986; **4**: 1162–70.

25 Henderson IC, Hayes DF, Gelman R. Dose-response in the treatment of breast cancer. A critical review. *Journal of Clinical Oncology* 1988; **6**: 1501–15.

26 Tannock IF, Boyd NF, De Boer G *et al*. A randomized trial of two dose levels of cyclophosphamide, methotrexate, and fluorouracil chemotherapy for patients with metastatic breast cancer. *Journal of Clinical Oncology* 1988; **6**: 1377–87.

27 Bremon A, Kerbrat P, Fumoleau P *et al*. Five-year follow-up results of a randomized trial testing the role of the dose intensity and duration of chemotherapy in node-positive premenopausal breast cancer patients. *Proceedings of the American Society of Clinical Oncology* 1996; **15**: 113 (abstract).

28 Bonneterre J, Roché H, Bremond A *et al*. A randomized trial of adjuvant chemotherapy with FEC 50 vs. FEC 100 for node-positive operable breast cancer: early report. *Proceedings of the American Society of Clinical Oncology* 1996; **15**: 104 (abstract).

29 Dimitrov N, Anderson S, Fisher B *et al*. Dose intensification and increased total dose of adjuvant chemotherapy for breast cancer: findings from NSABP B-22. *Proceedings of the American Society of Clinical Oncology* 1994; **13**: 64 (abstract).

30 Wood WC, Budman DR, Korzun AH *et al*. Dose and dose intensity of adjuvant chemotherapy for stage II, node-positive breast carcinoma. *New England Journal of Medicine* 1994; **330**: 1253–9.

31 Goldhirsch A, Gelber RD, Price KN *et al*. Effect of systemic adjuvant treatment on first sites of breast cancer relapse. *Lancet* 1994; **343**: 377–81.

32 Jaiyesimi IA, Budzar AU, Decker DA, Hortobagyi GN. Use of tamoxifen for breast cancer. Twenty-eight years later. *Journal of Clinical Oncology* 1995; **13**: 513–29.

33 Marini G, Murray S, Goldhirsch A *et al*. The effect of adjuvant prednisone combined with CMF on pattern of relapse and occurrence of second malignancies in patients with breast cancer. *Annals of Oncology* 1996; **7**: 245–50.

34 Harris JR, Hellman S, Henderson IC (eds) *Breast diseases*, 2nd edn. Philadelphia, PA: JB Lippincott, 1991.

35 Budzar AU, Gutterman JU, Blumenschein GR *et al*. Intensive postoperative chemoimmunotherapy for patients with stage II and stage III breast cancer. *Cancer* 1978; **41**: 1064–75.

36 Misset JL, Gil-Delgado M, Chollet P *et al*. Ten-year results of the French trial comparing adriamycin, vincristine, 5-fluorouracil and cyclophosphamide to standard CMF as adjuvant therapy for node-positive breast cancer. *Proceedings of the American Society of Clinical Oncology* 1992; **11**: 54 (abstract).

37 Fisher B, Redmond C, Wickerham DL *et al*. Doxorubicin-containing regimens for the treatment of stage II breast cancer. The National Surgical Adjuvant Breast and Bowel Project experience. *Journal of Clinical Oncology* 1989; **7**: 572–82.

38 Carpenter JT, Velez-Garcia E, Aron BS *et al*. Five-year results of a randomized comparison of cyclophosphamide, doxorubicin (adriamycin) and fluorouracil (CAF) vs. cyclophosphamide, methotrexate and fluorouracil (CMF) for node-positive breast cancer. *Proceedings of the American Society of Clinical Oncology* 1994; **13**: 62 (abstract).

39 Marty M, Bliss JM, Coombes RC *et al*. Cyclophosphamide, methotrexate, fluorouracil (CMF) vs. F-epirubicin-C (FEC) chemotherapy in premenopausal women with node-positive breast cancer. Results of a randomized trial. *Proceedings of the American Society of Clinical Oncology* 1994; **13**: 62 (abstract).

40 Fisher B, Brown AM, Dimitrov NV, *et al*. Two months of doxorubicin-cyclophosphamide with and without interval reinduction therapy compared with 6 months of cyclophosphamide, methotrexate, and fluorouracil in positive-node breast cancer patients with tamoxifen-non-responsive tumors: results from the National Surgical Adjuvant Breast and Bowel Project B-15. *Journal of Clinical Oncology* 1990; **8**: 1483–96.

41 Levine M, Bramwell V, Bowman D *et al*. CEF vs. CMF in premenopausal women with node-positive breast cancer. *Proceedings of the American Society of Clinical Oncology* 1995; **14**: 103 (abstract).

42 Fisher B, Dignam J, Wolmark N *et al*. Tamoxifen and chemotherapy for lymph-node-negative, estrogen-receptor-positive breast cancer. *Journal of the National Cancer Institute* 1997; **89**: 1673–82.

43 Osborne CK, Kitten L, Arteaga CL. Antagonism of chemotherapy-induced cytotoxicity for human breast cancer cells by antiestrogens. *Journal of Clinical Oncology* 1989; **7**: 710–17.

44 Moliterni A, Bonadonna G, Valagussa P *et al*. Cyclophosphamide, methotrexate and fluorouracil with and without doxorubicin in the adjuvant treatment of resectable breast cancer with one to three positive axillary nodes. *Journal of Clinical Oncology* 1991; **9**: 1124–30.

45 Bonadonna G, Zambetti M, Valagussa P. Sequential or alternating doxorubicin and CMF regimens in breast cancer with more than three positive nodes. Ten-year results. *Journal of the American Medical Association* 1995; **273**: 542–7.

46 American Society of Clinical Oncology Recommendations for the use of hematopoietic colony-stimulating factors: evidence-based clinical practice guidelines. *Blood* 1994; **12**: 2471–508.

47 Gianni AM, Bregni M, Siena S *et al*. Recombinant human granulocyte-macrophage colony-stimulating factor reduces hematologic toxicity and widens clinical applicability of high-dose cyclophosphamide treatment in breast cancer and non-Hodgkin's lymphoma. *Journal of Clinical Oncology* 1990; **8**: 768–78.

48 Peters WP, Ross M, Vredenburg JJ *et al*. High-dose chemotherapy and autologous bone marrow support as consolidation after standard-dose adjuvant therapy for high-risk breast cancer. *Journal of Clinical Oncology* 1993; **11**: 1132–43.

49 Gianni AM, Siena S, Bregni M *et al*. Efficacy, toxicity and applicability of high-dose sequential chemotherapy as adjuvant treatment in operable breast cancer with 10 or more axillary nodes involved. Five-year results. *Journal of Clinical Oncology* 1997; **15**: 2312–21.

50 Garcia-Carbonero R, Hidalgo M, Paz-Ares L *et al*. Patient selection in high-dose chemotherapy trials: relevance in high-risk breast cancer. *Journal of Clinical Oncology* 1997; **15**: 3178–84.

51 Crump M, Goss PE, Prince M, Girouard C. Outcome of extensive evaluation before adjuvant therapy in women with breast cancer and 10 or more positive axillary lymph nodes. *Journal of Clinical Oncology* 1996; **14**: 66–9.

52 Recht A, Come SE, Henderson IC *et al*. The sequencing of chemotherapy and radiation therapy after conservative surgery for early-stage breast cancer. *New England Journal of Medicine* 1996; **334**: 1356–61.

53 Overgaard M, Hansen PS, Overgaard J *et al*. Postoperative radiotherapy in high-risk premenopausal women with breast cancer who receive adjuvant chemotherapy. *New England Journal of Medicine* 1997; **337**: 949–55.

54 Ragaz J, Jackson SM, Le N *et al*. Adjuvant radiotherapy and chemotherapy in node-positive premenopausal women with breast cancer. *New England Journal of Medicine* 1997; **337**: 956–62.

55 Bonadonna G. Current and future trends in the multidisciplinary approach for high-risk breast cancer: the experience of the Milan Cancer Institute. *European Journal of Cancer* 1996; **32A**: 209–14.

56 Bonadonna G, Valagussa P, Zucali R, Salvadori B. Primary chemotherapy in surgically resectable breast cancer. *CA Cancer Journal for Clinicians* 1995; **45**: 227–43.

57 Bonadonna G, Valagussa P. Primary chemotherapy in operable breast cancer. *Seminars in Oncology* 1996; **23**: 464–74.

58 Fisher B, Gunduz N, Saffer EA. Influence of the interval between primary tumor removal and chemotherapy on kinetics and growth of metastases. *Cancer Research* 1983; **43**: 1488–92.

59 Holmgren L, O'Reilly MS, Folkman J. Dormancy of micrometastases: balanced proliferation and apoptosis in the presence of angiogenesis suppression. *Nature Medicine* 1995; **1**: 149–53.

60 Bonadonna G, Valagussa P, Brambilla C *et al*. Primary chemotherapy in operable breast cancer. Eight-year experience at the Milan Cancer Institute. *Journal of Clinical Oncology* 1998; **16**: 93–100.

61 Fisher B, Brown A, Mamounas E *et al*. Effect of preoperative therapy for primary breast cancer (BC) on local-regional disease, disease-free survival (DFS) and survival (S): results from NSABP B-18. *Proceedings of the American Society of Clinical Oncology* 1997; **16**: 126A (abstract).

62 Rowinsky EK, Eisenhauer EA, Chaudhry U *et al*. Paclitaxel (Taxol) Investigators' Workshop. *Seminars in Oncology* 1993; **20 (Supplement 3)**: 1–60.

63 Aapro MS, Lavelle F, Bissery MC *et al*. The impact of docetaxel (Taxotere) on current treatment. *Seminars in Oncology* 1995; **22 (Supplement 4)**: 1–33.

64 Abeloff MD, Hayes DF, Henderson IC *et al*. The current status of vinorelbine (Navelbine) in breast cancer. *Seminars in Oncology* 1995; **22 (Supplement 5)**: 1–87.

65 Gianni L, Munzone E, Capri G *et al*. Paclitaxel by 3-hour infusion in combination with bolus doxorubicin in women with untreated metastatic breast cancer. High antitumor efficacy and cardiac effects in a dose-finding and sequence-finding study. *Journal of Clinical Oncology* 1995; **13**: 2688–99.

66 Gusterson BA, Gelber RD, Goldirsch A *et al*. Prognostic importance of *c-erbB-2* expression in breast cancer. *Journal of Clinical Oncology* 1992; **10**: 1049–56.

67 Muss HB, Thor AD, Berr DA *et al*. *C-erbB-2* expression and response to adjuvant therapy in women with node-positive breast cancer. *New England Journal of Medicine* 1994; **330**: 1260–6.

68 Seidman AD, Baselga J, Yao TJ *et al*. Her-2/*neu* overexpression and clinical taxane sensitivity: a multivariate analysis in patients with metastatic breast cancer (MBC). *Proceedings of the American Society of Clinical Oncology* 1996; **15**: 104 (abstract).

69 Gianni L, Capri G, Mezzelani A *et al*. HER-2/*neu* duplication and response to doxorubicin/paclitaxel (AT) in women with metastatic breast cancer. *Proceedings of the American Society of Clinical Oncology* 1997; **16**: 139A (abstract).

21

Hormonal therapy for advanced breast cancer

ANTHONY HOWELL AND DAVID DeFRIEND

INTRODUCTION

A century has passed since Beatson first demonstrated that altering the female hormonal milieu by oophorectomy could produce tumour regression in women with advanced breast cancer.[1] At the time, the mechanism underlying such responses was not known. The term hormone was not coined until the following decade, and it would be many decades before the pivotal role of oestrogens and their mechanism of tumour stimulation would be recognized.

Although, our understanding of the exact relationship between hormones and breast cancer growth/progression still remains incomplete, a variety of endocrine treatment modalities have been introduced during the last century (Table 21.1), many of which share the common aim of reducing oestrogenic stimulation of the breast cancer cell. Three main treatment strategies have evolved in order to achieve this aim, namely ablative therapy, additive therapy and the use of oestrogen antagonists.

Ablative therapies inhibit oestrogen action by reducing oestrogen synthesis. This can be achieved by ablation of the glands responsible for oestrogen synthesis, by manipulation of the regulatory systems that control steroidogenesis, or by inhibition of the enzymes involved in steroidogenesis. In premenopausal women the principal site of oestrogen synthesis is the ovary but in post-menopausal women oestrogen production occurs predominantly in the adrenals and in peripheral fat. Oophorectomy, hypophysectomy and pharmacological castration using luteinizing-hormone-releasing

hormone (LHRH) analogues have thus all been used in premenopausal patients, whilst adrenalectomy and aromatase inhibitors have been employed in the treatment of post-menopausal patients.

Additive therapy with high pharmacological doses of oestrogens, androgens or progestins has been used mostly in post-menopausal patients. Because of the high incidence of side-effects associated with the use of oestrogens and androgens, the synthetic progestins, megestrol acetate and medroxyprogesterone acetate, are the only additive endocrine agents currently in common

Table 21.1 *The development of endocrine therapy, with date of first publication about each type of therapy shown (the 'pure' anti-oestrogens are currently in phase II clinical trial)*

Year	Type of therapy	First author
1896	Oophorectomy	Beatson
1922	Ovarian irradiation	De Courmelles
1939	Androgens	Ulrich
1944	Synthetic oestrogens	Haddow
1951	Progestins	Escher
1952	Pituitary irradiation	Douglas
1953	Adrenalectomy	Huggins
1953	Hypophysectomy	Luft
1971	Anti-oestrogens	Cole
1973	Aromatase inhibitors	Griffiths
1982	LHRH antagonists	Klijn
1987	Antiprogestins	Romieu
1995	'Pure' anti-oestrogens	Howell

Source: Howell A, DeFriend D, Anderson E. Mechanisms of response and resistance to endocrine therapy for breast cancer and the development of new treatments. *Rev Endocr Rel Cancer* 1993; **43**: 5–21.

use. Despite extensive clinical experience with these agents, their precise mechanisms of action are not well understood. However, they have been shown to have a number of potentially anti-oestrogenic effects *in vivo* and *in vitro*.[3] These include down-regulation of oestrogen-receptor expression in breast cancer cells, inhibition of pituitary/hypothalamic regulatory pathways controlling oestrogen synthesis, and elevation of serum levels of sex-hormone-binding globulin (SHBG), which consequently reduces the circulating levels of available oestrogen.[2]

Oestrogen antagonists inhibit the activity of oestrogen in target cells by competing directly with the natural ligand for oestrogen-receptor-binding. A number of non-steroidal and steroidal agents have been developed which exhibit anti-oestrogenic activity but, to date, only the triphenylethylene derivative tamoxifen has gained widespread international usage in the treatment of breast cancer.

Since nearly all endocrine therapies give equivalent rates and durations of response (Figure 21.1), the evolution of endocrine therapy has been driven by the need to reduce the toxicity/invasiveness of treatments, and to make them more widely applicable and easily administered. Thus aromatase inhibitors have replaced adrenalectomy, anti-oestrogens have replaced the more toxic high-dose oestrogens, and progestins have largely replaced androgens.

In this chapter, we shall review the results of current first- and second-line endocrine treatment of advanced breast cancer, examine the insights that can be gained from the clinic into the mechanisms underlying tumour response and resistance to endocrine therapy, and try to evaluate whether current results can be improved by the future introduction of new agents, at present undergoing laboratory and early clinical trials.

FIRST-LINE ENDOCRINE THERAPY

Following its first reported use in advanced breast cancer 25 years ago,[3] the anti-oestrogen tamoxifen has become widely accepted as the first-line endocrine treatment of choice for patients with advanced breast cancer, as a result of its equal efficacy and low toxicity compared to other available endocrine agents. The detailed results presented in this section are from a group of 431 patients with advanced breast cancer who were treated in the South Manchester Breast Unit with tamoxifen as first-line systemic therapy. They are presented here as being representative of the international clinical experience with tamoxifen which has been reviewed previously in an overview analysis by Patterson *et al*.[4]

Clinically, the outcome of endocrine therapy is evaluated by the response of the tumour (according to internationally accepted criteria, e.g. Hayward *et al*.[5]), the duration of response and the duration of survival. For patients treated with endocrine therapy, the duration of response/survival and the tumour oestrogen progesterone (OR/PgR)-receptor status of those who show disease stabilization (NC) for $\geq$ 6 months are not significantly different to those of women who show a partial response (PR).[6–8] As a result, stable disease responses of $\geq$ 6 months are now generally included when assessing the overall response rate to endocrine therapy.

Overall, approximately 50% of patients showed a response to first-line endocrine therapy with tamoxifen. The duration of response and overall survival of patients are shown in figure 21.2 according to response category. The median duration of response for all tamoxifen responders (CR+PR+NC) was 20 months. Both duration of response and overall survival were longer for complete responders (CR), but there were no significant differences in these parameters between partial responders and patients who showed disease stabilization. The median overall survival of tamoxifen responders and non-responders was 43 months and 14 months, respectively. Thus the response to first-line endocrine therapy selects a group of patients who will fare relatively well.[9]

A number of factors influence the overall response rate and the type and duration of response to tamoxifen. The

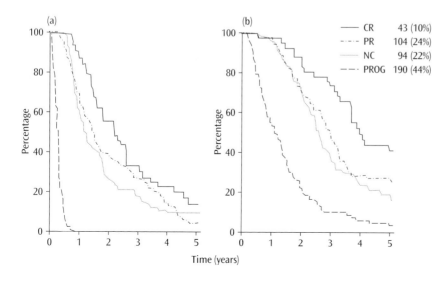

—— CR	43	(10%)
–·–· PR	104	(24%)
⋯⋯ NC	94	(22%)
– – PROG	190	(44%)

Figure 21.1 *Relationship between category of response and (a) time to progression and (b) survival from the start of treatment with tamoxifen in advanced breast cancer. CR, complete response; PR, partial response; NC, no change; PROG, progressive disease. The number of patients in each group (as a percentage of the total) is also shown.*

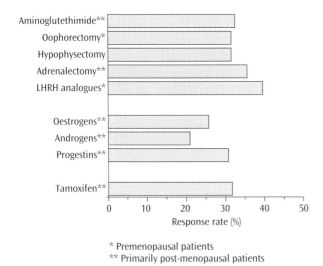

Figure 21.2 *Complete plus partial response rates of unselected patients with advanced breast cancer to various endocrine therapies. Adapted from Henderson (1991).[10]*

* Premenopausal patients
** Primarily post-menopausal patients

Table 21.3 *Response to tamoxifen by dominant site and number of disease sites in 431 evaluable patients with advanced breast cancer*

	Number of patients	Response* Progression (%)	NC (%)	PR (%)	CR (%)
Dominant site					
Soft tissue	215	32	27	24	17
Bone	98	52	19	27	2
Lung	98	58	13	24	5
Liver	20	70	10	20	0
Number of sites					
1	279	39	26	22	13
2	124	51	15	31	3
3	28	68	11	18	3

* Responses: NC, no change; PR, partial; CR, complete.

overall response rate was higher in patients with OR/PgR-positive tumours (Table 21.2), in patients with soft tissue/bone as opposed to visceral sites of disease, and in those with a lower tumour burden as indicated by fewer sites of disease (Table 21.3). In previous studies, increasing patient age, longer disease-free interval[4] and tumour expression of oestrogen-induced peptides such as pS2 have also been shown to predict the response,[11] while tumour expression of the epidermal growth factor receptor has been shown to be associated with tamoxifen resistance.[12]

Identification of factors which influence the type of response (i.e. CR vs. PR vs. NC) and the response duration is more difficult. Among our own patients, neither OR/PgR positivity nor absolute receptor levels appeared to influence the type or duration ($\leq$ or $>$ median) of response (Table 21.4). The type of response to tamoxifen did appear to be influenced by the predominant site of disease and by the number of disease sites present, but neither of these variables appeared to influence the response duration, which must be determined by other as yet unidentified factors that are intrinsic to the tumour or the tumour–host relationship.

SECOND-LINE ENDOCRINE THERAPY

Following failure of first-line endocrine therapy, 45% of our own patients received treatment with a second-line endocrine treatment. As with selection of first-line therapy, there appears to be little to choose between the available agents with respect to efficacy (Figure 21.3), and

Table 21.2 *Receptor positivity according to response category in 266 patients treated with tamoxifen as first therapy for advanced breast cancer (OR-positive is equivalent to 5 fmol/mg cytosol protein and PgR-positive to >15 fmol/mg cytosol protein): the NC category has similar receptor values to the other two response groups*

Response*	n (%)	OR-positive (%)	Median amount of OR (range) (fmol/mg)	PgR-positive (%)	Median amount of PgR (range) (fmol/mg)
CR	26 (10)	81	101 (0–1001)	50	8 (0–544)
PR	65 (24)	82	102 (0–914)	65	46 (0–1570)
NC	53 (20)	74	79 (0–833)	52	16 (0–1218)
Progression	122 (46)	51	6 (0–651)	36	0 (0–565)

* Responses: CR, complete: PR, partial: NC, no change.
OR, oestrogen receptor; PgR, progesterone receptor.
Source: *Endocr Rel Cancer* 1995; **2**: 131–9.

Table 21.4 *Responders to tamoxifen (CR plus PR plus NC): relationship between duration of response (above or below the median) and site of disease, number of disease sites and receptor content*

	Number of patients				
	Total	Response duration ≤ 453 days	(%)	Response duration > 453 days	(%)
Dominant site					
Soft tissue	109	51	(47)	58	(53)
Bone	45	25	(56)	20	(44)
Lung	36	17	(47)	19	(53)
Liver	8	6	(75)	2	(25)
Number of sites					
1	133	60	(45)	73	(55)
2	57	35	(61)	22	(39)
3	8	4	(50)	4	(50)

	Number of patients	Receptor content (median and range) (fmol)	
		Response duration ≤ 453 days	Response duration > 453 days
Oestrogen receptor	116	85 (0–833)	83 (0–914)
Progesterone receptor	117	18 (0–1570)	29 (0–742)

treatment choices are therefore governed by drug toxicity. Until recently, most clinicians have tended to favour one of the synthetic progestins, megestrol acetate or medroxyprogesterone acetate, the principal side-effects of which are weight gain and fluid retention (reported by 20–50% of patients), or the aromatase inhibitor aminoglutethimide, which is associated with lethargy and skin rashes (usually of a temporary nature, and reported by 30–50% of patients) and glucocorticoid suppression. The choice of second-line agent may well alter in the future as new less toxic/more selective aromatase inhibitors and pure, non-agonist anti-oestrogens (reviewed later in this chapter) become available.

The overall response rate to second-line endocrine therapy among our own patients, who received a variety of agents – predominantly synthetic progestins (75%) or aromatase inhibitors (15%) – was 40% (Table 21.5), with a median duration of response of 11 months. As with previous studies, the most important factor predicting response to second-line therapy was prior response to first-line therapy (Figure 21.3). Second-line response did appear to show some association with tumour OR status, but showed no apparent relationship to PgR status, a finding which is noteworthy, given the high proportion of our own patients who were treated with progestins.

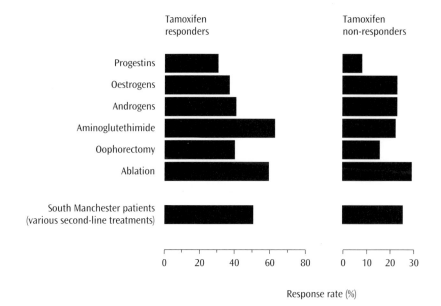

Figure 21.3 *Response rates of tamoxifen-responders and non-responders to second-line endocrine treatments. Adapted from Henderson (1991).*[10]

Table 21.5 *Response to second-line endocrine therapy for 126 evaluable patients*

Response*	n	(%)
CR	3	(2%)
PR	25	(20%)
NC	22	(17%)
Overall (CR + PR + NC)	50	(40%)
PD	76	(60%)

* Responses: CR, complete; PR, partial; NC, no change.

WITHDRAWAL RESPONSES (Table 21.6)

Withdrawal responses (WR) or 'rebound regressions' of breast cancer were first described in 1949 in a group of patients who had initially responded to androgens.[13] When disease progression eventually occurred, a further response was obtained after androgen treatment was stopped. WRs have subsequently been reported after cessation of treatment with other additive endocrine treatments, including oestrogens[14,15] and progestins.[16]

The first reported withdrawal response after cessation of tamoxifen was seen in a patient with parenchymal lung metastases.[22] When treated with tamoxifen, the growth rate of the lung secondaries increased but, after tamoxifen withdrawal, growth ceased and a partial remission occurred. Over the past decade a number of other case reports and small series of tamoxifen withdrawal responses have appeared in the literature.[20,21,23–25]

The overall rate of response to tamoxifen withdrawal has varied greatly between studies. In one early study no WRs were seen in 19 evaluated patients,[26] causing many clinicians to doubt that tamoxifen WRs were truly observable. However, more recent series containing larger numbers of patients have confirmed the validity of tamoxifen WRs. Canney et al. reported an unselected series of 61 consecutive patients in whom tamoxifen treatment failed, of whom 6 patients (9.8%) showed a WR.[20] In a more selected series of 65 patients from our own clinic who had relatively indolent progressive disease at the time of tamoxifen failure, 19 patients (30%) showed a response to tamoxifen withdrawal.[21] In both of these studies the majority of WRs were seen in patients who had originally responded to tamoxifen, and in those who relapsed with soft-tissue disease at the time of tamoxifen failure.

Because it may take many months for tamoxifen to be cleared completely from human breast cancer cells after cessation of treatment, and modern second-line endocrine agents are available which are both effective and safe, evaluation of WRs is useful and ethical for only a minority of patients who relapse on tamoxifen with very indolent progressive disease. However, tamoxifen WRs may be of greater importance in offering clues to the mechanisms underlying anti-oestrogen resistance in some patients.

IMPLICATIONS OF SECOND-LINE RESPONSES AND WITHDRAWAL RESPONSES

The demonstration that up to 50% of patients who respond to tamoxifen and subsequently relapse will respond to a second-line endocrine therapy clearly suggests that a significant proportion of tumours remain hormone responsive at the time of tamoxifen failure. The response rate varies little between different types of second-line treatment, many (if not all) of which appear likely to have antagonism of tumour stimulation by oestrogen as their pivotal effect. Second-line responses may therefore suggest that failure on first-line endocrine therapy occurs because the tumour becomes restimulated by an oestrogenic signal.

Published laboratory and clinical findings suggest two principal mechanisms by which oestrogenic restimulation might occur in tamoxifen-resistant tumours (summarized in Table 21.7). Although serum concentrations of tamoxifen and its principal metabolites have been shown to remain relatively stable during prolonged treatment periods,[27] there is preliminary evidence to suggest that intratumoral drug and metabolite levels may alter

Table 21.6 *Responses after withdrawal of oestrogens, androgens and tamoxifen*

Treatment	Number of patients					Reference
	WR	Total assessed	%*	Total study population	%†	
Androgens	7	11	64	Not known	—	Escher (1949)[13]
Oestrogens	9	14	64	100	9.0	Huseby (1954)[14]
Androgens and oestrogens	15	88	17	674	2.2	Kaufman and Escher (1961)[17]
Oestrogens	7	22	32	97	7.2	Baker and Vaitkevicius (1972)[18]
Oestrogens	8	32	25	83	9.6	Nesto et al. (1976)[19]
Tamoxifen	6	61	10	61	9.8	Canney et al. (1987)[20]
Tamoxifen	19	65	29	308	6.2	Howell et al. (1992)[21]

WR, withdrawal response.
* WR as a percentage of total number assessed.
† WR as a percentage of total study population.

Table 21.7 *Possible mechanisms of tumour resistance to tamoxifen*

- Inactivation of tamoxifen by intracellular degradation, intracellular sequestration to proteins other than OR, or increased drug exclusion from the cell, leaving receptors available for stimulation by endogenous oestrogens/inhibition by second-line endocrine agents[29,31]

- Increased metabolism of tamoxifen to oestrogenic metabolites and/or increased sensitivity to their agonist activity secondary to OR mutations/changes in post-receptor signalling[31–33]

- Acquisition of a hormone-independent phenotype

prior to tumour progression both in a nude mouse xenograft model of tamoxifen resistance[28] and in patients with advanced breast cancer,[29] resulting in reduced intra-tumoral levels of tamoxifen and its principal anti-oestrogenic metabolite, 4-hydroxytamoxifen. In addition, Pavlik *et al.* have suggested that there may be increased sequestration of tamoxifen away from ORs at other intracellular binding sites in tamoxifen-resistant breast tumours.[30] Overall, these changes in intracellular metabolism and sequestration might thus render OR more available for stimulation by endogenous oestrogens or inhibition by further endocrine therapies.

Altered intratumoral drug metabolism may also result in increased levels of oestrogenic tamoxifen metabolites within the cell, which may provide an exogenous source of OR stimulation.[28,29] Alternatively, changes in the OR protein resulting from point mutations,[34] or alterations in the post-receptor signalling pathway, may make the tumour cell more sensitive to the agonist effects of tamoxifen and its metabolites. In either case, cessation of tamoxifen therapy would remove a source of exogenous oestrogenic stimulation from the tumour. This may therefore explain why tamoxifen withdrawal responses occur.

In our own series of patients evaluated for withdrawal response, the majority of cases of WR were in patients who had initially responded to tamoxifen, but four WRs occurred in patients who had appeared resistant to tamoxifen *de novo*. This suggests that in some patients tamoxifen may be viewed as a tumour agonist from the outset of therapy, while in others it becomes an agonist after an initial period of antagonist activity. Such a change in activity might result from variations in sensitivity to tamoxifen between different clones of cells present in breast cancers, which are known to exhibit considerable tumour heterogeneity. As a result of the selective pressure of tamoxifen therapy, clones inhibited by the drug would regress, while those stimulated to proliferate would gradually grow out and become dominant, resulting in tumour progression. Withdrawal of tamoxifen would then result in removal of a growth stimulus from tamoxifen-stimulated clones, and would result in tumour regression and a withdrawal

response. With time, the original clonal balance within the tumour might be gradually restored, explaining the occasional clinical finding of second responses to tamoxifen (Figure 21.4). The hypothesis of clonal remodelling is currently unproven, but is supported by the results of *in vitro* studies with T47D cells[35] and tumour ploidy changes detected *in vivo*.[36,37]

Finally, it seems clear that a significant proportion of tumours express a hormone-independent phenotype after progression on tamoxifen, and fail to respond to subsequent second-line endocrine therapy. It must be assumed that growth and progression of these tumours is driven by alternative non-hormonal mitogens. Many tumours that exhibit endocrine resistance *de novo* and fail to respond to tamoxifen or second-line therapy lack measurable ORs. It is possible that the remainder which appear OR-positive express defective/non-functional forms of the receptor. Although changes in OR status between primary and metastatic breast tumours have been reported occasionally in patients subjected to serial biopsies,[38,39] there is little evidence that temporal changes in measurable OR status are responsible for tumour endocrine resistance after prior response to tamoxifen.[40] However, it is possible that, although measurable OR remains present, the development over time of mutated/non-functional OR variants may result in acquired hormone independence and tamoxifen resistance.

STRATEGIES FOR IMPROVING THE RESULTS OF ENDOCRINE THERAPY

The principal goals of future endocrine therapy should be to improve the rate and duration of response to treatment, to minimize toxicity and to optimize ease of

	Mrs A (age 54 years)		Mrs B (age 72 years)		Tumour clones
	Type	Months	Type	Months	
First response	CR	57	CR	27	(S) (I) (I) (I)
Withdrawal	NC	11	NC	20	(S) (S) (S) (I)
Second response	PR	7	PR	6	(S) (I) (I) (I)

Figure 21.4 *Repeat responses to tamoxifen in two patients. Both patients showed a complete response (CR) to tamoxifen, followed by a 'no change' (NC) response when tamoxifen was withdrawn after progression. Both patients had a partial remission (PR) when tamoxifen was reintroduced after a withdrawal response. We postulate that the balance between tamoxifen-inhibited (I) and tamoxifen-stimulated (S) clones changed during the course of treatment as shown.*

administration. There appears little prospect in the immediate future of rendering hormone-independent tumours responsive to current or new endocrine agents, although preliminary *in-vitro* studies have shown that it is possible to produce OR expression/hormone responsiveness in OR-negative human breast cancer cell lines by appropriate gene transfection.[41,42] However, for hormone-responsive tumours understanding the mechanisms by which resistance develops to particular treatments should permit the development of strategies to avoid it.

From the preceding discussion, it would appear that response results might be improved by using treatment regimes which produce more complete/durable inhibition of oestrogen production/action and avoid the possibility of iatrogenic stimulation of tumour growth. Logically, this might be achievable by:

- using combinations or sequences of existing endocrine treatment in order to prevent or delay the onset of resistance to individual agents; or
- developing new agents which are more potent inhibitors of endogenous oestrogen production or are purer/more potent antagonists of oestrogen at its receptor.

At present, data from trials where alternating or combined regimens of endocrine therapy have been used are disappointing and do not result in improved survival.

NEW ENDOCRINE AGENTS

The remainder of this chapter considers the efficacy and toxicity of newer endocrine therapies which are undergoing clinical trials but which are not yet (and may never be) commercially available. The three most active areas of clinical research at present are the new anti-oestrogens,

the new aromatase inhibitors and the antiprogestins. Other potential new modalities of endocrine therapy, such as vitamin D analogues, retinoids and somatostatin analogues, are not included because of the paucity of clinical results to date. Progestins and LHRH analogues are similarly excluded in view of the lack of new data concerning these agents.

ANTI-OESTROGENS

Two main avenues have been followed in order to attempt to improve on tamoxifen. One is to alter chemically the non-steroidal triphenylethylene ring structure of tamoxifen or to produce new ring structures (e.g. the benzothiaphenes) (Figure 21.5). The second is to produce growth-inhibitory steroidal analogues of oestrogen (Figure 21.6).

The two types of anti-oestrogen, namely steroidal and non-steroidal, appear to have different mechanisms of action which may account for the differences in their activity and side-effect profiles. The triphenylethylene anti-oestrogens bind to the oestrogen-binding sites of OR monomers, which then combine to form dimers. The process of dimerization is thought to facilitate binding of the OR to its specific oestrogen-response element (ORE) in the vicinity of oestrogen-regulated genes. Each receptor monomer contains two transcription-activating functions (TAFs), both of which are activated when oestrogen binds to the molecule, resulting in the range of gene transcription and gene repression responses that are associated with the effect of oestrogen. Tamoxifen binding to OR results in activation of TAF1 in a manner similar to the effect of oestrogen, but activation of TAF2 is abrogated by tamoxifen. Thus tamoxifen is a partial agonist because binding to OR results in the activity of TAF1, and it is an antagonist because it inhibits TAF 2.

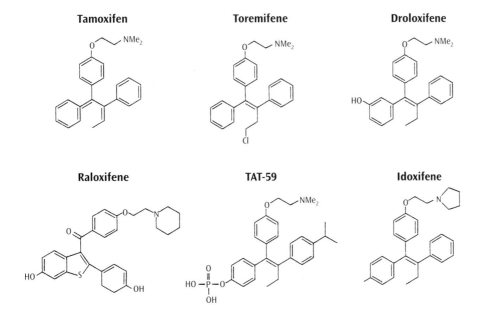

Tamoxifen

Toremifene

Droloxifene

Raloxifene

TAT-59

Idoxifene

Figure 21.5 *Structures of non-steroidal anti-oestrogens that are either clinically available or in clinical trial.*

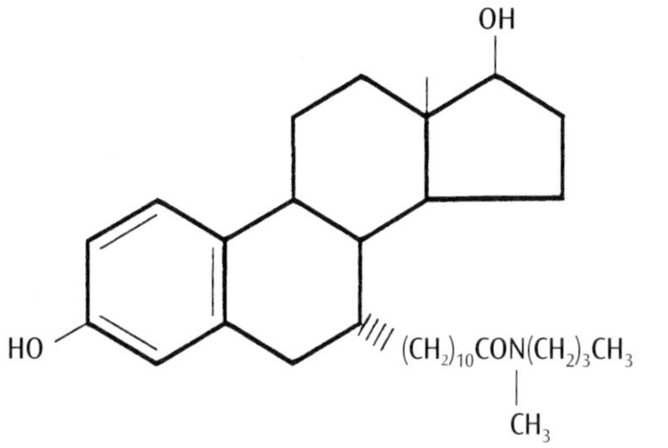

Figure 21.6 *Structures of the steroidal 'pure' anti-oestrogens ICI 164384 and ICI 182780.*

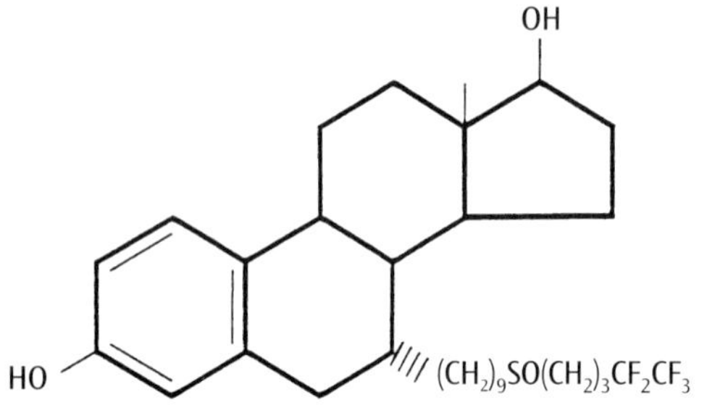

The interaction of steroidal anti-oestrogens with OR appears to be distinct from that of the non-steroidal compounds, but their precise action remains controversial. The specific anti-oestrogen ICI 182780 binds with high affinity to OR monomers, but binding of OR to OREs may be attenuated in its presence. This may be due to the long side-chain at the 7-alpha position of the molecule sterically inhibiting receptor dimerization,[43,44] or due to increased turnover and reduced nucleo-cytoplasmic shuttling of the receptor monomer producing dramatic reductions in the level of detectable OR molecules within cells exposed to the compound.[32,45] *In vitro* virtually no transcriptional activity of OR has been detected in cells treated with specific anti-oestrogens.

New non-steroidal anti-oestrogens (NSAEs)

Five NSAEs have completed their preclinical testing programme and are currently undergoing clinical trials (Figure 21.5). All of them are based on the triphenylethylene structure of tamoxifen, with the exception of raloxifene, which is a benzothiaphene. The clinical trial programmes of TAT-59, raloxifene and idoxifene are still in their early stages, whereas phase III trials of toremifene and droloxifene are currently in progress, comparing each agent with the best standard therapy (e.g. tamoxifen). The questions which need to be addressed in preclinical and clinical studies with new NSAEs are summarized in Table 21.8.

Table 21.8 *Assessment of non-steroidal anti-oestrogens (NSAEs)*

In the laboratory
  Oestrogen-receptor binding
  Tumour antagonism
  Peripheral antagonist/agonist ratio
  Alternative mechanisms of action
  Activity against tamoxifen-resistant cell lines

In the clinic
  First-line activity
  Activity in tamoxifen-resistant tumours
  Side-effect profile
  Utility of peripheral antagonist/agonist ratio
  Pharmacokinetics

New NSAEs – preclinical data

Preclinical studies should seek evidence of superiority over tamoxifen in one or more of the following areas: receptor binding, anti-tumour activity, balance between tumour antagonism and peripheral agonism, presence or absence of potentially useful alternative mechanisms of action, and activity against tamoxifen-resistant cells.

With the exception of toremifene, all of the NSAEs have greater binding affinities for OR than tamoxifen (Table 21.9). Some of the available data concerning their preclinical anti-tumour activity relative to tamoxifen against human mammary tumour cell lines (usually MCF-7 cells) grown either *in vitro* or as xenografts in athymic nude mice *in vivo* are summarized in Table 21.10. Data are also included for their activity against carcinogen-induced mammary tumours in rodents. In some studies no direct comparison with tamoxifen was made, and these are not cited. Toremifene and raloxifene appear to be less or equally active *in vitro* and *in vivo* compared to tamoxifen, whereas droloxifene TAT-59 and, to a lesser extent, idoxifene appear to be more active.

Although NSAE agonist activity may result in reduced anti-tumour efficacy, it may be beneficial with respect to the skeletal and cardiovascular systems, particularly when considering new agents for the adjuvant and chemoprevention arenas. The relative agonist/antagonist effects of the five non-steroidal anti-oestrogens in the

Table 21.9 *Binding to OR relative to tamoxifen and to oestrogen of NSAEs in clinical trial*

	Binding to OR relative to tamoxifen	Percentage binding to OR relative to oestrogen
Tamoxifen	—	5 (Kangas, 1986)[46]
Toremifene	× 1	5 (Kangas, 1986)[46]
Droloxifene	× 10	7.5 (Loser *et al.*, 1985)[47]
Raloxifene	?	>100 (Black *et al.*, 1983)[48]
TAT-59	× 10	10 (Toko, 1990)[49]
Idoxifene	× 2.5	12.5 (Chander *et al.*, 1991)[50]

Table 21.10 *Preclinical anti-tumour activity of non-steroidal anti-oestrogens compared to tamoxifen*

	Human cell lines *in vitro*	Human cell lines in the nude mouse	Carcinogen-induced rat tumours
Toremifene	< ×1	? NT	DMBA = tamoxifen[46]
Droloxifene	×10	>TAM	R3230AC >tamoxifen[47,51]
Raloxifene	?	NT	NMU <tamoxifen[52]
			DMBA <tamoxifen[53]
TAT-59	*c.* ×10	>TAM	DMBA >tamoxifen[49]
Idoxifene	×1.5	>TAM	NMU >tamoxifen[50]

NT, not tested against tamoxifen; DMBA, dimethylbenz(a)anthracene; NMU, nitrosomethylurea.

immature rat uterus assay are shown in table 21.11. Antagonist activity is assessed by the percentage reduction in weight of the oestrogen-primed uterus caused by the anti-oestrogen, whilst agonist activity is assessed by the percentage stimulation of uterine growth produced by the anti-oestrogen in the absence of oestrogen. In general, the new compounds have less agonist and more antagonist activity than tamoxifen, with raloxifene and idoxifene appearing to be the most antagonistic and least agonistic agents, respectively.

In experimental studies, high concentrations of non-steroidal anti-oestrogens cause cell death in OR-negative as well as OR-positive cell lines *in vitro*. The mechanism of this non-receptor-mediated cytotoxicity is not well understood, but may be related to calmodulin antagonism,[57] inhibition of protein kinase C activity, or as yet unidentified effects mediated via anti-oestrogen-binding sites which are found ubiquitously in cells irrespective of their OR status. The clinical importance of these non-OR-mediated effects is uncertain, although given the low level of efficacy of tamoxifen in patients with OR-negative disease, it seems unlikely to be highly significant. Nevertheless, there is interest in increasing the activity of NSAEs with respect to calmodulin antagonism, and idoxifene, for example, is four times more active as a calmodulin antagonist than tamoxifen.[57]

Table 21.11 *Appropriate agonist/antagonist activity of non-steroidal anti-oestrogens in the immature rat uterus assay*

	Agonism (%)	Antagonism (%)	Reference (first author)
Tamoxifen	50	50	Wakeling, 1991[54,55]
Toremifene	43	?	Kangas, 1986[46]
Droloxifene	35	*c.* 20	Loser, 1985[47]
			Eppenberger, 1991[56]
Raloxifene	5	83	Jones, 1984[53]
TAT-59	?	>TAM	Toko, 1990[49]
Idoxifene	15	85	Chander, 1991[50]

In-vitro evidence that a new NSAE is effective against tamoxifen-resistant cell lines would provide a rationale for further clinical evaluation in patients with tamoxifen-resistant tumours. Few data are currently available concerning the activity of the new NSAEs in tamoxifen-resistant cell lines, but Jarman (personal communication) has shown that idoxifene is 10 times more active against the tamoxifen-resistant cell line RL-3 than tamoxifen itself, and a clinical trial of this agent in patients who have failed tamoxifen treatment is currently in progress. Other clinical trials assessing cross-resistance of NSAEs are outlined below.

New NSAEs – clinical data

As judged by its receptor-binding, antitumour activity and agonist activity, toremifene appears to be very similar to tamoxifen in preclinical studies. Droloxifene appears to be much more active than tamoxifen in all three assays, although there are no data on whether it has alternative mechanisms of action or whether it is active in tamoxifen-resistant cell lines. We have been unable to find full reports of raloxifene. It appears to be highly active with regard to OR-binding and oestrogen antagonism in the rat uterus assay, but disappointing in animal model systems. Both TAT-59 and idoxifene appear to have excellent anti-oestrogen profiles. The question arises as to whether these preclinical data are reflected in the current clinical experience with each drug. Data on the first- and second-line activity, side-effect profile, peripheral antagonist/agonist ratios and the pharmacokinetics of the NSAEs are summarized below as far as they are known.

The results to date for NSAEs as first-line therapy for advanced disease trials are summarized in Table 21.12. All of the studies were performed in patients with

Table 21.12 *Results of studies using newer non-steroidal anti-oestrogens as first-line endocrine therapy for advanced breast cancer*

Drug	Dose (mg/day)	Number of patients	Response CR/PR (%)
Toremifene	20	14	21 (phase II trial)
	60	93	52 (summarized)
	240	38	68 (Valavaara, 1990)[63]
Toremifene	240	31	29 (phase III trial)
Tamoxifen	40	31	44 (Stenbygaard, 1993)[58]
Toremifene	60	221	21 (phase III trial)
	200	212	22 (Hayes, 1995)[59]
Tamoxifen	20	215	19 —
Droloxifene	20	84	30 (randomized)
	40	88	47 (phase II trial)
	100	96	44 (Rauschning, 1994)[65]
Raloxifene	Phase II studies in progress		
TAT-59	Phase II studies in progress		
Idoxifene	Phase II studies in progress		

tumours of positive or unknown OR status, and all patients were previously untreated with endocrine therapy for advanced disease. There were no significant differences in response rates between tamoxifen and toremifene in the randomized trials that have been published.[58,59] These data conflict with the findings of several earlier phase II studies, showing higher response rate for toremifene at doses of 60 mg and 240 mg per day,[60–64] which have not been seen in the phase III studies using comparable doses.

The results of a major international randomized phase II trial of droloxifene were reported recently.[65] Patients were randomized to receive 20, 40 or 100 mg of droloxifene daily. This study randomized a large number of patients and reported significantly higher response rates and significantly longer response durations at the two higher doses used, compared to the lower one (Table 21.12). Phase II studies with raloxifene and TAT-59 are in progress, but it is still too early for idoxifene to be assessed as a first-line agent.

Clinical evaluation of new NSAEs after tamoxifen failure (Table 21.13) is particularly interesting, as it demonstrates whether drugs which are thought to have similar mechanisms of action to tamoxifen exhibit cross-resistance or cross-sensitivity. With the exception of one small study,[66] the objective remission rate (CR + PR) with toremifene after tamoxifen failure has been ≤ 5% (Table 21.13), although a further unquantifiable group of patients appears to respond to toremifene with prolonged periods of disease stabilization. No responses were seen in a small study using raloxifene as second-line treatment,[67] but both tumour remissions and NC responses were obtained using droloxifene or idoxifene after tamoxifen failure, suggesting that 3-hydroxylation or 4-iodination of the tamoxifen molecule may produce non-cross-resistant NSAEs. However, the response rates observed were lower than expected for standard second-line therapy such as megestrol acetate, suggesting the existence of some degree of cross-resistance.

The more common side-effects of the new NSAEs and tamoxifen are compared in Table 21.14. No precise data are available for idoxifene and/or TAT-59. There appears to be little difference with regard to toxicity between tamoxifen and the new NSAEs. Apparent differences must be scrutinized for the assiduousness with which toxicity was sought and the size of the study (e.g. raloxifene data were based on only 14 patients).

All of the five new NSAEs exhibit agonist activity *in vivo*, since they reduce gonadotrophin levels and increase SHBG levels (with the possible exception of idoxifene). With the exception of raloxifene, there appear to be no data available on the effects of the new NSAEs on bone density, lipids and the endometrium. Raloxifene has equivalent activity to premarin on bone. It also reduces LDL-cholesterol levels significantly, but has no significant effect on HDL-cholesterol. Raloxifene also exhibits no apparent stimulatory effect on the endometrium,[74] and may therefore prove to be an attractive choice in the clinic, provided that evidence of adequate anti-tumour activity is forthcoming.

Table 21.13 *Response to NSAEs in tamoxifen-resistant breast cancer*

	Dose (mg)	Number of patients	CR + PR (%)	NC	Duration of NC	Author
Toremifene	200	9	33	35	(NK)	Ebbs, 1990[66]
	240	34	0	26	(5–27 months)	Jonsson, 1991[68]
	240	50	4	44	(> 2 months)	Pyrhonen, 1994[69]
	200	102	5	23	(median 7.8 months)	Vogel, 1993[70]
	240	23	0	22	(median 6.0 months)	Stenbygaard, 1993[58]
Droloxifene	100	26	15	19	(> 6.0 months)	Haarstad, 1992[71]
Raloxifene		14	0	NK		Lee and Buzdar, 1988[67]
Idoxifene*	20	14	14	21	(> 5/12 months)	Coombes et al., 1995[72]

* Given mainly as third-line endocrine therapy.
NK, not known.

Table 21.14 *Incidence of common side-effects with new NSAEs*

	Hot flushes (%)	Lassitude (%)	Nausea/ vomiting (%)	Author
Tamoxifen	30	10	10	Litherland and Jackson, 1988[73]
Toremifene	19	10	8	Valavaara, 1990[61,63]
Droloxifene	29	26	29	Rauschning and Pritchard, 1994[65]
Raloxifene	43	36	14	Lee and Buzdar, 1988[67]
Idoxifene	'similar to tamoxifen'			

Pharmacokinetic data for the new NSAEs are currently incomplete. Toremifene has similar pharmacokinetics to those of tamoxifen.[75] Idoxifene takes longer to reach steady-state concentrations (6–12 weeks) than tamoxifen, and has been shown to have a more prolonged terminal half-life of 23 days in patients on longer-term therapy.[72] Therapeutic levels of droloxifene are reached within the first day of therapy, compared to 11 days with tamoxifen. The terminal half-life of droloxifene is also short, at 25 hours,[76,77] and this drug may therefore be more suitable than tamoxifen when considering treatment regimes involving sequencing with other endocrine or cytotoxic therapies. The pharmacokinetics of raloxifene do not appear to have been published at the time of writing.

In summary, therefore, there is insufficient clinical data available at present to permit conclusions to be drawn as to whether any of the newer generation of NSAEs will supersede tamoxifen in the future. Large clinical studies with toremifene have borne out preclinical data suggesting that this agent has little or no advantage over tamoxifen as first-line therapy, and a high degree of cross-resistance with tamoxifen when investigated as second-line therapy. Droloxifene appears to be active in preclinical and early clinical studies, but as yet no clinical phase III data are available. Its short half-life may make it particularly useful in alternating drug schedules. Raloxifene appeared to be only weakly agonistic in the rat uterus assay but, paradoxically, has proved to be a clinically useful agent for the treatment of osteoporosis, and it also has a favourable effect on lipids.[78] Few clinical data are currently available on TAT-59, a Japanese NSAE, but preclinical studies suggest that it may be very active. Idoxifene has been specifically designed to be active in tamoxifen failure, and is currently undergoing clinical trial in this context. Its preclinical and early clinical activity appear promising.

Steroidal ('pure') anti-oestrogens

Substitutions of the oestrogen molecule at various positions can produce compounds with anti-oestrogenic activity.[54,79–82] Analysis of the structure–function relationship of these novel compounds revealed that the position, length and flexibility of the C7 side-chain were all important in determining agonist/antagonist behaviour.[83] In particular, it was found that OR-binding and biological activity reside almost exclusively in 7α- rather than 7β-isomers, and that pure anti-oestrogen activity is associated with overall side-chain lengths of 16–18 atoms.

The first compounds shown to be associated with pure antagonist profiles of activity were a group of 7α-alkylamide derivatives of oestradiol. The most potent of these compounds was N-n-butyl-N-methyl-11-(3,17 β-dihydroxyoestra-1,3,5(10)-trien-7α-yl)undecanamide (ICI 164384) (see Figure 21.6). This agent, which bears a methyl tertiary amide group on the C7 side-chain, came to be identified as a prototype pure anti-oestrogen, and it has been extensively evaluated in a wide range of oestrogen-responsive systems, including experimental breast cancer models.

Unfortunately, the potency of ICI 164384 in vivo was found to be too low for the compound to merit serious consideration as a candidate for clinical use, since very high doses were required to block oestrogen action completely. The search for more potent compounds which retained the pure anti-oestrogen profile of ICI 164384 led to the development of 7α-[9-(4,4,5,5,5-pentafluoropentylsulphinyl)nonyl]oestra-1,3,5,(10)-triene-3, 7β-diol (ICI 182780) (Figure 21.6). This agent differs from ICI 164384 in two key features of the 7α side-chain – the tertiary amide moiety of ICI 164384 is replaced by a sulphinyl group, and the terminal alkyl function is fluorinated to reduce the potential for metabolic attack. ICI 182780 is approximately five times more potent as an anti-oestrogen than ICI 164384 in vitro and approximately 10 times more potent in vivo.[84]

The oral bioavailability of ICI 182780 is low, and to date the compound has only been administered parenterally. Two formulations of ICI 182780 have been produced by Astra-Zeneca (formerly ICI) Pharmaceuticals for laboratory and clinical investigation – a short-acting formulation, ICI 182780 (SA), containing the active drug in a propylene-glycol based vehicle, and a long-acting formulation, ICI 182780 (LA), containing the active drug in a castor-oil-based vehicle.

This new generation of steroidal anti-oestrogens has been described as 'pure' or 'specific' anti-oestrogens, as they have shown little or no agonist activity in preclinical studies. For reasons of potency discussed above, clinical data are only available for ICI 182780. These and the relevant preclinical data are summarized in tables 21.15 and 21.16.

ICI 182780 binds to OR with the same affinity as oestrogen.[84] It is superior to tamoxifen with respect to growth inhibition of human breast cancer cell lines grown in vitro,[84] or as xenografts in nude mice in vivo.[85] In addition, ICI 182780 retains in-vitro activity vs. tamoxifen-resistant cell lines,[86–89] (Table 21.15), and also inhibits the clonogenic growth in vitro of breast cancer cells harvested directly from patients with metastatic disease at the time of clinical relapse on tamoxifen.[33]

Limited data are currently available from clinical studies (Table 21.16). In a phase I study, ICI 182780 was shown to inhibit tumour proliferation and significantly reduce tumour OR and PgR content when administered to post-menopausal patients for 1 week prior to primary breast cancer surgery.[32] Importantly, ICI 182780 has shown a high level of activity against tamoxifen-resistant advanced breast cancer in an ongoing phase II clinical trial, producing 7 partial responses and 6 stable disease responses in 19 patients entered.[7,92] As predicted from the nude mouse model,

Table 21.15 *Preclinical data concerning ICI 182780 in comparison with tamoxifen*

Assessment	Effect	Reference
Oestrogen-receptor binding	• Equal to oestrogen	Wakeling et al., 1991[84]
Tumour antagonism	• MCF-7 cells in vitro twice as active • MCF-7 cells in nude mice, growth suppressed twice as long • Animal tumours?	Wakeling et al., 1991[84] Osborne et al., 1995[85]
Peripheral antagonist/agonist ratio	• Immature rat uterus assay – complete antagonist. No agonist activity • Reduced cancellous bone in rats • No effect on bone in rats • No effect on gonadotrophins	Wakeling et al., 1991[84] Gallagher et al., 1993[90] Wakeling, 1993[86] Wakeling, 1992[91]
Alternative mechanisms of action	• None reported	
Activity against tamoxifen-resistant cell lines	• Yes	Lykkesfeldt et al., 1994[89] Coopman et al., 1994[88] Wakeling, 1993[86]

ICI 182780 administration has resulted in a particularly long duration of tumour suppression, such that the median duration of response has only just been reached after 23 months of treatment. Although the overall rate of response to ICI 182780 is not significantly greater, comparison of these results with a comparably selected group of 57 historical patients treated with megestrol acetate after tamoxifen failure suggests that the duration of the response to ICI 182780 may be almost twice as long as is seen with current second-line endocrine therapy.[93]

At the time of writing there are very preliminary data available concerning the activity of ICI 182780 at other central and peripheral oestrogen-target sites. Data from the short- and long-term dosing studies suggest an apparent absence of agonist or antagonist effects of ICI 182780 on the hypothalamus/pituitary gland and the liver, producing no significant changes in serum levels of gonadotrophins, lipids or SHBG.[7,32] Administration of the short-acting formulation of ICI 182780 to pre-menopausal women for 1 week prior to hysterectomy was associated with significant inhibition of uterine proliferation.[94] The longer-term effects of ICI 182780 on the genital tract of post-menopausal women have yet to be confirmed, although none of the patients in the phase II study reported vaginal discharge or dryness, and no apparent changes in endometrial thickness were seen in 5 patients in whom serial measurements were performed by ultrasound. As yet there are no clinical data on the effect of ICI 182780 on bone. As the limited data available from animal studies have been equivocal in this respect, demonstrating a lack of effect in one study[86,87] and a negative effect in a second study,[90] further clinical studies will be needed to clarify this issue. Clearly, specific antagonists such as ICI 182780 may be an important new approach to anti-oestrogen therapy. Overviews of the laboratory and clinical development of these compounds have been published recently.[95,96]

Table 21.16 *Clinical results with ICI 182780*

Assessment	Effect	Reference
Activity first line	• No studies • Reduces tumour proliferation and OR before surgery	 DeFriend et al., 1994a[32]
Activity in tamoxifen-resistant tumours	• PR 7/19(37%) NC6/19 (32%) • 19 patients treated • Median duration of response > 22/12 • Active in vitro	Howell, 1995a[92] Howell, 1996[7] DeFriend, 1994[33]
Side-effects	• None of note	Howell, 1995, 1996[8,92]
Peripheral antagonist/agonist ratio	• No effect on gonadotrophins or SHBG • Inhibition of endometrial proliferation • Bone – no data	Howell, 1996[8] Thomas et al., 1994[94]
Pharmacokinetics	• Given by monthly depot • Therapeutic levels present throughout month	Howell, 1996[7]

AROMATASE INHIBITORS

The structure of new aromatase inhibitors currently available for use in the clinic or undergoing clinical trials is shown in Figure 21.7. They fall into two major groups – non-steroidal and steroidal – each with different mechanisms of action.

Potency, selectivity and pharmacokinetics

Following the recognition that aminoglutethimide was a non-specific, reversible inhibitor of several cytochrome P450-dependent enzyme pathways, and that aromatase inhibition was prominent among these, the quest began for non-steroidal compounds that were both more selective and more potent. Pyridoglutethimide was an early example showing improved enzyme and pharmacological selectivity (no CNS effects), but only comparable potency. Like aminoglutethimide, pyridoglutethimide is a potent inducer of liver enzymes and enhances its own metabolism.

Fadrazole represented a major advance in potency (c. 500-fold) and selectivity, but the latter is not complete,

and 18-hydroxylase inhibition becomes apparent towards the upper end of the dose–response curve for aromatase inhibition in women. Vorozole, letrozole and anastrozole (all triazole derivatives) combine potency with high selectivity for aromatase, and have no discernible effects on adrenal function at the maximally effective aromatase-inhibiting doses. The latter three drugs have been shown to reduce circulating oestradiol levels in post-menopausal women to the limits of detection of the most sensitive assays currently available (see Table 21.17). Although intrinsically reversible as enzyme inhibitors, the long plasma half-lives of letrozole and anastrozole enable continuous enzyme inhibition to be achieved with simple once-daily dosing.

4-Hydroxyandrostenedione (Lentaron) was one of the first of the steroidal substrate analogues to be described, and is the first to have been developed to the stage of routine clinical use. It has high enzyme selectivity, but poor oral bioavailability due to high first-pass metabolism. It is therefore provided as a parenteral formulation for twice-monthly administration. Weak 'hormonal' (androgenic) effects in the form of gonadotrophin suppression are discernible in animals. In humans, lowering of serum SHBG levels has been observed, athough only after twice-

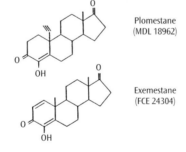

Figure 21.7 *New aromatase inhibitors.*

Table 21.17 *Suppression of serum oestradiol, oestrone and oestrone sulphate by second- and third-generation aromatase inhibitors*

	Dose (mg/day)	Oestradiol (% of baseline value)	Oestrone (% of baseline value)	Oestrone sulphate (% of baseline value)	Authors
Exemestane (FCE 24304)	25	28	35	39	Di Salle *et al.* 1994[97]
Pyridoglutethimide	1600	50	17	—	Dowsett 1991[98]
Fadrozole (CGS 16949A)	2–16	65	27	30	Santen 1989[99]
Vorozole (R83842)	5	11	45	31	Johnston *et al.*, 1994[100]
Letrozole (CGS 20267)	0.1–2.5	21*	21*	—	Iveson *et al.*, 1993[101]
Letrozole (CGS 20267)	0.1–5	<10*	<10*	<10*	Lipton *et al.*, 1990[102]
Anastrozole (ZD 1033)	1	15*	15*	8*	Plourde, 1994[103]

* At or below detection limit of assay.

daily oral dosing with large doses. Plomestane and exemestane represent second-generation steroidal-type inhibitors, and both offer the potential for oral dosing. All three steroidal compounds interact covalently with aromatase during the first oxidation cycle, and cause irreversible inhibition. This provides prolonged peripheral aromatase inhibition despite rapid plasma clearance of the drugs. The cross-reactivity of plomestane and its metabolites in oestrogen assays has complicated serum oestrogen measurements in trials and has slowed its development.

Clinical data

The results of many of the clinical trials with the new aromatase inhibitors reported to date are shown in Table 21.18. Except for the randomized trials, the response rates should be viewed with caution, as the response rate in small phase II studies can be greatly influenced by patient selection. With the exception of the trial comparing tamoxifen with fadrozole,[104] the new aromatase inhibitors have been tested as second- or third-line treatments in OR-positive or OR-unknown patients.

Three phase II trials of exemestane are currently ongoing in the USA and Europe in tamoxifen or megestrol acetate failures. In addition, a further European study is evaluating the activity of exemestane after aminoglutethimide failure. With the exception of the latter study,[105] data are not yet available.

Two dose-finding randomized phase II studies of pyridoglutethimide were reported recently which suggest that the optimal dose is 600 mg or 800 mg.[106,107] Fadrozole has been shown to be active after tamoxifen failure in a phase II study,[108] and to be equivalent in terms of efficacy and toxicity to tamoxifen in a European phase III study[104] (Table 21.18).

Vorozole has been shown to be active after tamoxifen failure,[100] and is now undergoing phase III evaluation vs.

Table 21.18 *Response rates in phase II and (where available) phase III studies with second- and third-generation aromatase inhibitors*

	Dose (mg/day)	Number of patients	CR+PR (%)	NC* (%)	Authors
Pyridoglutethimide	600	21	14	34 (?)	Schultz *et al.*, 1995[106]
	800	21	10	86 (?)	
	400	46	4	—	Harnett *et al.*, 1995[107]
	800	46	14	—	
Fadrozole†	1.4	80	23	45 (?)	Falkson *et al.*, 1992[108]
Fadrozole†	2	86	16	48 (?)	Thurlimann *et al.* 1996[104]
vs. tamoxifen	20	90	24	48 (?)	
Vorozole‡	1–5	24	33	17 (≥6/12)	Johnston *et al.*, 1994[100]
Letrozole‡	0.5–2	21	33	24 (≥3/12)	Iveson *et al.*, 1993[101]
Anastrozole†	1	135	10	24 (≥ 6/12)	Jonat *et al.*, 1996, 1997[109,110]
Anastrozole	10	118	13	21	
Megestrol acetate	160	125	13	22	

* Minimum duration of NC.
‡ Phase III study.
† Randomized phase II studies.

aminoglutethimide. Letrozole has also been shown to be active in two phase II studies,[101,102] and is undergoing phase III evaluation in a three-arm study comparing two dose levels of letrozole against megestrol acetate.

Two phase III studes of anastrozle (Arimidex) have been completed and preliminary results reported for each one.[109–111] The results of the European trial are shown in Table 21.18. In both studies anastrozole 1 mg or 10 mg daily was compared with megestrol acetate 160 mg. The lower dose of anastrozole (1 mg) proved sufficient to suppress serum oestradiol levels to below the detection limit of the assay used (3 pmol/L). The 10-mg dose was also evaluated on the basis that there may be some additional drug effect at the higher dose (e.g. suppression of intratumoral aromatase or additional depression of serum oestradiol levels (to well below the selection limits of most assays). Both trials were performed in patients who had failed tamoxifen and who had OR-positive or OR-unknown tumours. The two trials have produced identical results. There were no significant differences in response rates between the two doses of anastrozole, or between either dose of anastrozole and megestrol acetate. However, a major advantage of anastrazole was observed in its lack of propensity to cause weight gain, since more than 30% of patients treated with megestrol acetate experienced weight gain of ⩾ 5%, and more than 10% of patients experienced weight gain of ⩾ 10%.[109,110] Furthermore, the weight gain experienced with megestrol acetate increased over time (Figure 21.8). The once daily dosing and lack of

weight gain seen with anastrozole make it more attractive than megestrol acetate as a second-line endocrine agent, and identify it as a potential candidate for adjuvant therapy. The dose of anastrozole to be used in the clinic will be 1 mg daily.

None of the second- and third-generation aromatase inhibitors undergoing clinical trials appear to share the significant toxicity associated with aminoglutethimide. The major side-effects reported to date have been mild gastrointestinal disturbance and hot flushes, which together have been observed in approximately 40% of patients.[100,101,109,110,112]

ANTIPROGESTINS

Progestins are currently the most commonly used second-line endocrine therapy for advanced breast cancer.[2] Antiprogestins have been used in clinical trials for some years, but have not become serious contenders as standard treatment, mainly because of their toxicity and apparent low efficacy.

The precise mechanism whereby antiprogestins inhibit steroid-receptor-positive tumour cells is unclear. They may act as antiprogestins,[113] anti-oestrogens[114–116] or oestrogens.[117,118] The antiprogestins which have entered the clinic, namely mifepristone (RU 486) and onapristone (ZK 98299) (see Figure 21.9 and Table 21.19), also bind glucocorticoid (GR) and androgen receptors. In fact, the affinity of mifepristone for GR is more than three times that of dexamethasone. The newer antiprogestin ZK 98299 has only a 21% affinity for GR compared to dexamethasone, but also has a lower affinity for PgR. Newer compounds with higher affinity for PgR and lower affinity for GR are being developed (e.g. Org 31710).[119,120]

Recent studies using cells transfected with oestrogen and progesterone reporter vectors containing a variety of promotors and expression vectors for PgR (A and B isoforms) and OR have helped to elucidate one mechanism of action of antiprogestins. These experiments indicate that there is extensive inhibitory cross-talk between OR and PgR. Both progestins (RS020) and antiprogestins (mifepristone) were shown to act as potent ligand-dependent repressors of OR activity when bound to

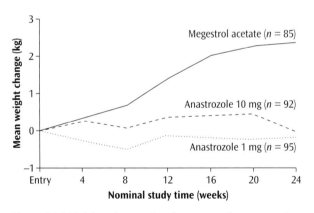

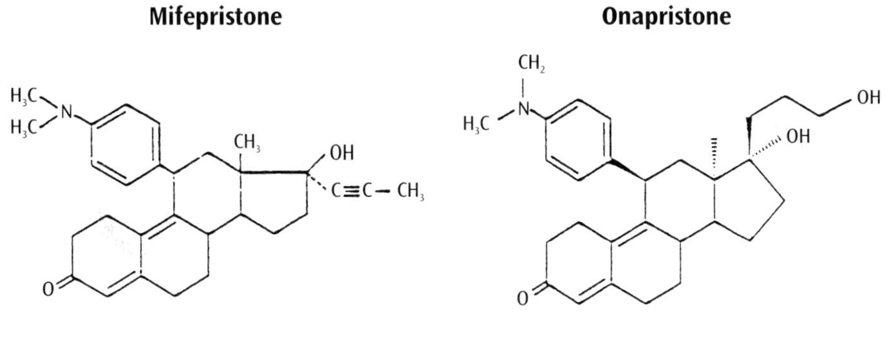

Figure 21.8 *Weight gain over time for megestrol acetate and anastrozole.*

Mifepristone

Onapristone

Figure 21.9 *Chemical structures of the anti-oestrogens mifepristone and onapristone.*

Table 21.19 *Preclinical studies with mifepristone and onapristone*

Assessment		Mifepristone (RU 486)	Onapristone (ZK 98299)
Receptor/activator binding		Binds PR and induces DNA binding	Binds PR, no DNA binding
Tumour antagonism	Cell lines	Inhibits MCF-7 (Bardon *et al.*, 1985)[122]	MCF-7 (Classen, 1993)[121]
	Nude mice	NT	T 61 (Schneider *et al.*, 1992)[123]
	Animal tumours	DMBA (Bakker *et al.*, 1989)[124]	DMBA induction
			NMU = tamoxifen (Schneider *et al.*, 1990)[125]
Peripheral antagonist/agonist ratio		NK	NK
Alternative mechanism of action		Non-competitive inhibitor of OR	Induction of differentiation (Michna *et al.* 1992)[126]
Activity against resistant cell lines		Active in E2-insensitive lines (Horwitz 1992)[127]	NK

NT, not tested; NK, not known.

either isoform of PgR.[128] Some studies indicate that ZK 98299 may act by blocking PgR binding to DNA,[129] but this mechanism of action remains controversial. Jeng *et al.*[118] demonstrated that mifepristone stimulated the growth of MCF-7 cells at a concentration of 10^{-6}M, an effect which appeared to be potentially oestrogenic, as it could be blocked by 40H-tamoxifen and ICI 164384.

Whatever their mechanism of action, mifepristone and onapristone inhibit the proliferation of human PgR-positive mammary tumour cell lines,[122] the growth of human tumour cell xenografts in nude mice,[123] and the growth of carcinogen-induced animal tumours.[124,125] In addition, mifepristone has been shown to be active in oestradiol-insensitive cell lines.[127] One further action which is of interest is the demonstration that ZK 98299 can induce differentiation in human mammary cancer cell lines.[126,130]

Mifepristone was initially tested clinically in tamoxifen-resistant advanced breast cancer, but only a few responses were seen[131,132] (Table 21.20). In order to test mifepristone under the best possible circumstances, Perrault *et al.*[133] examined its efficacy in patients with PgR-positive tumours previously untreated with endocrine therapy. Unfortunately, the response rate was low (9% CR + PR), and 59% of patients reported lethargy. Onapristone has shown activity in phase II trials (Table 21.20), but has been withdrawn from further clinical development because of induction of abnormal liver function tests. It would appear therefore that further development of antiprogestin therapy must await the availability of more specific and less toxic compounds.

SUMMARY AND CONCLUSIONS

Endocrine therapy for breast cancer remains one of the best tolerated and least toxic systemic treatments available for any human malignancy. The ability to conduct extensive evaluations of conventional and new agents over the years in the advanced breast cancer clinic has allowed clinicians to gain insights into the mechanisms underlying response and resistance to these agents, and has enabled them to select out suitable agents with proven efficacy and safety records for evaluation in the adjuvant and chemoprevention settings.

At the time of writing, there is an exciting selection of new endocrine agents at various stages of clinical development. It remains to be seen whether any of these new agents will prove more active than tamoxifen in advanced disease, or as safe as tamoxifen in adjuvant usage. To date, none of the new non-steroidal anti-oestrogens have shown unequivocal evidence of improved efficacy in the clinic to mirror their improved profiles over tamoxifen in preclinical studies. The specific steroidal anti-oestrogen, ICI 182780, looks very promising, but is still at a relatively early stage in its developmental programme. The new aromatase inhibitors are likely to prove equal to tamoxifen for the

Table 21.20 *Response to antiprogestins in clinical studies*

Drug	Dose (mg/day)	Number of patients	CR+PR (%)	NC (duration) (%)	Author
Mifepristone	200	22	18	?	Romieu *et al.* 1987[131]
Mifepristone	200	11	9	?	Klijn *et al.*, 1989[132]
Mifepristone*	200	22	9	41 (?)	Perrault *et al.*, 1996[133]
Onapristone	100	90	10	42 (>3/12)	Schering, 1994[134]

* Previously untreated for advanced disease and PR-positive.

treatment of advanced disease, but it is disappointing that improved oestrogen suppression has not so far led to improved efficacy. At present, the antiprogestins appear disappointing, and we will need to wait a considerable time for proposed new agents now awaiting preclinical testing to reach the clinic.

Considering that it was originally developed as an antifertility treatment, it is somewhat ironic that the complex range of activity which tamoxifen exhibits, and which made it unsuitable for antifertility purposes, may by serendipity have made it an almost ideal adjuvant endocrine treatment, combining reasonable anti-oestrogenic, anti-tumour activity with beneficial oestrogenic, cardio- and osteo-protective effects. There is no doubt that, despite the scientific and developmental effort that underlies the production of the newer agents discussed above, tamoxifen is likely to prove a very difficult drug to surpass in the adjuvant setting. Similarly, it will be many years before any of the new agents will have been demonstrated to have the high levels of long-term safety that must be demanded of potential candidate drugs for use in chemoprevention studies.

REFERENCES

1 Beatson G. On the treatment of inoperable cases of carcinoma of the mamma: suggestions for a new method of treatment with illustrative cases. *Lancet* 1896; **ii**: 104–7.
2 Lundgren S. Progestins in breast cancer treatment. A review. *Acta Oncol* 1992; **31**: 709–22.
3 Cole MP, Jones CT, Todd ID. A new anti-oestrogenic agent in late breast cancer. An early clinical appraisal of ICI46474. *Br J Cancer* 1971; **25**: 270–5.
4 Patterson JS. Clinical aspects and development of antioestrogen therapy: a review of the endocrine effects of tamoxifen in animals and man. *J Endocrinol* 1981; **89** (**Supplement**): 67P–75P.
5 Hayward JL, Carbone PP, Heuson JC, Kumaoka S, Segaloff A, Rubens RD. Assessment of response to therapy in advanced breast cancer: a project of the Programme on Clinical Oncology of the International Union Against Cancer, Geneva, Switzerland. *Cancer* 1977; **39** 1289–94.
6 Howell A, Wakeling AE. Steroid and peptide hormones and growth factors. *Cancer Chemother Biol Response Modif* 1988; **10**: 117–28.
7 Howell A, DeFriend DJ, Robertson JF *et al.* Pharmacokinetics, pharmacological and anti-tumour effects of the specific anti-oestrogen ICI 182780 in women with advanced breast cancer. *Br J Cancer* 1996; **74**: 300–8.
8 Howell A, Dowsett M. Recent advances in endocrine therapy of breast cancer. *BMJ* 1997; **315**: 863–6.
9 Howell A, Anderson E, Blamey R *et al.* The primary use of endocrine therapies. *Recent Results Cancer Res* 1998; **152**: 227–44.
10 Henderson 1991
11 Schwartz LH, Koerner FC, Edgerton SM *et al.* pS2 expression and response to hormonal therapy in patients with advanced breast cancer. *Cancer Res* 1991; **51**: 624–8.
12 Nicholson RI, McClelland RA, Finlay P *et al.* Relationship between EGF-R, c-erbB-2 protein expression and Ki67 immunostaining in breast cancer and hormone sensitivity. *Eur J Cancer* 1993; **29A**: 1018–23.
13 Escher GC. Clinical improvement of inoperable breast carcinoma under steroid treatment. 92–99. Chicago: Proceedings of the First Conference on Steroid Hormones and Mammary Carcinoma. The Therapeutic Trials Committee of the Council of Pharmay Chemistry of American Medical Association (GENERIC), 1949.
14 Huseby RA. The use of estrogen in the treatment of advanced breast cancer. In: Segaloff A (ed.) *Breast Cancer – The Second Biennial Louisiana Cancer Conference*. St Louis, MS: CV Mosby, 1958; 206–16.
15 Lewison, Trimble & Ganelin (1956)
16 Howell A, DeFriend DJ, Anderson E. Mechanisms of response and resistance to endocrine therapy for breast cancer and the development of new treatments. *Rev Endocr Rel Cancer* 1993; **43**: 5–21.
17 Kaufman and Escher 1961
18 Baker LH and Vaitkevicius VK. Reevaluation of rebound regression in disseminated carcinoma of the breast. *Cancer* 1972; **29**: 1268–71.
19 Nesto *et al.* (1976)
20 Canney PA, Griffiths T, Latief TN, Priestman TJ. Clinical significance of tamoxifen withdrawal response (letter). *Lancet* 1987; **1**: 36.
21 Howell A, Dodwell DJ, Anderson H, Redford J. Response after withdrawal of tamoxifen and progestogens in advanced breast cancer. *Ann Oncol* 1992; **3**: 611–17.
22 Legault-Poisson S, Jolivet J, Poisson R, Beretta-Piccoli M, Band PR. Tamoxifen-induced tumor stimulation and withdrawal response. *Cancer Treat Rep* 1979; **63**: 1839–41.
23 Stein W, Hortobagyi GN, Blumenschein GR. Response of metastatic breast cancer to tamoxifen withdrawal: report of a case. *J Surg Oncol* 1983; **22**: 45–6.
24 Rudolph 1986
25 Belani CP, Pearl P, Whitley NO, Aisner J. Tamoxifen withdrawal response. Report of a case. *Arch Intern Med* 1989; **149**: 449–50.
26 Beex L, Pieters G, Smals A, Koenders A, Benraad T, Kloppenborg P. Tamoxifen versus ethinyl estradiol in the treatment of postmenopausal women with advanced breast cancer. *Cancer Treat Rep* 1981; **65**: 179–85.
27 Langan-Fahey SM, Tormey DC, Jordan VC. Tamoxifen metabolites in patients on long-term adjuvant therapy for breast cancer. *Eur J Cancer* 1990; **26**: 883–8.
28 Osborne CK, Coronado E, Allred DC, Wiebe V, DeGregorio M. Acquired tamoxifen resistance: correlation with reduced breast tumor levels of tamoxifen and isomerization of trans-4-hydroxytamoxifen. *J Natl Cancer Inst* 1991; **83**: 1477–82.
29 Osborne CK, Wiebe VJ, McGuire WL, Ciocca DR, DeGregorio MW. Tamoxifen and the isomers of 4-hydroxytamoxifen in

tamoxifen-resistant tumors from breast cancer patients. *J Clin Oncol* 1992; **10**: 304–10.

30 Pavlik EJ, Nelson K, Srinivasan S *et al*. Resistance to tamoxifen with persisting sensitivity to estrogen: possible mediation by excessive antiestrogen binding site activity. *Cancer Res* 1992; **52**: 4106–12.

31 Simon 1984

32 DeFriend DJ, Anderson E, Bell J *et al*. Effects of 4-hydroxytamoxifen and a novel pure antioestrogen (ICI 182780) on the clonogenic growth of human breast cancer cells *in vitro*. *Br J Cancer* 1994; **70**: 204–11.

33 DeFriend DJ, Howell A, Nicholson RI *et al*. Investigation of a new pure antiestrogen (ICI 182780) in women with primary breast cancer. *Cancer Res* 1994; **54**: 408–14.

34 Jiang SY, Langan-Fahey SM, Stella AL, McCague R, Jordan VC. Point mutation of estrogen receptor (ER) in the ligand-binding domain changes the pharmacology of antiestrogens in OR-negative breast cancer cells stably expressing complementary DNAs for OR. *Mol Endocrinol* 1992; **6**: 2167–74.

35 Graham ML, Smith JA, Jewett PB, Horwitz KB. Heterogeneity of progesterone receptor content and remodeling by tamoxifen characterize subpopulations of cultured human breast cancer cells: analysis by quantitative dual parameter flow cytometry. *Cancer Res* 1992; **52**: 593–602.

36 Baildam AD, Zaloudik J, Howell A, Barnes DM, Moore M, Sellwood RA. Effect of tamoxifen upon cell DNA analysis by flow cytometry in primary carcinoma of the breast. *Br J Cancer* 1987; **55**: 561–6.

37 Baildam AD, Zaloudik J, Howell A *et al*. DNA analysis by flow cytometry, response to endocrine treatment and prognosis in advanced carcinoma of the breast. *Br J Cancer* 1987; **55**: 553–9.

38 Kamby C, Rasmussen BB, Kristensen B. Oestrogen receptor status of primary breast carcinomas and their metastases. Relation to pattern of spread and survival after recurrence. *Br J Cancer* 1989; **60**: 252–7.

39 Kamby C, Ejlertsen B, Andersen J *et al*. Body size and menopausal status in relation to the pattern of spread in recurrent breast cancer. *Acta Oncol* 1989; **28**: 795–9.

40 Robertson JF, Cannon PM, Nicholson RI, Blamey RW. Oestrogen and progesterone receptors as prognostic variables in hormonally treated breast cancer. *Int J Biol Markers* 1996; **11**: 29–35.

41 Jordan VC. Third Annual William L. McGuire Memorial Lecture. 'Studies on the estrogen receptor in breast cancer' – 20 years as a target for the treatment and prevention of cancer. *Breast Cancer Res Treat* 1995; **36**: 267–85.

42 Jordan VC. Tamoxifen: toxicities and drug resistance during the treatment and prevention of breast cancer. *Annu Rev Pharmacol Toxicol* 1995; **35**: 195–211.

43 Fawell SE, White R, Hoare S, Sydenham M, Page M, Parker MG. Inhibition of estrogen receptor-DNA binding by the 'pure' antiestrogen ICI 164,384 appears to be mediated by impaired receptor dimerization. *Proc Natl Acad Sci USA* 1990; **87**: 6883–7.

44 Fawell SE, Lees JA, White R, Parker MG. Characterization and co-localization of steroid binding and dimerization activities in the mouse estrogen receptor. *Cell* 1990; **60**: 953–62.

45 Dauvois S, White R, Parker MG. The antiestrogen ICI 182780 disrupts estrogen receptor nucleocytoplasmic shuttling. *J Cell Sci* 1993; **106**: 1377–88.

46 Kangas 1986

47 Loser *et al*. 1985

48 Black *et al*. 1983

49 Toko 1990

50 Chander *et al*. 1991

51 Kawamura 1991

52 Gottardis and Jordan 1987

53 Jones 1984

54 Wakeling AE, Bowler J. Development of novel oestrogen-receptor antagonists. *Biochem Soc Trans* 1991; **19**: 899–901.

55 Wakeling AE. Regulatory mechanisms in breast cancer. Steroidal pure antiestrogens. *Cancer Treat Res* 1991; **53**: 239–57.

56 Eppenberger 1991

57 Hardcastle IR, Rowlands MG, Houghton J *et al*. Rationally designed analogues of tamoxifen with improved calmodulin antagonism. *J Med Chem* 1995; **38**: 241–8.

58 Stenbygaard LE, Herrstedt J, Thomsen JF, Svendsen KR, Engelholm SA, Dombernowsky P. Toremifene and tamoxifen in advanced breast cancer – a double-blind cross-over trial. *Breast Cancer Res Treat* 1993; **25**: 57–63.

59 Hayes DF, Van Zyl JA, Hacking A *et al*. Randomized comparison of tamoxifen and two separate doses of toremifene in postmenopausal patients with metastatic breast cancer. *J Clin Oncol* 1995; **13**: 2556–66.

60 Valavaara R, Tuominen J, Johansson R. Predictive value of tumor estrogen and progesterone receptor levels in postmenopausal women with advanced breast cancer treated with toremifene. *Cancer* 1990; **66**: 2264–9.

61 Valavaara R. Phase II trials with toremifene in advanced breast cancer: a review. *Breast Cancer Res Treat* 1990; **16 (Supplement)**: S31–S35.

62 Valavaara R, Pyrhonen S, Heikkinen M *et al*. Safety and efficacy of toremifene in breast cancer patients. A phase II study. *J Steroid Biochem* 1990; **36**: 229–31.

63 Valavaara R. Phase II experience with toremifene in the treatment of OR-positive breast cancer of postmenopausal women. *Cancer Invest* 1990; **8**: 275–6.

64 Valavaara R. Tuominen J, Toivanen A. The immunological status of breast cancer patients during treatment with a new antiestrogen, toremifene. *Cancer Immunol Immunother* 1990; **31**: 381–6.

65 Rauschning W, Pritchard KI. Droloxifene, a new antiestrogen: its role in metastatic breast cancer. *Breast Cancer Res Treat* 1994; **31**: 83–94.

66 Ebbs SR, Roberts J, Baum M. Response to toremifene (Fc-1157a) therapy in tamoxifen failed patients with breast cancer. Preliminary communication. *J Steroid Biochem* 1990; **36**: 239.

67 Lee and Buzdar 1988

68 Jonsson 1991

69 Pyrhonen 1994

70 Vogel 1993

71 Haarstad 1992

72 Coombes RC, Haynes BP, Dowsett M *et al.* Idoxifene: report of a phase I study in patients with metastatic breast cancer. *Cancer Res* 1995; **55**: 1070–4.

73 Litherland and Jackson 1988

74 Draper MW, Flowers DE, Neild JA, Huster WJ, Zerbe RL. Antiestrogenic properties of raloxifene. *Pharmacology* 1995; **50**: 209–17.

75 Wiebe VJ, Benz CC, Shemano I, Cadman TB, DeGregorio MW. Pharmacokinetics of toremifene and its metabolites in patients with advanced breast cancer. *Cancer Chemother Pharmacol* 1990; **25**: 247–51.

76 Tanaka Y, Sekiguchi M, Sawamoto T *et al.* Pharmacokinetics of droloxifene in mice, rats, monkeys, premenopausal and postmenopausal patients. *Eur J Drug Metab Pharmacokinet* 1994; **19**: 47–58.

77 Grill HJ, Pollow K. Pharmacokinetics of droloxifene and its metabolites in breast cancer patients. *Am J Clin Oncol* 1991; **14** (**Supplement 2**): S21–S29.

78 Draper MW, Flowers DE, Huster WJ, Neild JA, Harper KD, Arnaud C. A controlled trial of raloxifene (LY139481) HCI: impact on bone turnover and serum lipid profile in healthy postmenopausal women. *J Bone Miner Res* 1996; **11**: 835–42.

79 Wakeling AE, Bowler J. ICI 182,780, a new antioestrogen with clinical potential. *J Steroid Biochem Mol Biol* 1992, **43**: 173–7.

80 Levesque C, Merand Y, Dufour JM, Labrie C, Labrie F. Synthesis and biological activity of new halo-steroidal antiestrogens. *J Med Chem* 1991; **34**: 1624–30.

81 Claussner A, Nedelec L, Nique F, Philibert D, Teutsch G, Van d V. 11 Beta-amidoalkyl estradiols, a new series of pure antiestrogens. *J Steroid Biochem Mol Biol* 1992; **41**: 609–14.

82 Auger S, Merand Y, Pelletier JD, Poirier D, Labrie F. Synthesis and biological activities of thioether derivatives related to the antiestrogens tamoxifen and ICI 164384. *J Steroid Biochem Mol Biol* 1995; **52**: 547–65.

83 Bowler J, Lilley TJ, Pittam JD, Wakeling AE. Novel steroidal pure antiestrogens. *Steroids* 1989; **54**: 71–99.

84 Wakeling AE, Dukes M, Bowler J. A potent specific pure antiestrogen with clinical potential. *Cancer Res* 1991; **51**: 3867–73.

85 Osborne CK, Coronado-Heinsohn EB, Hilsenbeck SG *et al.* Comparison of the effects of a pure steroidal antiestrogen with those of tamoxifen in a model of human breast cancer. *J Natl Cancer Inst* 1995; **87**: 746–50.

86 Wakeling AE. Are breast tumours resistant to tamoxifen also resistant to pure antioestrogens? *J Steroid Biochem Mol Biol* 1993; **47**: 107–14.

87 Wakeling AE. The future of new pure antiestrogens in clinical breast cancer. *Breast Cancer Res Treat* 1993; **25**: 1–9.

88 Coopman P, Garcia M, Brunner N, Derocq D, Clarke R, Rochefort H. Anti-proliferative and anti-estrogenic effects of ICI 164,384 and ICI 182,780 in 4-OH-tamoxifen-resistant human breast-cancer cells. *Int J Cancer* 1994; **56**: 295–300.

89 Lykkesfeldt AE, Madsen MW, Briand P. Altered expression of estrogen-regulated genes in a tamoxifen-resistant and ICI 164,384 and ICI 182,780 sensitive human breast cancer cell line, MCF-7/TAMR-1. *Cancer Res* 1994; **54**: 1587–95.

90 Gallagher A, Chambers TJ, Tobias JH. The estrogen antagonist ICI 182,780 reduces cancellous bone volume in female rats. *Endocrinology* 1993; **133**: 2787–91.

91 Wakeling AE. Steroid antagonists as nuclear receptor blockers. *Cancer Surv* 1992; **14**: 71–85.

92 Howell A, DeFriend D, Robertson J, Blamey R, Walton P. Response to a specific antioestrogen (ICI 182780) in tamoxifen-resistant breast cancer. *Lancet* 1995; **345**: 29–30.

93 Robertson *et al.* 1995

94 Thomas EJ, Walton PL, Thomas NM, Dowsett M. The effects of ICI 182,780, a pure anti-oestrogen, on the hypothalamic-pituitary-gonadal axis and on endometrial proliferation in pre-menopausal women. *Hum Reprod* 1994; **9**: 1991–6.

95 Nicholson RI, Gee JM, Manning DL, Wakeling AE, Montano MM, Katzenellenbogen BS. Responses to pure antiestrogens (ICI 164384, ICI 182780) in estrogen-sensitive and -resistant experimental and clinical breast cancer. *Ann N Y Acad Sci* 1995; **761**: 148–63.

96 Nicholson RI, Gee JM, Bryant S *et al.* Pure antiestrogens. The most important advance in the endocrine therapy of breast cancer since 1896. *Ann N Y Acad Sci* 1996; **784**: 325–35.

97 Di Salle E, Ornati G, Paridaens R, Coombes RC, Lobelle JP, Zurlo MG. Preclinical and clinical pharmacology of the aromatase inhibitor exemestane (FCE 24304). In: Motta M, Serio M (eds) *Sex hormones and antihormones in endocrine dependent pathology: basic and clinical aspects.* Amsterdam: Elsevier, 1994:303–9.

98 Dowsett 1991

99 Santen 1989

100 Johnston SR, Smith IE, Doody D, Jacobs S, Robertshaw H, Dowsett M. Clinical and endocrine effects of the oral aromatase inhibitor vorozole in postmenopausal patients with advanced breast cancer. *Cancer Res* 1994; **54**: 5875–81.

101 Iveson TJ, Smith IE, Ahern J, Smithers DA, Trunet PF, Dowsett M. Phase I study of the oral nonsteroidal aromatase inhibitor CGS 20267 in postmenopausal patients with advanced breast cancer. *Cancer Res* 1993; **53**: 266–70.

102 Lipton A, Harvey HA, Demers LM *et al.* A phase I trial of CGS 16949A. A new aromatase inhibitor. *Cancer* 1990; **65**: 1279–85.

103 Plourde 1994

104 Thurlimann B, Beretta K, Bacchi M *et al.* First-line fadrozole HCI (CGS 16949A) versus tamoxifen in postmenopausal women with advanced breast cancer. Prospective randomised trial of the Swiss Group for Clinical Cancer Research SAKK 20/88. *Ann Oncol* 1996; **7**: 471–9.

105 Thurlimann B, Castiglione M, Hsu-Schmitz SF *et al*. Formestane versus megestrol acetate in postmenopausal breast cancer patients after failure of tamoxifen: a phase III prospective randomised cross-over trial of second-line hormonal treatment (SAKK 20/90). Swiss Group for Clinical Cancer Research (SAKK).

106 Schultz *et al*. 1995

107 Harnett *et al*. 1995

108 Falkson G, Raats JI, Falkson HC. Fadrozole hydrochloride, a new nontoxic aromatase inhibitor for the treatment of patients with metastatic breast cancer. *J Steroid Biochem Mol Biol* 1992; **43**: 161–5.

109 Jonat W, Howell A, Blomqvist C *et al*. A randomised trial comparing two doses of the new selective aromatase inhibitor anastrozole (Arimidex) with megestrol acetate in postmenopausal patients with advanced breast cancer. *Eur J Cancer* 1996; **32A**: 404–12.

110 Jonat W. Clinical overview of anastrozole – a new selective oral aromatase inhibitor. *Oncology* 1997; **54 (Supplement 2)**: 15–18.

111 Buzdar A, Jonat W, Howell A *et al*. Anastrozole, a potent and selective aromatase inhibitor, versus megestrol acetate in postmenopausal women with advanced breast cancer: results of overview analysis of two phase III trials. Arimidex Study Group. *J Clin Oncol* 1996; **14**: 2000–11.

112 Thurlimann B. Hormonal treatment of breast cancer: new developments. *Oncology* 1998; **55**: 501–7.

113 Baulieu EE. RU 486 (mifepristone). A short overview of its mechanisms of action and clinical uses at the end of 1996. *Ann N Y Acad Sci* 1997; **828**: 47–58.

114 McDonnell DP, Goldman ME. RU486 exerts antiestrogenic activities through a novel progesterone receptor A form-mediated mechanism. *J Biol Chem* 1994; **269**: 11945–9.

115 Kraus WL, Montano MM, Katzenellenbogen BS. Identification of multiple, widely spaced estrogen-responsive regions in the rat progesterone receptor gene. *Mol Endocrinol* 1994; **8**: 952–69.

116 Kraus WL, McInerney EM, Katzenellenbogen BS. Ligand-dependent, transcriptionally productive association of the amino- and carboxyl-terminal regions of a steroid hormone nuclear receptor. *Proc Natl Acad Sci USA* 1995; **92**: 12314–18.

117 Jeng MH, ten Dijke P, Iwata KK, Jordan VC. Regulation of the levels of three transforming growth factor beta mRNAs by estrogen and their effects on the proliferation of human breast cancer cells. *Mol Cell Endocrinol* 1993; **97**: 115–23.

118 Jeng MH, Langan-Fahey SM, Jordan VC. Estrogenic actions of RU486 in hormone-responsive MCF-7 human breast cancer cells. *Endocrinology* 1993; **132**: 2622–30.

119 Kloosterboer HJ, Schoonen WG, Deckers GH, Klijn JG. Effects of progestagens and Org OD14 in *in vitro* and *in vivo* tumor models. *J Steroid Biochem Mol Biol* 1994; **49**: 311–18.

120 Kloosterboer HJ, Deckers GH, Schoonen WG. Pharmacology of two new very selective antiprogestagens: Org 31710 and Org 31806. *Hum Reprod* 1994; **9 (Supplement 1)**: 47–52.

121 Classen 1993

122 Bardon S, Vignon F, Chalbos D, Rochefort H. RU486, a progestin and glucocorticoid antagonist, inhibits the growth of breast cancer cells via the progesterone receptor. *J Clin Endocrinol Metab* 1985; **60**: 692–7.

123 Schneider MR, Michna H, Habenicht UF, Nishino Y, Grill HJ, Pollow K. The tumour-inhibiting potential of the progesterone antagonist onapristone in the human mammary carcinoma T61 in nude mice. *J Cancer Res Clin Oncol* 1992; **118**: 187–9.

124 Bakker GH, Setyono-Han B, Portengen H, de Jong FH, Foekens JA, Klijn JG. Endocrine and antitumor effects of combined treatment with an antiprogestin and antiestrogen or luteinizing hormone-releasing hormone agonist in female rats bearing mammary tumors. *Endocrinology* 1989; **125**: 1593–8.

125 Schneider MR, Michna H, Nishino Y, el Etreby MF. Antitumor activity and mechanism of action of different antiprogestins in experimental breast cancer models. *J Steroid Biochem Mol Biol* 1990; **37**: 783–7.

126 Michna H, Gehring S, Kuhnel W, Nishino Y, Schneider MR. The antitumor potency of progesterone antagonists is due to their differentiation potential. *J Steroid Biochem Mol Biol* 1992; **43**: 203–10.

127 Horwitz KB. The molecular biology of RU486. Is there a role for antiprogestins in the treatment of breast cancer? *Endocr Rev* 1992; **13**: 146–63.

128 Kraus WL, Weis KE, Katzenellenbogen BS. Inhibitory cross-talk between steroid hormone receptors: differential targeting of estrogen receptor in the repression of its transcriptional activity by agonist- and antagonist-occupied progestin receptors. *Mol Cell Biol* 1995; **15**: 1847–57.

129 Sartorius CA, Groshong SD, Miller LA *et al*. New T47D breast cancer cell lines for the independent study of progesterone B- and A-receptors: only antiprogestin-occupied B-receptors are switched to transcriptional agonists by cAMP. *Cancer Res* 1994; **54**: 3868–77.

130 Michna H, Nishino Y, Neef G, McGuire WL, Schneider MR. Progesterone antagonists: tumor-inhibiting potential and mechanism of action. *J Steroid Biochem Mol Biol* 1992; **41**: 339–48.

131 Romieu G, Maudelonde T, Ullmann A *et al*. The antiprogestin RU486 in advanced breast cancer: preliminary clinical trial. *Bull Cancer* 1987; **74**: 455–61.

132 Klijn JG, de Jong FH, Bakker GH, Lamberts SW, Rodenburg CJ, Alexieva-Figusch J. Antiprogestins, a new form of endocrine therapy for human breast cancer. *Cancer Res* 1989; **49**: 2851–6.

133 Perrault D, Eisenhauer EA, Pritchard KI *et al*. Phase II study of the progesterone antagonist mifepristone in patients with untreated metastatic breast carcinoma: a National Cancer Institute of Canada Clinical Trials Group study. *J Clin Oncol* 1996; **14**: 2709–12.

134 Schering 1994

Improving the quality of care for breast cancer patients

22

Variation in practice and health-care delivery of surgical management of primary breast cancer

ROBERTO GRILLI AND ALESSANDRO LIBERATI

INTRODUCTION

Research findings show that many patients fail to receive what should be considered the best treatment option for their condition according to the available evidence, and that physicians' opinions vary greatly with regard to what constitutes the best course of action for many clinical indications. As a consequence, the patterns of care for specific patient categories differ widely both across and within countries.[1–4]

Geographical variation in health services delivery has become one of the strongest motives for those who claim that more rationality is needed in the practice of medicine. It has also become the factor that often dominates apart from those suggested by scientific evidence in affecting medicine at the microclinical level.

In this paper we report on a systematic review of the literature aimed at addressing the following questions.

- What is the available evidence for variation in clinical practice styles with regard to the surgical management of breast cancer patients?
- What is the available evidence on the relationship between organizational aspects (e.g. degree of specialization, hospital or surgeon caseload) of health services and the surgical management of breast cancer?

These reviews have recently been conducted in the framework of a project funded by the UK Department of Health,[5] aimed at providing evidence-based guidelines to purchasers on defining the best configuration of health services for breast cancer patients.

For the purposes of that project, a literature search was undertaken using Medline and Embase, including papers that met the following inclusion criteria:

- publication between 1980 and 1995;
- provision of objective (i.e. not self-reported) measures of variation in the process of surgical care for breast cancer patients. In particular, studies had to provide, at the very minimum, information on the overall rate of use of specific surgical procedures, together with their range;
- information on comparisons of the surgical management of breast cancer provided by centres/clinicians and different degrees of specialization, or of centres/clinicians and different caseloads.

Overall, of a total of 190 papers identified, 6 studies were available to answer the question related to variation in clinical practice, and 11 and 9 studies were available to answer the questions concerning the relationship between surgical management and specialization, and between surgical management and caseload, respectively.

EVIDENCE OF VARIATION IN THE SURGICAL MANAGEMENT OF BREAST CANCER

In this section, the findings from the studies retrieved will be presented and analysed using the three basic concepts of *needs, demands* and *supply* as a frame of reference. These concepts will be operationally defined as 'ability to benefit from health care' (need), 'explicit request by patient for health care' (demand) and 'provision of health services' (supply). Using such a conceptual framework, the 'optimal' rate of use can be regarded as that at which the three factors are in equilibrium.

Summary of the evidence

The general characteristics and results of the 6 studies identified[6-11] are outlined in Table 22.1. Five of them focused on the use of breast-conserving procedures, and one study[9] dealt with the rate of appropriate use of different surgical interventions.

In all of the studies considered there was evidence of variation in the use of breast-conserving surgery (BCS), regardless of the type of study design, its methodological quality and the level of analysis (i.e. whether it was at the level of states, counties/provinces or individual hospitals). It is worth noting that these studies were conducted in different settings, and in the context of different countries adopting various models of health service provision and with different characteristics in terms of access to services. The amount of variation for studies on BCS, expressed with the Estremal Quotient (EQ) (the ratio of the highest to the lowest rate) ranged from 1.95[11] to 7.64.[8] Although the results are presented in Table 22.1 as crude (i.e. non-standardized) rates, together with their range,

in all of the studies the degree of variation was greater than would be expected by chance alone, even after adjusting for the potential confounding of patient characteristics and other factors.

Interpretation of the evidence

Only the findings from the Italian study,[9] which specifically assessed the appropriateness of surgical management for breast cancer, clearly identified a quality-of-care problem. All of the other available studies of variation in the use of BCS provided information which only suggests but does not confirm the possible existence of a quality problem. In fact, before concluding that variation in the delivery of conservative surgical procedures represents poor quality of care, we need to assess to what extent the observed variation truly represents a mismatch between the provision (i.e. supply) of a specific intervention and the patient's health needs (i.e. their 'ability to benefit from the intervention') and demands (i.e. the 'explicit request by the patient for health care').

NEED

We defined need as the ability of patients to benefit from BCS. This obviously requires a definition of which

Table 22.1 *General characteristics and results of studies on geographical variation in the surgical management of breast cancer*

Author, country and year of publication	Source of patients identification	Number of patients identified and aspect of care	Rates at the level of:	Mean rate of use (range)	Amount of variation EQ*
Nattinger et al., USA, 1992[6]	Administrative databases	36 982 Use of BCS in patients over 65 years of age	11 North American states	11.2% (3.5–21.2%)	6.06
Farrow et al., USA, 1992[7]	Population-based cancer registry	18 399 Use of BCS	9 North American states	22% (1983–1984) (9.2–32.1%) 33% (1985–86) (19.6%–41.5%)	3.49 2.12
Iscoe et al., Canada, 1994[8]	Population-based cancer registry	14 570 Use of BCS	38 counties of Ontario	52.6% (11–84%)	7.64
Scorpiglione et al., Italy, 1995[9]	Consecutive admissions at participating hospitals	1724 Appropriate use of surgical procedures	8 Italian regions	63% (52–88%)	1.62
Grilli and Repetto, Italy, 1995[10]	Administrative databases	3736 Use of BCS	11 geographical areas of one region	45% (29–60%)	2.07
Sainsbury et al., UK, 1995[11]	Population-based cancer registry	27 216 Use of BCS	16 districts	10% (2–25%) (1978) 55% (40–78%) (1992)	12.5 1.95

* EQ, ratio of highest rate/lowest rate.

patients can benefit (i.e. are eligible to do so) from the procedure.

It is known from clinical trials that a number of clinical characteristics are likely to affect patient eligibility for BCS, including: tumour size, its location within the breast, the breast/lesion ratio and the stage of the former.[12] It has been estimated that about 50% of women with breast cancer could be eligible for BCS.[13] Ideally, potential differences in these factors should be accounted for in studies of geographical variation, as the observed variation could depend on differences in patient characteristics (i.e. case mix) across the areas, and on the subsequent differences in perception of benefits (especially cosmetic ones) by doctors.

Usually the data on which these studies are based (i.e. claims and hospital discharge data) do not provide all of the detailed information on patients' clinical characteristics that would be needed. However, it is generally believed that variations cannot really be accounted for by differences in patient characteristics. When the rates of use are compared across relatively large geographical areas, it is in fact difficult to imagine major imbalances in the distribution of patients' characteristics across the units of comparison. This is at least partially confirmed if one considers the studies in which the analysis of variation in use was restricted to patients with localized (i.e. stage I or II) breast cancer.[6,7] The degree of variation was still substantial, confirming the hypothesis that differences in the clinical characteristics of patient populations are not likely to be the major determinant of variation. This does not mean that individual physicians do not take clinical factors into account when deciding what surgical approach to adopt in their individual patients. Rather, it suggests that when provider behaviour is analysed in aggregate, the picture that emerges resembles a more 'prevailing behaviour' that is not as strictly related to patients' clinical factors as one would assume.

What is likely to vary across the areas is the extent to which patients' clinical and sociodemographic characteristics influence physicians' decisions. For example, there is some evidence that the age of the patient influences physicians' attitudes to BCS.[14–17] However, the findings of the available studies on variation in use are not particularly consistent with regard to the role of patient age. This is probably because the study populations were different (in the studies in the USA the analysis was restricted to Medicare patients, and thus to individuals over 65 years of age), or perhaps because physicians' attitudes towards the age of the patient vary from one country to another. In the two studies in which patients of different ages were included, younger patients were more likely to receive BCS than their older counterparts in the Italian study[10] but not in the Canadian one.[8]

To investigate whether such a relationship exists, data from physicians' surveys[18–22] can also be used. In two such studies conducted in Italy[18] and the USA,[19] in which physicians' attitudes towards BCS were elicited through postal questionnaires presenting clinical scenarios, doc-

tors were consistently more likely to opt for BCS in younger than in older women.

Apart from age, patient ethnic origin and social status are other potential modifying factors which have been investigated. In one of the two US studies,[6] based on Medicare data, black race was an important predictor of use of BCS, with black women showing a 20% lower likelihood (95% CI: 30–10%) of undergoing this procedure. However, in the other study[7] race was not associated with BCS.

A further, although indirect, indication of the role of social status emerges from the Italian study, in which rates of BCS were significantly higher in private clinics that were not linked to the national health service. After controlling for age, women receiving care at private centres had a higher probability of receiving BCS (OR: 1.59; 95% CI: 1.20–2.08) than those who were seen at private institutions.[10] In these hospitals, care is either paid for directly by patients or paid indirectly through their own private insurance. It is reasonable to assume that women seeking care in these centres are likely to be of higher social status than those admitted to public hospitals, where care is free at the point of consumption.

Physicians' personal characteristics have also been studied by means of opinions/attitude surveys. It has been found that female and younger physicians show a more favourable attitude towards BCS than their male and older peers.[18–21]

The potential role of physicians' attitudes has rarely been considered in studies on variation, which have been mostly based on general information derived from administrative databases. One attempt at an in-depth analysis of the relationship between utilization and doctors' personal characteristics was made in an Italian study.[23] Hospitals were grouped according to the mean age of the surgical staff and the proportion of female physicians in surgical wards, the hypothesis being that hospitals with younger surgeons and a higher proportion of female surgeons on the staff would have a higher rate of BCS. However, this hypothesis was only partially confirmed. The rates of BCS were indeed related to the proportion of female surgeons on the staff (the rate of use of conservative surgery was 16%, 20% and 31% in centres with 0%, < 20% and 20–50% female surgeons, respectively; $P=0.003$, but no association was found with age of the surgical staff.[23] Furthermore, the amount of observed variation between centres that could be attributed to physicians' personal characteristics was modest.

However, the limited data available do support the hypothesis that physicians use different criteria when defining women who are eligible for BCS, and these criteria extend much further than patients' clinical characteristics and sociodemographic factors. Furthermore doctors' personal characteristics appear to play a role in the way in which the results of clinical research are incorporated into clinical practice.

DEMAND

Only by being fully informed about the benefits and risks of BCS may women truly participate in the decision-making process and express their preferences. Indeed, the concept of demand has to do with the patient's awareness that the benefit which can be obtained from the procedure actually meets her preferences.

Overall, data on women's preferences for BCS are scarce, but they indicate that even when fully informed, not all patients would choose BCS.[24,25] This is not entirely surprising, considering that conservative surgery has certain features which could be perceived as disadvantages by some women. For example, radiotherapy treatment after surgery is required and, more importantly, BCS may expose patients to a higher rate of local relapses compared to mastectomy if post-operative treatment is delivered suboptimally. When patients' preferences for BCS and mastectomy were assessed using a quantitative approach (i.e. measuring utilities),[26] the results were consistently in favour of BCS, but with only a modest difference, suggesting that breast preservation is important, but it is not the only factor that women take into account.

What therefore is the role of patient preferences in determining the observed variation in the use of BCS? In cases where patients are fully informed, and their preferences are elicited, there is some evidence that BCS is more frequently used. In an American study comparing rates of use of BCS across states, the highest rate was found in the state where a specific law requires physicians to provide their patients with full information about the alternative treatment options for breast cancer surgery.[6] Additional evidence that indirectly supports the role of patient preferences comes from studies conducted in Italy, where the highest rate of use of BCS was found in private hospitals.[10] As care in these centres is paid for by patients, the social status of the latter is likely to differ from that of those patients who are admitted to public hospitals. Higher social status (which in turn correlates with higher level of education) may also possibly be associated with greater patient awareness of different treatment options. Indeed, patient–physician relationships do differ when patients pay out of their own pocket. Patients are admitted to private centres by their private physicians with whom they may already have discussed their treatment preferences.

Further evidence confirming the relationship between BCS and socio-economic indicators comes from the study by Lazovich et al.,[14] where data from a population-based cancer registry showed that the frequency of this procedure was higher among better educated women.

Although none of these hypotheses are yet supported by 'hard data', we can infer from the available studies that women's preferences are likely to influence patterns of BCS use. However, the relative importance of all of these factors still needs to be better assessed.

SUPPLY

Supply refers to the availability of the specific resources/services necessary for the delivery of a given intervention. Of the three factors discussed here, it is unquestionably the easiest to explore. Therefore it is not surprising that a great deal of attention has been focused on exploring the relationship between availability of services and BCS frequency.

The availability of radiotherapy facilities is indeed a key issue when it comes to evaluating the extent to which specific resources affect the use of the procedure. However, the empirical evidence does not appear so clear-cut, as both positive and negative studies can be found.

The Italian and Canadian studies mentioned previously found no relationship between BCS use and the availability of radiotherapy.[8,10] This, at least in the case of the Italian study, may reflect the setting in which the study was conducted. In Italy, in fact, the distribution of radiotherapy wards/services was quite even, with generally more uniform availability compared to the rest of the country. Another study that included a more heterogeneous sample of eight Italian regions, which differed widely with regard to availability of radiotherapy facilities, showed that the lowest rate of BCS use was found where fewer services were available.[11] Findings from US studies are consistent in this respect.[6,7,14] Lazovich et al. observed that limited availability of radiotherapy facilities was an independent predictor of lower use of BCS (OR: 0.39; 95% CI: 0.33–0.45)[14] and Nattinger et al.[6] showed that the availability of an in-house radiotherapy facility was related to a higher rate of use.

Geographical location (i.e. urban vs. rural) is another factor that has been found to be related to BCS use. However, it is not clear whether location should be interpreted as a factor related to hospital characteristics (thus being related to the availability of specific facilities) or to the features of the hospital's catchment area (which may vary in their social characteristics according to the location of the centre). In a US study,[6] a trend was found in the rates of BCS use across the metropolitan areas, according to the size of their population. Women who were treated at hospitals located in metropolitan areas with >1 000 000 residents were approximately twice as likely (OR: 2.1; 95% CI: 1.9–2.4) to undergo BCS than those treated at hospitals in areas with >100 000 inhabitants. Patients admitted to centres located in areas with intermediate population size (i.e. 100 000–1 000 000) showed intermediate values for likelihood of receiving BCS (OR: 1.3; 95% CI: 1.2–1.5).

This finding is also supported by the study conducted in Italy (in the region of Lombardia).[10] It also suggests that women who are admitted to centres located in the capital of each province are more likely to receive BCS (OR: 1.54; 95% CI: 1.37–1.69). However, a similar finding did not emerge from the Canadian study.[8]

EVIDENCE FOR THE RELATIONSHIP BETWEEN ORGANIZATIONAL CHARACTERISTICS AND SURGICAL MANAGEMENT OF BREAST CANCER

In the following section, the available findings from the studies providing information on the relationship between breast cancer surgery and health services organization will be presented and analysed. All of the studies in this area were observational,[6,8,10,11,17,21–31] and their quality was assessed with regard to methodological rigour and strength of design and analysis. In particular, the extent to which the populations under study were truly comparable was the most important quality aspect considered. In the framework of observational research, it can be obtained through the adoption of a rigorous process of patient identification, the avoidance of 'selection bias' through the analyses, and by satisfactorily accounting for the effects of potential confounding factors.

Thus, according to our quality criteria, observational studies of good quality (i.e. where comparability of the population was likely to be achieved) were classified as Grade II (assuming that the highest theoretical score – Grade I – would have been assigned to randomized studies, had they been available). Studies of adequate methodological quality were classified as Grade III, and those of poor quality as Grade IV.

Summary of the evidence

A total of 10 observational studies[6,8,10,11,17,21–31] (see Table 22.2) provided information on the impact of specialization on the process of surgical care for breast cancer. Specialization was defined variably, either at the level of centres or at the level of individual clinicians. Furthermore, in most studies some proxy definitions of specialization were considered, such as hospital teaching status or hospital size (assuming that teaching

Table 22.2 *Results from studies on the impact of specialization on the surgical management of breast cancer*

Author and year of study	Grade of evidence	Definition of specialization	Aspect of care	Results	P-value
Nattinger *et al.*, 1992[6]	II	Teaching status	Use of BCS	OR: 1.4 95% CI: 1.3–1.5	Statistically significant
Satariano *et al.*, 1992[17]	II	Hospital size	Use of BCS+radiotherapy	OR: 2.13 95% CI: 1.73–2.62	Statistically significant
Iscoe *et al.*, 1994[8]	II	Teaching status	Use of BCS	57% vs. 50%	Not statistically significant
Lee-Feldstein *et al.*, 1994	II	Teaching status	Use of BCS	60% vs. 25%	Not reported
Grilli and Repetto, 1995[16]	II	Hospital size	Use of BCS	OR: 0.77 95% CI: 0.67–0.87	Statistically significant
GIVIO 1986[27]	III	Presence of oncology department/ward	Use of BCS in patients aged <50 years	38% vs. 19%	Not reported
Samet *et al.*, 1994[30]	III	Presence of a cancer centre in patient's area of residence	Use of BCS in localized breast cancer	Residents in areas with a cancer centre had higher probability of receiving BCS *OR: 1.24 95% CI: 1.12–1.37*	Statistically significant
Scorpiglione *et al.*, 1995[9]	III	Presence of oncology department/ward	Inappropriate use of Halsted mastectomy	OR: 0.34 95% CI: 0.20–0.50	Statistically significant
Grilli *et al.*, 1995[10]	III	Hospital size	Inappropriate use of Halsted mastectomy	OR: 0.6 95% CI: 0.43–0.83	Statistically significant
Scorpiglione *et al.*, 1995[9]	III	Teaching status	Inappropriate use of Halsted mastectomy	OR: 0.40 95% CI: 0.30–0.60	Statistically significant
Foster *et al.*, 1995[31]	III	Teaching status	Use of BCS	73% vs. 22%	$P<0.0001$
Studnicki *et al.*, 1993[29]	IV	Teaching status	Use of BCS	57.6% vs. 16.8%	$P=0.001$

institutions and larger hospitals have a higher degree of specializaton).

Overall, the results obtained were in favour of specialized clinicians/centres (however defined) and, with few exceptions, were statistically significant. Two Italian observational studies showed that specific surgical procedures for breast cancer, namely breast-conserving surgery (BCS) and Halsted mastectomy, were more common in centres with and without oncology departments/wards available, respectively.[9,27] This result is confirmed by the findings from the study by Samet et al.,[30] in which residents of areas with cancer centres were more likely to undergo a breast-conserving procedure. Conservative surgical procedures in general were also more frequently used in patients who were treated at teaching or larger hospitals. With a few exceptions,[8] a strong association was found between hospital teaching status/size and higher use of BCS.

With regard to the relationship between surgical management and centre's/clinician's case volume,[8,9,17,28,32,37] the results are summarized in Table 22.3.

Overall, with the exception of the study by Iscoe et al.,[8] hospital or health services provider case volume was related to the rate of provision of breast-conserving surgery for breast cancer patients, regardless of how 'high volume' – in terms of patients cared for per year – was defined. Ferguson et al. compared surgeons treating more than 5 patients per year,[33] while other researchers used a higher cut-off point – either > 50 patients/year[14] or > 20 patients/year.[37] The '20-patient' cut-off value was also used by Grilli et al. to define caseload at the hospital level.[18] In terms of results, Satariano et al.,[17] Ferguson et al.,[33] and Hill et al.[37] found that patients cared for by providers with a higher case volume were more likely to undergo this procedure. Byrne et al. reported the same finding,[35] but their results failed to reach the level of statistical significance. Grilli et al., consistently observed an inverse relationship between hospital case volume and the likelihood of using inappropriately radical surgical procedures,[28] while Scorpiglione et al. did not find any relationship between hospital caseload and appropriateness of the surgical management of breast cancer.[9] However, most of the studies considered only the *proportion* of patients receiving breast-conserving surgery, and only the two Italian studies[9,28] used the *appropriateness* of the surgical procedures adopted.

Interpretation of the evidence

The observational studies considered in this review are generally consistent in supporting the view that specialization and a higher caseload have an impact on the process of surgical care for breast cancer patients. However, they must be interpreted cautiously. The great majority of the studies merely compared specialists with non-specialists (or centres/clinicians with a different caseload) with regard to the rate of breast-conserving surgery, which is assumed to be a good indicator of quality of care, and generally found higher rates in specialized centres. However, conservative surgery is not expected to lead to higher survival rates, and whether evidence of higher rates of use of this procedure should be regarded as an indicator of better quality of care depends on the extent to which the use of this procedure actually reflects patient preferences. In general, only very limited attempts have been made to assess the quality of care and compare centres'/clinicians' performance using process indicators that more directly relate the performance of specific procedures to patients' clinical needs. For example, only two studies specifically considered the appropriateness of use of surgical procedures in the management of breast cancer patients.[9,28]

It is also important to stress the relatively limited quality of the existing evidence and the susceptibility of observational studies to bias when attempts to ensure true comparability of the patient populations (i.e. those cared for by specialized and non-specialized centres, respectively) to be studied were not made reliably.

CONCLUSIONS

Variation in BCS use is interesting both in itself and as a general indicator of the complex relationship between clinical research, physicians' behaviour, features of health service organization and patient preferences.

Overall, we can conclude that there is good evidence for the existence of wide variation in clinical practice with respect to the surgical management of breast cancer patients, and reasonable evidence (i.e. from Grade II observational studies) that specialization and higher caseload, defined at the level of individual clinicians or centres, are associated with higher rates of use of breast-conserving surgery.

Whether these findings indicate that breast cancer patients should be referred to specialized centres, and that the latter should have a minimum annual case volume to ensure good quality of care, is dependent on the extent to which performance of BCS can be regarded as an indicator of quality of care. However, no single study has considered the role of patient preference in the provision of BCS, and only a few have addressed the surgical management of breast cancer by focusing on the appropriateness of use of surgical interventions, and not merely looking at rates of utilization of a single procedure.

The lessons to be learned from this review also extend beyond the specific problem of breast-conserving surgery.

From the viewpoint of health services research, the analysis of practice variation has been a very fertile area, stimulating interest in quality and, more recently, appropriateness of care. A number of studies have been published since the completion of this systematic review,[38–45]

Table 22.3 *Results from studies on the relationship between case volume and surgical management of breast cancer*

Author	Grade of evidence	Aspect of care	Case volume defined at the level of:	Case volume treated as:	Results
Hand et al.[24]	II	Axillary dissection in stage I–II breast cancer patients	Hospitals	Continuous variable	No association was found
Satariano et al.[17]	II	Use of BCS in stage I node-negative breast cancer	Surgeons	Categorical variable: comparison between ≤ 50 patients/year and > 50 patients/year	Patients treated by surgeons with > 50 patients/year were more likely to receive BCS OR: 1.28; 95% CI: 1.03–1.58)
Ferguson et al.[33]	II	Use of BCS	Surgeons	Categorical variable: comparison between ≤ 5 patients/year and > 5 patients/year	Range of BCS use from 0 to 20% for surgeons with ≤ 5 patients/year, 35% for those with < 5 patients/year (P=0.001)
Iscoe et al.[8]	II	Use of BCS	Hospitals	Categorical variable: comparison between 1–15 patients, 16–40 patients, 41–120 patients and >120 patients over the study period	No relationship was found between hospital caseload and use of BCS
Byrne et al.[35]	II	Use of BCS in breast cancer	Surgeons	Continuous variable	Slope of linear regression between number of patients per surgeon and number of BCS performed = 0.16 (P = 0.67)
Scorpiglione et al.[9]	III	Appropriate use of surgical procedures in breast cancer	Hospitals	Categorical variable: comparison between centres with ≤ 20/year, 21–30/year, 31–50/year and > 50/year surgeries performed over the study period	No relationship was found between rate of appropriateness of the use of surgical interventions and hospital caseload
Miransky et al.[32]	IV	Use of radical surgical interventions	Hospitals	Categorical variable: comparison between small centres (contributing ≤ 25 patients to the study sample), medium centres (contributing 26–45 patients to the study sample), medium-large centres (contributing 46–65 patients to the study sample) and large centres (contributing > 65 patients to the study sample)	Medium-large and large centres used radical and extended radical interventions less often (1.5% and 4.4%, respectively vs. 12.2% and 21.6% for medium and small hospitals, respectively; $p<0.001$). All of the comparisons were adjusted for age and stage of disease
Grilli et al.[16]	IV	Inappropriate use of Halsted mastectomy	Hospitals	Categorical variable: comparison between 1–10 patients/year (reference category), 11–20 patients/year and >20 patients/year	Centres with higher volume were less likely to offer Halsted mastectomy: >20 patients/year: OR: 0.36 (95% CI: 0.23–0.55); 11–20 patients/year: OR: 0.82 (95% CI: 0.51–1.32)
Hill et al.[37]	IV	Use of BCS	Surgeons	Categorical variable: comparison between 1–4 patients/year (reference category), 5–10 patients/year, 11–19 patients/year and >20 patients/year	Likelihood of BCS for surgeons with: 5–10 patients/year: OR: 0.59 (95% CI: 0.34–1.01); 11–19 patients/year: OR: 0.77 (95% CI: 0.46–1.31); >20 patients/year: OR: 1.76 (95% CI: 1.10–2.83)

but none of them have yielded findings that alter the conclusions drawn here.

However, most research has been strictly quantitative, and only very limited attention has been paid to the more qualitative aspects of physicians' attitudes and beliefs, patients' preferences and expectations, and the interactions between all of these factors. In this sense, the findings reviewed in this chapter could be seen as ample documentation that, even in an area where a substantial body of research has been carried out, our knowledge is still fairly limited with regard to the true relevance and impact (especially in terms of patients' psychosocial outcomes) of variation in practice.

REFERENCES

1 McPherson K, Wennberg JE, Hovind OB, Clifford P. Small-area variations in the use of common surgical procedures: An international comparison of New England, England and Norway. N Engl J Med 1982; 307: 1310–4.

2 Chassin MR, Brook RH, Park RE et al. Variations in the use of medical and surgical services by the Medicare population. N Eng J Med 1986; 314: 285–90.

3 Folland S, Stano M. Small area variations: a critical review of propositions, methods, and evidence. Med Care Rev 1990; 47: 419–65.

4 Naylor CD, Ugnat AM, Weinkauf D, Anderson GM, Wielgolsz A. Coronary artery bypass grafting in Canada: what is its rate of use? Which rate is right? Can Med Assoc J 1992; 146: 851–9.

5 Improving outcomes in breast cancer: review of the research evidence. Centre for Reviews and Dissemination Report 7. York: University of York, 1996.

6 Nattinger AB, Gottlieb MS, Veum J, Yahnke D, Goodwin JS. Geographic variation in the use of breast-conserving treatment for breast cancer. N Engl J Med 1992; 326: 1102–7.

7 Farrow DC, Hunt WC, Samet JM. Geographic variation in the treatment of localized breast cancer. N Engl J Med 1992; 326: 1097–101.

8 Iscoe NA, Goel V, Wu K et al. Variation in breast cancer surgery in Ontario. Can Med Assoc J 1994; 150: 345–52.

9 Scorpiglione N, Nicolucci A, Grilli R et al. Appropriateness and variation of surgical treatment of breast cancer in Italy: when excellence in clinical research does not match with generalized good quality care. J Clin Epidemiol 1995; 48: 345–52.

10 Grilli R, Repetto F. Variation in use of breast-conserving surgery in Lombardia, Italy. Int J Technol Assess Health Care 1995; 11: 733–40.

11 Sainsbury R, Haward B, Rider L, Johnston C, Round C. Influence of clinician workload and patterns of treatment on survival from breast cancer. Lancet 1995; 345: 1265–70.

12 Mueller CB. Valid alternatives in the management of early breast cancer. Ac Surgery 1987; 20: 183–216.

13 Mueller CB. Lumpectomy: who is eligible? Surgery 1986; 100: 584–5.

14 Lazovich D, White E, Thomas DB, Moe RE. Under-utilization of breast-conserving surgery and radiation therapy among women with stage I or II breast cancer. J Am Med Assoc 1991; 266: 3433–8.

15 Greenfield S, Bianco DM, Elashoff RM et al. Patterns of care related to age of breast cancer patients. J Am Med Assoc 1987; 257: 2766–70.

16 Grilli R, Alexanian AA, Apolone G et al. Trends in patterns of care for breast cancer in Italy (1979–1987). Tumori 1990; 76: 184–9.

17 Satariano ER, Swanson M, Moll PP et al. Nonclinical factors associated with surgery received for treatment of early-stage breast cancer. Am J Public Health 1992; 82: 195–8.

18 Liberati A, Apolone G, Nicolucci A et al. The role of attitudes, beliefs and personal characteristics of Italian physicians in the surgical treatment of early breast cancer. Am J Public Health 1991; 81: 38–42.

19 Liberati A, Bradford Patterson W, Biener L, McNeil BJ. Determinants of physicians' preferences for alternative treatments in women with early breast cancer. Tumori 1987; 73: 601–9.

20 GIVIO (Interdisciplinary Group for Cancer Care Evaluation) Survey of treatment of primary breast cancer in Italy. Br J Cancer 1988; 57: 630–4.

21 Belanger D, Moore M, Tannock I. How American oncologists treat breast cancer: an assessment of the influence of clinical trials. J Clin Oncol 1991; 9: 7–16.

22 Grilli R, Apolone G, Marsoni S et al. The impact of patient management guidelines on the care of breast, colorectal and ovarian cancer patients in Italy. Med Care 1991; 29: 50–63.

23 Grilli R, Scorpiglione N, Nicolucci A et al. Variation in use of breast surgery and characteristics of hospitals' surgical staff. Int J Qual Health Care 1994; 3: 233–8.

24 Fallowfield LJ, Hall A, Maguire GP, Baum M. Psychological outcomes of different treatment policies in women with early breast cancer outside a clinical trial. BMJ 1990; 301: 575–80.

25 Udaya Kumar TM, Al-Asadi A, Mosley JG. Which women prefer which treatment for breast cancer? Breast 1992; I: 193–5.

26 Hall J, Gerard K, Salked G, Richardson J. A cost utility analysis of mammography screening in Australia. Soc Sci Med 1992; 34: 993–1004.

27 GIVIO (Interdisciplinary Group for Cancer Care Evaluation) Diagnosis and first-line treatment of breast cancer in Italian general hospitals. Tumori 1986; 72: 273–83.

28 Grilli R, Mainini F, Penna A et al. Inappropriate Halsted mastectomy and patient volume in Italian hospitals. Am J Public Health 1993; 83: 1762–4.

29 Studnicki J, Shapira DV, Bradham DD, Clark RA, Jarrett A. Response to the National Cancer Institute Alert. The effect of practice guidelines on two hospitals in the same medical community. Cancer 1993; 72: 2986–992.

30 Samet JM, Hunt WC, Farrow DC. Determinants of receiving breast conserving surgery. The Surveillance, Epidemiology, and End Results Program, 1983–1986. *Cancer* 1994; **73**: 2344–51.

31 Foster RS, Farwell ME, Costanza MC. Breast-conserving surgery for breast cancer: patterns of care in a geographic region and estimation of potential applicability. *Ann Surg Oncol* 1995; **2**: 275–80.

32 Miransky J, Kerner JF, Sturgeon SR *et al*. A comparison of primary breast cancer management in small, intermediate and large community hospitals and a comprehensive cancer center. In: Engstrom PF, Anderson PN, Mortenson LE (eds) *Advances in cancer control: epidemiology and research*. New York: Liss AR, 1984: 87–96.

33 Ferguson CM, Feinstein AC, Pendergrast WJ. Determinants of primary therapy of early stage breast cancer. *J MAG* 1990; **79**: 351–4.

34 Hand R, Sener S, Imperato J, Chmiel JS, Sylvester J, Fremgen A. Hospital variables associated with quality of care for breast cancer patients. *J Am Med Assoc* 1991; **266**: 3429–32.

35 Byrne MJ, Jamrozik K, Parsons RW *et al*. Breast cancer in Western Australia in 1989. II. Diagnosis and primary treatment. *Aust N Z J Surg* 1993; **63**: 624–9.

37 Hill DJ, White VM, Giles GG, Collins JP, Kitchen PRB. Changes in the investigation and management of primary operable breast cancer in Victoria. *Med J Aust* 1994; **161**: 110–22.

38 Elward KS, Penberthy LT, Bear H, Swartz DM, Boudreau RM, Cook SS. Variation in the use of breast-conserving therapy for Medicare beneficiaries in Virginia: clinical, geographic and hospital characteristics. *Clin Perform Qual Health Care* 1998; **6**: 63–9.

39 Guadagnoli E, Weeks JC, Shapiro CL, Gurwitz JH, Borbas C, Soumerai SB. Use of breast-conserving surgery for treatment of stage I and stage II breast cancer. *J Clin Oncol* 1998; **16**: 101–6.

40 Moritz S, Bates T, Henderson SM, Humphreys S, Michell MJ. Variation in management of small invasive breast cancers detected on screening in the former south east Thames region: observational study. *BMJ* 1997; **315**: 266–72.

41 Craft PS, Primrose JG, Lindner JA, McManus PR. Surgical management of breast cancer in Australian women in 1993: analysis of Medicare statistics. *Med J Aust* 1997; **166**: 626–9.

42 Polednak AP. Predictors of breast-conserving surgery in Connecticut, 1990–1992. *Ann Surg Oncol* 1997; **4**: 259–63.

43 Morris J, McNoe B, Eldwood JM, Packer S. Breast cancer surgery in New Zealand: consensus or variation? *N Z Med J* 1997; **110**: 53–6.

44 Hislop TG, Olivotto IA, Coldman AJ *et al*. Variations in breast conservation surgery for women with axillary lymph node negative breast cancer in British Columbia. *Can J Public Health* 1996; **87**: 390–4.

45 Albain KS, Green SR, Lichter AS *et al*. Influence of patient characteristics, socio-economic factors, geography, and systemic risk on the use of breast-sparing treatment in women enrolled in adjuvant breast cancer studies: an analysis of two intergroup trials. *J Clin Oncol* 1996; **14**: 3009–17.

23

Linking research to the management of breast cancer

J BUNKER

The management of breast cancer is based on an incomplete but rapidly expanding knowledge of its underlying pathophysiology, as previous chapters have outlined. We have seen that, as understanding improves, so also does rational treatment. The efficacy of new treatments has been extensively assessed in randomized clinical trials, with new evidence appearing monthly. The results of trials world-wide are made available electronically, and are collated and analysed almost continuously, the resultant 'overview' being updated and published at regular and frequent intervals. However, the implementation of these results in the care of patients has been disappointingly slow and variable in quality. Why is this?

BACKGROUND AND THEORY

Much of medical care is still provided without reliable evidence of its efficacy. When reliable evidence has been obtained, usually in randomized clinical trials, it may be several years before it is made available to clinicians in review articles and meta-analyses, textbooks or 'clinical alerts' such as the *Physician Data Query* (*PDQ*) published by the National Cancer Institute. Even when evidence of efficacy has been clearly established, and such evidence is readily available, its implementation by clinicians often falls far short of what could be achieved, and we are left with the problem of how to get information to practising physicians in a form that they can apply.

The transition from science to patient care begins with basic research and proceeds through clinical trials, culminating in clinical implementation. This process of dissemination involves many intermediate steps. Starting with basic research, it progresses through the formulation of clinical hypotheses, testing hypotheses in clinical

trials, analysing for statistical significance, often re-analysing by meta-analysis, assessing the magnitude of effect for clinical significance, formulating clinical policy, and finally introducing research findings into clinical practice. In the past, many of these steps have been skipped, hypotheses have been proposed with or without an experimental basis, and research findings have been implemented with or without clinical trials.

The transition from basic research to clinical implementation is a fragile one, with potential weaknesses at every step. Basic research is often incomplete or inadequate, hypotheses are accordingly uncertain, and clinical trials may lead to ambiguous conclusions. The strengths and weaknesses of such trials are well known and have been discussed fully in previous chapters. However, it is the final step that is least successful. New medical knowledge, even when fully validated, is disseminated only slowly among clinicians,[1] and it is rarely provided in a form that is readily adapted to the realities of clinical decision-making.

The clinical decision is consequently often a poor reflection of the science on which it is presumably based. To understand why this is so, it is necessary first to understand how and when information or knowledge is incorporated into the rules of thumb and guidelines on which clinicians generally rely when making therapeutic decisions. Weed, quoting Whitehead, states that 'it is a misconception, particularly among educated people, that we can think about what we are doing at the time that we are doing it in a complex task'.[2] Doctors rarely have the time to undertake a thorough review of the relevant literature when facing a new and complex clinical problem, and then to create a fresh plan on the basis of this. As a result, their decisions are usually based on analyses and planning that they (or others) have carried out in advance.

Therapeutic strategies are mapped out beforehand, and from these strategies relatively simple decision rules are derived. These decision rules are yesterday's imprecise rules of thumb and tomorrow's 'evidence-based' guidelines.

Thus the scientific information available at the time of therapeutic decision-making consists largely of prepackaged rules of thumb, and guidelines distilled from 'textbooks, journal articles, speeches, letters to the editor, pronouncements by department chairpersons, and conversations in hospital cafeterias'.[3] The rules of thumb are as reliable or unreliable as the evidence on which they are based. In the past, that evidence has usually been woefully inadequate, as Paul Beeson concluded in his examination of the scientific basis for the recommendations in the first edition of Cecil's *Textbook of Medicine*.[4] Today, the continuous stream of new and effective therapies documented in clinical trials holds promise that guidelines can be introduced on a firm scientific basis.[5]

Current guidelines that are evidence based represent a major advance over earlier implicit rules of thumb. Science-based guidelines are indeed a good way to provide information to assist the clinician in making therapeutic decisions. However, they have only taken us half-way towards the goal of medical practice linked directly to the relevant scientific evidence. The prospects for such an ideal linkage of science with practice, together with an outline of how it will work, have been described by a number of the practitioners of the new 'medical informatics'.

McDonald and Barnett, writing in 1990, expressed the hope that

> some day physicians may be able to access data for a specific patient, summarize the collective experience with similar patients in the institution or even in numerous locations, consult knowledge bases of expert opinions, and search the medical literature. Thus, physicians of the future could find all the information they need linked in one seamless web, available at any time through their medical-record workstations.[6]

More recently, Lau and Chalmers have spelled out the scenario in greater detail.

> [doctors] will approach computer terminals or use their computerized workpads to enter orders into the hospital's computer...most hospital computer information systems will have the capacity to integrate the different facets of patient care, medical records, laboratory data, ordering, therapeutic tracking, patient physiological monitoring and other relative functions. As doctors enter the therapeutic orders, they will be reminded by the computers that it has been more than a certain period of time since they last reviewed the Online Therapeutic Manual for treatments...and that several new studies have been published since....[The doctor can then] ask the computer to display the current recommendations and the evidence on which the recommendations were

based, together with a ranking of the reliability of the clinical evidence.[7]

The Lau and Chalmers scenario is already a reality in a variety of settings. One of these, an experimental system known as 'ONCOCIN', was developed in the early 1980s at Stanford University to assist oncologists in managing chemotherapy of patients in clinical trials.[8] ONCOCIN and similar information systems were initially developed to aid the implementation of complex research protocols, but they are also valuable for creating non-experimental registries or databases. Randomized clinical trials, while clearly the 'gold standard', are not the only source of important outcome data, and there is a substantial body of methodological research into the use of non-experimental data,[9] including registries and data-banks,[10] for this purpose. Registries have a long track record with regard to administrative and epidemiological studies of malignant disease. More recently, registries have been increasingly used to complement randomized clinical trials, or as an alternative methodology.[11,12]

As an illustration of the effective integration of registries with clinical trials, haematologists in northern England, covering a population of 3.1 million, enter all new cases of haematological malignancy into their leukaemia registry. The full patient population has thus become 'available for study, but also all haematologists have a hands-on role in the production and development of the data',[13] with the expectation of 'a greater effect on clinical practice and therefore on patient care...because each participant has some ownership of the data and is able to compare local practice through locally generated data with that of other centres'.[14]

An important function of the condition-specific registry is the routine monitoring or audit of adherence to protocol or guidelines. The resultant information

> provides individual units with information about their practice and indicates aspects of practice where care of patients...does not meet...standards and where patients are getting less than the best available treatment. On reviewing the audit data, it may become apparent that not all aspects of care outlined by the guidelines are considered ideal, and these guidelines may need to be reviewed and form the basis of new research or audit approach.[14]

How, in the light of experience obtained with information systems elsewhere in oncology and in medicine generally, can we improve knowledge about breast cancer management among doctors? Why, in the first place, should there be such a need? The treatment of breast cancer has been at least as widely assessed in randomized clinical trials as any other medical condition. The complexity of the resultant data is, in itself, part of the difficulty. The database is simply too large to be assimilated easily into the practice of the occasional surgeon, oncologist or institution. Compounding the difficulty for the non-specialist, the data consist of a body of knowledge that is constantly shifting – a 'moving target' – as new clinical trials continue to generate new data.

Not surprisingly in view of such complexity, the guidelines that have emerged from clinical trials and meta-analyses of breast cancer have been implemented with varying degrees of success. Hospitals and institutions that treat larger numbers of patients with breast cancer are more likely to follow guidelines[15] and report better outcomes.[16–19] These are the institutions that have the capacity to integrate outcome data into day-to-day therapeutic decisions, a process Weed has termed 'knowledge coupling'.[2] Their function as skilled recipients of information input from clinical trials is essential to the success of knowledge coupling.

The provision of an optimal information system for breast care management for clinicians presents both difficulties and unusual opportunities. A wealth of evidence for the efficacy of therapeutic options, continually updated by ongoing randomized clinical trials, is already well established. Yet to be implemented, however, and now urgently needed, is a registry that includes all new patients as they enter treatment. Such a registry will serve as an ongoing record of success in implementing the results of clinical trials as they emerge, and as a source of hypotheses for testing in the laboratory and for new treatments to be tested in clinical trials. Equally importantly, the registry would provide a comprehensive record of accumulated experience as a first approximation of answers to the very large numbers of questions that have not yet been addressed in clinical trials.

The resulting information system will represent a great improvement in the potential to apply advances in breast cancer research to patient care, but it will not dictate the clinical decisions that doctors must take. There will always be a need for clinical judgement that only doctors can make – interpretation of the research data, collaboration with colleagues in setting personal and institutional guidelines, determining their relevance to each individual patient and adapting the clinical decision to patient preference. Information systems do not tell the doctor what to do – they merely provide better data with which to inform the decision process.

REFERENCES

1 Fineberg HV. Effects of clinical evaluation on the diffusion of medical technology. In: *Assessing medical technologies*. Washington, DC: Committee for Evaluating Medical Technologies in Clinical Use, Institute of Medicine, National Academy Press, 1985.

2 Weed LL. *Knowledge coupling: new premises and new tools for medical care and education*. New York: Springer-Verlag, 1991.

3 Eddy DM. The art of diagnosis: solving the clinicopathological exercise. *N Engl J Med* 1982; **306**: 263–8.

4 Beeson PB. Changes in medical therapy during the past half century. *Medicine* 1980; **59**: 79–99.

5 Haynes RB. Some problems in applying evidence in clinical practice. *Ann N Y Acad Sci* 1993; **703**: 210–24.

6 McDonald CJ, Barnett GO. Medical records systems. In: Shortliffe EH, Perreault LE (eds) *Medical informatics*. Reading, MA: Addison-Wesley, 1990.

7 Lau J, Chalmers TC. The rational use of therapeutic drugs in the 21st century. *Int J Technol Assess Health Care* 1995; **11**: 509–22.

8 Shortliffe EH. Clinical decision-support systems. In: Shortliffe EH, Perreault LE (eds) *Medical informatics: computer applications in health care*. Reading, MA: Addison-Wesley, 1990.

9 Sechrest L, Perrin E, Bunker J (eds) *Research methodology: strengthening causal interpretations of non-experimental data*. Washington, DC: US Department of Health and Human Services, 1990.

10 Burdick E, McPherson M, Mosteller F (eds) The contribution of medical registries to technology assessment. *Int J Technol Assess Health Care* 1991; **7**: 123–202.

11 Hlatky MA, Califf RM, Harrell FE Jr, Lee KL, Mark DB, Pryor DB. Comparison of predictions based on observational data with results of randomized controlled clinical trials of coronary artery bypass surgery. *J Am Coll Cardiol* 1988; **11**: 237–45.

12 Klawansky S, Berkey C, Shah N, Mosteller F, Chalmers TC. Survival from localized breast cancer: variability across trials and registries. *Int J Technol Assess Health Care* 1993; **9**: 539–53.

13 Anonymous. From research to practice. *Lancet* 1994; **344**: 417–18.

14 Proctor SJ. Why clinical research needs medical audit. *Qual Health Care* 1993; **2**: 1–2.

15 Sainsbury R, Haward B, Rider L, Johnston C, Round C. Influence of clinician workload and patterns of treatment on survival from breast cancer. *Lancet* 1995; **345**: 1265–70.

16 Hand R, Sener S, Imperato J, Chmiel JS, Sylvester J, Fremgen A. Hospital variables associated with quality of care for breast cancer patients. *J Am Med Assoc* 1991; **266**: 3429–32.

17 McFall SL, Warnecke RB, Kaluzny AD, Aitken M, Ford L. Physician and practice characteristics associated with judgements about breast cancer treatment. *Med Care* 1993; **32**: 106–17.

18 Stiller CA. Centralised treatment, entry to trials and survival. *Br J Cancer* 1994; **70**: 352–62.

19 Basnett I, Gill M, Tobias JS. Variations in breast cancer management between a teaching and a non-teaching district. *Eur J Cancer* 1992; **28A**: 1945–50.

24

What can patients contribute to the design of clinical trials?

HAZEL THORNTON

Yet all experience is an arch wherethrough
gleams that untravelled world, whose margin fades
For ever and for ever when I move.
(Tennyson, *Ulysses*)

INTRODUCTION

The patient, the keystone in this arch of our experience of clinical trials, can bring a perspective that is both unique and valuable as we all travel this exploratory road.

We can look to the early fifteenth century to see the benefits of interdisciplinary collaboration in the discovery of perspective,[1] when the mathematical laws applied by the architect Brunelleschi were used by the young genius Masaccio in one of the first paintings to employ these mathematical rules: 'The Holy Trinity, the Virgin, St John and Donors'. The very subject, combining architectural features to frame and give grandeur to the main subject of the picture, and placing those features in an archway to enhance the message of the central character, brought fresh illumination to an often treated subject. The patient's perspective can, I believe, similarly bring a new perspective and fresh illumination to an oft-treated subject, by contributing to the design of clinical trials.[2] Masaccio – which means 'clumsy Thomas' – brought about a revolution in painting by the sincerity and clarity of his new method of communication. The revolutionary concept that patients, the 'clumsy

Thomas's', could contribute to the design of clinical trials is surely worthy of examination by the 'doubting Thomas's' of the profession in their pursuit of excellence and improvement!

Sir Kenneth Calman, the UK Chief Medical Officer, in an editorial in the *Lancet*,[3] referred to 'the inhumanity of medicine'[4] when he emphasized the importance of the study of the arts by medical students. He observes that the study of literature is one route into ethics. Might courses in 'medical humanities' go some way towards addressing the serious deterioration in the sensitivity of medical students that has been identified by Hébert *et al*.?[5] They produced evidence that the ethical sensitivity of medical students increases in the first and second years, but decreases such that fourth-year students identify fewer issues than those entering medical school. Calman emphasized the need for total involvement, which must come from the humanity of practitioners, in both medicine and arts. I believe we need both total involvement and wider involvement to encourage and keep alive the humanity of practitioners of clinical trials, in order to take account of more than the scientific requirement of trial protocols. Active rather than passive, patients can help to fulfil this role.[6–9]

Richard Horton, the editor of the *Lancet*, has introduced features on art and poetry because he believes that 'the unifying science of medicine is an inclusive art of interpretation.'[10] One such feature, namely an attempt at diagnosis of Masaccio's cripple written by

Espinel,[11] demonstrated the power of observation which has spanned the centuries by this examination of Massacio's art in which Espinel 'observed, reflected and interpreted'. The centuries are also spanned by Espinel's observation that Masaccio, by mathematically ordering our observations, introduced method to art, accomplishing this wonder of 'illusion with science', but also portraying people anatomically correctly and psychologically individualized. Is there not a broader lesson here for trialists? Espinel rated Masaccio's art as having made a major contribution to the history of neurological science and of medicine. He asks that, like the giants Leonardo da Vinci, Michelangelo, Raphael, Andrea del Sarto and Fra Angelico, we learn from him when we have patients to see. He concludes: 'With Masaccio's cripple we experience the science, the art and the values of medicine.'

MEANS AND METHODS

It was the affirmation of my belief in the power of observation in both art and science,[2] particularly as applied to my own experience of being invited to join the UK Ductal Carcinoma *In Situ* trial,[12,13] and my growing conviction of the benefits that the involvement of patients could bring to the design stage of trials (thus bringing the added illumination of another perspective, and the consideration of qualitative as well as quantitative aspects), that led to increasing opportunities both to advocate and to implement these ideas. Patients can encourage and be involved in the development and application of method to the art of combining the value judgements they bring to propositions with the scientific aspects in the design of trials, thus enabling a more sensitively devised and presented hypothesis.

I, as a patient, have had to engage in an analysis of ideas and a study of methods in order to be able to contribute to this pursuit of quality in research by engagement in dialogue with the profession,[14–19] where the main tool is the randomized controlled trial. Inevitably, this has resulted in 'a knowledge base in excess of the average patient', as the Third Report on Breast Cancer Services from the Health Committee of the House of Commons expressed it.[2] They went on to say 'but we believe that this kind of patient advocacy by a small group of well-informed patients is far preferable to little or no patient involvement at all.' It concluded in its Summary of Conclusions and Recommendations that 'We believe that patient involvement at all stages of a trial, including the initial design, *is essential*, and that initiatives such as the Consumers' Advisory Group for Clinical Trials (CAG-CT) are to be welcomed.'

The establishment of this Group was a direct consequence of the vision of partnership that I described in my view of 'The patient's role in research' at the *Lancet* Challenge of Breast Cancer Conference in Brugge in April 1994.

Brugge was a landmark – a watershed in my involvement. In my paper I described my vision of the ideal of profession and patient working collaboratively in breast cancer research from the design stage onwards, thereby facilitating a new attitude in which research is not *imposed* on the patient, but is a shared responsibility where the patient can contribute a freshness of observation. As Professor Michael Baum has said when speaking of this establishment of the CAG-CT:[20]

It has to be perceived that the women or consumers themselves have a stake in the clinical trial, and that the questions we address and the method of addressing these questions has been scrutinised and perhaps modified by these special interest groups.

There is a further advantage to the notion of women 'having a stake in the clinical trial', which is that we shall also want to see disseminated and implemented the improvements in treatments demonstrated by such trials, particularly if we have shared the responsibility of helping to devise and present trial questions. To quote Baum again: 'Only by this kind of partnership can we reverse the trend to "rightism" and protect ourselves from the ill-informed attacks from the self-appointed armchair ethicists.'

DISSEMINATION AND IMPLEMENTATION OF EVIDENCE-BASED MEDICINE

Patients who have had a stake in clinical trials will want to ensure that evidence gained from clinical trials is incorporated rapidly into medical practice. Iain Chalmers, Director of the UK Cochrane Centre, (the NHS Research and Development centre established to facilitate and co-ordinate the preparation, maintainance and dissemination of systematic reviews of the effects of health care), graphically describes a patient's initiative in seeking for herself specific evidence-based medicine (when it seemed likely that she was again about to give birth prematurely).[21] He expressed his frustration at the length of time it can take for the relevant Royal College to recommend Units to 'consider the use of such therapy.' He asks the following pertinent question: 'At what time in the past twenty years [since that particular evidence was produced] will it be judged to be negligent not to have administered steroids when there were no clear contraindications?' The wide involvement of patients in the perinatal field has led the way, and demonstrates the benefits that profession/patient collaboration can bring.

The UK Cochrane Centre (UKCC) is one of several Cochrane Centres around the world that provides the infrastructure for co-ordinating the Cochrane Collaboration, one of its roles being to assemble and manage the parent database from which The Cochrane Database of Systematic Reviews (CDSR) is derived. Their literature makes it clear that staff at the UKCC have a particular interest in exploring how to involve consumers in the work of the Cochrane Collaboration, and the aim of the Consumer Network within the Collaboration is to involve consumers at every level of activity. Individual Review Groups formed to prepare systematic reviews of all of the various aspects of health care have consumer members, and the Breast Cancer Review Group is no exception. Thus the mechanism is already in place for patient contribution both to advocate for quality research worthy of inclusion in systematic reviews, and to ensure the early implementation of research findings. There is thus a logic in patient involvement from start to finish!

Quality – 'constant as the northern star' (from Shakespeare's *Julius Caesar* III, i, 59) – must be our 'true-fix'd' objective! It needs to be as true-fixed as the vanishing point for the converging lines of all the perspective lines that need to be drawn, so that we may define this research picture as skilfully as Masaccio might have done to encompass the science, the art and the values of medicine. The involvement of patients brings a new dynamism to the activity, and even introduces tensions. This must be viewed as desirable (as in any struggle) to ensure a vigorous contribution which is never complacent, self-satisfied or self-congratulatory, but is constantly alert to the benefits of new input, as it might equally be to discordant content. Only in this way will a striving to seek balance occur and a tendency towards establishing new dogmas be avoided.

WHY?

Before attempting to consider *what* patients can contribute to the design of clinical trials, or even going on to explain *how* they can do this, it is necessary to consider *why* they should want to contribute in this way. What is the motivation? A life-threatening diagnosis and an incomprehensible invitation to join a trial can be a very strong incentive.

> Beside, incentives come from the soul's self;
> The rest avail not.
> (R Browning, *Andrea del Sarto*)

Let me say immediately that I believe we all have a moral responsibility to promote any strategem which we have identified that will lead to an improvement in the quality of research and better use of resources, whoever we might be and wherever we might live. First-hand experience of being invited to join a contentious trial can be a remarkably potent spur!

> Now spurs the lated traveller apace,
> To gain the timely inn.
> (W Shakespeare, *Macbeth* III, iii, 6)

To come closer to realizing that noble precept, there is no substitute for a personal confrontation at a traumatic moment, a personal experience at a moment of vulnerability, followed by a burning desire to understand from a position of ignorance a proposition that demands acceptance or rejection within a stated time! To accept or refuse an invitation to help to evaluate a treatment for a life-threatening illness is not something that can be brushed lightly aside. Indeed, it is likely to monopolize one's waking thoughts! Not only does the proposition seem to the patient at that moment to be a gross intrusion both on their life and on the intimate physician/patient relationship,[13] but it is also aggravating and frustrating not to be able to assemble information on a complicated issue in order to be able to make a decision on the matter.

It was this frustration, aggravation and incomprehension which ultimately led me to the belief that, as there was obviously a pressing need to produce evidence about the efficacy of medical interventions, the choice, framing and presentation of those research questions should be a joint responsibility of the inviter and the invitee. A trial question devised and framed *solely* by the medical profession and thus *imposed* on the patient would be likely to encounter resistance. Low accrual figures support this contention.[22] I repeat my rhetorical questions:[23] 'But was the struggle not for *all* of us? Should we not *all* be involved? Were we not *all* potential patients? How effective and efficient is this epic struggle in achieving the progress that is sought?'

I can surely do no better than Professor William Silverman, who quotes in his book *Human Experimentation – a Guided Step into the Unknown*[24] from Henry G Sigerist, who wrote in *Medicine and Human Welfare* more than 50 years ago:

> The people's health is the concern of the people themselves. They must want health. They must struggle for it and plan for it. Physicians are merely experts whose advice is sought in drawing up plans and whose co-operation is needed in carrying them out. No plan, however well designed and well intentioned, will succeed if it is imposed on the people. The war against disease and for health cannot be fought by the physician alone. It is a people's war in which the entire population must be mobilised permanently.

Not only does this notion of joint responsibility seem right and proper to me, but it appears to possess certain advantages in terms of contributing from first hand to mounting a successful enterprise.[25] It is right and proper that we should all be involved in defining this research process, which in the UK utilizes resources provided by public funding and charitable donations in an activity which is for the good of society as a whole.

It also seemed that there was a moral obligation for me to identify a perceived shortcoming and to attempt to offer ideas for improvement of the UK DCIS trial, which could be judged to be financially expensive and profligate in its use of resources when assessed against the wider harm/benefit ratio for all potential breast cancer patients. This is the antithesis of distributive justice if we consider that it might also be a positive contributor to harm,[26] at the expense perhaps of benefits to those patients with more advanced disease.

The UK DCIS trial, at six times the average cost for trials,[27] could be the focus point for an even wider consideration of resource use in the treatment of breast cancer as a whole where, we are informed,[12] the necessity to research DCIS management arose because of the enormously increased incidence from about 1% pre-screening to 20.1% in 1994/1995 in the UK.[28] There is this extraordinarily unbalanced use of resources in breast cancer, with £37 million spent annually on screening (which has its own research budget that is larger than that for the rest of breast cancer), with its dubious and contentious harm–benefit ratio.[29] It also incurs six times the average cost to determine the management of a non-invasive cancer, where only 1 in 4 cases will ever progress to an invasive cancer, compared to the resources available for treating symptomatic breast cancers, and the extra resource use involved,[30,31] In view of the above considerations, it seems immensely advantageous to have the benefit of the observations of the 'users', who will certainly not lose sight of the objective, but will stand well back from this canvas to ensure that aberrant lines which do not converge at the vanishing point are brought to attention for evaluation, to be discarded if they are found wanting.

What is 'the objective'? It must surely be to improve the morbidity and mortality of women with breast cancer. Those involved in screening have a tendency to focus on their target to 'reduce mortality by 25% by the year 2000'. Advocating 2-year, two-view, increased age-range screening to achieve a decrease in mortality with even more massive resource use further unbalances this equation by increasing morbidity, anxiety and psychological effects.[32,33]

The medical profession gave me the 'breast cancer patient' label. I have reservations about the nomenclature, have supported suggestions for a revised nosology,[34,35] and have also thoroughly considered the implications.

Inevitably, therefore, my attention was initially on the UK DCIS trial, which provided a perfect testing ground for such activity. It was by compulsive examination of this protocol that I cut my teeth in attempting to engage in dialogue with the Chairman and all of the members of its working party.

Study of the progression of this exchange provides a fascinating insight into subtleties – the attitudes, beliefs and expectations of the profession when it is in dialogue with 'a patient' concerning a particular trial protocol. It took considerable persistence to arrive at the acceptance of the ideality that my motivation for attempting to engage in debate was not personal, but was due to the fact that I believed that my observations and criticisms could

make a valuable contribution to the analysis and determination of why this trial was so contentious and unpopular both with the profession and with prospective participants.[36–42] It was also to justify my belief that my own moral responsibility lay not in joining the trial,[43,44] but in convincing the profession of the value of my type of input in improving trial quality (in terms of both content and presentation).

It follows that those in the profession who understood the ethical implications of my contention should likewise feel compelled to debate, engage in dialogue and develop the idea.[14,16,17,19] Having done so and identified with this discovery, it also followed that for them to ignore it would be insupportable and irreconcilable with their avowed belief in the development of the randomized controlled trial as a means to progress.[23]

Neither patients nor profession are a homogenous entity. This was amply borne out by the individuality of the responses I received from the 11 eminent members of that working party! The responses varied from total silence to total engagement.

It became apparent to me through this exercise that the acceptance of a new idea is entirely dependent on the attitude of those involved. There could be no imposition of my ideas – only recognition followed by acceptance. It is said that if one wishes to convert, one must be equally ready to be converted! However, it was evident from my limited experience that if there was to be a sharing of responsibility in the design of trials, a new attitude towards research would need to be cultivated in both professionals and the lay public. In the UK, there is currently a wide range of attitudes, with the extremes in the public ranging from those who believe they are guinea-pigs to those who are keen to become involved. In the profession, attitudes vary from those who believe that consumer involvement provides a fresh and different perspective to guide the application of scientific principles in trial methodology, to those who positively exclude people such as myself from scientific meetings, believing them to be the preserve of:

> medical and nursing personnel and scientists, all specialising in treatment of breast cancer. It [the meeting] is for presentation of research data, whether clinical or laboratory, and is not open to any other registrants, so I am afraid I cannot offer you a place at the meeting (unpublished personal correspondence, name withheld).

However, attitudes are subject to constant change according to many influences, and can vary from place to place and from one time to another. We all have the privilege of modifying our ideas according to influences: 'Progress is impossible without change: and those who cannot change their minds cannot change anything' (George Bernard Shaw). This whole activity of mine sprang from a traumatic experience. Albert Schweitzer, when discussing the influence people had had on his life, said he thought that 'we all live, spiritually, by what others have given us in the significant hours of our life.'[45] As Michael Baum wrote when describing my own experience when I was 'forced to contemplate the scientific process': 'This experience has in a perverse way been invigorating and has opened up vast new perspectives for her personal experience.'[19] Since then, the numerous opportunities, both provided and self-sought, for the sharing of that experience have, I believe, opened up perspectives undreamed of at the time when that was written for my debating adversaries as well.

> There are more things in heaven and earth, Horatio,
> Than are dreamt of in your philosophy.
> (W Shakespeare, *Hamlet* I, v, 166)

Attitudes have changed since my first involvement, and I believe that the CAG-CT will contribute towards bringing about a change in attitude to research for the better, by giving a very loud signal that the public have a stake in research,[20] and by offering an interface for enabling their responsibility to be exercised.

The questions I had raised with the trial working party led on eventually to a wider examination of these issues by, and dialogue with, the UK Co-ordinating Committee for Cancer Research (UKCCCR). My own involvement and – by implication then – acceptance demonstrated that there *was* benefit in the patient's viewpoint – even an individual one! How many more valuable insights and what wealth of material could there be waiting to be tapped from other like-minded individuals?[7–9,35,46]

CONSUMERS' ADVISORY GROUP FOR CLINICAL TRIALS

To explore this possibility, the Consumers' Advisory Group for Clinical Trials (CAG-CT), a small mixed group of professionals and patients established specifically to improve the quality of breast cancer research, met for the first time in September 1994. It immediately began work on a draft feasibility study on the use of hormone replacement therapy (HRT) in symptomatic women with breast cancer.[47] The following year the CAG-CT was awarded a much coveted National Health Service Research and Development (NHS R&D) grant to implement its project which was entitled 'Using a Consumers' Advisory Group to increase accrual into clinical trials – a study of the process and outcomes of involving patients in the design of randomized clinical trials.'

If we are to obtain answers to the many questions that exist with regard to breast cancer, we need to accrue participants quickly if we are to continue to pinpoint the small treatment differences that go towards improving quality of life and mortality. Currently accrual levels are low, and yet it is not considered acceptable to put pressure on patients to join trials. We might question the boundaries between bland presentation, enthusiastic presentation, persuasion and coercion. This is because most trials are currently unilaterally designed by the profession. If it were to be perceived by everyone that research is a necessary, constantly ongoing process of refinement in which we *all* have a stake, and if it were perceived that it was being planned collaboratively, there would be no need for such reticence. I believe it is not always appreciated by the general public that research is a step-by-step process – an ongoing process. The media are constantly reinforcing the notion that research takes place by 'breakthroughs', and that there is an ultimate magic answer which we shall one day find! We need a new confidence which only a collaborative effort can bring. There is no room for adversarial or confrontational attitudes when we all ought to have the same goal, namely to improve the morbidity and mortality of women with breast cancer.

At an early CAG-CT meeting I opened by stating the following:

> Every member of this committee comes bringing their wisdom and experience to bear, forgetting how we have acquired it or what means we have at our disposal for our own growth, and that our purpose round this table is to forget, firstly, who we are and who the others are and focus impersonally on the matters in hand. We come, each with our unique experiences, to lay them down in parallel in an attempt to improve the content and methods of achieving the best from the hypothesis of this study, so that the trial which comes out of it is the best we can manage. Because we only have hindsight and imperfect knowledge, it will not be perfect – all we are trying to do is make it *better*. Our main aim is to reduce morbidity and mortality in women with breast cancer: all other aims are subsidiary to this.

The ethos of our group is that we act in an iterative fashion. When considering a study, the joint objective of us all and the means of achieving it are first approximated as closely as possible. Then, by adjustment and tuning of input (with rejection or acceptance), we may more carefully, by a wider consideration of all of the relevant matters (to both profession and patient) reach agreement on a more finely tuned, jointly acceptable study. This process of moulding a feasibility study will lead to a multi-centre trial which will have been formulated to the best of our abilities by the profession, with women, for women. This will only be achieved by a balanced 'give and take' – an iterative type of action, with respect and deference, but with equal weight.

Our aims are as follows:

1 to attempt to assist the profession in providing *quality* studies which, because they have been planned in a spirit of co-operation between the professionals (who provide the expertise) and lay people (who comment on the relevance and presentation), will accrue more rapidly and thus provide the desperately needed answers more quickly;

2 to ensure that the questions being addressed by trial protocols are worthwhile and *relevant* to patients' needs, and that they merit assessment by trials;

3 to participate in considering which outcomes should be used to assess the effects of different treatments;

4 to assess whether the questions being addressed by the method outlined will provide *reliable* evidence that will be of value to people;

5 to advise how best to present such a hypothesis so that it:
- appeals to people so that they want to participate;
- presents the hypothesis to them in a clear, understandable way;
- provides sufficient information clearly, so that they can make a proper decision;
- clearly indicates the need to resolve the uncertainty being addressed;
- clearly conveys that this must be done within a trial discipline;

6 by these means of co-operation and shared responsibility, to demonstrate a new attitude to research which is not *imposed* on the patient, but which has been devised and executed as an expression of the appreciation of the ideal that, as this research is *for* the patients, the latter have been allowed to exercise their responsibility by participating in the defining and planning of trials which might more clearly express their desired outcomes, thereby providing trials in which they will be pleased to participate.

Our primary objective is 'to initiate, promote, facilitate and produce quality research that meets the needs and interests of health professionals, patients and public.'

In our brief existence we have used methods pragmatically to suit the time and money available and the circumstances, on a voluntary basis, employing our expertise as lay people with 'a knowledge base in excess of the average patient'[48] to provide (on invitation), at very short notice, collated comments on draft protocols. We have offered collated comments which have been discussed and recollated, and on occasion we have declined to comment retrospectively. Our first funded project, 'Using a Consumers' Advisory Group to increase accrual into clinical trials', used the Focus Group method[49] to tap into a relatively small number of eager and far from passive women who responded from support groups nationwide to our enquiry for women to become involved so that we might explore and identify key concerns about the use of HRT by breast cancer patients, and related topics.

This latter method of working has the advantage of being endlessly repeatable in breast cancer research, as well as for other conditions and in other places, and it addresses the problem of representativeness. The CAG-CT will be flexible and responsive, devising and developing methods as it grows in partnership.

The CAG-CT, with a mix of professionals and patients on its Executive, may thus be viewed as the corpus callosum of the cerebrum conveying afferent and efferent impulses in a lively body of activity, where all parts contribute to the general good, 'that there should be no schism in the body' (The New Testament, I Corinthians 12.25).

I am convinced that this is an idea right for its time, which is already being welcomed both in the UK and in other countries that are emulating what we are doing – and it will sink or swim by the rightness of what we are trying to do. I advocated it because I believe it is the right way to go, not because I had any aspirations to achieve it. Indeed, I vigorously resisted people who urged me to 'lead a group'. But how could I refuse when given the opportunity to turn vision into reality? I still do not believe that *I* have the answers or the abilities to achieve the reality, nor do I have the means, resources or facilities to do this. However, I have also seen that in my whole involvement in these dilemmas and problems it has been by asking questions, debating and laying out ideas that changes have come about, and by the involvement of others who *are* able to supply the means and the expertise, and who recognize the vision I have tried to describe. At our first meeting of the CAG-CT I said I was convinced that if we all went home that day and did not meet again it would not stop the tide of feeling that was turning against 'rightism' to a recognition of the need only to claim rights by fulfilling responsibilities. My dialogue with others in other countries indicates that they believe we are leading the way in an approach that involves collaborative working. I believe we must continue to provide that example.

At Brugge I suggested (quoting from Peter Medawar) that:[50]

> patients can provide the encouragement for the tolerance of different kinds of scientists: the collectors, classifiers and compulsive tidiers-up; those with the temperaments of detectives or of explorers; those who are artists or artisans; the poet scientist, the philosopher scientist and the mystic.

Looking at breast cancer research from a patient's point of view, I have been forgiven my ignorance, and it proved relatively easy to rush in where angels feared to tread.[51]

OBSERVATION ON TRIAL METHODOLOGY

Patients can contribute to identifying why a series of trials which are available in an institution, and which may be offered to patients, experiences very variable problems of accrual. These problems need to be identified and classified in order to avoid unnecessary wastage of manpower time, patient participation, resources and, above all, time taken to obtain data. Time spent on identification of factors that are likely to result in failure to accrue is time well spent. The solutions to the problems identified may require a radical shift of thought away from the notion that consent is 'to protect the patient's interests' or even 'to protect the doctor from litigation' to a recognition that there is no *single* solution to this problem,[52] but that the likely remedies aimed at increasing patient participation in trials need to be specifically tailored. Protection of both the patient's interests and the doctor's likelihood of litigation could thus be at least partly achieved.

Many of these problems might be better identified by the patient, who is, largely unaware of the value of their instinctive reactions to a particular proposition to enter a trial that has been put to them. Perhaps it should be obligatory to find out from each and every patient at the time of invitation their reasons for refusing. Then, in a manner which leads them to believe that even their *refusal* has value and meaning, it would be possible to go towards mitigating the guilt engendered in many thinking patients who have been told, and believe, that they may have a *moral obligation to enter trials!*[43,44] Perhaps it could be countered by the suggestion that the professionals have a moral obligation to find out why their patients have refused to join a trial. However, two suppositions concerning the moral obligations of both parties in this contract must be founded on total commitment to the notion that therapeutic trials are necessary for determining the way forward, and based on reasonable understanding.

SUPPORT AND INFORMATION ORGANIZATIONS

There is a variety of both patient self-help support groups and other support/information organizations, and it is probably desirable that this should be so. One of the most frequent needs identified by patients is for adequate information.[7–9] If the patient is to be well served in this respect, it would seem essential for there to be firstly recognition that this is so, and then collaboration between these various organizations and the professionals in order to monitor the quality of material available and to press for systems to provide adequate and consistent information and health education.[53,54]

When considering these various organizations, it might be helpful to think of them in a 'structural–functionalist' manner as postulated by Talcott Parsons[55] when considering the structure and function of institutions, such as the family, organized religion and medicine, within society. He likened society to a living organism in which each part contributes to the functioning of the whole. Older well-founded support and information organizations may have an observable pattern of evolution, progress, regression or dissolution, dependent on their ability to adapt to changing circumstances and needs. There can be a tendency for instant

resistance to influences. Defence mechanisms are then instantly brought into play to self-protect, rather than seeking to accommodate or adapt to new conditions. There is surely a need for diversity of effort and provision, but at the same time it is essential for all of these groups or organizations to observe the need for a certain uniformity of quality and content in their provision of information, and to be aware of the need for a unity of aim, namely to improve the lot of women with breast cancer and to collaborate to that end, rather than to compete.

I believe that there is a gross misconception in the minds of some people concerning the word 'Research'. To many it denotes a world of white coats in light and airy laboratories, with intense young research assistants endlessly pipetting pretty coloured liquids into a rack of phials, fostered no doubt by the inevitable background scenes during the reporting on television news of the latest breakthrough in cancer! Such a picture offers no scope for understanding that this glamorous and suitably photogenic activity is only one part of that activity which is labelled 'Research', much as the word 'Engineer' can convey a mental picture of anyone from a grubby mechanic under a car to a hard-hatted executive with his entourage visiting some vast civil engineering project!

This network of involved people – professionals, organizations and patients – with the unbalancing of the old notions of paternalism challenged by the current vogue for consumer involvement, might be in danger of loss of equilibrium which urgently needs to be addressed. What may be needed is an atmosphere of 'outreach', to avoid the tendency of any of the parties to *fight* criticism out of concern to maintain their position, which results in non-growth and is death to progress.[19]

How then can we change a culture, influence attitudes, educate and find practical ways of incorporating the ideas of those who want to take a share of the responsibility and improve the quality and speed of research? We need to ensure that the scientific process *is* open to welcome dissenting voices for, as Professor Michael Baum stated,[19] 'without dissent there can be no progress.' I cannot resist citing another quotation from that same paper: 'Impeding medical research, no less than performing it, has ethical consequences. Not to act is to act.' This applies to all of us – each and every part of that network – professionals, support and information organizations and patients!

EDUCATION AND COMMUNICATION

The need for education of the healthy public about research concepts has been identified.[43] There is often poor understanding by the lay person of research concepts, typified by the response of the man who was asked how he viewed his chance of winning the lottery. 'Well, it's fifty/fifty, isn't it? Either I win or I lose!', he said.

Earlier in the century, a good classical education was regarded as the proper foundation for a career in most walks of life. Current strategems in the UK, such as the establishment of a Chair for the Public Understanding of Science at Oxford, currently held by Professor Richard Dawkins, and the formation of the Committee on the Public Understanding of Science, currently chaired by Professor Lewis Wolpert, perhaps reflect a recognition of the need to deal with the aftermath of this attitude, which has in part brought about the current dichotomy between art and science, and the generally poor levels of understanding of scientific concepts.

One of the main problem areas when seeking informed consent is *randomization*. Schulz,[56] when considering subversion of the randomization process by the professionals, said 'Randomised controlled trials (RCT) are anathema to the human spirit; we must acknowledge the human elements of this important scientific process.' Schulz was discussing the empirical evidence that inadequate methodological approaches in controlled trials, particularly the subversion of randomization by trialists by exploiting inadequate treatment allocation concealment (so that they might express *their* treatment preferences) yielded larger treatment effects by comparison with trials with adequately concealed allocation.[57] Resultant bias due to inadequate treatment assignment methods was identified nearly 20 years ago,[58] as was commented upon in the *Lancet*.[59]

There is evidence that the rationale for trials, and concepts such as randomization, consent and equipoise, are poorly understood by patients.[46] There is also evidence that the medical profession has methodological problems with randomization. These two pieces of information are rather alarming when considered together in terms of the likely effects of introduction of bias, thus influencing the quality of evidence obtained. It is these problems which have led to the strenuous examination of trial methodology and patient preferences, with proposals being put forward to address these problems.[59-62] It seems to me that some of these proposals for dealing with this intense dislike of randomization, which have been criticized for being ethically dubious, have been because these practical suggestions address the *symptoms*, rather than the *cause* as identified by Schulz et al.[57] The statistical aspects of using single and double randomized consent designs also need to be considered. These aspects have been examined in some detail by Altman et al., together with the ethical issues that are raised by these different methods.[63]

These findings reinforce the need for wider education about research and the sharing of responsibility in helping to design quality trials. I had felt, before I recently became aware of Schulz and Chalmers' empirical evidence of bias and the dimension of methodological quality associated with estimates of treatment effects in controlled trials,[57] that the *imposition* by the professionals of trials on a public with poor understanding of the concept was

unbalanced. However, this was based on the assumption that trials were being conducted according to the rules, and that 'compliance' and 'pleasing the doctor' were judgements of *patients'* behaviour. Schulz's revelation of 'non-compliance' and 'pleasing the patient' entirely alters that balance when considering poor accrual, making poor accrual even worse if the rules have been disregarded by the professionals in practising trials. I believe that a realistic assessment of *all* methodological shortcomings is essential, with involvement of lay people in the debate to find better ways of conducting quality research whilst at the same time heeding everyone's preferences. This would demand better education not only of the lay public, but evidently also of the professionals, about the basic concepts of the research process and the need for its rigorous implementation. As Clare Bradley has stated, 'We must abandon illusions of being able to evaluate treatments in isolation from the users of the treatments.'[64]

UNDERSTANDING

The strategem employed by Gallo et al.[59] with surrogate patients attending a scientific exhibition who were young, educated and healthy, and who had been able to study a poster display on the stand clarifying the basic principles of clinical research, demonstrated this difficulty of lack of understanding by even surrogate patients. The clinician speaking to a patient in the 'real' setting[65] may attempt to assess the level of understanding of his or her patient, and may even believe that he or she has been reasonably successful, but it has been shown that optimism may prevail here.[66] This doubt about the level of understanding, which will obviously vary from one patient to another, is a crucial factor which needs to be taken into account before we go on to suggest remedies such as those proposed by Gallo et al. in their paper. This will do little to address the non-compliance of clinicians, deny eligible patients balanced and full information, delay results and, of particular importance, conceal the necessity for restraint and discipline in the evaluation of new treatments before they become generally available.[65] I believe that the most potent remedy for increasing accrual into trials is a greater appreciation by potential patients of the need for research,[2] which is after all to everyone's benefit. To side-step this problem by suggesting ethically dubious devices for circumventing the difficulty is a short-term, short-sighted proposal which could set back progress if it led to an ultimate loss of confidence in methods of seeking consent.[17,19,67]

I believe therefore that the first, fundamental and priority requirement is education of the public and the fostering of a new attitude which holds that research is a *joint* activity where the participation of the patient throughout is as necessary as the participation of the professional – the equivalent of bottoms on seats for those promoting concerts or plays! Research should be an equally collaborative activity, with an eager public demanding a quality product *which has been devised with their requirements in mind*.[67] This can only be provided if those requirements for total outcome are known. If the stated aims of a trial do not coincide with the preferred aims of the patient,[68,69] it is to be expected that patients will not accrue. Should we attempt to define whether such preferences are rational or irrational? After all, it is possible to fly in the face of reason, logic and confirmed data for hidden reasons which relate to a person's set of values, their circumstances, their personality, and their upbringing and culture as well as their (to others) irrational prejudices![13] Perhaps it is their privilege so to decide, without too much criticism by unaware professional practitioners.[70] Flexibility of trial treatment options and the methodology which catered for such prejudices, although probably requiring greater numbers of participants to give a power to detect, might possibly be offset by increased speed of accrual and a more specific result.

The reasons for poor accrual cannot be considered globally for all trials – parameters for their application need to be drawn. At the same time, hand in hand with that requirement is the need to consider different types of randomization which might be suitable in particular circumstances, together with different types of consent for different types of trials[52,65] and, at the same time, different levels of consent for different types of people within a single trial,[65] predetermined by sensitive questioning. For example, it is quite probable that individual patients being approached for entry to a trial will range from those who declare 'I would like to leave it to you, doctor!' to the awkward ones (like myself)[71] who are eternally seeking to acquire enough wisdom and understanding to arrive at the moment when they can declare a decision in the matter! It is apparent that both the information needs and the amount of clinician time could be extremely different in these two extreme scenarios, but the probable level of explanation that is needed – whether a plain outline of the options only is all that is needed, or a detailed explanation – if determined at the beginning, would save a great deal of time and anguish for everyone. If this flexibility of approach was to be coupled with a flexibility of options within the trial design to cater for prejudices of various kinds, and was offered to prospective participants in a trial which reflected their own perceived desire for outcome,[68,69] in an atmosphere of collaboration and desire to seek improvement of our knowledge base, recognized and understood, perhaps we should achieve much better accrual rates.

It is fortunate that there is now a history of this activity from which we may learn. How brave are the pioneers of any new venture, uncertain how to proceed for the best, with their burning enthusiasm to find the opportunity to test their hypotheses! We are taught to learn from history. Perhaps this really means that we need a breadth of approach – recognition of the need to modify with the benefit of hindsight, which also marvels on recalling the achievements of the past. Consent and randomization which might be deemed to be acceptable at the gestation period of a trial protocol[72] might, on completion of accrual of reporting of the findings, be criticized for being ethically dubious.[73] Hindsight is always so much easier than foresight!

Techniques, fashions, prevailing attitudes and the novelty of a procedure, set against the prevailing activity of the time, dictate the reactions which decide the methods. The obvious illustration here is the trial of mastectomy vs. lumpectomy plus radiation.[74] At the time it could logically be argued by the profession that, since patients with breast cancer received one treatment or the other arbitrarily according to the surgeon whom they happened to consult, and were *not* asked for their consent, it should surely not be deemed necessary to ask patients who were randomly allocated, not by which consulting-room door they happened to walk through, but by computer? During the previous two decades, the perception of the general public had been that the former allocation method was acceptable but the latter was degrading and reduced people to the level of human 'guinea-pigs' – a view that is difficult to comprehend today. Yet this media-fuelled horror story led to the demand for informed consent 'to protect the patient' (also useful later on 'to protect the doctor') in a blanket manner. The variety and complexity of trials on offer in this decade perhaps demand a degree of sophistication in determining levels of consent and randomization procedures of which we have only become aware because of the history of trials, which is now extensive enough in the breast cancer field to provide a testing ground for newer theories – not only in this field, but also elsewhere in other specialties. This is a typical illustration of the familiar 'swing of the pendulum' from 'nothing' to 'all', and now the consideration of a middle ground of various permutations of possibilities!

It could be that we also need to examine perceptions of categories of patient according to the labels which they are given, which seem to denote the requirement for a particular course of action which may not necessarily be valid, and which should be accommodated. The course of cancer is notoriously unpredictable, yet protocols have to be formulated to suit different categories of patients, determined by a series of labels which are then reflected in the inclusion/exclusion criteria. Feasibility studies can show these criteria to be unrealistic and in need of modification. These unpredictable areas and difficulties in defining 'eligibility' may also relate in part to the characteristics of patients which are *not* considered, such as their tendency to optimism or pessimism, their faith in conventional medicine (or their preference for avoiding it if at all possible), their level of confidence in themselves and in the available treatments, their level of gullibility and their personal philosophy, the blunters and monitors,[75–77] and the risk-takers and risk-avoiders.[78]

FRAMING OF INVITATION – ETHICAL CONSIDERATIONS AND IMPLICATIONS

The mode of presentation of information affects the proportion of risk-takers and risk-avoiders, and is an *ethically significant act*.[79,80] As Tversky summarizes:

> The psychological principles that govern the perception of decision problems and the evaluation of probabilities and outcomes produce predictable shifts of preference when *the same problem is framed in different ways*. The dependence of preferences on the formulation of decision problems is a significant concern for the theory of rational choice.

Trialists thus need to be aware that the manner in which they present information, including the presentation of probabilities and likelihoods, will affect people's decisions. The findings indicate that choices involving gains are often *risk averse* and choices involving losses are often *risk-taking*. It follows that the way in which the proposition is framed will affect the numbers who accept or refuse. It also follows that if the proposition is *incomplete*, the subject's decision will be affected, particularly if there is a sequential or contingent decision to be made which is further complicated by value-laden components. Worry can be manipulated by the labelling of outcomes (e.g. '20% gain, 80% loss', 'or 30% survival, 70% mortality').

There are obvious scientific reasons for labelling women as pre- or post-menopausal (whether natural or induced), with the age of 50 years being cited as the dividing line. Patients younger than this may not only have different therapeutic responses because of their hormonal profile, but are likely to have different circumstantial pressures and responsibilities. On the other hand, we tend to assume that patients in their seventies have a different attitude to life, with a much smaller likelihood of responsibility for others, yet a moment's reflection will lead us to conclude that these are convenient assumptions which enable us to group people into convenient categories so that we may apply eligibility criteria to them.[81] These notions of categorization probably lead to a tendency to make assumptions in terms of, for instance, the degree of aggressiveness that they might be prepared to suffer for minimal survival gains, and thus also to steer them towards the *type of trial for which we believe they might be eligible for*. Again, if these preconceptions are inaccurate, we may be faced with a mismatch of aims,[68,69] by offering trials which do not accord with the patient's own preferred outcome. This possibility, if valid, would need to be addressed by a better understanding of patient preferences[80,82–85] and a greater flexibility of the trial options on offer. And it is *the patient* who can help to provide the insight and views to form the information base which will guide us towards a greater sophistication of permutations of methods of consent, presentation, randomization and acceptable trial options.[2]

There are many other rate-limiting factors – practical, organizational, political and economic – which require the application of solutions of a very different kind. Nevertheless, in a world of finite resources, and building on an already sophisticated system of therapeutic research, we need to be sensitive to the climate in which we work and seek to offer and educate about the need for research methodologies which, in themselves, demonstrate a responsiveness and adaptability for the benefit of the central figure and focus for all of these efforts, namely the patient – who can make a very valuable contribution to the design of trials.

> For I dipt into the future, far as human eye could see,
> Saw the vision of the world, and all the wonder that would be.
> (Tennyson, *Lockeley Hall*, 1.119)

REFERENCES

1 Gombrich EH. *The story of art*. London: Phaidon Press Ltd.
2 Thornton H. The patient's role in research. In: Health Committee Third Report Breast Cancer Services. London: HMSO, 1995: 112–14.
3 Calman K, Down R. Why arts courses for medical curricula? *Lancet* 1996; **347**: 1499–500.
4 Weatherall D. *BMJ* 1994; **39**: 24–31.
5 Hebert C, Meslin EM, Dunn EV. Measuring the ethical sensitivity of medical students: a study at the University of Toronto. *J Med Ethics* 1992; **18**: 142–7.
6 Thornton H. 'Passive patient' or 'involved participant'? *Newsletter of British Psychosocial Oncology Group* 1995.
7 National Cancer Alliance *'Patient-centred cancer services?' What patients say*. 1996.
8 Consumers' Advisory Group for Clinical Trials. *Patients' views of participating in a pilot study of HRT use after breast cancer*. 1996.
9 Consumer's Advisory Group for Clinical Trials. *The views of women in breast cancer support groups on a proposed clinical trial of HRT use after breast cancer*. 1996.
10 Horton R. The interpretative turn. *Lancet* 1995; **346**: 3.
11 Espinel. C.H. Masaccio's cripple: a neurological syndrome. Its art, medicine, and values. *Lancet* 1995; **346**: 1684–6.
12 Working party of the Breast Cancer Trials Co-ordinating Sub-Committee on Cancer Research (BCTCS). *Protocol of the UK Randomised Trial for the Management of Screen-Detected Ductal Carcinoma in Situ (DCIS) of the Breast*. UKCCCR, 1989.
13 Thornton HM. Breast cancer trials: a patient's viewpoint. *Lancet* 1992; **339**: 44–5.
14 Baum M, Houghton J. Confirmed dissent and informed consent. *Eur J Cancer* 1993; **29A**: 295–6.
15 Thornton H. UK DCIS Trial – time for review? *Eur J Cancer* 1993; **29A**: 428–9.
16 Fentiman IS, Joslin CAF. The defence of the UK DCIS trial. *Eur J Cancer* 1993; **29A**: 430.

17 Gillon R. Recruitment for clinical trials: the need for public professional co-operation. *J Med Ethics* 1994; **20**: 3–5.

18 Thornton H. Clinical trials – a brave new partnership? *J Med Ethics* 1994; **20**: 19–22.

19 Baum M. Clinical trials – a brave new partnership: a response to Mrs Thornton. *J Med Ethics* 1994; **20**: 23–5.

20 Baum M. The ethics of randomised controlled trials. *Eur J Surg Oncol* 1995; **21**: 136–9.

21 Chalmers I. Underuse of antenatal corticosteroids and future litigation. *BMJ* 1993; **341**: 699.

22 Slevin M, Mossman J, Bowling A *et al.* Volunteers or victims: patients' views of randomised cancer clinical trials. *Br J Cancer* 1995; **71**: 1270–4.

23 Thornton H. *The patient's involvement and informed consent.* Paper presented at British Oncological Association Joint Meeting, Cardiff. Published in Appendix 4, King's Fund Report to the NHS. Professional attitudes and attributes to support the strategic objectives of the NHS. London: King's Fund, 1996.

24 Silverman WS. *Human experimentation – a guided step into the unknown.* Oxford: Oxford University Press, 1985.

25 Thornton H. Understanding 'informed consent'. *Lancet* 1995; **346**: 1047.

26 Thornton H. Screening for breast cancer. Recommendations are costly and short-sighted. *BMJ* 1995; **310**: 1002.

27 Houghton J. Paper presented at Meeting of the British Oncological Association and British Oncology Data Managers Association. 1994.

28 *NHS Breast Screening Programme. Review 1996.* Sheffield.

29 Skrabanek P. Mass cancer screening in women: more harm than benefit? In: Stoll BA (ed.) *Social dilemmas in cancer prevention.* Macmillan Press, Scientific and Medical, 1989.

30 Skrabanek P. The cost-effectiveness of breast cancer screening. *Int J Technol Assess Health Care* 1991; **7**: 633–5.

31 Lidbrink E. *Mammographic screening for breast cancer. Aspects of benefits and risks.* Stockholm: Gotab, 1995.

32 Field S, Michell MJ, Wallis MGW, Wilson ARM. What should be done about interval breast cancers? *BMJ*; **310**: 203–4.

33 Thornton H. Economy, equity, efficiency, effectiveness: the NHS breast screening programme from the patient's perspective. In: *Clinician in management.*

34 Foucar E. Carcinoma *in-situ* of the breast: have pathologists run amok? *Lancet* 1996; **347**: 707–8.

35 Thornton H. Randomised clinical trials: the patient's point of view. In: Silverstein MJ, Lagios MD, Poller DN, Recht A (eds) *Ductal carcinoma* in situ *of the breast. A diagnostic and therapeutic dilemma.* Baltimore, MD: Williams and Wilkins, 1996.

36 Thornton H. Preventive radiotherapy for early breast cancer? *Radiother Today* 1992; **58**.

37 Thornton H. The luck of the draw. *Nurs Times* 1992; **88**.

38 Thornton H. A sacrifice for others? Ethical dilemmas surrounding the UK randomised trial for the management of screen-detected ductal carcinoma *in situ* of the breast. *Prof Nurse* 1993.

39 Thornton H. A patient's viewpoint on current DCIS trials. *Clin Oncol* 1993; **5**: 313.

40 Joslin CAF. The patient's view of breast cancer trials. *Lancet* 1992; **339**: 314.

41 Thornton H. Ductal carcinoma of the breast. *Lancet* 1992; **339**: 1420.

42 Recht A. Radiotherapy and ductal carcinoma of the breast. *Lancet* 1992; **340**: 312.

43 Baum M. New approach for recruitment into randomised controlled trials. *Lancet* 1993; **341**: 812–13.

44 Thornton H. Whose interest? Patient's or researcher's? *Bull Med Ethics* 1993.

45 Schweitzer A. *Memories of childhood and youth.* 1925.

46 Social Science Research Unit, University of London. *Women's views of breast cancer treatment and research.* London: KKS Printing, 1994.

47 Marsden J, Sacks NPM, Whitehead MI, Crook D. Protocol for randomized clinical trial of hormone replacement therapy (HRT) in symptomatic patients with previous breast cancer – a feasibility study.

48 *Health Committee Third Report on Breast Cancer Services. Vol. I. Involving patients in research.* London: HMSO, 1995.

49 Morgan DL. *Focus groups as qualitative research.* London: Sage Publications, 1988.

50 Medawar P. '*Pluto's republic*'. Oxford: Oxford University Press, 1982.

51 Pope A. *An essay on criticism.*

52 Tobias JS, Houghton J. Is informed consent essential for all chemotherapy studies? *Eur J Cancer* 1994; **30A**: 897–9.

53 BMA Medical Book Competition Awards: Patients Information Award 1997.

54 Centre for Health Information Quality (CHIQ) *Topic Bulletin 1. Good-quality evidence-based information comprises three basic elements.* CHIQ, 1997.

55 Parsons T. *The social system.* London: Routledge and Kegan Paul, 1951.

56 Schulz KF. Subverting randomisation in controlled trials. *J Am Med Assoc* 1995; **274**: 1456–8.

57 Schulz KF, Chalmers I, Hayes RJ, Altman DG. Empirical evidence of bias. Dimensions of methodological quality associated with estimates of treatment effects in controlled trials. *J Am Med Assoc* 1995; **273**: 408–12.

58 Chalmers TC, Celano P, Sacks HS, Smith H. Bias in treatment assignment in controlled clinical trials. *N Engl J Med* 1983; **309**: 1358–61.

59 Gallo C, Perrone F, De Placido S, Giusti C. Informed versus randomised consent to clinical trials. *Lancet* 1995; **346**: 1060–4.

60 Olschewski M, Schleurlen H. Comprehensive cohort study: an alternative to randomised consent design in a breast preservation trial. *Methods Inf Med* 1985; **24**: 131–4.

61 Bradley C. Designing medical and education intervention studies: a review of some alternatives to conventional randomized controlled trials. *Diabetes Care* 1993; **2**: 509–18.

62 Gore SM. The consumer principle of randomisation. *Lancet* 1994; **343**: 58.

63 Altman DG, Whitehead J, Parmar MKB, Stenning SP, Fayers PM, Machin D. Randomised consent designs in cancer clinical trials. *Eur J Cancer*; **31A**: 1934–44.

64 Bradley C. Clinical trials – time for a paradigm shift? *Diabetic Med* 1988; **5**: 107–9.

65 Thornton H, Baum M. The ethics of clinical trials – the 'forbidden fruit' phenomena. *Breast* 1966; **5**: 1–4.

66 Simes RJ, Tattersall MHN, Coates AS, Raghaven D, Solomon HJ, Smartt H. Randomised comparison of procedures for obtaining informed consent in clinical trials of treatment for cancer. *BMJ* 1986; **293**: 1065–8.

67 Thornton H. Understanding informed consent. *Lancet* 1995; **346**: 1047.

68 Thornton H. Patient's preferences and randomised trials. *Lancet* 1994; **344**: 689.

69 Widder J. Randomising means, not aims, in clinical trials. *Lancet* 1994; **343**: 359.

70 Veatch RM. *Abandoning informed consent. Hastings Center Report*. 1994.

71 Wellisch D. Commentary. In: Silverstein MJ (ed.) *Ductal carcinoma* in situ *of the breast*. Baltimore, MD: Williams and Wilkins, 1997.

72 Wald NJ, Murphy P, Major P, Parkes C, Townsend J. Frost C. UKCCCR multi-centre randomised controlled trial of one- and two-view mammography in breast cancer screening. *BMJ* 1995; **311**: 1189–93.

73 Thornton H. Informed consent/mammography. *BMJ* 1996; **312**.

74 Fisher B, Montague E, Redmond C *et al*. Comparison of radical mastectomy with alternative treatments for primary breat cancer: a first report of results from a prospective randomised controlled trial. *Cancer* 1977; **39**: 2827–39.

75 Andrew JM. Recovery from surgery, with and without preparatory instruction for three coping styles. *J Person Soc Psychol* 1970; **15**: 223–6.

76 Miller SM. When is a little information a dangerous thing? Coping with stressful events by monitoring versus blunting. In: Levine S, Ursin H (eds) *Coping and health*. New York: Plenum Press, 1980: 145–69.

77 Steptoe A, O'Sullivan. Monitoring and blunting coping types in women prior to surgery. *Br J Clin Psychol* 1986; **25**: 143–4.

78 Siminoff LA, Fetting JH. Factors affecting treatment decisions for a life-threatening illness: the case of medical treatment of breast cancer. *Soc Sci Med* 1991; **32**: 813–18.

79 Tversky A, Kahneman D. The framing of decisions and the psychology of choice. *Science* 1981; **211**: 453–8.

80 McNeil BJ. Values and preferences in the delivery of health care. In: *Assessing medical technology*. 535–41.

81 Hickish TF, Smith IE, Ashley G, Middleton G. *Lancet* 1995; **346**: 580.

82 Silverman WA. Patients' preferences and randomised trials. *Lancet* 1994; **343**: 1586.

83 Silverman WA, Altman DG. Patient preferences and randomised trials. *Lancet* 1996; **347**: 171–4.

84 Brewin CR, Bradley C. Patient preferences and randomised clinical trials. *BMJ* 1989; **299**: 313–15.

85 Russell I. Evaluating new surgical procedures. *BMJ* 1995; **311**: 1243–4.

25

Variation in the management of breast cancer – does it matter, some possible causes, and what can be done

IAN BASNETT

INTRODUCTION

Breast cancer is an important public health problem, representing just under one-fifth of all female cancers and 570 000 new cases in the world each year. Although the incidence increases with age, it is the commonest cause of death in women aged 40–50 years. The UK has the highest age-standardized incidence and mortality in the world, and the incidence is increasing.[1] Although important variations in care may only make a *moderate* contribution to variations in survival (perhaps 5% or so improved 5-year survival),[2,3] they could have a major public health impact. That is to say nothing of the potential morbidity and opportunity cost of inappropriate interventions. This is of particular concern in the UK, as data from the EUROCARE I and EUROCARE II studies suggest that survival rates following diagnosis are well below the European average (6–8% below the average 5-year relative survival for 1985–1989)[4,5] (also discussed on BBC TV *Panorama* programme, *The Breast Cancer Lottery*, broadcast on 21 March 1994). The authors point out that these comparisons rely on registry data which is incomplete, and it is likely that survival has improved in the 1990s in England. The reasons for this difference may include poorer access to high-quality care, or delayed diagnosis, and further research is in progress to investigate this.

I shall argue that variation in care exists across many interventions and that it is a persistent international feature in breast cancer care. I shall also discuss whether at times it represents poor care, and whether care changes and at what speed, together with the range of interventions available to improve care.

VARIATION AS A GENERAL ISSUE

Variation in care has been observed and researched for many years. Nearly 150 years ago, Jarvis in the USA noted a threefold variation between counties in rates of use of the state lunatic asylum, and in the UK in 1856 William Guy observed that the hospitalization rates in King's College Hospital, London, ranged from 325 in 1000 in St Mary le Strand to 1 in 1000 in Marylebone. Glovers' observations that Kent County overall had the same tonsillectomy rate as the UK, but that one district was double that and another three times the rate, led him to conclude that 'there is a tendency for the operation to be performed as a routine prophylactic ritual for no particular reason with no particular result'.[6]

There is now a very substantial international literature describing variations in the management of illness and how they might be addressed.[6–17] In their review of literature on variations in hospital admission, Saunders et al.[6] quote over 350 references, the majority relating to elective surgery, and many studies have been based on a limited number of surgical procedures.[18]

Differences in the rates or types of interventions and their outcomes may reflect random variation or errors either in the data or in the data-collection process. For example, variations in outcome found with cancer registry data may have artefactual explanations such as cancer registration completeness, exclusions and notifi-cations at death, demographic explanations or social class.[19] There are also methodological difficulties in studying small area variations.[20,21] However, appropriate study design and use of statistics can surmount many of these problems.[22] Of course, there may be quite appropriate variation between centres due to differences in local need and case-mix, and very often this is more difficult to detect, especially with routine data. This is particularly likely when data are analysed by institution. Patient choice is also an appropriate reason for variation or deviation from accepted standards.

In their review of variation in hospital admissions, Saunders et al.[6] discuss the possible contributory factors and their influence. They conclude that need and demand play a minor role. The available evidence suggests that differences in morbidity contributed to the variation in a few cases but do not explain the majority, especially where there is greater clinical uncertainty. In contrast, supply factors were thought to have played a substantial role in the majority of studies in which they were investigated. For example, in the UK, renal dialysis rates were found to vary with the distance from units.[23] Previous studies of the impact of supply variables had led to two new laws being proposed. Lewis[24] adapted Parkinson's law as 'patient admissions for surgery expand to fill beds, operating suites and surgeon's time'. Meanwhile, 'Roemer's law' related hospital utilization to the supply of physicians.[25]

The third variable that Saunders et al. investigated was clinical decision-making. They also found this to be a major contributory factor with regard to a very wide range of medical problems. Quite considerable variation between clinicians or areas may occur when there are alternative procedures with similar outcomes, and many of the studies on women with breast cancer have examined variation in the use of breast-conserving and radical surgery. Wennberg and others have written extensively on this.[17,26–29] Not surprisingly, the role of clinical decision-making is greatest when clinical uncertainty exists.[10,29,30]

Variation is inappropriate if it represents over- or underuse of an intervention, deprives patients of choice, or if it is likely to produce an adverse outcome. Too often there is very substantial variation in the face of clinical uncertainty, suggesting that clinical preference, training, habit or prejudice is the deciding factor. There are also examples of deviations from accepted research-based guidelines, and clearly these raise serious questions about the standards of care.

VARIATION IN THE MANAGEMENT OF BREAST CANCER

I shall now address the question of whether variation in care exists with regard to the management of breast cancer, and whether it means sub-standard care.

Many of the studies of variation review the use of breast-conserving surgery vs. more extensive surgery. The belief that breast-conserving surgery with local radiotherapy and mastectomy offered equivalent survival was confirmed by randomized controlled trials published in Europe in the early 1980s,[31,32] and then in the USA in 1985.[33] In 1985 and 1986 consensus statements in the USA and the UK accepted the appropriateness of breast-conserving surgery.[34,35] Although some of the US data were later found to be falsified,[36] this did not affect the main conclusion, and an international overview supported the equivalence of breast-conserving surgery with radiotherapy and more radical surgery.[37] It is estimated that 50–60% of cases of breast cancer are suitable for breast-conserving surgery.[38,39]

Clinicians' views on treatment

A number of studies have detected uncertainty and variation between clinicians in how they state they would manage breast cancer (see Table 25.1).

A 1983 UK postal survey of surgeons in the UK found no consensus about the treatment of primary breast cancer, with varying patterns of use of surgery, radiotherapy and adjuvant chemotherapy. The authors concluded that surgeons do not follow the results of trials, but use their own treatments.[40] Again in the UK, in 1986 a survey of radiologists reported substantial variation in the radiotherapy regimes they said they would apply to a variety of clinical vignettes, including breast cancer.[41] A survey of surgeons found that those in the north of England were more likely to recommend mastectomy, as compared to breast-conserving surgery, in a hypothetical clinical situation.[42] In the USA, Tarbox et al. found that 56% of surgeons either did not believe that radical mastectomy and breast-conserving surgery were equivalent (preferring the former), or steered women towards radical mastectomies.[43] Again in the USA, in a survey of doctors' recommended management of breast cancer (excluding oncologists), there was variation both between clinicians and from National Institutes of Health (NIH) guidelines.[46]

Standing in contrast to the studies described above is a later study from New Zealand, in which most surgeons stated that their practice was in line with published guidelines with regard to the likelihood of using breast-conserving surgery in appropriate cases.[47] Evidence on actual practice is not quoted, and would be interesting. A study from the south-eastern Netherlands also shows consensus developing.[48] It compares the results of a survey of surgeons in 1987, in which only 43% of surgeons stated that they were willing to use breast-conserving surgery for small tumours, with one in 1995 when 93% of surgeons said they would use this approach. They use cancer registry data to demonstrate a substantial increase in the use of breast-conserving surgery between 1984 and 1989.

Table 25.1 *Selected surveys of physicians' stated practice in the management of breast cancer*

Study	Year published (commonly 2 years after survey)	Country	Findings
Gazet et al.[40]	1985	UK	Varying patterns of surgery, radiotherapy and chemotherapy, not always following the results of trials
Priestman et al.[41]	1989	UK	Varying patterns of radiotherapy
Morris[42]	1992	UK	Surgeons varied in their stated use of mastectomy
Tarbox et al.[43]	1992	USA	Many surgeons either did not believe radical mastectomy and breast-conserving surgery are similar, or steered women towards the former
Morris et al.[44,45]	1989 + 1992	UK	Increase in practice and staff in line with consensus guidelines including use of breast-conserving surgery
McFall et al.[46]	1994	USA	Variation between clinicians and from guidelines
Morris et al.[47]	1997	New Zealand	Much-stated practice in breast-conserving surgery in line with guidelines
Voogd et al.[48]	1997	The Netherlands	The proportion of surgeons willing to undertake breast-conserving surgery for small tumours increased from 43% in 1987 to 90% in 1995

Variation in treatment

Given the variation in physicians' stated treatments, it is not surprising to find that a large number of studies from different countries have demonstrated variation in the management of breast cancer (see Table 25.2).

Bunker observed that the rates of breast surgery in the USA in the mid-1960s, in common with other surgical interventions, were almost twice those in England and

Wales.[7] Greenberg and Stevens found much the same during the 1970s,[49] together with substantial changes in the type of mastectomy. In both countries there was a trend away from radical mastectomies. In the USA, extended simple and modified radical mastectomy became the most common form of management. In the UK, simple mastectomies remained the most common approach.[49] The authors speculate that some of the difference in overall rates may have been due to unnecessary

Table 25.2 *Selected studies showing substantial variation in the management of breast cancer*

Study	Years in which patients were treated	Country	Findings
Bunker, 1970[7]	Mid-1960s	USA/UK	Higher rates of breast cancer surgery in the USA
Greenburg and Stevens, 1986[49]	1970s	USA/UK	Higher rates of surgery in the USA. More extensive surgery in the USA
Farrow et al., 1992[50]	Mid-1980s	USA	Large geographical variation in the use of breast-conserving surgery (9–32%)
Nattinger et al., 1992[51]	1986	USA	Large geographical variation in the use of breast-conserving surgery (4–21%)
Osteen et al., 1992[52]	1985–1988	USA	Large variation in the use of partial mastectomies (11–40%)
Lee-Feldstein et al., 1994[53]	1988–1990	USA	Variation between hospitals in the use of breast-conserving surgery for localized disease in one county (30–50%)
Izuo and Ishida, 1994[54]	1991	Japan	Geographical variation in the use of breast-conserving surgery (6–17%)
Sainsbury et al., 1995[55]	1978–1992	UK	Variation between districts in breast-conserving surgery, radiotherapy, chemotherapy and hormonal manipulation
Grilli and Repetto, 1995[56]	1990 and 1991	Italy	Variation in the use of breast-conserving surgery (29–60%)
Goel et al., 1997[57]	1991	Canada	Variation in the use of breast-conserving surgery (44–68% in node-negative women) and radiotherapy

surgery in the USA. During the mid-1980s, the rates of breast-conserving surgery in the USA ranged from 9.2% to 32% of operations for breast cancer, a finding which was not explained by demographic factors.[50] Similar variation was found in a study conducted during 1986,[51] and another study conducted in Orange County between 1988 and 1990 found that more than 50% of women with localized disease received breast-conserving surgery at teaching hospitals, compared to 30% at non-teaching hospitals.[53] Farrow et al. also demonstrated variation according to ethnic group, with black women in some areas less likely to undergo radiotherapy after breast-conserving surgery.[50]

In the UK in the Yorkshire region, cancer registry data were used to review 27 000 women who were treated between 1978 and 1992. Substantial variation in management was observed between districts in breast-conserving surgery, radiotherapy, chemotherapy and hormonal manipulation. The variation in the use of mastectomy was large and unrelated to the availability of radiotherapy – the districts at the extremes of the range occupied that position year on year.[55] In Japan, a survey of the Institutes of the Japanese Breast Cancer Society found variation between areas in the use of breast-conserving surgery in 1991, from 6.1% to 17.1% of surgery, with inner cities and urban areas having higher rates.[54] Similarly, Osteen et al.[52] reported on treatment in 587 hospitals in the USA and found large differences in the use of partial mastectomies across the regions, ranging from 11.5% to 40.2%. This study was hospital

based and had a relatively low response rate, with a large number of unidentified cases at the hospitals. However, the variation is still striking. More recently, Goel et al.[57] reported substantial variation between two provinces in Canada in 1991. Breast-conserving surgery was used in 44% of cases in British Columbia and in 68% of cases in Ontario. Curiously, in those cases radiotherapy was undergone by only 76% of patients in Ontario and 92% in British Columbia. In 1990 and 1991, similar variation in the use of breast-conserving surgery was observed in Lombardia in Italy.[56]

Variation from 'good care'

Numerous studies have demonstrated variation between centres. As I have argued above, variation is important if patients are being denied a choice and treated according to prejudice, or if there is over- or under-use of an intervention. There is an opportunity cost attached to unnecessary treatment or investigations, and those resources could be deployed elsewhere with more effect. However, variation is clearly of most importance when it represents sub-standard care and is likely to affect the outcome – with deviations from accepted standards. This may be measured in a number of ways, including patient satisfaction, physical or psychological morbidity, health status, recurrence rates and mortality.

The majority of studies review the process of care against accepted evidence, and for the most part I have

Table 25.3 *Selected studies showing variation from 'agreed standards of good care' for breast cancer*

Study	Years in which patients were treated	Country	Findings
Samet et al., 1986[62]	1969–1982	USA	Older patients receiving less appropriate treatment
Greenfield et al., 1987[63]	1980–1982	USA	Older patients receiving less appropriate treatment
Kosecoff et al., 1990[64]	1977–1979 + 1980–1981	USA	Variation from two 1979 NIH consensus conference recommendations and little change following the conference
McCarthy and Bore, 1991[65]	1986	UK	Variation from King's Fund Consensus recommendations at one hospital
Tarbox et al., 1992[43]	1986–1990	USA	'Under-use' of breast-conserving surgery
Basnett et al., 1992[66]	1982–1986	UK	Variation from King's Fund Consensus recommendations and between hospitals
Nicolucci et al., 1993[67]	1988–1989	Italy	'Under-use' of breast-conserving surgery, and older patients receiving less appropriate treatment
Alexanian et al., 1993[68]	1986–1988	Italy	'Under-use' of breast-conserving surgery
Richards et al., 1995[69]	1984–1988	UK	Inappropriate variation in axillary sampling and adjuvant therapy
Sainsbury et al., 1995[3,55]	1978–1992	UK	Deviation from accepted standards, including the use of chemotherapy
Young et al., 1996[70]	1986–1990	USA	'Under-use' of radiotherapy after lumpectomy
Moritz et al., 1997[39]	1991–1992	UK	Variation in breast-conserving surgery, axillary surgery, little use of chemotherapy and under-use of radiotherapy

taken deviations from those to represent poor care. It might be argued that good clinical care explains the treatment options and women can then choose on the basis of their personal and social circumstances and beliefs. Particularly where treatments are equivalent (e.g. breast-conserving surgery vs. extensive surgery), this may explain some of the variation that is observed. Unfortunately, only a limited number of studies have looked at the provision of adequate information and choice.[58]

Only a limited number of studies have examined variation in outcome, and they have concentrated on survival,[3,53,59–61] but variation from measures of process associated with good care might be considered an important indicator (see Table 25.3).

In 1992, Tarbox et al. commented on the relative under-utilization of breast-conserving surgery in Colorado from 1986 to 1990, when 72% of women underwent modified radical mastectomy for T1 tumours.[43] This was despite evidence that these were equivalent treatments (see above), and that the stated preference of a sample of healthy women was breast-conserving surgery.[71]

A retrospective survey of management in 63 hospitals within 8 regions of Italy found substantial deviations from accepted standards. Over one-third of surgical operations were inappropriate, with over-use of radical surgery and under-use of limited surgery in appropriate cases.[67] Age was a major influence on clinicians' behaviour, with elderly patients being likely to have a less intensive diagnostic work-up, and undergoing more inappropriate surgery. Coexistent diseases did not explain this. This confirmed earlier findings in the USA by Greenfield et al.[63] and Samet et al.,[62] although the latter did not adjust for coexistent disease. A review of the surgical management of 1300 women recruited into a trial of follow-up regimes between 1986 and 1988 found that 51% of women with cancers suitable for breast-conserving surgery actually underwent such surgery.[68] Women were more likely to undergo extensive breast surgery if they were treated by hospitals in southern Italy or hospitals without radiotherapy equipment, or if they were over 50 years of age, had a lower level of education, did not have tumours in the upper-outer quadrant of the breast, or had positive axillary nodes.

A number of studies in the UK have detected deviations in care from accepted standards, as well as between centres. In the mid-1980s, deviations from the standards in the King's Fund consensus statement were reported.[35,65] A subsequent study reported differences between a teaching and non-teaching centre, and deviations from the consensus statement and emerging research.[66] Although based on hospital attendees, there were marked differences in diagnostic procedures, the proportion of women undergoing breast-conserving surgery (at its highest 75% at the teaching centre vs. 33% at the non-teaching centre) and the use of adjuvant therapy,

which was used more frequently in the teaching centre. Only 12% of women were being entered into clinical trials, which is a low figure given the continuing uncertainty in a number of clinical areas and the number of trials in progress. A retrospective review of a sample of 334 women treated in south-east England in 1990 revealed low levels of axillary surgery (46%), and once again only a small proportion of women (5%) were being entered into clinical trials.[72] A study in one region in south-east England has also demonstrated variation between centres, and deviation from good practice in the management of 1812 women treated between 1984 and 1988, particularly in relation to the use of axillary surgery and adjuvant systemic therapy.[69] A later study in the same area, which examined screen-detected cancer presenting between 1991 and 1992, found wide variation in mastectomy rates and axillary sampling, and widespread use of tamoxifen, although little use of chemotherapy and under-use of radiotherapy.[39] In the Yorkshire region, Sainsbury et al.[55] noted deviations from accepted standards, including variation in the use and under-use of chemotherapy in node-positive premenopausal women. Studies have demonstrated the frequent use of staging procedures such as bone scans,[66,72] although in the UK they are not indicated routinely.

In a case-note review, the management of over 550 women who had breast cancer treated in Washington State in the 1970s and early 1980s was compared with two of the 1979 NIH consensus conference's recommendations, namely treating early breast cancer with axillary dissection and total mastectomy (evidence of the equivalence of breast-conserving surgery with radiotherapy had not yet emerged), and separating diagnostic biopsy from treatment, enabling another discussion of the treatment options with the patient ('two-step procedure'). There were only small movements towards those recommendations.[64] Although the researchers also documented an increase in the use of pectoral muscle-conserving operations, this was probably part of an earlier trend. Among their conclusions they suggest that the quality of care in the treatment and diagnosis of breast cancer still needs to be addressed. The other evidence about sub-standard care reinforces this conclusion. Young et al.[70] found under-use of radiotherapy after lumpectomy between 1986 and 1990 was related to insurance type (45% of women on Medicaid underwent radiotherapy, 78% for those with private insurance and 88% for Medicare recipients), although this may have been a confounder for other factors such as patient characteristics, as the benefits offered did not vary significantly.

Variation in outcome

In Orange County, among women treated between 1988 and 1990, better survival was seen at larger hospitals and teaching hospitals compared to smaller hospitals and

HMO[a] hospitals,[53] although a later study found outcomes within two large HMOs were at least equal to fee-for-service settings.[74] Other studies have demonstrated improved survival with treatment by clinicians treating a larger volume of women, or surgeons designated as 'specialists'. An observational analysis of the outcome of nearly 13 000 women, treated with curative intent in Yorkshire between 1979 and 1988, demonstrated considerable variation in survival between surgeons, and examined to what extent these differences could be explained by treatment differences and surgeon's caseload.[3] Clinical caseload was related to survival and was not explained by other factors. Women seen by consultants managing more than 30 women with breast cancer per year fared better than those treated by consultants with lower caseloads. Specific treatments were also important explanatory variables; 20% of the variation was associated with less use of chemotherapy and 6% was associated with less use of hormone therapy. A substantially improved survival with increasing volumes was found by Roohan et al.[61] in a study of 50 000 women treated between 1984 and 1989. With increasing numbers of women operated on, the survival improved across very low-, low-, medium- and high-volume providers in New York State. The survival was 60% better in high-volume providers (those seeing more than 150 operations a year), compared to low-volume providers (those seeing 10 or fewer operations a year). A study in the west of Scotland examined the survival of 3786 women with breast cancer treated by specialist vs. non-specialist surgeons, and found it was substantially better for women treated by specialist surgeons. The 5-year survival rate was 9% higher, the 10-year survival rate was 8% higher and there was a reduction in risk of dying of 16% after adjusting for the main prognostic factors.[60] Both UK studies suffered from incomplete and possibly biased ascertainment of the main prognostic factors, hampering complete adjustment for selective referral or more thorough assessment of stage. Baum suggested that the survival advantage was implausibly large given the relatively small improvements in survival produced by adjuvant therapy in trials (around 5%).[2] However, the studies suggest that organizational factors have an important influence on survival.

WHY DO THESE VARIATIONS EXIST?

Clinicians' characteristics, beliefs and advice

As described above, one possible explanation for variation between centres is differences in clinical view. This is easily understood in the case of variation in the use of breast-conserving surgery, where in terms of survival the outcome can be similar to that achieved by radical surgery. Furthermore, the paradigm many surgeons had learned was 'Halstedian', so had taught that breast cancer was a local disease requiring extensive excision. Physicians are influenced by their own local communities, making 'clusters' of practice styles more likely.[75]

A study in Canada in 1985 compared physicians who still recommended modified radical mastectomy (30%) with those who recommended less aggressive surgery (69%) for a hypothetical stage I patient.[76] They found no significant differences in most physician characteristics. There were also no differences in the estimated survival, the importance of treatment goals, involvement in clinical trials or acceptance of their importance. However, the 'modified radical group' expressed more scepticism about the ability to generalize from clinical trials.

Ignorance or mistrust of research findings was also found in a survey of Colorado surgeons, where contraindications were quoted that had no basis in fact.[43] In total, 22% of surgeons stated that they did not believe breast-conserving surgery and mastectomy were equivalent treatments. Despite believing they were equivalent, a further 34% influenced patients towards having radical mastectomies. In a postal survey conducted in 1986 and 1987 of Italian physicians' preferred treatment of four clinical scenarios of early breast cancer, a smaller proportion (9%) of the use of radical surgery could be explained by ignorance or distrust of recent trials.[77] The authors postulated that the majority of differences between physicians who preferred breast-conserving or radical surgery could be explained by their speciality, and their views on the role that patients should have in determining treatment. They concluded that factors other than scientific findings guide many doctors in their decision-making!

McFall et al. found (see above) that the clinicians who were more likely to make decisions in line with the NIH consensus conferences were those who participated in the networks associated with cancer and who saw more women with breast cancer, not those in solo practice and younger practitioners.[46]

Burns et al. used videos of clinical scenarios played by actors to assess the role of clinician characteristics.[78] They found specialty, length of time in practice and fear of malpractice influenced evaluation and treatment of breast cancer in older women. They only studied male physicians.

In a study in Italy, centres with a higher proportion of female surgeons were found to be more likely to use breast-conserving treatment, although this only explained a minority of the variation.[79]

---

[a] HMOs or Health Maintainance Organizations usually accept responsibility for a defined population and undertake to provide care for them for an agreed amount of money. The five distinguishing characteristics of HMOs are an enrolled population, responsibility for delivering necessary medical care within a fixed budget, low or no financial barriers to enrollee use, risk-sharing by the providers, not just the insurer, and voluntary choice of plan.[73]

The organization of care

Bunker postulated that the higher rates of mastectomy observed in the USA were attributable to the enthusiasm for different procedures in the surgical literature.[7] However, he concludes that the fundamental differences in the payment and organization of care underlie variation between health-care systems. Montini and Ruzek suggested that the higher payment which surgeons received for more extensive surgery under the fee-for-service system in the USA may have influenced their advice.[80] In a study of women treated in 1986 that found substantial variation in the use of breast-conserving surgery, radiotherapy on site was associated with a greater use of breast-conserving surgery.[51] Also so associated was the presence of a cancer centre, teaching status or affiliation and hospitals with more beds or Medicare throughput. These findings persisted in a later study.[81,82] The availability of radiotherapy has not been found to be related to the use of breast-conserving surgery in other studies.[56]

In the USA, Hand et al. found variation in the degree of compliance with clinical standards.[83] An urban setting, small hospitals and marginal reimbursement explained a significant amount of the variation between hospitals in meeting standards related to hormone-receptor status and the appropriate use of radiotherapy. The authors conclude that there is 'a group of urban hospitals, generally small and marginally reimbursed, where comprehensive diagnosis and treatment of breast cancer are not obtained'. A study conducted between 1986 and 1990 in south-western Pennsylvania found variation according to hospital type, the use of breast-conserving surgery being higher at metropolitan teaching and urban community hospitals than at sole community hospitals, although hospital size, teaching status and radiation facilities were not predictors.[70] As described above, in Japan increased use of breast-conserving surgery was associated with inner cities and urban areas, although no adjustment was made for confounders such as stage or the availability of radiotherapy.[54] Larger hospitals and teaching hospitals were associated with better survival in Orange County.[53] A difference between teaching and non-teaching hospitals has not been reported by other studies.[3,70]

Treatment by surgeons designated as specialist because of their known interest was shown to have an important effect, as described above.[60] As the authors point out, this is probably at least in part due to better access to adjuvant therapy, as well as surgery. The observational study from the Yorkshire region described above found an association between consultant caseload and outcome.[3]

Women's age

Age alone has been found to affect the treatment that women receive, with older women less likely to receive breast-conserving treatment.[50,62,63,67,68,70] Hillner et al. reported that older women were less likely to receive hormone therapy or radiotherapy after controlling for clinical and other factors.[84] Lichter suggests that there is a strong age bias against the use of lumpectomy in older women, and irradiation may be withheld.[85] Ayanian and Guadagnoli's review reached a similar conclusion.[86]

Race and ethnicity

There is a suggestion from some studies that race may play a role in the treatment undergone by women, although it has not always been possible to perform satisfactory adjustment for confounding factors. Nattinger et al. found that black women were less likely to undergo breast-conserving surgery,[51] and although Farrow et al. did not confirm this,[50] they found that black women in some areas were less likely to undergo radiotherapy after breast-conserving surgery. Other studies have found that black women are less likely to undergo surgery after controlling for stage.[87] Ayanian and Guadagnoli have reviewed a number of studies of the effect of race and ethnicity.[86] They conclude that there is some evidence that black women are less likely than white women to undergo breast-conserving surgery, and that they are less likely to receive radiotherapy after breast-conserving surgery.

Women's choice

Particularly where there is an equivalence of outcome, as with mastectomy and breast-conserving surgery, women's choice may explain some of the variation observed. At least one study has found the psychological outcome of women undergoing mastectomy and breast conservation in the UK to be similar.[58] We also know that not all women will opt for breast-conserving surgery, given a choice.[88] Assuming that women are fully aware of the options, concerns about recurrence, radiotherapy or the inconvenience of radiotherapy could all influence them to have a mastectomy.

Selective referral

The effect of selective referral should also be considered when studying variation and its significance. For example, if – following discussion with a patient – the primary care physician knows that her preference is for mastectomy, they may refer her to a particular surgeon knowing that he or she almost always performs mastectomy for breast cancer. In this context, some of the variation might actually be patient choice. This effect is very difficult to test for using secondary data.

CAN CARE BE IMPROVED?

In 1991, in comparison to an earlier survey in 1985, a significantly higher proportion of surgeons said that they would perform breast-conservation surgery, would discuss reconstructive surgery and had access to a counsellor or specialist nurse.[44,45] Surgeons also said that they were more willing to discuss treatment options when there was a choice. A similar increase in willingness to use breast-conserving surgery was found in The Netherlands, supported by data showing an increase in its use for small tumours – from 31% in 1984 to 60% in 1989.[48]

In the USA a substantial change from using radical mastectomy to modified radical mastectomy was noted during the 1970s,[89] and a significant increase in the use of breast-conserving surgery was documented in the Detroit area during the 1980s.[90] Farrow et al. reported increases in the use of breast-conserving surgery between 1983 and 1986 in nine areas of the USA, although only to a maximum of 43% in one area, and the areas maintained their relative rankings in frequency of use.[50] However, using US national Medicare data, only a minimal increase was found in women aged 65–79 years between 1986 and 1990. New England ranked highest at 25%.[82] An increase from 35% to 42% was found in all women in south-eastern Pennsylvania over the same time period.

In Japan, trends towards more breast-conserving surgery were observed between 1989 and 1991.[54]

In the UK, between 1982 and 1986 the proportion of women undergoing breast-conserving surgery increased from 35% to 75% and from 17% to 43% in a teaching and non-teaching centre, respectively. Over the same time period, the proportion of women having aspiration cytology increased considerably, particularly at the teaching centre.[66] Richards et al. demonstrated an increase in the use of breast-conserving surgery during 1984 and 1988 in south-east England in women under 50 years of age. Mastectomy rates fell from 52% to 28%.[69] In the UK Yorkshire region, between 1978 and 1992 the mastectomy rate fell from 70% to 44%, the use of adjuvant chemotherapy rose from 5% to 19%, and hormone therapy rose from 19% to 80%.[55] There was an increase in breast-conserving surgery to over 50% on average, although the districts maintained their overall rankings in its use, as in the USA.[50]

In Australia, the proportion of women undergoing breast-conserving surgery increased from 22% in 1986 to 42% in 1990.[91] The proportion undergoing chemotherapy did not change, but the proportion receiving endocrine therapy increased from 20% to 40%.

Thus change does occur, but perhaps the issue is the pace of change and whether for some clinicians there is any change at all.[85]

WHAT CAN BE DONE TO IMPROVE CARE?

How can variation in care and poor care be addressed? After all, some of the evidence has been around for a long time. Guidelines, consensus statements and meta-analyses continue to be produced.[34,35,92–96]

Guidelines

The evidence that producing guidelines alone improves treatment is poor. As described above, Kosecoff et al. examined whether the 1979 NIH Consensus Conference had influenced practice in Washington State, and the results were depressing. Examples abound from other fields. The release of authoritative consensus guidelines had only a limited influence on Caesarean section rates.[97] Traditional continuing medical education and dissemination of printed materials also seemed to have little or no effect.[27] However, an overview of 59 rigorous evaluations of guidelines found that they could improve practice.[98] The likelihood of their being effective was increased according to the development, dissemination and implementation strategies used (See Table 25.4).

Audit and information

As part of the 1990 UK NHS reforms, all doctors were required to audit their practice.[99] The evidence of the success of this initiative in improving care is mixed.[100–102] A review of 36 published studies of interventions or audits designed to influence clinical care found that providing feedback to clinicians can produce change.[103] Change was most likely if the feedback of information was part of a strategy to target decision-makers who had already agreed to review their practice.

Table 25.4 *Likelihood of guidelines being effective*

Probability of being effective	Development strategy	Dissemination strategy	Implementation strategy
High	Internal	Specific education intervention	Patient-specific reminder
Above average	Intermediate	Continuing education	Patient-specific feedback
Below average	External, local	Mailing targeted groups	General feedback
Low	External, national	Publication in journal	General reminder

Source: Grimshaw and Russell, 1993.[98]

In the USA the National Cancer Institute issued information in 1988 about the efficacy of adjuvant therapy for node-negative breast cancer (a Clinical Alert summarizing findings prior to publication). This increased the use of adjuvant therapy, although this study did not provide data on whether the increase was sustained.[104] In Ontario, a substantial increase in the use of breast-conserving surgery was observed shortly after the publication of the National Surgical Adjuvant Breast and Bowel Project (NSABP) B-06 trial in 1985.[105]

A project in the North Thames Region in the UK has developed guidelines with local clinicians and research leaders, promulgated these and is working with the Thames Cancer Registry to feed back data about clinicians' care prospectively. The results of a pilot study have been encouraging.[106]

Financial incentives and the health-care system

In the USA in particular, financial incentives and disincentives and protocols for care have been introduced. However, the emphasis has largely been on achieving more cost-effectiveness and cost control.[107] Health care in the USA is *substantially changing*, as fee-for-service medicine is being replaced by managed health care in its various forms.[b] It is estimated that approximately 75% of employer-sponsored care is now in some form of managed health care, and Medicaid and Medicare are increasingly being provided via managed care plans. We await further evidence of the effect this has on the quality of care. In their review, Luft and Miller concluded that studies of managed care plans demonstrated better quality as often as they did worse.[108] However, they did raise concerns about patients with chronic illness, and pointed out that the majority of the studies pre-dated 1992, when there were further cost cuts. The empirical evidence on breast cancer treatment is limited, and some studies have found poorer outcomes and others better ones.[53,74,109,110] A few studies have shown improved mammography rates within managed care,[109] but there is anecdotal evidence about inappropriately shortening lengths of stay – so-called 'drive-through' mastectomies, and concern about decreasing access to trials.[111] Perhaps there should be most concern about the large and growing number of transient or permanently uninsured (≥40 million) and the under-insured. Patients without private health insurance have been found to have worse survival from breast cancer than those who are privately insured.[112]

In the study in Lombardia, after controlling for other factors, breast-conserving surgery was found to be more likely to be performed in private institutions (i.e. paid for out of pocket by patients) than in the public hospitals.

This may be an effect of the level of education of the women concerned, clinicians being more open to these patients' views.[56]

Although financial incentives have been shown to change practice in the UK, concern has been expressed that they may have the negative effect of discouraging clinicians from thinking about their practice.[113]

The 1990 UK National Health Service (NHS) reforms created a purchaser/provider split. Health authorities who previously had management responsibility for hospitals and community services became purchasers of care. They were responsible for the health of the local population and were allocated a budget to purchase health care, as were GP practices who opted for fundholder status. Although in principle the new arrangements provided a powerful lever for change, the main preoccupations were related to finance and activity, and an early commentator suggested any improvements were mainly in the efficiency of services rather than in appropriateness.[114] Reviews of the reforms have suggested limited evidence of benefit.[115–118] The Labour Government's reforms, set out in *The New NHS: Modern, Dependable*, emphasize quality of care, and a new National Institute for Clinical Excellence has been created to set standards, as well as a Centre for Health Improvement to enforce them.[119] The impact on clinical practice has yet to be seen, but there is a renewed emphasis on reducing variation and improving the quality of care, building on the work begun by the Chief Medical Officer in reviewing cancer services (see below).

Research and development and evidence-based care

A further potentially important influence is the research and development programme within the UK NHS.[120] It aims to create a health service in which decisions are based on evidence, including improving the implementation of research in practice. Internationally, the Cochrane Collaboration is producing systematic reviews of the effects of health care, as is the York Centre for Reviews and Dissemination in the UK.[121] Together with continuing medical education for clinicians, these initiatives could play an important role in improving care. The increasing adoption of 'evidence-based medicine', a clinical learning strategy developed at the McMaster Medical School in Canada in the 1970s, may have an important role. Evidence-based medicine aims to ensure that clinical decisions are based on critically appraised research findings,[122] and in the USA in 1991 the ACP Journal Club was initiated to provide clinicians with the evidence that they need.[123] A similar journal, *Evidence-Based Medicine*, has been published in the UK.[124]

---

[b] Managed care has varying definitions, but it usually refers to a plan which has at least some of the following features; access to specialists through gatekeepers; management of the care provided by guidelines/utilization review, etc.; channelling patients to 'network providers'; providers assuming some financial risk – usually by being paid monthly fees per enrollee, irrespective of the care provided. Most are for profit.

Opinion leaders

In an editorial in the *Mayo Clinic Proceedings* in 1994, Lichter points again to variation in the use of lumpectomy and radiation rather than mastectomy, and asks that physicians embrace findings of previous research. Research findings may contribute to changing practice, but the views of influential local colleagues – the so-called opinion leaders – are thought to be an important influence.[27,75,125]

Media coverage and consumer pressure

Media coverage of hysterectomy was thought to have resulted in lower rates of this operation in a canton in Switzerland by increasing patients' understanding.[126] Consumer pressure may be particularly important in the USA, perhaps because consumerism is more of a way of life there. Montini and Ruzek describe the influence of the women's health movement,[80] and the US National Breast Cancer Coalition has achieved considerable success in involving consumers in research and policy formation.[127] In the UK, the UK National Breast Coalition has been formed, and consumer pressure was one of the primary influences in the production of *Changing Childbirth* in the UK, which proposed more flexible and responsive care in childbirth.[128] Also in the UK the Macmillan Cancer Relief Fund responded to public concern by producing a self-help leaflet for women describing how to ensure that they obtain appropriate care.[129] In America and Italy there is evidence that education plays a role in the choice of the type of surgery that women undergo,[51,68] and it is likely that consumer pressure will play an increasingly important role in improving services in the future.

Legislation

Partly as a result of consumer pressure, in the USA a number of states have introduced legislation pertaining to breast cancer. Some legislation has responded specifically to concerns about access to expensive treatments for advanced breast cancer, such as bone-marrow transplantation, whilst other measures required the physician to disclose all of the options available for treatment of breast cancer. A study of the effect of the latter legislation, using the rates of breast-conserving surgery, found that its introduction produced only a transient increase in the use of breast-conserving surgery.[81] However, the law has been used in some cases, and in the USA a number of HMOs have been successfully sued for denying access to treatment for advanced breast cancer, such as autologous bone-marrow transplantation.[109]

Other interventions to improve care

A systematic review of trials of interventions to improve the effectiveness or efficiency of health-care delivery found that educational material, conferences, outreach visits, local opinion leaders, patient-mediated interventions, audit and feedback, reminders, marketing, multi-faceted interventions and local consensus processes could all improve practice if used appropriately.[130] Many of these were echoed in reviews by Eisenberg from the USA,[131] who discussed the effects of education, feedback, participation, administrative changes, incentives and penalties, and others who have reviewed the role of quality programmes, continuing education and medical informatics, all of which are developing.[107] Reviews of the evidence for the effectiveness of both continuing medical education and clinical support systems (computer programs offering advice on the management of a patient given clinical data) suggest that in many cases they can improve physician performance.[132,133]

The organization of care

A number of studies have addressed the relationship between the organization of care and its quality. Studies have found that larger hospitals and those with academic affiliations were associated with higher rates of breast-conserving surgery, measures of better care or better outcomes.[51,53,54,70,83]

A world-wide review of observational studies examined whether centralized treatment or entry into a trial improved survival for a number of cancers, including five studies of breast cancer.[59] The review found that specialist centres, larger numbers and treatment according to protocols, usually within trials, was often linked to better survival. Treatment by specialist surgeons and surgeons or providers treating larger volumes of cases has been associated with better outcomes, probably because of better access to adjuvant therapy.[3,60,61] Sainsbury *et al.* concluded that patients with breast cancer should only be dealt with by clinicians who see more than 30 new cases per year, and who have the full range of treatment options available within a multidisciplinary setting.[3]

The suggestion that outcome improves when more cases are treated is reinforced by the findings of studies of other diseases and procedures.[134–138] However, many of the studies were of a limited number of conditions and procedures, the relationship is not consistent for all conditions or procedures, and few of them separated the volume of work at an institution from the expertise or volume of work of an individual clinician or team. The associations found in these studies are not necessarily causal – they could be confounded by factors which are difficult to measure, (e.g. the case-mix or the experience and quality of clinicians). More widespread use of assessment procedures at 'centres' may artefactually improve the stage-specific survival. In the review by Stiller,[59] larger-volume centres did not consistently have better outcomes for breast cancer. In the Yorkshire region,[3] tumour grade was only known in 53% of patients, and the relationship between case volume and outcome is almost certainly more complex.[139] It is also difficult to separate cause and effect in case volume outcome studies (i.e. to what extent a larger volume is a result of better outcomes rather than its cause). It might be anticipated that outcome would be more likely to be related to volume when procedures or treatments demand a degree of technical skill, decision-making or co-ordination with others, and they have considerable risks or the capacity to improve outcomes significantly. Whether outcome can be improved by concentrating care on fewer sites, thereby increasing the volume per clinician or centre, is a complex issue, and there is limited evidence that increasing case volume alone will improve care.[140]

In the UK, recognizing that not all patients might be gaining access to a uniformly high standard of care, and that there were variations in outcome, an Expert Advisory Group was set up to review cancer services. After consulting on an initial draft, the Chief Medical Officers for England and Wales published the findings of the review.[141] The report proposes three integrated levels of care. Primary care will be the focus, and cancer units and centres will be developed from existing hospitals. Cancer units will possess the skills and facilities to manage the commoner cancers, and cancer centres will have expertise in the management of all cancers, including the rarer ones. The intention is to build a network of expertise on cancer care, and to address the apparent variation in outcome. The effects of this policy remain to be seen, but the limited evidence from breast cancer and elsewhere suggests that improving the integration of care with specialist services and the increased adoption of common treatment guidelines could improve standards. Expert guidance on the organization and clinical care of individual cancers has now begun to be produced. Breast cancer was the first,[142] and health authorities and clinicians have started to act on this guidance.

CONCLUSIONS

Variations in care for breast cancer are persistent and international. This is particularly the case where there is uncertainty or equivalence of outcome, but many studies have demonstrated deviations from clinically effective care. The factors contributing to this are complex and interrelated. When a fully informed patient exercises her choice, even if that deviates from clinical guidance, it is difficult to describe this as poor care. However, it seems unlikely that such situations account for all of the variation and deviation from good care that is observed, even allowing for selective referral.

The evidence appears to suggest that the role of the physician in influencing treatment options is important, so remedies should aim to enable physicians to provide better, more appropriate advice. From the many reviews of changing practice described above, it is clear that a wide range of interventions is available. Furthermore, the

likelihood of improving care is greatly increased if clinicians are committed to change and more than one intervention is used. It is likely that a variety of strategies are required.[125]

Changing the organization of care may improve care by making facilities more available, ensuring that clinicians can work in networks and teams and directing patients towards those which provide better-quality care. With regard to breast cancer, which is a relatively common malignancy, important organizational considerations include access to facilities such as mammography/ultrasound, cytology, counselling and radiotherapy (not necessarily on site), and the ability to achieve teamwork among clinicians involved in the management of breast cancer, including multidisciplinary assessment.[95] In each locality the benefits of centralizing services, with better access to specialist facilities, need to be balanced against ease of access for patients. It may be that, in some areas, easy access to facilities and teamwork cannot be achieved without increasing the numbers seen at some units at the expense of others. However, any such moves should be driven by the requirement to access facilities easily and to ensure that clinicians can build networks and develop common protocols. Although centralizing care may in some cases be a proxy for better care, as described above the relationship is complex.

In order to increase the influence of clinical trials, the results should be presented in a more accessible form, which could incorporate individual patient characteristics.[76] Improvements in knowledge of the management of breast cancer can only come from well-designed studies. A low rate of participation in clinical trials has been reported by numerous authors,[40,41,72] and given the uncertainties that still exist in the management of breast cancer, only by increasing participation rates can we improve our knowledge. However, equally important is an improvement in the effectiveness of the use of our existing knowledge. After all, should the treatment that women receive depend on the prejudices of their physicians, or on their age, education, race or the area in which they live?

ACKNOWLEDGEMENTS

Although responsibility for the contents of this chapter rests entirely with me, I would like to thank Professor Klim McPherson, Dr Ann McPherson and Dr Mark McCarthy for reading earlier versions of this chapter, and Jonathan Geach for his assistance in tracing references.

REFERENCES

1 McPherson K, Steel CM, Dixon JM. ABC of breast diseases. Breast cancer – epidemiology, risk factors and genetics. *BMJ* 1994; **309**: 1003–6.

2 Baum M. Specialist surgeons and survival in breast cancer. Large differences in survival are not explained. *BMJ* 1996; **312**: 1155.

3 Sainsbury R, Haward R, Rider L, Johnston C, Round C. Influence of clinician workload and patterns of treatment on survival from breast cancer. *Lancet* 1995; **345**: 1265–70.

4 Quinn MJ, Martinez-Garcia C, Berrino F. Variations in survival from breast cancer in Europe by age and country, 1978–1989. In: Coebergh J, Sant M, Berrino F, Verdecchia A (eds) *Survival of adult cancer patients in Europe diagnosed from 1978–1989*: the Eurocare II study. *Eur J Cancer* 1998; **34**: 2137–278.

5 Berrino F, Sant M, Verdecchia A, Capocaccia R, Hakulinnen T, Esteve J (eds). *Survival for cancer patients in Europe. The Eurocare study*. Lyon: IARC, 1995.

6 Saunders D, Coulter A, McPhearson K. *Variations in hospital admission rates: a review*. London: King's Fund, 1989.

7 Bunker JP. Surgical manpower, A comparison of operations and surgeons in the United States and in England and Wales. *N Engl J Med* 1970; **282**: 135–44.

8 Wennberg J, Gittelsohn A. Small-area variations in health care delivery. *Science* 1973; **142**: 1102–8.

9 McPherson K, Strong PM, Epstein A, Jones L. Regional variations in the use of common surgical procedures within and between England and Wales, Canada and the United States of America. *Soc Sci Med* 1981; **3**: 273–88.

10 McPherson K, Wennberg JE, Hovind OB, Clifford P. Small-area variations in the use of common surgical procedures: an international comparison of New England, England and Norway. *N Engl J Med* 1982; **307**: 1310–14.

11 Roos NP, Roos LL. Surgical rate variations: do they reflect the health or socio-economic characteristics of the population? *Med Care* 1982; **20**: 945–58.

12 Paul-Shaheen P, Clark JD, Williams D. Small-area analysis: a review and analysis of the North American literature. *J Health Politics Policy Law* 1987; **12**: 741–809.

13 Burns AK, Cwalina V, Hohenthaner D, Guntow C, Behney CJ, Herdman RC. *Research on geographic variations in physician patterns*. Staff paper prepared by the Health Program Office of Technology Assessment, Congress of the USA, 1987.

14 Ham C. *Health care variations: assessing the evidence*. Research Report No. 2. London: King's Fund Institute, 1988.

15 Ryan M, Mooney G. *Research in medical practice variations: where now? A paper for debate*. Aberdeen: University of Aberdeen, Economics Research Unit, 1991.

16 Ontario Ministry of Health (1994)

17 Wennberg JE, Cooper MA and other members of the Dartmouth Atlas of Healthcare Working Group. *The Dartmouth Atlas of Healthcare in the United States*. American Hospital Association, 1996.

18 Newton JN, Seagrott V, Goldacre M. Geographical variation in hospital admission rates: an analysis of workload in the Oxford region, England. *J Epidemiol Commun Health* 1994; **48**: 590–5.

19 Schrijvers CTM, Mackenbach JP. Cancer patient survival by socioeconomic status in seven countries; a review for six common cancer sites. *J Epidemiol Commun Health* 1994; **48**: 441–6.

20 Diehr P. Small area statistics: large statistical problems. *Am J Public Health* 1994; **74**: 313–14.

21 Detsky A. Regional variation in medical care. *N Engl J Med* 1995; **333**: 589–90.

22 McPherson K. Variations in hospitalisation rates: why and how to study them. In: Ham C (ed.) *Health care variation: assessing the evidence*. London: King's Fund Institute, 1988.

23 Dalziel M, Garrett C. Intraregional variation in treatment of end-stage renal failure. *BMJ* 1987; **294**: 1382–3.

24 Lewis CE. Variations in the incidence of surgery. *N Engl J Med* 1969: 880–84.

25 Roemer M. Hospital utilization and the supply of physicians. *J Am Med Assoc* 1961; **178**: 989–93.

26 Wennberg J, Gittelsohn A. 1982

27 Lomas J. *Teaching old (and not so old) docs new tricks: effective ways to implement research findings*. McMaster University for Health Economics and Policy Analysis Working Paper 93–4, April 1993.

28 Roos 1984

29 Wennberg JE. Dealing with medical practice variations. A proposal for action. *Health Affairs* 1984; **3**: 6–33.

30 Eddy DM. Variations in physician practice: the role of uncertainty. *Health Affairs* 1984; **3**: 72–89.

31 Veronesi *et al.* 1981

32 Sarazin *et al.* 1984

33 Fisher *et al.* 1985.

34 NIH 1985

35 King's Fund Forum. Consensus development conference: treatment of primary breast cancer. *BMJ* 1986; **293**: 946–7.

36 Rennie D. Breast cancer: how to mishandle misconduct. *J Am Med Assoc* 1994; **271**: 1205–7.

37 Early Breast Cancer Trialists' Collaborative Group. Effects of radiotherapy and surgery in early breast cancer. An overview of the randomised trials. *N Engl J Med* 1995; **333**: 1444–55.

38 Muller CB. Lumpectomy: who is eligible? *Surgery* 1986; **100**: 584–5.

39 Moritz S, Bates T, Henderson SM, Humphreys S, Mitchell MJ. Variation in management of small invasive cancers detected on screening in the former South-East Thames Region: observational study. *BMJ* 1997; **315**: 1266–72.

40 Gazet J, Rainsbury RM, Ford HT, Powles TJ, Coombes RC. Survey of treatment of primary breast cancer in Great Britain. *BMJ* 1985; **290**: 1793–5.

41 Priestman TJ, Bullimore JA, Godden TP, Deutsch GP. The Royal College of Radiologists Fractionation Survey. *Clin Oncol* 1989; **1**: 39–46.

42 Morris J. Regional variation in the surgical treatment of early breast cancer. *Br J Surg* 1992; **79**: 1312–13.

43 Tarbox B, Rockwood JK, Abernatty CN. Are modified radical mastectomies done for T1 breast cancers because

of surgeon's advice or patient's choice? *Am J Surg* 1992; **164**: 417–22.

44 Morris J, Royle G, Taylor I. Changes in the surgical management of early breast cancer in England. *J R Soc Med* 1989; **82**: 12–14.

45 Morris J, Farmer A, Royle G. Recent changes in the surgical management of T$_{1//2}$ breast cancer in England. *Eur J Cancer* 1992; **28A**: 1709–12.

46 McFall SL, Warnecke RB, Kaluzny AD, Aitken M, Ford L. Physician and practice characteristics associated with judgements about breast cancer treatment. *Med Care* 1994; **32**: 106–17.

47 Morris *et al.* (1997)

48 Voogd AC, Repelaer van Driel OJ, Roumen RM, Crommelin MA, van Beek MW, Coebergh JW. Changing attitudes towards breast-conserving treatment of early breast cancer in the south-eastern Netherlands: results of a survey among surgeons and a registry-based analysis of patterns of care. *Euro J Surg Oncol* 1997; **23**: 134–8.

49 Greenburg ER, Stephens M. Recent trends in breast surgery in the United States and the United Kingdom. *BMJ* 1986; **292**: 1487–91.

50 Farrow DC, Hunt William C, Samet JM. Geographic variation in the treatment of localized breast cancer. *N Engl J Med* 1992; **326**: 1097–101.

51 Nattinger AB, Gottlieb MS, Veum J, Yahnke D, Goodwin JS. Geographic variation in the use of breast-conserving treatment for breast cancer. *N Engl J Med* 1992; **326**: 1102–7.

52 Osteen RT, Steele GD, Menck HR, Winchester DP. Regional differences in surgical management of breast cancer. *CA Cancer Clin* 1992; **42**.

53 Lee-Feldstein A, Anton-Culver H, Feldstein P. Treatment differences and other prognostic factors related to breast cancer survival. *J Am Med Assoc* 1994; **371**: 1163–8.

54 Izuo M, Ishida T. Changing practices in the surgical treatment of breast cancer in Japan: a nationwide survey by the Japanese Breast Cancer Society. *Jpn Surg Today* 1995; 133–6.

55 Sainsbury R, Rider L, Smith A, MacAdam A. Does it matter where you live? Treatment variation for breast cancer in Yorkshire. *Br J Cancer* 1995; **71**: 1275–8.

56 Grilli R, Repetto F. Variation in use of breast-conserving surgery in Lombardia, Italy. *Int J Technol Assess Health Care* 1995; **11**: 733–40.

57 Goel V, Olivotto I, Hislop TG, Sawka C, Coldman A, Holowaty EJ. Patterns of initial management of node-negative breast cancer in two Canadian provinces. *Can Med Assoc J* 1997; **156**: 25–35.

58 Fallowfield LJ, Hall A, Maguire P, Baum M. Psychological outcomes of different treatment policies in women with early breast cancer outside a clinical trial. *BMJ* 1990; **301**: 575–80.

59 Stiller CA. Centralised treatment, trial entry and survival. *Br J Cancer* 1994; **70**: 352–62.

60 Gillis CR, Hole DJ. Survival outcome of care by specialist surgeons in breast cancer: a study of 3786 patients in the west of Scotland. *BMJ* 1996; **312**: 145–8.

61 Roohan PJ, Bickell NA, Baptiste MS, Therriault GD, Ferrara EP, Siu AL. Hospital volume differences and five-year survival from breast cancer. *Am J Public Health* 1998; **88**: 454–7.

62 Samet J, Hunt WC, Key C, Humbol CG, Goodwin JS. Choice of cancer therapy varies with age of patient. *J Am Med Assoc* 1986; **266**: 3385–90.

63 Greenfield S, Blanco DM, Elashoff RM, Gonz PA. Patterns of care related to age of breast cancer patients. *J Am Med Assoc* 1987; **257**: 2766–70.

64 Kosecoff J, Kanouse DE, Brook RH. Changing practice patterns in the management of primary breast cancer: consensus development program. *Health Serv Res* 1990; **25**: 809–23.

65 McCarthy M, Bore J. Treatment of breast cancer in two teaching hospitals: a comparison with consensus guidelines. *Eur J Cancer* 1991; **27**: 579–82.

66 Basnett I, Gill M, Tobias JS. Variations in breast cancer management between a teaching and a non-teaching district. *Eur J Cancer* 1992; **28A**: 1945–50.

67 Nicolucci A, Mainini F, Penna A *et al.* The influence of patient characteristics on the appropriateness of surgical treatment for breast cancer patients. *Ann Oncol* 1993; **4**: 133–40.

68 Alexanian AA, Scorpiglione N, Apolone G *et al.* Breast cancer surgery in 30 Italian general hospitals. *Eur J Surg Oncol* 1993; **19**: 1232–9.

69 Richards MA, Wolfe CDA, Tilling K, Barton J, Bourne IIM. Variations in the management and survival of women under 50 years with breast cancer in the South East Thames Region. *Br J Cancer* 1995; **73**: 751–7.

70 Young *et al.* 1996

71 Valanis B, Rumpler C. Healthy women's preferences in breast cancer treatment. *J Am Med Wom Assoc* 1982: **37**: 311–6.

72 Chouillet AM, Bell CMJ, Hiscox JG. Management of breast cancer in southeast England. *BMJ* 1994; **308**: 168–71.

73 Luft H. How do health maintenance organizations achieve their savings? *New Engl J Med* 1978; **298**: 1336–43.

74 Potosky AL, Merrill R, Riley GF *et al.* Breast cancer survival and treatment in health maintenance organization and fee-for-service settings. *J Natl Cancer Inst* 1997; **89**: 1683–91.

75 Greer AL. The state of the art versus the state of the science. The diffusion of new technologies into practice. *Int J Technol Assess Health Care* 1988; **4**: 5–26.

76 Deber RB, Thompson GG. Who still prefers aggressive surgery for breast cancer? Implications for the clinical applications of clinical trials. *Arch Intern Med* 1987; **147**: 1543–7.

77 Liberati A, Apolone G, Nicolucci A *et al.* The role of attitudes, beliefs and personal characteristics of Italian physicians in the surgical treatment of early breast cancer. *Am J Public Health* 1990; **81**: 38–42.

78 Burns RB, Freund KM, Moskowitz MA. Physician characteristics: do they influence the evaluation and treatment of breast cancer in older women? *Clin Stud* 1997; **103**: 263–9.

79 Grilli R, Scorpiglione N, Nicolucci A *et al*. Variation in use of breast surgery and characteristics of hospitals' surgical staff. *Int J Qual Health Care* 1994; **6**: 233–8.

80 Montini T, Ruzek S. Overturning orthodoxy: the emergence of breast cancer treatment policy. *Res Soc Health Care* 1989; **8**: 3–32.

81 Nattinger AB, Hoffmann R, Shapiro R, Gottlieb MS, Goodwin JS. The effect of legislative requirements on the use of breast-conserving surgery. *N Engl J Med* 1996; **335**: 1035–40.

82 Nattinger AB, Gottlieb MS, Hoffman R, Walker A, Goodwin J. Minimal increase in breast-conserving surgery from 1986 to 1990. *Med Care* 1996; **34**: 479–89.

83 Hand *et al*. 1991

84 Hillner BE, Penberthy L, Desch CE, McDonald MK, Smith TJ, Retchin SM. Variation in staging and treatment of local and regional breast cancer in the elderly. *Breast Cancer Res Treat* 1996; **40**: 75–86.

85 Lichter AS. *Non-mastectomy therapy for breast cancer: where do we go from here?* Ann Arbor, MI: Department of Radiation Oncology, University of Michigan, 1994.

86 Ayanian JZ, Guadagnoli E. Variations in breast cancer treatment by patient and provider characteristics. *Breast Cancer Res Treat* 1996; **40**: 65–74.

87 Bain RP, Greenburg RS, Whitaker JP. Racial differences in survival of women with breast cancer. *J Chroni Dis* 1986; **39**: 631–42.

88 Fallowfield L. Offering choice of surgical treatment to women with breast cancer. *Patient Educ Couns*, 1997; **30**: 209–14.

89 Kleinman JC, Machlin SR, Madans J, Makuc D, Feldman JJ. Changing practice in the surgical treatment of breast cancer. The national perspective. *Med Care* 1983; **21**: 1232–42.

90 Swanson GM, Satariano ER, Satariano WA, Osuch JR. Trends in conserving treatment of invasive carcinoma of the breast in females. *Surgery Gynaecol Obstetrics* 1990; **171** 465–71.

91 Hill DJ, White VM, Giles GG, Collins JP, Kitchen PRB. Changes in the investigation and management of primary operable breast cancer in Victoria. *Med J Aust* 1994; **161**: 110–22.

92 Early Breast Cancer Trialists' Collaborative Group. Systemic treatment of early breast cancer by hormonal, cytotoxic or immune therapy. *Lancet* 1992; **339**: 1–15, 71–84.

93 National Co-ordination Group for Surgeons Working in Breast Cancer Screening. *Quality assurance for surgeons in breast screening. NHS Breast Screening Programme 1992*.

94 Forza Operativa Nazionale sul Carcinoma Mammario. *I tumori della mammella. Protocollo di trattamento. Progetto Finalizzato 'Oncologia'*, 2nd edn. Milan: CNR, 1981.

95 British Breast Group. Report of a Working Party. *Provision of breast services in the UK: the advantages of specialist breast units*. London: British Breast Group, 1994.

96 British Association of Surgical Oncologists 1994

97 Lomas J, Anderson G, Pierre K, Vayda E, Enkin M, Hannah W. Do practice guidelines guide practice? The effect of a consensus statement on the practice of physicians. *N Engl J Med* 1989; **321**: 1306–11.

98 Grimshaw JN, Russell IT. Effect of clinical guidelines on medical practice: a systematic review of rigorous evaluations. *Lancet* 1993; **342**: 317–22.

99 Department of Health. *Medical audit in the hospital and community health services*. London: Department of Health, 1991.

100 Kerrison S, Packwood T, Buxton M. *Medical audit, taking stock*. London: King's Fund Centre, 1993.

101 Royal College of Physicians. *Medical audit: a second report*. London: Royal College of Physicians, 1993.

102 Robinson M. Evaluation of medical audit. *J Epidemiol Commun Health* 1994; **48**: 435–40.

103 Mugford M, Banfield P, O'Hanlon M. Effects of feedback of information on clinical practice: a review. *BMJ* 1991; **303**: 398–402.

104 Johnson TP, Ford L, Warnecke RB *et al*. Effect of a National Cancer Institute clinical alert on practice patterns. *J Clin Oncol* 1994; **12**: 1783–8.

105 Iscoe NA, Naylor CD, Williams JI *et al*. Temporal trends in breast cancer surgery in Ontario: can one randomized trial make a difference? *Can Medi Assoc J* 1994; **150**: 1109–15.

106 Bell CMJ, Ma M, Campbell S, Basnett I, Pollock A, Taylor I. The use of local guidelines and region-wide audit to improve the management of breast cancer. *BMJ* 1998.

107 Budd J, Dawson S. *Influencing clinical practice: implementation of R+D results. Report for the R+D Priority Working Group North West Thames Regional Health Authority*. London: The Management School, Imperial College of Science, Technology and Medicine, 1994.

108 Luft HS, Miller RH. Does managed care lead to better or worse quality of care? *Health Affairs* 1997; **16**: 5–25.

109 Haas B. The effect of managed care on breast cancer detection, treatment and research. *Nurs Outlook* 1997; **45**: 167–72.

110 Amster *et al*. 1994

111 Jenks S. Does managed care jeopardise cancer research? *J Natl Cancer Inst* 1995; **87**: 1102–6.

112 Ayanian JZ, Kohler BA, Abe T, Epstein AM. The relation between health insurance coverage and clinical outcomes among women with breast cancer. *N Engl J Med* 1993; **329**: 326–31.

113 Stocking B. Promoting change in clinical care. *Qual Health Care* 1992; **1**: 56–60.

114 Gill M. Purchasing for quality still in the starting blocks? *Qual Health Care* 1993; **2**: 179–82.

115 Robinson R, Le Grand J (eds). *Evaluating the NHS reforms*. London: King's Fund Institute, 1994.

116 Coulter A. Evaluating general practice fundholding in the UK. *Eur J Public Health* 1995; **5**: 233–9.

117 Dixon J, Glennester H. What do we know about fundholding in general practice? *BMJ* 1995; **311**: 727–30.

118 Le Grand J, Mays N, Mulligan J-A (eds). *Learning from the NHS internal market: a review of the evidence*. London: King's Fund, 1998.

119 Department of Health. *The new NHS: modern, dependable*. London: Department of Health, 1997.

120 Department of Health. *Research for health*. London: Department of Health, 1991.

121 Sheldon T, Chalmers I. The UK Cochrane Centre and the NHS Centre for Reviews and Dissemination: respective roles within the information strategy of the NHS R+D programme, co-ordination and principles underlying collaboration. *Health Econ* 1994; **97**: 11–25.

122 Rosenburg W, Donald A. Evidence-based medicine: an approach to clinical problem-solving. *BMJ* 1995; **301**: 1122–6.

123 Haynes RG. *The origins and aspirations of the ACP Journal Club*. ACP Journal Club, 1991.

124 Davidoff F, Haynes B, Sackett D, Smith R. Evidence-based medicine. *BMJ* 1995; **301**: 1085–6.

125 Haines A, Jones R. Implementing the findings of research. *BMJ* 1994; **308**: 1488–92.

126 Domenighetti G *et al*. *Reducing hysterectomies: the mass media*. Paper given at Copenhagen Conference on Regional Variations, November 1986.

127 National Breast Cancer Coalition. *Call to action – first quarterly newsletter*. Washington, DC: National Breast Cancer Coalition, 1994.

128 Department of Health. *Changing childbirth. Report of the Expert Maternity Group*. London: HMSO, 1993.

129 Macmillan Cancer Relief Fund. *Breast cancer: how to help yourself*. London: Macmillan Cancer Relief Fund, 1994.

130 Oxman A. *No magic bullets. A systematic review of 102 trials of interventions to help health-care professionals deliver services more effectively or efficiently. Report prepared for North East Thames Regional Health Authority R+D programme*. 1994.

131 Eisenberg J. *Doctors' decisions and the costs of medical care: the reasons for doctors' practice patterns and ways to change them*. Ann Arbor, MI: Health Administration Press, 1986.

132 Davis DA, Thomson MA, Oxman AD, Haynes BR. Evidence for the effectiveness of continuing medical education. A review of 50 randomized controlled trials. *J Am Med Assoc* 1992; **268**.

133 Johnston ME, Langton K, Haynes B, Mathieu A. The effects of computer-based clinical decision support systems on clinical performance and patients outcome: a critical appraisal of research. *Ann Intern Med* 1994; **120**: 135–42.

134 Hannan EL, Kilburn H, Bernard H, O'Donnell JF, Lucacik G, Shields EP. Coronary artery bypass surgery: the relationship between in-hospital mortality rate and surgical volume after controlling for clinical risk factors. *Med Care* 1991; **29**: 1094–107.

135 Luft HS, Bunker JP, Enthoven AC. Should operations be regionalised? The empirical relation between surgical volume and mortality. *N Engl J Med* 1979; **301**: 1364–9.

136 Showstack JA *et al*. Association of volume with outcome of CABG surgery: scheduled vs nonscheduled operations. *J Am Med Assoc* 1987; **257**: 785–9 [erratum, *J Am Med Assoc* 1987; **257**: 2438].

137 Farley D, Ominkowski R. Volume–outcome relationship and in-hospital mortality: the effect of changes over time. *Med Care* 1992; **30**: 77–94.

138 Houghton A. Variation in outcome of surgical procedures. *Br J Surg* 1994; **81**: 653–60.

139 Anon. Specialisation, centralised treatment and patient care. *Lancet* 1995; **345**: 1251–2.

140 NHS Centre for Reviews and Dissemination. *Relationship between volume and quality of health care: a review of the literature*. York: University of York, 1995.

141 Department of Health. *A policy framework for commissioning cancer services, prepared by the Expert Advisory Group on Cancer to the Chief Medical Officers of England and Wales*. London: Department of Health, 1995.

142 Department of Health. *Improving outcomes for breast cancer*. London: Department of Health, 1996.

26

Measuring quality of life in patients treated for breast cancer

ALAN COATES

INTRODUCTION

Quality of life is difficult if not impossible to define in any absolute sense. It may be viewed from an individual or from a societal perspective, but its application to patient care is almost exclusively focused on the individual. Clearly, many factors other than health or disease may influence the quality of an individual's life. The term 'health-related quality of life' has been used to emphasize this distinction, and it is in this sense that I shall use the term here. Quality of life has come to represent a useful shorthand for a spectrum of essentially subjective aspects of an individual's experience of a disease and its treatment. Although concern about these aspects of patient care has always been part of good medical practice, it is only by the introduction of measurements of quality of life that this dimension of the study of disease and treatment has been able to move from the anecdotal into the scientific sphere. What we study about quality of life is to a very real extent limited to what we can measure. Such measurements have only been developed over the last two decades. Many are in the form of simple questionnaires, scarcely more than variants of the everyday question 'How are you?' which is used in virtually every patient encounter. Perhaps surprisingly, the scores derived from these simple measurement instruments have proved to be useful in a number of ways. This usefulness is the essential justification for the ongoing interest by clinicians in the measurement of quality of life.

Quality of life may be used as an endpoint by which to judge the efficacy of a treatment, or in the comparison of two competing treatments. In this role, quality of life may be the dominant endpoint, if other outcomes such as survival duration are either not greatly or rather similarly affected by the treatments under consideration. Alternatively, it may stand as an adjunct to other endpoints, as for example if a treatment which achieves longer survival duration incurs significantly greater subjective morbidity. Quality-of-life measures are not conceptually identical to the utility coefficients used in decision analysis, but qualitatively they fulfil much the same role in this situation.[1]

A second quite distinct application which has emerged for quality-of-life measures is as a prognostic factor for survival. This has been empirically observed in many studies, not limited to breast cancer, but usually involving patients with sufficient metastatic disease to cause symptoms. The predictive value of quality-of-life scores has proved to be independent of other clinically recorded prognostic factors. It is of course possible that the quality-of-life scores merely reflect the progress of the underlying disease (although more accurately than is otherwise achievable). An alternative explanation, which is equally consistent with the data, would be that the perception of better quality of life actually prolongs survival. This possibility has led to the development of several prospective trials of psychological interventions aimed at evaluating the prolongation of survival through improvement of quality of life.

MEASUREMENT INSTRUMENTS

As in all spheres of scientific measurement, quality-of-life scales should be reliable and valid. Reliability is the measure of the extent to which a scale is free from random error, so that it yields essentially the same result in the same situation. If we use a ruler to measure the length of a piece of string, do we obtain – at least very nearly – the same answer each time? For single-item quality-of-life scales this may be assessed, just as for the measurement of the piece of string, by repeated measurement over time (test–retest). Multi-item scales may also be assessed by the degree of their internal consistency, which is frequently measured by a statistical test known as Cronbach's alpha.

Reliability alone is not enough, unless what we are measuring is worth measuring. We may obtain the same answer each time, but what does the answer actually mean? Suppose, for example, that we had really measured the piece of string in order to predict the frequency at which it would vibrate in a musical instrument. We might call the concept 'pitch', and imagine that we had a useful measure of pitch from the ruler. Indeed, to some extent we would be right, but if we had completely ignored the tension in the string we might find that the measurements of length, no matter how reliable, were disappointing in their ability to predict pitch, because an important extra dimension had been overlooked. Validity is the term used for the extent to which a given quality-of-life scale actually measures the concept it is intended to measure. A full discussion of the various assessments of validity is beyond the scope of this chapter. Validation of a quality-of-life scale is never absolute or complete, but evidence of validity can be gleaned from the plausibility of the instrument itself, the comparison of the scores obtained with some previously established 'gold standard', the differences in scores between groups that would be expected to be different, and the general usefulness of the instrument as it is applied in practical situations. The question of validation of quality-of-life instruments has been extensively considered by many groups.[2–11]

The first quantitative studies of quality of life in breast cancer used linear analogue self-assessment (LASA) scales.[12–14] Each scale consists of a horizontal line, usually about 10 cm long, labelled to represent a concept, such as 'Physical well-being'. The ends of the line are labelled with adjectives describing the extremes of the concept – in this case 'good' at one end and 'lousy' at the other. The patient is invited to mark the line at some point between the extremes which represents her assessment of the concept as it applies to her during a defined time period, such as the previous week or the period since she last completed such an assessment. The line can then be measured from either end. Measurements from the 'bad' end represent quality of life more directly, in that higher scores indicate that the mark was made further from the bad end and thus represent better quality of life. However, in some studies the measurement is taken from the 'good' end of the line, and the measure is thus one of how far the patient's assessment departs from the good extreme, rather akin to toxicity scales in which higher scores conventionally represent greater toxicity. These scales are still in use,[15,16] and have proved comparable to more complex instruments in assessment of mood in cancer patients.[17] The LASA technique is used in several instruments,[3] including the International Breast Cancer Study Group quality-of-life instrument,[18] which is available in 13 languages, and the Functional Living Index-Cancer (FLIC) scale.[11]

A different approach to quality-of-life assessment was taken by Spitzer et al.[19] They developed and validated a 5-item questionnaire, the quality-of-life index (QLI), which was designed to be completed by the physician, not the patient. Although the bulk of opinion favours patient self-assessment,[20] the QLI has proved to be a robust measure of quality of life, giving results closely similar to those obtained by patient self-assessment.[21–24] This scale has also been used in terminal care.[25]

The European Organization for Research and Treatment of Cancer (EORTC) has a major interest in the development of quality-of-life measures and their application in clinical trials. They have adopted a modular approach,[4] with key areas common to many cancers being included in a core questionnaire, while aspects relevant to a particular cancer type are included as separate modules.[26] The core questionnaire, known as the QLQ-C30,[27] is a multi-dimensional 30-item questionnaire. It evolved from an earlier 36-item scale, first to a 30-item scale (version 1), then to the QLQ-C30 (+3), and then back to a 30-item instrument (Version 2). Version 3 is currently being tested. The core questionnaire produces scores for five functional scales (physical functioning, role functioning, emotional functioning, cognitive functioning and social functioning), a global health status/QL scale, symptom scales for fatigue, nausea, vomiting and pain, and single-item questions covering other symptoms. The core questionnaire is available in 24 languages. Disease-specific modules have been developed for lung, breast, colorectal and oesophageal cancer.

Other instruments suitable for assessment of quality of life in patients with breast cancer include the Functional Assessment of Cancer Therapy (FACT) scale, which consists of a general scale and several disease-specific sub-scales, including a scale for breast cancer.[28] Several general scales may also be relevant to particular studies. These include the Hospital Anxiety and Depression (HAD) scale,[29] the Rotterdam Symptom Checklist,[7] the SF12[30] and the Profile of Mood States (POMS). The POMS consists of 65 five-point adjective rating scales designed to assess transient mood states in medical and research settings.[31] The impact of breast cancer and its treatment on women's sexual function may be assessed by the Sexual Activity Questionnaire.[32]

QUALITY OF LIFE IN METASTATIC DISEASE

Metastatic breast cancer is not curable by any currently available therapy. Initially, most patients should receive endocrine therapy.[33] Because toxicity is low, the quality-of-life implications of such treatment are seldom clinically of great concern. After the failure of endocrine therapy, a trial of cytotoxic chemotherapy is frequently undertaken. Cytotoxic therapy for metastatic breast cancer is toxic but frequently effective, at least in terms of reducing tumour volume. There is little evidence that it prolongs survival. The main justification for cytotoxic therapy must therefore be the hope that it may control or reverse the progress of the disease. This in turn may offer improved quality of life compared to a purely symptomatic conservative palliative approach. There is now good evidence that this can be achieved. The evidence comes from prospective randomized clinical trials of cytotoxic therapy, which include direct measurement of quality of life.

Because of the perceived toxicity of cytotoxic therapy, the Australian New Zealand Breast Cancer Trials Group decided in 1981 to conduct a trial of an intermittent therapy policy. This policy was compared to the standard approach of continuing therapy until the disease progressed. In the intermittent therapy arm, treatment was discontinued after three cycles (9–12 weeks) of therapy, and was only re-introduced when the disease progressed. The hope was that the short course of therapy would control the symptoms of disease, and the treatment-free interval would avoid unnecessary treatment toxicity and thus afford a better net quality of life. It was clearly necessary to include quality-of-life measurement among the trial endpoints. The instruments chosen were five of the LASA scales originally used by Priestman and Baum,[14] and the Spitzer QLI.[19] Contrary to the hope which guided its design, this trial showed clearly superior quality of life with continuous rather than intermittent therapy.[24] Quality of life improved with both treatment policies during initial chemotherapy, which was common to both groups. Thereafter, patients assigned to continuous therapy showed a further improvement in quality of life, while those assigned to intermittent therapy showed deterioration in quality of life. Improvement in quality of life was linked to objective tumour response, which was significantly better on the continuous therapy. Time to disease progression and survival were also significantly better on the continuous therapy.[34] Two chemotherapy regimens were tested, namely a combination of doxorubicin and cyclophosphamide and a combination of cyclophosphamide, methotrexate and 5-fluorouracil (CMF) with high-dose prednisone. The effect was similar with both regimens.

At the same time, Tannock et al.[35] conducted a randomized trial of standard vs. half-dose CMF cytotoxic therapy in a similar attempt to reduce morbidity. Quality of life was assessed by a panel of LASA questions. Again, the more intensive therapy yielded superior objective outcomes, and a trend towards better quality of life. It would appear that, in both of these trials, the efficacy of the treatment in controlling symptomatic metastatic disease was more than enough to outweigh the associated toxicity.

A subsequent trial from the Australian New Zealand Breast Cancer Trials Group randomized patients to initial full-dosage combination CMF with prednisone (CMFP) or to single-agent mitozantrone, a drug chosen as a potentially less morbid alternative. In this trial, patients were crossed over to the alternative regimen after disease progression. CMFP was associated with a superior tumour response rate and time to first disease progression, but differences in survival were not significant.[36] Quality-of-life endpoints other than alopecia and nausea again favoured the more effective and more toxic therapy. These findings are entirely consistent with the original observation of Priestman et al.[37] that the factor which most influenced improvement in quality of life was the achievement of a tumour response, rather than the type of therapy used to achieve it.

QUALITY OF LIFE AS A PROGNOSTIC FACTOR

As evidence to support the validity of quality-of-life scores, several groups have investigated the relationship between quality of life and subsequent survival. In Australian New Zealand Breast Cancer Trials Group study ANZ 8101, it was noted that both the baseline quality-of-life scores and subsequent changes in scores were significantly predictive of subsequent survival.[23,24,34,38] This association persisted in multivariate analyses allowing for other significant recorded disease and patient characteristics (performance status and liver, brain and node metastases). The LASA scores for physical well-being and the Spitzer QLI remained significant predictors of survival independent of these conventional factors. When included together, both remained independently significant (although performance status did not). This finding indicated that patient self-assessment of physical well-being and physician assessment of QLI measure different aspects of prognostic information. Furthermore, they include the prognostic information conveyed by conventional recording of similar concepts on a performance status scale.[23,38]

The relationship between quality of life and prognosis is not unique to breast cancer. Similar associations have been observed in patients with metastatic malignant melanoma,[22] lung cancer,[39–41] and in populations of adult patients with a variety of advanced malignancies.[42,43,44] These studies have used different quality-of-life instruments. The reason for the predictive value of quality-of-life scores is unclear. It is entirely possible that quality of life merely captures prognostically important information about the status of the underlying disease more precisely than conventional medical recording. If this simple explanation were true, recording of quality-of-life information would still be a useful exercise. Another more intriguing possibility is that perceived quality of life actively influences prognosis. Put another way, this alternative postulates that patients live longer because they feel better, rather than merely feeling better because their disease is such that they are destined to live longer. If quality of life actively promotes survival, it is a possibility, although not a necessary corollary, that interventions aimed at improved quality of life might lead to prolongation of survival. This is a testable hypothesis. Several randomized trials testing such interventions are in progress, as described below.

Some preliminary evidence may support the simpler explanation. The association between Spitzer QLI and prognosis in both breast cancer[23,24] and melanoma[22] was analysed in more detail. The QLI consists of five questions, each of which is answered on a 3-point scale. These questions measure the patient's ability to work, to undertake self-care, their general health, the level of support provided by others, and their outlook. Conventionally, the sum of these five scores is used as the QLI. The scores on the five separate questions were analysed for their separate prognostic significance in univariate and multivariate analyses in order to determine which questions carried most prognostic information for survival. In the breast cancer study, QLI data at randomization were available for 240 women, and in the melanoma study for 150 patients, including 104 males and 48 females. In each data set, the total QLI score at the time of entry to the study and each of its five components was a significant predictor of subsequent survival duration in univariate analyses. The only exception was the question on perceived support, which was significant among the melanoma patients but not among those with breast cancer. Multivariate models containing all five questions were performed separately in each clinical trial data set. In these analyses, only the scores from the question relating to health remained independently significant. This would seem to imply that the main prognostic value of the QLI lies in its ability to describe the general health of the patient. Correspondingly, concepts such as support and outlook appeared to be of lesser importance, conveying no independent prognostic information.

QUALITY OF LIFE DURING ADJUVANT THERAPY

Adjuvant systemic therapy for early breast cancer differs in several important ways from treatment of metastatic disease. The trauma of initial diagnosis is usually more recent, and cure is still a real possibility. Most impor-

tantly, there is by definition no detectable residual cancer, and therefore the trade-off seen in metastatic disease, whereby the alleviation of tumour-associated symptoms may outweigh treatment toxicity, cannot apply here. Adjuvant chemotherapy clearly improves disease-free and overall survival,[45] and may have contributed to the recent reduction in breast cancer mortality.[46] Nevertheless, there is still a real need to decide whether or not to give toxic but potentially effective treatment, particularly chemotherapy.

Adjuvant therapy trials require large numbers of patients and substantial follow-up. Thus although the need for incorporation of quality-of-life endpoints has been evident for many years, results from trials incorporating direct quality-of-life measurement have only recently become available. Q-TWiST was developed to provide an alternative methodology for considering quality-of-life concepts in adjuvant therapy. This technique can be used even if quality of life has not been directly measured, as the impact of quality of life on outcome can be modelled.

In the Q-TWiST model,[47,48] the time from randomization (or initiation of treatment) is partitioned into three intervals. The time during toxic therapy (if given) is denoted by TOX. The period after recovery from the toxicity and before disease recurrence is called TWiST (time without symptoms or toxicity). Finally, the period after recurrence (if any) is referred to as REL. The follow up period is truncated in those patients who are not known to have died. TWiST is assigned a relative value of 1.0. The relative values of TOX and REL can be set to any desired level between 0 and 1. Assigning a value of 0 implies that such periods are of no value. A value of 1.0 would imply that the period should be valued equally with TWiST. The coefficients are denoted by U_t and U_r, respectively. The quality-adjusted score is then the sum of the period in TWiST and the discounted value obtained by multiplying the periods in TOX and REL by their respective coefficients, according to the following formula:

$$Q\text{-}TWiST = U_t\ TOX + TWiST + U_r\ REL.$$

Two treatment groups from a clinical trial can then be compared as follows. The average lengths of TOX, TWiST and REL are recorded for each group. Various values may then be considered for U_t and U_r. In some situations, one therapy will yield superior results regardless of the assumptions made about the coefficients. The superiority of one treatment is then evident, regardless of the utilities assigned to TOX and REL. In other situations it is possible to define threshold values of U_t and U_r which result in overall equivalence of Q-TWiST between the two treatments. This approach has recently been applied to the data from the Early Breast Cancer Trialists' Collaborative Group (EBCTCG) overview.[45] The particular comparison was between endocrine and chemo-endocrine adjuvant therapies for post-menopausal women with early breast cancer. Within the available follow-up period, plausible values of the coefficients U_t and U_r led to the conclusion that the two treatment approaches resulted in very similar quality-adjusted survival.[49]

The International Breast Cancer Study Group (IBCSG) recently reported two large adjuvant clinical trials which incorporated direct patient self-assessment of quality of life.[15] The question was whether the survival benefits were worth the adverse effects on quality of life.[50] Patient self-assessment of quality of life during adjuvant therapy was used to help to answer this question. Quality-of-life instruments used in these studies comprised three single-item LASA scales for physical well-being, mood and appetite, a psychological adjustment to chronic illness (PACIS) scale,[51] and an adjectival checklist to assess mood.[52] Baseline scores were available for 1248 (85%) of the 1461 evaluable premenopausal patients in IBCSG trial VI, and for 998 (83%) of the 1202 analysable post-menopausal patients in IBCSG trial VII.

Among premenopausal patients, there were significant associations between quality-of-life scores and some biological prognostic factors, in that LASA mood scores were lower in patients with oestrogen-receptor-negative than in those with oestrogen-receptor-positive tumours ($P=0.0009$). Similarly, both mood and PACIS scores became significantly worse as the number of involved axillary lymph nodes increased. These analyses were exploratory, and may merely reflect patients' knowledge of the factors concerned, but an association between oestrogen-receptor status and survival may be an intrinsic biological association.[53] Older patients (> 60 years) reported better emotional well-being ($P = 0.009$), mood ($P = 0.007$) and PACIS scores ($P = 0.001$) than younger post-menopausal patients. Among post-menopausal patients, baseline quality-of-life scores were not affected by oestrogen-receptor status or by the number of nodes involved.

There was a significant improvement in all quality-of-life score measures during the first 18 months of treatment ($P = 0.04$ for physical well-being, $P \leqslant 0.0001$ for all other scales). This applied within each treatment group. After all of the treatment groups had completed therapy, there was no significant difference among the treatment groups for any quality-of-life scale.

In IBCSG trial VII, no group of patients was undergoing cytotoxic treatment at the 6-month assessment. This provided an assessment of the impact of reintroduction of delayed CMF, since two treatment groups received treatment at 9 months. Patients assigned this delayed single cycle of CMF reported poorer quality of life, but individual scale differences were not significant. The adverse effect of delayed chemotherapy on quality of life was more pronounced among patients who had not previously undergone chemotherapy. These patients showed good recovery after the initial adverse impact of the cycle at 9 months. Their PACIS scores at 12 and 15 months

were similar to those for patients who did not receive delayed CMF therapy.

The effect of tumour recurrence was partially studied in 365 patients in trial VI and 257 patients in trial VII who had disease recurrence within the first 2.5 years. In total, 133 patients in trial VI and 90 patients in trial VII completed quality-of-life assessment both within 6 months before and 3 months after the date of recurrence. In each trial there was a significant decrease in all quality-of-life scores following recurrence, the magnitude of which was similar to the degree of improvement seen in non-relapsing patients over the first 18 months. This decline in quality of life was independent both of the time from randomization at which the patient's disease recurred, and of whether the patient had received chemotherapy at the last assessment before recurrence.

Patients' quality-of-life scores varied according to the duration and timing of chemotherapy. In premenopausal patients, the duration of initial CMF had a clear impact on patients' adjustment. Among post-menopausal patients, three cycles of early chemotherapy were associated with a mild and transient impairment of patients' quality of life. These results seem to be clinically plausible. These trials are the first large-scale adjuvant trials with both pre-recurrence and post-recurrence quality-of-life data. They represent a first step towards recording patients' self-assessment of the subjective consequences of therapy and of disease recurrence. This should aid the evaluation of the TOX and REL phases of the Q-TWiST model.

These studies showed that, although adjuvant chemotherapy had a measurable adverse impact on patient perception of quality of life, this impact was transient, and it was less substantial than the process of adaptation to the disease. Moreover, after completion of cytotoxic treatment, there was no lasting adverse effect, and patients' quality of life was indistinguishable regardless of the earlier therapy they had received. These findings should help to dispel some excessive fears associated with adjuvant chemotherapy, and should encourage patients and clinicians to use effective adjuvant therapy for early breast cancer.

IS TOXIC THERAPY WORTHWHILE FROM THE VIEWPOINT OF THE PATIENT?

Another approach to evaluating the patient's view on whether adjuvant therapy is worthwhile is to ask patients with experience of the treatment what degree of benefit they consider would justify the toxicity involved. Between November 1986 and December 1987, women who had received standard cytotoxic chemotherapy were studied. Planned treatment had to have included at least three 28-day cycles of CMF as adjuvant treatment after local treatment for operable breast cancer. These patients were interviewed in order to determine the degree of benefit that they considered would make such treatment worthwhile. Of 129 patients considered for participation, 104 patients completed the initial interview. Of these, 65 patients completed a retest interview. This was done in order to assess the reliability of the estimates. The interviews were conducted by two observers who were not connected with the patients' treatment, and they were held at least 3 months after completion of chemotherapy.

The basic approach of the study was to establish the patient's opinion of what additional period of survival with treatment would be worthwhile to justify the adverse experience of the treatment they had received. Patients were presented with hypothetical scenarios of the following general form:

> Suppose that without treatment you would live 5 years. Based on your experience of chemotherapy, what period of survival would make 6 months of initial treatment worthwhile?

Cards bearing alternative answers were presented until the patient considered the period offered to be of roughly equal value to the 5 years without treatment. A similar sequence was then followed to establish equivalence to an expectation of 15 years' survival without treatment, perhaps appropriate to low-risk node-negative patients.

Survival-rate questions were essentially similar to the time trade-off approach, but expressed the outcome of treatment in terms of the percentage likelihood of remaining alive at 5 years. The percentage selected as equivalent to 65% untreated was referred to as SR65, and that equivalent to 85% untreated as SR85. The major finding was that a large majority of the patients felt that relatively modest improvements in survival duration or in the percentage of 5-year survival would justify 6 months of the treatment they had received. This was true both for the optimistic scenarios, with untreated survival set at 15 years or 5-year survival at 85%, and for the less favourable scenarios, with untreated expectations of 5 years and 65%, respectively. Most patients would accept treatment in return for a 1-year survival increment. This was true both from 5 years to 6 years (77% acceptance) and from 15 years to 16 years (61% acceptance). When asked about survival percentages, the women indicated that they would accept treatment for a 2% improvement in survival probability, either from 65% to 67% (53% acceptance) or from 85% to 87% (54% acceptance). In the light of the EBCTCG overview,[45] differences of this magnitude appear to be reasonably achievable for many patient groups.

CAN QUALITY OF LIFE BE MEASURED EFFECTIVELY IN EVERYDAY PRACTICE?

Most of the results described so far have been derived from prospective clinical trials. Studies of this nature demand considerable logistic support. The International Group for Quality of Life in Oncology wanted to assess the feasibility of quality-of-life measurements in everyday clinical oncology practice. They used the EORTC QLQ-C30 questionnaire to study a total of 735 patients from 12 institutions in 10 countries. The largest number of patients (n305) had breast cancer. Other diagnoses were non-small-cell lung cancer (85 patients), small-cell lung cancer (45 patients), head and neck cancers (82 patients), gastrointestinal cancers (47 patients), acute leukaemias (42 patients), other haematological malignancies (65 patients) and cancer at other sites (64 patients). To minimize logistic demands, the only follow-up information required was the date and cause of death, or the fact that a patient was alive at the defined date of analysis. The association between quality-of-life scores and subsequent survival duration was defined in the protocol as the major endpoint of the study. All of the QLQ-C30 scales, and the single-item scores for questions 29 and 30, were significantly predictive of subsequent survival duration in univariate analyses. The patient factors that were significantly related to survival duration were age and performance status. Allowing for these non-quality-of-life variables, the social functioning and global scales and the single-item scores for overall physical condition and overall quality of life were independently significant prognostic factors for survival duration.

Among patients with solid tumours, the best set of non-quality-of-life variables predictive of survival was PS, liver and brain metastases. Again, after allowing for these variables, the social functioning and global scales and the questions on overall physical condition and overall quality of life remained independently significant prognostic factors for survival.

The success of the study demonstrated the feasibility of collecting quality-of-life data in a very broad range of oncology patients. The study clearly demonstrated that, just as in the more closely defined clinical trial situation, the quality-of-life scores provided independent additional information about prognosis. This should encourage measurement of quality of life in routine patient care.

SELECTING A QUALITY-OF-LIFE INSTRUMENT

Interest in quality-of-life measurement is clearly and appropriately increasing. Many researchers designing treatment trials will wish to include quality-of-life endpoints, and some clinicians may wish to do so outside the trial setting. Selection of an appropriate instrument is crucial to success.[6] Because of the complexity of developing and validating new instruments, it is almost always better to select an existing well-characterized quality-of-life scale. The choice will be guided by the question being asked, the resources available and the experience of the group. International studies will be limited to those scales available in the relevant languages. The International Breast Cancer Study Group scales and the EORTC QLQ-C30 are good choices for this purpose. It is important to remember that cultural as well as linguistic differences may complicate interpretation of multi-national studies.[18] Other general-purpose questionnaires suitable for consideration include the FACT,[28] the FLIC,[11] the Rotterdam Symptom Checklist[7] and the SF12.[30] Selection will depend on prior familiarity with one or other technique, and the extent to which each questionnaire samples the areas of interest in the particular clinical or research context.

PSYCHOSOCIAL INTERVENTIONS

As noted above, studies are in progress to assess the potential for therapies aimed at improving quality of life in order to ascertain whether they also improve survival. Preliminary studies have demonstrated an association between psychological response to cancer and survival,[54,55] and noted prolonged survival in patients receiving psychological support in breast cancer[56] and melanoma.[57] Rational design of psychological interventions aimed at prolonging survival would be aided by better definition of the detailed psychosocial factors that are most closely associated with survival.

CONCLUSIONS

Quality-of-life measures are clearly established as useful endpoints by which to compare and assess alternative treatments for breast cancer. The scores obtained also carry powerful independent prognostic information for survival. Methods of measurement are now well established, practical, valid and reliable. Quality of life is an integral part of the modern assessment of breast cancer.

REFERENCES

1 Hürny C, van Wegberg B, Bacchi M et al. Subjective Health Estimations (SHE) in patients with advanced breast cancer: an adapted utility concept for cancer clinical trials. Br J Cancer 1998; 77: 985–91.

2 Derogatis LR, Spencer PM. Psychometric issues in the psychological assessment of the cancer patient. Cancer 1984; 53: 2228–34.

3 Selby P, Robertson B. Measurement of quality of life in patients with cancer. Cancer Surv 1987; 6: 521–43.

4 Aaronson NK, Bullinger M, Ahmedzai S. A modular approach to quality of life assessment in cancer clinical trials. Recent Results Cancer Res 1988; 111: 231–49.

5 Donovan K, Sanson-Fisher RW, Redman S. Measuring quality of life in cancer patients. J Clin Oncol 1989; 7: 959–68.

6 Cella DF, Tulsky DS. Measuring quality of life today: methodological aspects. Oncology 1990; 4: 29–38.

7 de Haes JCJM, van Knippenberg FCE, Neijt JP. Measuring psychological and physical distress in cancer patients: structure and application of the Rotterdam Symptom Checklist. Br J Cancer 1990; 62: 1034–8.

8 Butow PN, Coates AS, Dunn S et al. On the receiving end. IV. Validation of quality of life indicators. Ann Oncol 1991; 2: 597–603.

9 Bjordal K, Kaasa S. Psychometric validation of the EORTC core quality of life questionnaire, 30-item version, and a diagnosis-specific module for head and neck cancer patients. Acta Oncol 1992; 31: 311–21.

10 Gill TM, Feinstein AR. A critical appraisal of the quality of quality-of-life measurements. J Am Med Assoc 1994; 272: 619–26.

11 Schipper H, Clinch J, McMurray A et al. Measuring the quality of life of cancer patients: the functional living index – cancer: development and validation. J Clin Oncol 1994; 2: 472–83.

12 Aitken RCB. Measurement of feelings using visual analogue scales. Proc R Soc Med 1969; 62: 989–96.

13 Baum M, Ebbs SR, Fallowfield LJ et al. Measurement of quality of life in advanced breast cancer. Acta Oncol 1990; 29: 391–5.

14 Priestman TJ, Baum M. Evaluation of quality of life in patients receiving treatment for advanced breast cancer. Lancet 1976; 1: 899–901.

15 Hürny C, Bernhard J, Coates AS et al. Impact of adjuvant therapy on quality of life in women with node-positive operable breast cancer. Lancet 1996; 347: 1279–84.

16 Bernhard J, Hürny C, Coates AS et al. Quality of life assessment in patients receiving adjuvant therapy for breast cancer: the IBCSG approach. Ann Oncol 1997; 8: 825–35.

17 Hürny C, Bernhard J, Coates AS et al. Responsiveness of a single-item indicator versus a multi-item scale: assessment of emotional wellbeing in an international breast cancer trial. Med Care 1996; 34: 234–48.

18 Bernhard J, Hürny C, Coates AS et al. Applying quality of life principles in international cancer clinical trials. In Spiker B (ed.) Quality of life and pharmacoeconomics in clinical trials, 2nd edn. Philadelphia, PA: Lippincott-Raven Publishers, 1996; 693–705.

19 Spitzer WO, Dobson AJ, Hall J et al. Measuring the quality of life of cancer patients: a concise QL-Index for use by physicians. J Chron Dis 1981; 34: 585–97.

20 Slevin ML, Plant HJ, Lynch D et al. Who should measure quality of life, the doctor or the patient? Br J Cancer 1988; 57: 109–12.

21 Coates AS, Gebski V. On the receiving end. VI. Which dimensions of quality of life scores carry prognostic information? Cancer Treat Rev 1996; 22: 63–7.

22 Coates AS, Thomson D, McLeod GR et al. Prognostic value of quality of life scores in a trial of chemotherapy with or

without interferon in patients with metastatic melanoma. *Eur J Cancer* 1993; **29A**: 1731–4.

23 Coates AS, Gebski V, Signorini D *et al*. Prognostic value of quality-of-life scores during chemotherapy for advanced breast cancer. Australian New Zealand Breast Cancer Trials Group. *J Clin Oncol* 1992; **10**: 1833–8.

24 Coates AS, Gebski V, Bishop JF *et al*. Improving the quality of life in advanced breast cancer. A comparison of continuous and intermittent treatment strategies. *N Engl J Med* 1987; **317**: 1490–5.

25 Addington-Hall JM, MacDonald LD, Anderson HR. Can the Spitzer quality of life index help to reduce prognostic uncertainty in terminal care? *Br J Cancer* 1990; **62**: 695–9.

26 Sprangers MAG, Cull A, Bjordal K *et al*. The European Organization for Research and Treatment of Cancer approach to quality of life assessment: guidelines for developing questionnaire modules. *Qual Life Res* 1993; **2**: 287–95.

27 Aaronson NK. Quality of life research in cancer clinical trials: a need for common rules and language. *Oncology* 1990; **4**: 59–66.

28 Cella DF, Tulsky DS, Gray G *et al*. The Functional Assessment of Cancer Therapy Scale: development and validation of the general measure. *J Clin Oncol* 1993; **11**: 570–9.

29 Zigmund AS, Snaith RP. The Hospital Anxiety and Depression Scale. *Acta Psychiatr Scand* 1983; **67**: 361–70.

30 Ware JE, Kosinski M, Keller SD: A 12-item short-form health survey: construction of scales and preliminary tests of reliability and validity. *Med Care* 1996; **34**: 220–33.

31 McNair DM, Lorr M, Droppleman LF. *EITS manual for the profile of mood states*. San Diego, CA: EITS, 1971.

32 Thirlaway K, Fallowfield LJ, Cuzick J. The Sexual Activity Questionnaire: a measure of women's sexual functioning. *Qual Life Res* 1996; **5**: 81–90.

33 Australian New Zealand Breast Cancer Trials Group. A randomized trial in postmenopausal patients with advanced breast cancer comparing endocrine and cytotoxic therapy given sequentially or in combination. *J Clin Oncol* 1986; **4**: 186–93.

34 Coates AS, Byrne M, Bishop JF *et al*. Intermittent versus continuous chemotherapy for breast cancer (letter). *N Engl J Med* 1988; **318**: 1468.

35 Tannock IF, Boyd NF, DeBoer G *et al*. A randomized trial of two dose levels of cyclophosphamide, methotrexate and fluorouracil chemotherapy for patients with metastatic breast cancer. *J Clin Oncol* 1988; **6**: 1377–87.

36 Simes RJ, Gebski V, Coates AS *et al*. Quality of life on single agent mitozantrone versus cyclophosphamide, methotrexate, 5-fluorouracil, prednisone for advanced breast cancer. *Proc Annu Meet Am Soc Clin Oncol* 1994; **13**: 73 (abstract).

37 Priestman TJ, Baum M, Jones V *et al*. Comparative trial of endocrine versus cytotoxic treatment in advanced breast cancer. *BMJ* 1977; **1**: 1248–50.

38 Coates AS, Forbes JF, Simes RJ. Prognostic value of performance status and quality-of-life scores during chemotherapy for advanced breast cancer. The Australian New Zealand Breast Cancer Trials Group (letter). *J Clin Oncol* 1993; **11**: 2050.

39 Kaasa S, Mastekaasa A, Lund E. Prognostic factors for patients with inoperable non-small-cell lung cancer, limited disease. The importance of patients' subjective experience of disease and psychosocial well-being. *Radiother Oncol* 1989; **15**: 235–42.

40 Ganz PA, Lee JJ, Siau J. Quality of life assessment. An independent prognostic variable for survival in lung cancer. *Cancer* 1991; **67**: 3131–5.

41 Ruckdeschel JC, Piantodosi S. Quality of life assessment in lung surgery for bronchogenic carcinoma. *Theor Surg* 1991; **6**: 201–5.

42 Dancey J, Zee B, Osoba D *et al*. Quality of life scores: an independent prognostic variable in a general population of cancer patients receiving chemotherapy. *Qual Life Res* 1997; **6**: 151–8.

43 Coates AS, Porzsolt F, Osoba D. Quality of life in oncology practice: prognostic value of EORTC QLQ-C30 scores in patients with advanced malignancy. *Eur J Cancer* 1997; **33**: 1025–30.

44 Wilsoff F, Hjorth M. Health-related quality of life assessed before and during chemotherapy predicts for survival in multiple myeloma. *Br J Haematol* 1997; **97**: 29–37.

45 Early Breast Cancer Trialists' Collaborative Group. Systemic treatment of early breast cancer by hormonal, cytotoxic or immune therapy. 133 randomised trials involving 31 000 recurrences and 24 000 deaths among 75 000 women. *Lancet* 1992; **339**: 1–15, 71–85.

46 Beral V, Hermon C, Reeves G *et al*. Sudden fall in breast cancer death rates in England and Wales. *Lancet* 1995; **345**: 1642–3.

47 Gelber RD, Goldhirsch A. A new endpoint for the assessment of adjuvant therapy in postmenopausal women with operable breast cancer. *J Clin Oncol* 1986; **4**: 1772–9.

48 Goldhirsch A, Gelber RD, Simes RJ *et al*. Costs and benefits of adjuvant therapy in breast cancer: a quality-adjusted survival analysis. *J Clin Oncol* 1989; **7**: 36–44.

49 Gelber RD, Cole BF, Goldhirsch A *et al*. Adjuvant chemotherapy plus tamoxifen compared with tamoxifen alone for postmenopausal breast cancer: meta-analysis of quality-adjusted survival. *Lancet* 1996; **347**: 1066–71.

50 Quality of life and clinical trials (editorial). *Lancet* 1995; **346**: 1–2.

51 Hürny C, Bernhard J, Bacchi M *et al*. The Perceived Adjustment to Chronic Illness Scale (PACIS): a global indicator of coping for operable breast cancer patients in clinical trials. *Support Care Cancer* 1993; **1**: 200–8.

52 Zersen DV. Clinical self-rating scales (CSRS) of the Munich Psychiatric Information System (PSYCHIS Muenchen). In: Sartorius N, Ban TA (eds) *Assessment of depression*. Berlin: Springer, 1986: 270–303.

53 Razavi D, Farvacques C, Delvaux N. Psychosocial correlates of oestrogen and progesterone receptors in breast cancer. *Lancet* 1990; **335**: 931–3.

54 Greer S. Psychological response to cancer and survival. *Psychol Med* 1991; **21**: 43–9.

55 Greer S, Morris T, Pettingale KW *et al*. Psychological response to breast cancer and 15-year outcome (letter). *Lancet* 1990; **335**: 49–50.

56 Spiegel D, Bloom JR, Kraemer HC *et al*. The effect of psychosocial treatment on survival of patients with metastatic breast cancer. *Lancet* 1989; **2**: 888–91.

57 Fawzy FI, Fawzy NW, Hyun CS *et al*. Malignant melanoma. Effects of an early structured psychiatric intervention, coping and affective state on recurrence and survival 6 years later. *Arch Gen Psychiatry* 1993; **50**: 681–9.

27

Hormone replacement therapy and breast cancer risk

CHRISTOBEL MARY SAUNDERS

Twenty million prescriptions for hormone replacement therapy (HRT) were dispensed in the USA in 1986,[1] and it has been shown that up to 60% of women aged 50–64 years in the USA have taken non-contraceptive sex hormones.[2] In the UK this figure is probably nearer 15%,[3] but it seems to be rising. The benefits of HRT in terms of decreasing the mortality and morbidity from cardiovascular and bone disease, as well as providing dramatic improvement of menopausal symptoms, are well known. The safety of taking HRT in relation to breast cancer risk both for healthy women and for those who have had breast cancer is controversial. The aim of this chapter is to examine some of the evidence for the possible detrimental effect of exogenous sex hormones on the breast, and attempt to put into perspective the risks and benefits of HRT both in healthy post-menopausal women and in those who have previously had breast cancer.

INTRODUCTION

The climacteric is the phase of a woman's life when ovarian function declines, leading to a complete cessation in her menstrual periods, this point in time being described as the menopause. The median age of the menopause is 50.8 years, but the climacteric frequently begins 2–3 years before this. The endocrine consequences of the menopause are a fall in ovarian oestradiol production, as well as a deficiency in corpus luteal progesterone secretion. Gonadotrophin secretion rises markedly in an attempt to drive the failing ovaries, but plasma oestradiol levels will finally fall to a sufficiently low level that

endometrial proliferation ceases and amenorrhoea ensues.

Oestrogens were first used therapeutically in 1938 by Bishop to treat the symptoms of menopause in women who had undergone an oophorectomy. Since the 1950s their use has escalated, both for the treatment of menopausal symptoms and as prophylaxis against cardiovascular disease and osteoporosis in women with either a premature or natural menopause. These diseases currently affect approximately 10 million women in the UK over the age of 50 years, and this number is set to increase with the rise in female life expectancy – currently 82 years.[4] At the same time, there has been virtually no change in the average age at which the menopause is reached. Although probably only about 10% of women between the ages of 45 and 65 years use HRT, over 50% of post-menopausal women doctors in this age group have used it, suggesting that the frequency of use in the general population is likely to increase.[5] Concurrent with this increasing use of exogenous oestrogen and progesterone has been a clearer knowledge of their effects, both physiologically and pathologically. In particular, the *in-vitro* effects of oestrogens in promoting the growth of various human cancers, including endometrial and breast cancer, have become well recognized.

Oestrogens were in fact the first substance originating in the body to be implicated as a cause of cancer. Their influence on breast cancer was noted as long ago as 1896 by Beaston, who reported the beneficial effects of oophorectomy in advanced breast cancer.[6] This influence of natural oestrogen on the development of breast cancer has now been established both epidemiologically and experimentally,[7,8] and is highlighted by most of the risk factors for carcinoma of the breast, including female sex, early menarche, late menopause and obesity in post-menopausal women, all of which have in common the prolonged exposure of the breast tissue to unopposed circulating oestrogens. Hormone replacement therapy is administered either as oestrogen only (ORT) or as oestrogen combined with cyclical progestin (HRT), so it is important to elucidate the effects of both of these hormones on the human breast. There are, of course, many other endogenous hormones, such as prolactin, which may be important in the development of breast cancer, but their role is less certain.

It can be seen that an increase in the use of HRT coupled with an increase in our knowledge of the effects of sex hormones on breast tissue makes it imperative to assess the potential risks of the use of these compounds in healthy women, and to scrutinize any evidence for a role that these hormones may have in the development of breast cancer.

THE BIOLOGICAL EVIDENCE

Proliferative change in the normal female pre-menopausal breast is largely controlled by circulating levels of endogenous oestrogen and progesterone, although other substances (e.g. prolactin and growth factors) also play an important role.[9] There is a change in this proliferative activity during the menstrual cycle, with the highest indices of proliferation being on day 21 and the lowest on day 7 of the cycle, although all of the indices fall off with age.[10] It is suggested that this may either be due to a delayed priming effect by oestrogen in the first half of the cycle, with no progesterone effect, or it may reflect progesterone's ability to increase the responsiveness of breast epithelial cells to growth-stimulating peptide hormones.[11] Studies of breast tissue in cell-culture systems have also confirmed this stimulatory effect of sex hormones.[12] In a prospective study of endogenous oestrogens and hormonal cancer, it was found that women who subsequently develop breast cancer had increased levels of oestrone, oestradiol, free oestradiol and decreased SHBG-bound oestradiol.[13] The role of *exogenous* hormones in either normal or malignant breast epithelium is less well understood.

Animal and tissue culture studies strongly suggest that exogenous oestrogens may induce or promote the development of breast cancer.[14,15] The most likely mechanism by which oestrogen acts is as a promoter in previously transformed breast cancer cells, thus stimulating the growth of established tumours. It is doubtful whether it acts as an actual carcinogen. Longman and Beuhring have shown that exogenous oestrogen (of a dose and type similar to that found in the oral contraceptive pill) differentially stimulates cultures of malignant and non-malignant breast epithelial cells, so that the growth rate of the malignant cells exceeds that of the others, suggesting that exogenous oestrogen could be a promoter of already transformed cells, rather than the initiator of the transforming event.[15]

The effect of progestagens on the development of breast cancer is less clear. There is little laboratory evidence that progestagens can promote carcinogenesis, but their effects on already established breast cancer cell lines have been studied. Some studies suggest that progestagens given alone may stimulate growth of breast cancer cells,[12,16] possibly via regulation of the EGF receptor, and others suggest that progestagens may exert an additive effect with oestrogen on the stimulation of breast cancer growth.[17] However, most workers have shown that in both oestrogen-dependent human breast cancer cells[18] and anti-oestrogen-resistant, oestrogen-receptor-negative human breast cancer cell lines,[19] growth can be inhibited by progestagens. This inhibitory effect has been shown *in vitro* both at physiological doses in normal human breast epithelial cells,[20] and at high doses as found in the combined oral contraceptive pill and combined hormone replacement therapy.[15]

Progesterone and progestins have been shown to be anti-oestrogenic – they lower blood oestrogen levels,[21] decrease oestrogen receptor levels, as shown by a progressive fall in oestrogen-receptor levels in fibroadenomas removed in the luteal phase of the menstrual cycle,[22] and increase synthesis of 17β-hydroxysteroid dehydrogenase, which catalyses the conversion of oestradiol to the less active oestrone.[23] *In-vitro* experiments with pharmacological doses of megestrol acetate and progesterone demonstrate that they also have an oestrogen-independent direct inhibitory effect on breast cancer cells.[18,19]

There is abundant clinical evidence that progestagens may be inhibitory to breast cancer cells. In patients with advanced breast cancer treated with mixed oestrogen agonists and antagonists such as tamoxifen – who are no longer responsive to this treatment – there is a tumour response rate of approximately 30% if these relapsed patients are subsequently given high-dose progestagen.[24,25] A proposed mechanism for this is that progesterone stimulates the terminal differentiation of breast epithelial cells, thus making them less susceptible to mitogenesis.[17]

The *in-vivo* effects of these hormones are difficult to study, so indirect epidemiological methods have been employed in an attempt to demonstrate a causal relationship between exogenous hormone administration and breast cancer.

THE EPIDEMIOLOGICAL EVIDENCE

The premise that prolonged exposure of the breast tissue to exogenous oestrogen may promote the growth of an epithelial tumour has raised concerns about the safety of administering exogenous hormones to otherwise healthy women in the form of contraceptives or HRT. In the absence of any prospective randomized trial data, epidemiologists have undertaken numerous case–control and cohort studies looking at the association between exogenous hormones and breast cancer risk.[26–37]

However, both case–control and cohort surveys suffer from a number of inherent methodological problems which may bias their results. Cohort studies look at a large number of women over time, and try to match their health outcome with differences recorded between the women, including their use of oestrogen therapy. Despite the large numbers of subjects, there are relatively few who develop breast cancer, so the differences between those who do and those who do not may be spurious. In case–control studies, women with proven breast cancer (cases) are compared with demographically similar women without the disease (controls), and their past and present use of exogenous hormones are compared. Often the accuracy of the subject's memory is poor and she can remember neither when nor which hormones she used, if any at all. This recall is somewhat improved if women are interviewed personally and shown packets of the drugs, or if drug-history records are consulted. Of course, formulations and patterns of use have changed considerably over time, making interpretation difficult. For example, most HRT studies look at use of the oestrogen-only formulations, few of them look at combined preparations, and the only study which did show that these increased risk had only 10 patients with breast cancer.[27] Another confounding factor is a spuriously high detection rate of breast cancer in women using exogenous hormones, because they are screened more frequently than the general population.[4] Counterbalancing this bias is an artificially low true association due to the fact that women with breast cancer or those judged to be at high risk would not be prescribed these drugs. Finally, one must question whether women who are prescribed HRT for severe menopausal symptoms constitute a special group with a hormone environment that increases their susceptibility to the development of breast cancer.

Only one study was prospective, and it looked at 84 pairs of long-term institutionalized patients.[38] This study has been updated,[39] and the data suggest that 22 years' administration of HRT does not increase the incidence of breast cancer.

As shown in Figure 27.1, case–control and cohort studies have yielded inconsistent results,[40] leading to considerable confusion about the best advice to give to women who wish to use HRT. In any decision, both the risks and the benefits of treatment for the individual must be weighed up before an informed decision can be taken. Table 27.1 illustrates the benefits of HRT, whilst the risks include a small increase in the incidence of breast cancer and a significant increase in the incidence of endometrial carcinoma in those women with an intact uterus who have used oestrogen-only preparations. A prospective study of 8881 post-menopausal women by Henderson et al. showed that, overall, the all-cause mortality of women who had ever used oestrogen replacement therapy was

Study	Relative risk and confidence intervals			
Case control	1	2	3	4
Ross, 1980	***[1.1]****			
Hoover, 1981	***[1.4]***			
Hulka, 1982		***[1.6]********		
Brinton, 1986	*[1.0]*			
Wingo, 1987	*[1.1]*			
Rohan, 1988	*****[0.9]**			
Kaufman, 1988	**[1.2]*			
Bergkvist, 1989	*[1.1]**			
La Vecchia, 1990	**[1.3]*****			
Cohort				
Gambrell, 1983	*[0.7]*			
Mills, 1989		****[1.7]********		
Dupont, 1989	**[1.0]*			
Colditz, 1990	*[1.4]*			
Hunt, 1990	***[1.0]*			

Figure 27.1 Hormone replacement therapy and breast cancer risk.

20% lower than that of an age-matched population, and mortality decreased with duration of use.[45] This reduction in overall mortality was largely due to a fall in cardiovascular deaths, but a small reduction in cancer deaths was also seen. It has been estimated that the cost-effectiveness of treating menopausal symptoms is comparable to that of a GP giving advice to stop smoking, and 10 years of treatment (in terms of QALYs) is less than one-third as costly as coronary artery bypass for severe angina (E Daly et al., 1994; personal communication). A larger trial under the auspices of the Women's Health Initiative to look at all endpoints of HRT use, is now in progress.

FORMULATIONS

Hormone replacement therapy is most commonly administered via the oral route, but the oestrogen component may also be delivered by subcutaneous implant, transdermal patch, vaginal cream or vaginal ring, thus avoiding some of the problems of poor patient compliance – with oral preparations there is less than 40%

Table 27.1 Benefits of HRT

Immediate benefits
  Reversal of menopausal symptoms
  Reversal of atrophic changes in vagina
  Reversal of emotional and psychological upset

Long-term benefits
  Reduction in coronary artery disease[41,42]
  Reduction in osteoporosis[43]
  Reduction in incidence of ovarian cancer[3]
  Possible reduction in incidence of colon cancer[44]
  Improvement in skin elasticity

compliance at 9 months,[46] – and first-pass liver metabolism of oral oestrogens. A combination oestrogen and progestagen transdermal patch has been developed.[47]

Oestrogens may be administered as synthetic preparations such as ethinyl oestradiol or natural oestrogens, most commonly conjugated equine oestrogen. Although the latter are considerably less potent, they do produce a more physiological serum profile than synthetic oestrogens, and are particularly valuable in HRT because they are thought to be less thrombogenic.

Most of the 20 or so HRT preparations available will deliver the equivalent of 0.625 mg of natural conjugated oestrogen per day.[48] This dose of oestrogen will produce a low serum oestradiol level similar to that found in the early follicular phase of the menstrual cycle, and a total dose of oestrogen throughout the cycle of one-third of that found in premenopausal women.[17]

Many HRT preparations also contain progestagens, and this is essential if the woman still has an intact uterus, as they act as an effective protection against the development of endometrial cancer by reversing the cell proliferation caused by the oestrogen component of HRT.[49] The association between unopposed oestrogen in HRT and endometrial cancer was first noted in the 1970s, and epidemiological data puts this increased risk at 4–8 times the background incidence of endometrial cancer.[50] This was found to be both dose and duration dependent.[51,52] Exogenous oestrogens do not appear to increase the risk of cervical cancer.[53]

The addition of progestagens for part of the cycle can decrease premalignant endometrial hyperplasia from 15–30% to 0% in women using unopposed oestrogens, and has been shown to reduce the incidence of endometrial carcinoma to below that of the untreated population.[3] However, it has always been thought that the addition of progestagens in HRT would diminish their protective effects on the cardiovascular system and produce symptoms of depression, anxiety and irritability. Evidence suggests that the addition of progestagens does not alter the beneficial cardiovascular effects.[41] It has been shown that a combined HRT regime will lower blood cholesterol and low-density lipoprotein, and in a cohort study by Falkeborn et al.[55] the relative risk of acute myocardial infarction in combined HRT users was 0.53 – a similar value to that in users of ORT. Moreover, progestagens do not appear to diminish the positive benefits on osteoporosis,[43] and may in fact enhance these by increasing bone mineral mass.[56]

The progestagen component of HRT is usually in the form of norgestrel 0.15 mg or norethisterone 1 mg per day. However, the plasma levels of progestagen will be enormously variable among individuals treated with the same dose, due to vagaries of absorption and metabolism. The progestagen dosage is currently adjusted by noting withdrawal bleeding patterns. If a woman starts to bleed after completion of the usual 12 days of progestagen, she is likely to have uterine histological features suggestive of maximal endometrial protection, whereas if she bleeds before the 12-day course has been completed she is likely to require an increase in progestagen dose.[57]

BREAST CANCER RISK

As described above, HRT usually produces a serum oestradiol level of about one-third of that found in premenopausal women. Unlike the uterus, where even this low level of unopposed oestrogen will cause maximal epithelial cell proliferation, the induction of breast epithelial cell division will be minimal, as in the early follicular phase of the menstrual cycle.[17]

Four recent meta-analyses, conducted in 1991, 1992 and 1997[1,40,58,59] evaluated all of the published studies of the association between HRT and breast cancer – that is, over 50 studies in total. It may be argued that pooling the results from a wide variety of study types is of dubious validity, but in the absence of a large randomized trial it provides the largest possible database. The reviews conclude that there is an overall relative increased risk of 1.02 for each year of use (i.e. a 2% higher risk of developing breast cancer for women on HRT). The confidence intervals of most of the studies include unity. This figure is sufficiently small not to be of importance in most cases when making a decision as to whether to start a woman on HRT. However, a number of studies[26–29] do suggest that certain subgroups of women may be at higher risk than others. These may include women with a family history of breast cancer (where the addition of HRT will increase their risk over and above the increase due to their family history), women who have undergone a normal (rather than surgical) menopause, those currently on HRT rather than previous users,[37,59] suggesting that HRT is only important in the later stages of carcinogenesis, and those with established proliferative benign breast disease or previous cancer (the latter will be examined in more detail later). Some studies suggest that women with a lower body-mass index are at higher risk.[59] In addition, sub-group analyses, which of course have weaker power, suggest that some treatment factors may be associated with a higher relative risk of developing breast cancer.[29,34,59] These include a high dose of oestrogen (over 0.625 mg per day), prolonged duration of treatment (over 5 years, although the risk drops to normal 5 years after cessation of use),[59] and possibly the type of oestrogen used, oestradiol being associated with a higher risk than the more commonly used natural conjugated equine oestrogens. Newer agents such as livial have not been assessed.

The prognosis for women who are diagnosed as having breast cancer whilst on HRT seems to be better, with tumours presenting at a less advanced stage, as shown in Figure 27.2. This may be due to a variety of factors, including increased breast surveillance and screening.[59–61]

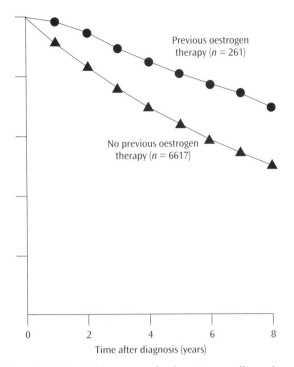

Figure 27.2 *Survival in women after breast cancer diagnosis.*

Thus in summary HRT does not significantly increase the risk of developing breast cancer in most women, although there is some evidence that high doses of oestrogens used for a prolonged period, and especially in certain high-risk groups, may cause a small but significant increase in the incidence of breast cancer. However, due to a better prognosis in these women, the overall mortality from breast cancer in women who use HRT appears to be no worse than that in those who do not.

Figure 27.3 illustrates some of the risks and benefits of HRT. Paradoxically, it may be possible to develop an agent which has the benefits of HRT, whilst at the same time helping to prevent breast cancer.

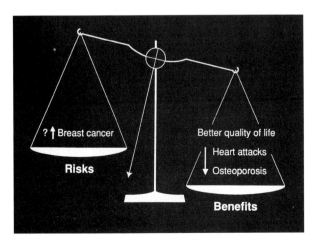

Figure 27.3 *Some risks and benefits of hormone replacement therapy.*

HORMONE REPLACEMENT THERAPY AFTER BREAST CANCER

Conventionally, the use of hormone replacement therapy in women who have had breast cancer has been discouraged because of the theoretical risks of oestrogen stimulation of any residual cancer cells, or stimulation of cells which have undergone partial malignant transformation. However, there is no scientific evidence that HRT does adversely affect the chance of recurrence. In fact, the limited clinical studies conducted to date have shown no deleterious effect on mortality or time to recurrence.[62–65] This can also be inferred from indirect evidence of the effect of oestrogen on the growth of breast tumours, such as the better prognosis from breast cancer in premenopausal women with higher levels of endogenous oestrogen,[66] the better prognosis of women diagnosed with breast cancer whilst on HRT, including those with screen-detected cancers,[67–69] and the similarity in survival of age- and stage-matched women with gestational breast cancer (and thus presumably high levels of sex hormones) to those with breast cancer unrelated to pregnancy.[70] Oral contraceptives do not appear to influence the risk of breast cancer unless they are used at a young age before the first full-term pregnancy, further providing indirect evidence of a lack of direct effect of oestrogen.[71]

Most patients with breast cancer are post-menopausal, and many of those who present premenopausally are rendered menopausal by their treatment. Many of these women will suffer considerable symptoms, and it has been clearly demonstrated that women with early ovarian failure secondary to cancer therapy have a high rate of sexual dysfunction and psychological distress.[72] A large proportion of breast cancer survivors will go on to succumb to cardiovascular disease, leading some to speculate that the improvement in survival mediated by chemotherapy may be negated by inducing more cardiovascular disease.[73] According to our current clinical practice, if the patient's quality of life (as assessed by her doctor and herself) is being severely affected by menopausal symptoms, or if she is at high risk of, for example, osteoporosis, initial treatment may be with a non-hormonal compound such as clonidine or a low-dose progestagen. If the patient's symptoms are still not relieved, then the short-term use of HRT, in combination with tamoxifen, is justified. A number of guidelines have been published for clinicians and patients regarding this subject.[74,75] Certainly it would seem that even if HRT did increase the growth of breast cancer, this would be detected early during follow-up.[76]

Whilst it may at first sight seem illogical to combine an oestrogen with an anti-oestrogen such as tamoxifen, it is now well established that tamoxifen has both oestrogen agonist and antagonist actions. Tamoxifen exerts its action not only via the oestrogen receptor, but via a number of other oestrogen-independent pathways such as induction of the tumour suppressor transforming growth factor beta from stromal cells.[77] The concern that oestrogen may antagonize the effect of tamoxifen, perhaps by competitive binding to the oestrogen receptor, is unlikely given that tamoxifen is just as efficacious in premenopausal women,[78] and indeed causes hyperoestrogenaemia.[79] Further development of selective oestrogen receptor modulators (SERMs), which mimic some but not all agonist properties of oestrogen in different tissues, may provide a new approach to HRT.[80]

Women who have had breast cancer are recommended a combination hormone therapy which includes progesterone. This will reduce the risk of the patient developing subsequent endometrial carcinoma, and will prevent the potentially dangerous 'unopposed oestrogen environment' which some have suggested may contribute to the stimulation of tumour growth.[81] It may even be of therapeutic benefit to the patient in terms of *decreasing* the likelihood of recurrence.[81]

More information is required both on the biological effects of HRT on breast tumours and on the clinical effects of prescribing HRT to women who have had breast cancer.[82] One area which urgently requires clarification is the effect of HRT on the mammographic appearance of the breast, and whether detection of breast cancer may be impaired by HRT.[83,84]

A prospective trial of HRT use in women who have had breast cancer is required to redress this situation. There is much interest in setting up this kind of study on a large scale, and in the USA a trial of this nature was set up in 1992 by the MD Anderson Hospital in Houston. The investigators in this study have found that, although the theoretical interest in this trial is high, the practicalities of participant recruitment are somewhat different. In fact, only 17% of women eligible for the study have been recruited, due to lack of interest (38% of cases), fear (33%), the fact that they were already on HRT (12%) or other reasons (17%). They found the profiles of all of these women to be similar in terms of both disease characteristics and demographics, and thus state that this may be an important consideration when designing trials of this kind.[85] Although the results of this study are still awaited, no events have been detected at 20 months. In this country, some pilot studies are being undertaken to address some specific issues. One such pilot study (J Marsden, personal communication) is being run both to evaluate the feasibility of a larger study, and to look at quality-of-life endpoints when using HRT in a group of women who have had breast cancer – ultimately a more useful endpoint than any presumably very small differences in survival rates.

Thus, in summary, the risks of providing HRT to women who have had breast cancer and have severe menopausal symptoms is unproven, whereas the benefits in terms of quality of life and reduction of morbidity and mortality from cardiovascular disease are very real. There

may even be beneficial effects with regard to suppression of breast cancer recurrence. The controversies which remain are listed in Table 27.2.

Table 27.2 *Factors which remain controversial*

Latency
High-risk groups
Chemoprevention
HRT after breast cancer

REFERENCES

1 Steinberg KK, Thacker SB, Smith SJ et al. A meta-analysis of the effect of estrogen replacement therapy on the risk of breast cancer. *J Am Med Assoc* 1991; **265**: 1985–90.
2 Weiss NS. *Case–control studies of exogenous hormones in relation to breast cancer in women conducted in Western Washington*. Paper presented at the Royal Society of Medicine Symposium on HRT and Breast Cancer, September 1991.
3 Wardle PG, Padwick ML. Hormone replacement therapy. *Hosp Update* 1992; **18**: 443–54.
4 Baber RJ, Studd JWW. Hormone replacement therapy and cancer. *Br J Hosp Med* 1989; **41**: 142–9.
5 Isaacs AJ, Britton AR, McPherson K. Utilisation of hormone replacement therapy by women doctors, *BMJ* 1995; **311**: 1399–401.
6 Beaston GT. On the treatment of inoperable cases of the mamma: suggestions for a new method of treatment with illustrative cases. *Lancet* 1896; **ii**: 104–65.
7 Kelsey JL. A review of the epidemiology of human breast cancer. *Epidemiol Rev* 1979; **1**: 74–109.
8 Moore DH, Moore CT. Breast cancer – etiological factors. *Adv Cancer Res* 1983; **40**: 189–253.
9 Anderson TJ, Ferguson DJP, Raab GM. Cell turnover in the 'resting' human breast: influence of parity, contraceptive pill, age and laterality. *Br J Cancer* 1982; **46**: 376–82.
10 Potten CS, Watson RJ, Williams GT et al. The effect of age and menstrual cycle upon proliferative activity of the normal human breast. *Br J Cancer* 1988; **58**: 163–70.
11 Murphy LJ, Sutherland RL, Stead B, Murphy LC, Lazarus L. Progestin regulation of epidermal growth factor receptor in human mammary carcinoma cells. *Cancer Res* 1986; **46**: 728.
12 McManus MJ, Welsch CW. The effect of oestrogen, progesterone, thyroxine and human placental lactogen on DNA synthesis of human breast ductal epithelium maintained in athymic nude mice. *Cancer* 1984; **54**: 1920–7.
13 Toniolo PG, Levitz M, Zeleniuch-Jacquotte A et al. A prospective study of endogenous estrogens and breast cancer in postmenopausal women. *J Natl Cancer Inst* 1995; **57**: 190–7.
14 International Agency for Research on Cancer. Monograph on evaluation of the carcinogenic risk of chemicals to

humans. II. Sex hormones. *IARC Monogr Eval Carcinog Risks Hum* 1979; **21**: 1–515.

15 Longman OM, Beuhring GC. Oral contraceptives and breast cancer. *Cancer* 1987; **59**: 281–7.

16 Klijn JGM, de Jong FH, Bakker GH, *et al.* Antiprogestins, a new form of endocrine therapy for human breast cancer. *Cancer Res* 1989; **49**: 2851–6.

17 Key TJA, Pike MC. The role of oestrogens and progestagens in the epidemiology and prevention of breast cancer. *Eur J Clin Oncol* 1988; **24**: 29–43.

18 Allegra JC, Kiefer SM. Mechanisms of action of progestational agents. *Semin Oncol* 1985; **12** (**Supplement 1**): 3–5.

19 Horwitz KB, Freidenberg GR. Growth inhibition and increase of insulin receptors in anti-oestrogen-resistant T47D human breast cancer cells by progestins: implications for endocrine therapies. *Cancer Res* 1985; **45**: 167–73.

20 Gompel A, Malet C, Spritzer P, Lalardrie J-P, Kuttenn F, Mauvais-Jarvis P. Progestin effect on cell proliferation and 17-hydroxysteroid dehydrogenase activity in normal human breast cells in culture. *J Clin Endocrinol Metab* 1986; **63**: 1174–80.

21 Mauvais-Jarvis P, Kuttenn F, Gompel A. Estradiolprogesterone interaction in normal and pathological cells. *Ann N Y Acad Sci* 1986; **464**: 152–67.

22 Kuttenn F, Fournier S, Durand JC, Mauvais-Jarvis P. Estradiol and progesterone receptors in human breast fibroadenomas. *J Clin Endocrinol Metab* 1981; **52**: 1225–9.

23 Fournier S, Kuttenn F, De Cicco F *et al.* Estradiol 17β-hydroxysteroid dehydrogenase activity in human breast fibroadenomas. *J Clin Endocrinol Metab* 1982; **55**: 428–33.

24 DeLena M, Brambilla C, Valagussa P, Bonadonna G. High-dose medroxyprogesterone acetate in breast cancer resistant to endocrine and cytotoxic treatment. *Cancer Chemother Pharmacol* 1979; **2**: 175–80.

25 Mouridsen HT, Paridaens R. Advanced breast cancer – new approaches to treatment: workshop report. *Eur J Cancer Clin Oncol* 1988; **24**: 95–8.

26 Mills PK, Beeson L, Phillips RL, Fraser GE. Prospective study of exogenous hormone use and breast cancer in seventh-day adventists. *Cancer* 1989; **64**: 591–7.

27 Adami H, Persson I, Hoover R, Schaire C, Bergkvist L. Risk of breast cancer in women receiving HRT. *Eur J Cancer* 1988; **44**: 833–9.

28 Hunt K, Vessey M, McPhearson K. Mortality in a cohort of long-term users of hormone replacement therapy: an updated analysis. *Br J Obstet Gynaecol* 1990; **976**: 1080–6.

29 Brinton LA, Hoover R, Fraumeni J. Menopausal oestrogens and breast cancer risk: an experimental case–control study. *Br J Cancer* 1986; **54**: 825–32.

30 Colditz GA, Stampfer MJ, Willett WC, Hennekens CH. Prospective study of oestrogen replacement therapy and risk of breast cancer in post-menopausal women. *J Am Med Assoc* 1990; **264**: 2648–53.

31 Rosner B, Speizer FE. Prospective study of oestrogen replacement treatment and the risk of breast cancer in post-menopausal women. *J Am Med Assoc* 1991; **264**: 2648–53.

32 Wingo PA, Layde PM, Lee NC, Rubin G, Ory HW. The risk of breast cancer in post-menopausal women who have used oestrogen replacement therapy. *J Am Med Assoc* 1987; **257**: 209–15.

33 La Vecchia, DeCarli A, Parazihni F, Gentile A, Liberati C, Franceschi S. Noncontraceptive oestrogens and the risk of breast cancer in women. *Int J Cancer* 1986; **38**: 853–8.

34 Ross RK, Paganini-Hill A, Gerkins VR *et al.* A case–control study of menopausal oestrogen treatment and breast cancer. *J Am Med Assoc* 1986; **243**: 1635–9.

35 Hulka BS, Chambless LE, Deubner DC, Wilkinson WE. Breast cancer and oestrogen replacement therapy. *Am J Obset Gynaecol* 1982; **143**: 638–44.

36 Colditz GA, Hankinson SE, Hunter DJ *et al.* The use of estrogens and progestins and the risk of breast cancer in post-menopausal women. *N Engl J Med* 1995; **332**: 1589–93.

37 La Vecchia C, Negri E, Franceschi S *et al.* Hormone replacement treatment and breast cancer risk: a co-operative Italian study. *Br J Cancer* 1995; **72**: 244–8.

38 Natchigall LE, Natchigall RH, Natchigall RD, Beckman EM. Estrogen replacement therapy. II. Prospective study of relationship to carcinoma and cardiovascular and metabolic problems. *Obstet Gynecol* 1979; **54**: 74–9.

39 Natchigall MJ, Smilen SW, Natchigall RD, Natchigall RH, Natchigall LE. Incidence of breast cancer in a 22-year study of women receiving estrogen-progestin replacement therapy. *Obstet Gynecol* 1992; **80**: 827–30.

40 Dupont WD, Page DL. Menopausal estrogen replacement therapy and breast cancer. *Arch Intern Med* 1991; **151**: 67–72.

41 The Writing Group for the PEPI Trial. Effects of estrogen or estrogen/progestin regimens on heart disease risk factors in postmenopausal women. *J Am Med Assoc* 1995; **274**: 199–208.

42 Stampfer MJ, Colditz GA, Willett WC *et al.* Postmenopausal estrogen therapy and cardiovascular disease: 10-year follow-up from the Nurses' Health Study. *N Engl J Med* 1991; **325**: 756–62.

43 Cauley JA, Seeley DG, Ensrud K, Ettinger B, Black D, Cummings SR. Estrogen replacement therapy and fractures in older women. *Ann Intern Med* 1995; **122**: 9–16.

44 Calle EE, Miracle-McMahill HL, Thun MJ, Heath CW Jr. Estrogen replacement therapy and risk of fatal colon cancer in a prospective cohort of post-menopausal women. *J Natl Cancer Inst* 1995; **87**: 517–23.

45 Henderson BE, Paganini-Hill A, Ross RK. Decreased mortality in users of estrogen replacement therapy. *Arch Intern Med* 1991; **151**: 75–82.

46 Ravinkar VA. Compliance with hormone therapy. *Am J Obstet Gynaecol* 1987; **156**: 1332–4.

47 Whitehead MI, Fraser D, Schenkel L, Crook D, Stevenson JC. Transdermal administration of oestrogen/progestagen hormone replacement therapy. *Lancet* 1990; **335**: 807–11.

48 Mashchak CA, Lobo RA, Donozo-Takano R *et al*. Comparison of pharmacokinetic properties of various oestrogen formulations. *Am J Obstet Gynaecol* 1982; **144**: 511.

49 Persson I, Adami HO, Bergkvist L *et al*. Risk of endometrial cancer after treatment with oestrogens alone or in conjunction with progestagens: results of a prospective study. *BMJ* 1989; **298**: 147–51.

50 Notelovitz M. Estrogen replacement therapy: indications, contraindications and agent selection. *Am J Obstet Gynecol* 1989; **161**: 1832–9.

51 Gray LA, Christopherson WM, Hoover RN. Estrogens and endometrial carcinoma. *Obstet Gynecol* 1977; **49**: 385–9.

52 Mack TM, Pike MC, Henderson BE *et al*. Estrogens and endometrial cancer in a retirement community. *N Engl J Med* 1976; **294**: 1262–7.

53 Parazzini F, La Vecchia C, Negri E *et al*. Case–control study of oestrogen replacement therapy and risk of cervical cancer. *BMJ* 1997; **315**: 85–7.

54 MacLennan AH, MacLennan A, O'Neill S *et al*. Oestrogen and cyclical progestogen in postmenopausal hormone replacement therapy. *Med J Aust* 1992; **157**: 167–70.

55 Falkeborn M, Persson I, Adami H-O *et al*. The risk of acute myocardial infarction after oestrogen and oestrogen-progestogen replacement. *Br J Obstet Gynaecol* 1992; **99**: 821–8.

56 Christiansen C, Riis BJ, Nilas L *et al*. Uncoupling of bone formation and resorption by combined oestrogen and progestagen therapy in postmenopausal osteoporosis. *Lancet* 1985; **2**: 800–1.

57 Padwick ML, Pryse-Davies J, Whitehead MI. A simple method for determining the optimal dosage of progestin in post-menopausal women receiving oestrogens. *N Engl J Med* 1986; **315**: 930–2.

58 Siller-Arenas M, Delgado-Rodriguez M, Rodigues-Canteras R, Bueno-Cavanillas A, Galvez-Vargas R. Menopausal hormone replacement therapy and breast cancer: a meta-analysis. *Obstet Gynecol* 1992; **72**: 286–94.

59 Collaborative Group on Hormonal Factors in Breast Cancer. Breast cancer and HRT: collaborative re-analysis from 51 epidemiological studies of 52 705 women with breast cancer and 108 411 women without breast cancer. *Lancet* 1997; **350**: 1047–59.

60 O'Connor IF, Shembekar MV, Shousha S. Breast carcinoma developing in patients on hormone replacement therapy: a histological and immunohistological study. *J Clin Pathol* 1998; **51**: 935–8.

61 Gapstur SM, Morrow M, Sellars TA. Hormone replacement therapy and risk of breast cancer with a favourable histology: results of the Iowa Women's Health Study. *J Am Med Assoc* 1999; **281**: 2091–7.

62 Stoll BA. Hormone replacement therapy in women treated for breast cancer. *Eur J Clin Oncol* 1989; **55**: 1909–13.

63 Wile AG, Opfell DA, Margileth DA, Hoda AC. Hormone replacement therapy does not affect breast cancer outcome. *Proc Am Soc Clin Oncol* 1991; **10**: 58.

64 Eden JA, Bush T, Nand S, Wren BG. The Royal Hospital for Women Breast Cancer Study: a case-controlled study of combined continuous hormone replacement therapy amongst women with a personal history of breast cancer. *Med J Austr* 1995.

65 De Saia PJ, Odicino F, Grosen EA *et al*. HRT in breast cancer. *Lancet* 1993; **342**: 1232.

66 Adami HO, Malker B, Holmberg L *et al*. The relation between survival and age at diagnosis in breast cancer. *N Engl J Med* 1986; **315**: 337–42.

67 Bergkvist L, Adami HO, Perssom I, Bergstrom R, Krusemo UB. Prognosis after breast cancer diagnosis in women exposed to estrogen and estrogen-progestogen replacement therapy. *Am J Epidemiol* 1992; **130**: 221–8.

68 Harding C, Knox WF, Faragher EB, Baildam A, Bundred NJ. Hormone replacement therapy and tumour grade in breast cancer: prospective study in screening unit. *BMJ* 1996; **312**: 1646–7.

69 Bilimoria MM, Winchester DJ, Sener SF, Motykie G, Sehgal UL, Winchester DP. Estrogen replacement therapy and breast cancer: analysis of age of onset and tumor characteristics. *Ann Surg Oncol* 1999; **6**: 200–7.

70 Saunders CM, Baum M. Breast cancer and pregnancy: a review. *J R Soc Med* 1993; **86**: 162–5.

71 Wingo PA, Lee NC, Ory HW *et al*. Age-specific differences in the relationship between oral contraceptive use and breast cancer. *Cancer* 1993; **71**: 1506–17.

72 Moadel AB, Ostroff JS, Lesko LM, Bajorunas DR. Psychosexual adjustment among women receiving hormone replacement therapy for premature menopause following cancer treatment. *Psychooncology* 1995; **4**: 273–82.

73 Cobleigh MA, Berris RF, Bush T *et al*. Estrogen replacement therapy in breast cancer survivors. *J Am Med Assoc* 1994; **272**: 540–5.

74 Saunders CM. *Hormone replacement therapy and breast cancer*. London: Royal Marsden Hospital, 1993.

75 Eden JA. Oestrogen and the breast. 2. Management of the menopausal woman with breast cancer. *Med J Aust* 1992; **157**: 247–50.

76 McNeil C. ERT for breast cancer survivors: a hot debate runs on little data. *J Natl Cancer Inst* 1996; **87**: 1047–50.

77 Bhutta A, MacLennan K, Flanders K *et al*. Induction of transforming growth factor B1 in human breast cancer *in vivo* following tamoxifen treatment. *Cancer Res* 1992; **52**: 4261–4.

78 Early Breast Cancer Trialists' Collaborative Group. Systemic treatment of early breast cancer by hormonal, cytotoxic or immune therapy. *Lancet* 1992; **339**: 1–15, 71–85.

79 Sawka CA, Pritchard KI, Paterson AHG *et al*. Role and mechanism of action of tamoxifen in premenopausal women with metastatic breast cancer. *Cancer Res* 1986; **46**: 3152–6.

80 Baynes KC, Compston JE. Selective oestrogen receptor modulators: a new paradigm for HRT. *Curr Opin Obstet Gynecol* 1998; **10**: 189–92.

81 Stoll BA. Hormone replacement therapy for women with a past history of breast cancer. *Clin Oncol* 1990; **2**: 309–12.

82 Anonymous. Treatment of estrogen deficiency symptoms in women surviving breast cancer. Part 2. Hormone replacement therapy and breast cancer. *Oncology* 1999; **13**: 245–257.

83 Laya MB, Larson EB, Taplin SH, White E. Effect of estrogen replacement therapy on the specificity and sensitivity of screening mammography. *J Natl Cancer Inst* 1996; **88**: 643–9.

84 Harvey JA. Use and cost of breast imaging for postmenopausal women undergoing hormone replacement therapy. *Am J Roentgenol* 1999; **172**: 1615–19.

85 Vassilopoulou-Sellin R, Klein MJ. Estrogen replacement therapy after treatment for localized breast cancer. *Cancer* 1996; **78**: 1043–8.

28

Breast cancer and pregnancy

CHRISTOBEL MARY SAUNDERS

INTRODUCTION

'Gestational' breast cancer encompasses this disease diagnosed during pregnancy or lactation, including up to 1 year postpartum. Of those women diagnosed as having breast cancer, this will be associated with pregnancy in about 3% of cases,[1-3] making it the second most common gestational cancer after cervical cancer. The prevalence of this may increase as many women delay their pregnancies until a later age.[4] The current average age for development of gestational breast carcinoma is 32–38 years.[5]

In some developing countries and other areas such as the Middle East, breast cancer, although rare, is a predominantly premenopausal disease, and so may be seen relatively more frequently in association with pregnancy.[6]

The juxtaposition of these two life-changing events can produce huge problems for the patient, her family and her carers, in terms of both medical treatment (of the mother and fetus) and psychological morbidity. Medical knowledge in this area often seems to be based more on rumour than on fact,[7] the individual physician's experience will usually be limited to very few cases, and so the advice given may be insufficient and inaccurate.

Pregnancy subsequent to breast cancer occurs in about 7% of women who remain fertile after treatment for this disease, yet it is not well understood, and the situation is often poorly managed. It is not known whether the improving mortality rates in young women seen in many countries[8] will increase the number that go on to subsequent pregnancy.

PATHOLOGY AND BIOLOGY OF GESTATIONAL BREAST CANCER

Although breast cancer diagnosed during pregnancy or in the immediate postpartum period is designated a 'gestational' carcinoma, in terms of tumour development it is likely that it in fact arose long before the pregnancy. Conversely, it may be assumed that a proportion of pregnant women will have undiagnosed carcinoma which does not manifest itself until some years later. Indeed, a diagnosis of breast cancer less than 2 years after having given birth is associated with a particularly poor prognosis, irrespective of the tumour stage.[9,10]

Thus it is not surprising that the pathology of these tumours is identical to that of tumours which occur in non-pregnant premenopausal women. This includes a reported incidence of inflammatory breast cancer in most studies of 1.5–4%,[11] and a relatively high proportion of oestrogen-receptor-negative and progesterone-receptor-negative tumours.[12] Some recent studies have shown a preponderance of inflammatory tumours[13] and oestrogen-receptor negativity.[6]

It should be noted that the ligand-binding oestrogen-receptor assay, which depends upon the availability of unbound receptor, can be deceptive in the presence of high circulating levels of oestradiol, as these can saturate all of the available oestrogen-receptor sites, leading to false-negative results. Unbound oestrogen must therefore be removed with dextran-charcoal or immunohistochemical assays employed. False-negative oestrogen-receptor data may also occur in the presence of raised oestrogen and progesterone levels, due to down-regulation of the oestrogen receptor.

However, in 1963 Bunker and Peters showed no objective response to oophorectomy, suggesting that these tumours are in fact functionally oestrogen-receptor-negative.[2]

In terms of tumour biology, there are a host of factors which suggest that gestational tumours should behave aggressively, and that their growth will be accelerated. These include the enormous variations in serum hormone levels in pregnant women, particularly increases in serum oestrogen, progestagen and placental hormones which are known to stimulate normal breast epithelial turnover and may stimulate tumour growth.[14] Prolactin, the levels of which are enormously elevated in pregnancy and lactation, is experimentally a promoter of tumour growth.[15] Conversely, some pregnancy-induced hormones may inhibit mammary carcinogenesis and tumour growth, such as human chorionic gonadotrophin[16] and relaxin.[17]

There is also an altered immune response during pregnancy, with a decrease in cell-mediated immunity, which could promote tumour spread.[18] Tumours arising in other immunosuppressed patients demonstrate more differentiated characteristics – for example, loss of HLA Class I or II antigens – and it has been suggested that this may render the tumour more resistant to chemotherapy.[19] However, little clinical evidence has been found for any effect of these factors.

In terms of the metastatic distribution of gestational breast tumours, this appears to be the same as for the majority of mammary carcinomas. Although there are a number of cases in the literature of metastasis to the placenta, there have been no reports of metastatic breast cancer in the fetus.[20] This has been reported in melanoma and choriocarcinoma.

ASSOCIATION OF BREAST CANCER AND PREGNANCY

Between 1 and 3 in every 10 000 pregnancies will be complicated by breast cancer,[21] and traditional teaching stated that the concurrence of these events heralded a grave prognosis. In 1880, Samuel Gross described 'it's growth [as] wonderfully rapid and its course excessively malignant'. Haagenson declared that no patient with breast cancer diagnosed during pregnancy should undergo surgery, as they were incurable.[22] He did, however, revise this statement when some patients survived 5 years after his diagnosis.[23] This obsolete dogma seems to have lodged itself in the medical psyche despite the lack of supporting evidence.

In fact, a recent survey of general practitioners, obstetricians and surgeons in the UK[7] found considerable confusion, with differing opinions on both the incidence and the prognosis of gestational breast cancer and its treatment. In this study, none of the general practitioners who were canvassed had experience of treating this condition, although all hospital practitioners had managed these patients. All GPs and surgeons thought that pregnancy conferred a worse prognosis, and none of them believed that diagnostic delay contributed to the poor outcome. Most surgeons also believed that subsequent pregnancy promotes recurrence. Obstetricians' perceptions were varied, whilst most GPs professed (very honestly!) ignorance on much of the subject, and certainly there was no consensus in any group (Figure 28.1).

If scrutinized, few of these beliefs stand up to the present evidence. The incidence of breast cancer occurring during pregnancy is of the same frequency as in

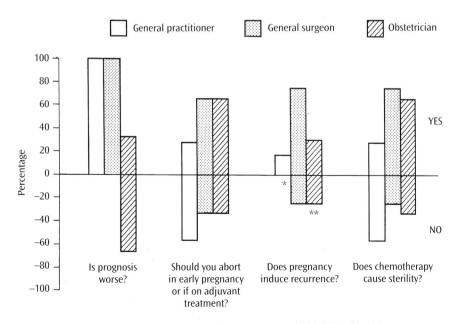

*83% of GPs did not know
**45% of obstetricians did not know

Figure 28.1 *Clinicians' current opinions on breast cancer and pregnancy. Reproduced from a survey by Saunders and Baum.[7]*

non-pregnant premenopausal women.[7] However, the prognosis for these patients is considerably worse,[3,11] with both an excess of node-positive tumours and more locally advanced and metastatic disease at presentation. In one analysis by Ribeiro *et al.*,[24] 72% of patients diagnosed during pregnancy had involved lymph nodes, and only 37% survived 5 years. Petrek showed that 50% of tumours in non-pregnant women were less than 2 cm in diameter, whilst only 30% in pregnant women were this small.[25] Nugent suggested that the poor prognosis may be due to the relative young age of these patients,[12] and certainly patients under the age of 33 years have a particularly poor outcome.[26] This poor outlook does *not* seem to be a result of inherently poor prognostic features of the tumour, nor of any deficient host response. Indeed it would seem counter-intuitive that these tumours present in an 'aggressive' state and then attain the same 'treatability' as tumours in non-pregnant women. Peters[27] has clearly shown that age- and stage-matched pregnant and non-pregnant patients have similar overall and recurrence-free survival (see Figure 28.2), and Petrek[25] has also confirmed a similar 5-year survival for pregnant and non-pregnant women, as does a study from the Memorial Sloane Kettering Hospital in New York, which showed an equal survival in early-stage breast cancer in women under the age of 30 years.[28] A recent paper by Guinee *et al.*[29] has challenged this view. This multinational group found the relative risk of death from breast cancer diagnosed during pregnancy to be 2.83 (1.24–6.45) when adjusted for tumour size, lymph-node status and treatment. However, this was based on only 15 women diagnosed

during pregnancy who went on to delivery, and 11 women undergoing termination of the pregnancy, which may have contributed to the poorer prognosis. A French case–control study[13] which included 154 women with pregnancy-associated breast cancer has also demonstrated a worse outcome when adjusted for stage and grade of tumour. The prognosis was also poorer for those who had been pregnant in the 36 months prior to diagnosis.

Thus it must be concluded that pregnant women present later than their non-pregnant counterparts,[30] but that most studies appear to demonstrate an equal age- and stage-matched survival.

Table 28.1 shows the survival data for many published studies to date. Survival is not related to the stage of pregnancy at presentation,[24] although it does appear to be worse if the diagnosis is made later in pregnancy,[1,27] as the disease is often more advanced.

DIAGNOSIS AND INVESTIGATION OF GESTATIONAL BREAST CANCER

Diagnosis

It seems clear that there is a delay in the diagnosis and treatment of pregnant patients of anything up to 1 year.[30] Byrd *et al.* quote a 6-month delay (75% due to doctors).[31] In a small series of 19 patients, diagnosis was delayed by between 2 and 16 months in 11 of the patients.[32] In a study by Ribeiro *et al.*,[24] there was a mean duration of symptoms of 10 months, and Bunker and Peters found that only 7% of pregnant women were treated within 1 month of detection of their breast lump.[2] The reasons for this are less clear, as most pregnant women will undergo a breast examination at least once. Even so, 90% of women will detect the breast lump themselves.[33] It is possible that the normal physiological changes during pregnancy may mask a mass, but it is also likely that any lump which is detected will be attributed to lactational change and not promptly investigated. It would thus seem important to examine the patient's breasts at the start of her pregnancy, and any abnormality that is found should be treated according to the same objective criteria as in any other patient, noting that the differential diagnosis may include galactocoele, inflammatory conditions, localized infarcts and fibroadenomas, which can enlarge rapidly during pregnancy (see Table 28.2). In up to 30% of cases of gestational carcinoma there is coincident pathology such as lactational mastitis,[31] and any abscess cavity should be biopsied.

Investigation

Investigation of breast symptoms should follow a similar pattern to that for any patient – that is a clinical history and examination followed by radiological screening

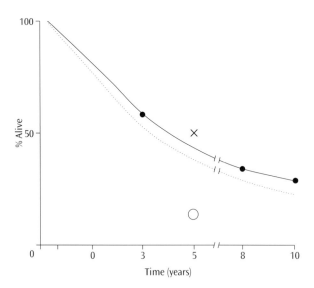

Figure 28.2 *Survival curves of 221 patients with gestational breast cancer and 221 non-pregnant age- and stage-matched women. X, those with mammary cancer in first half of pregnancy who survived 5 years after treatment. ○, those with mammary cancer in second half of pregnancy who survived 5 years after treatment. Reproduced from Anderson JM. Mammary cancers and pregnancy. BMJ 1979; **1**: 1124–7.*

Table 28.1 *Retrospective analyses of survival data for operable gestational breast cancer**

Reference	Year	n	Node-positive (%)	5-year survival N−	5-year survival N+	10-year survival N−	10-year survival N+
73	1937	92	85	62	6	40	3
1	1955	27	59	73	6	26	0
31	1962	28	60	100	29		
27	1968	60	65	62	23	45	12
30	1973	48	81	56	18	22	13
11	1978	121				22	
12	1985	19	74	100	50		
43	1985	24	71	86	31		
24	1986	121	72	79	37		
74	1988	35		15			
75	1989	65	59	71	27	48	0
25	1991	56	61	82	47		
76	1992	192		65		55	
29	1994	26	55	40			
28	1996	22		73			
6	1996	28	90	57			
13	1997	154		44			

N−, node-negative; N+, node-positive.

* A number of problems inherent in these analyses include differences in staging systems (some may include non-operable patients), treatment differences (particularly in studies spanning long periods of time), and inclusion of a wide variety of patients, including pregnant and lactating women and those up to 1 year postpartum.

(mammography or ultrasound) and tissue sampling (fine-needle aspiration cytology, core-cut biopsy or excision biopsy).

Mammography may be contraindicated because of a very small potential risk to the fetus, and because of poor definition in dense breasts. Max and Klamer found that in only 25% of pregnant patients could the carcinoma be detected mammographically, and even in non-pregnant women under 35 years of age with breast cancer, in only 50% of cases could the lesion be seen on mammogram.[34] Ultrasound is useful for distinguishing cystic from solid lesions, but even with the advent of colour Doppler images it is not diagnostic for cancer.

This makes the tissue sampling of breast lumps in young women even more vital. Fine-needle aspiration cytology is useful, but the cytopathologist must be aware that the patient is pregnant or lactating, as diagnostic difficulty may be encountered.[35,36] Breast epithelial cells from patients during the gestational period demonstrate features similar to those found in malignancy, such as nuclear pleomorphism, nucleolar hypertrophy and a

Table 28.2 *Differential diagnosis of breast lumps in pregnancy*

Galactocoele

Abscess

Fibroadenoma (rapidly enlarging)

Infarct

Carcinoma

decrease in cell aggregation. These may exist without the typical lactational changes, and thus lead to considerable confusion. The use of flow cytometry may help to clarify this picture.

If excisional or incisional biopsy is indicated, it must be noted that haematoma and infection rates are liable to be high, and it may be advisable to suppress lactation and give prophylactic antibiotics. These complications are especially likely if the biopsy is from a more central area of the breast.

Staging investigations in early breast cancer have been largely abandoned,[37] but if they are indicated, most may be performed safely. If X-rays are required, it is advisable to restrict the total radiation dose to less than 10 cGy (a chest X-ray results in exposure of about 0.008 cGy and a pelvic X-ray about 0.04 cGy). Liver ultrasound is considered safe, and even a bone scan may be performed as long as the patient is well hydrated and catheterized to ensure prompt excretion of the Tc-99 methylene diphosphonate radioactive isotope. However, since in most cases the results of this investigation will not alter the management of the patient, it may be wise to delay the procedure until after delivery, if it is done at all.

When analysing the results of serum liver function tests, it must be remembered that alkaline phosphatase levels may be elevated by pregnancy.

Magnetic resonance imaging (MRI) appears to be both safe and accurate, can be used both for imaging the breast and for diagnosis of bone, liver, lung and brain metastases, and may thus be a useful alternative to CT scanning.

TREATMENT

Treatment during pregnancy

Treatment of gestational breast cancer, although essentially the same as for all premenopausal patients with breast cancer, involves not only the patient but also the fetus, and indeed the whole family, and thus entails a balance of care.

In addition to medical decisions, there may be ethical and legal implications of treatment of the mother if that treatment adversely affects fetal outcome.[38] The obligation of the pregnant woman to maintain the best possible *in-utero* environment for her unborn child is considerably less clear if this impinges on her own prognosis. This remains a controversial subject, and is best tackled by open discussion of the risks and benefits of treatment both to the mother and to the fetus.

The patient should start treatment immediately after diagnosis unless she is only a few weeks from full term, in which case a planned delivery may be carried out first. Termination of pregnancy is not routinely indicated and confers no survival advantage – the disease is usually hormone insensitive – unless the carcinoma is rapidly progressive, if chemotherapy is indicated in the first trimester, or if conception occurs during radiotherapy.[12,24,25,39] Thus 'therapeutic' abortion is a misnomer.[38] In the words of Byrd *et al.*[31] 'in the face of general enthusiasm for terminating the pregnancy, we believe the evidence is that the cancer should be terminated.' Ultimately, it must be the decision of the patient and her partner, taking into consideration both treatment factors and the possibility of a shortened life expectancy.

Some authors suggest that the rate of spontaneous abortions in these patients is increased,[24] although it is not clear whether this is solely treatment related, or whether it is also a factor in the mother's illness.

Surgery

Surgery is usually the first-line treatment, and the preferred surgical option is mastectomy and axillary clearance, with the option of breast reconstruction after the pregnancy. Anaesthesia is generally safe during pregnancy as long as consideration is given to the increase in blood volume and coagulability, positional hypotension, decreased lung function and delayed gastric emptying, and fetal monitoring during anaesthesia may be advisable.[40]

Mastectomy is the commonest surgical option, as this aims to avoid the need for radiotherapy. Conservative surgery and radiotherapy offer a similar outcome in terms of maternal survival in non-pregnant patients, but this may not be the case in pregnant women, where the anatomy of the breast, which consists of large inter-anastomosing ducts, may predispose to local recurrence after conservative surgery.[4]

Breast reconstruction, if considered, should be performed at a later date when the patient is no longer pregnant or lactating.

Radiotherapy

Radiotherapy to the breast during pregnancy is not recommended because of the risks of the fetus. The main human data on the effects of radiation in pregnancy are from the Hiroshima and Nagasaki atomic bombs, where it was found that an air dose of 1–9 cGy during weeks 6 to 11 of gestation caused an 11% microcephaly rate (as opposed to 4% in non-irradiated fetuses), whereas an air dose of over 100 cGy caused 100% abnormalities.[41]

The scatter dose to the fetus can be accurately calculated, and the risk is both dose and trimester dependent and related to the energy of the radiation, the field size and the position of the center of the field.[41] Thus whilst a first-trimester fetus is still in the true pelvis and will receive, with shielding, only 0.2–0.3% of the total tumour radiation dose, a fetus near gestation may receive 4% of the dose (Figure 28.3). However, most serious fetal damage occurs during organogenesis in the first trimester, especially with regard to the brain, skeleton and eyes. In the third trimester, fetal defects are less likely, although there is a theoretical risk of childhood cancer.[42] Donegan reports a risk of leukaemia at 10 years after a 2-cGy exposure of 1 in 2000 vs. 1 in 3000 in unexposed subjects.[43] At the pre-implantation stage there is likely to be an 'all-or-nothing' effect. This is illustrated in Figure 28.4.

The internal scatter dose to the fetus via the mother's tissues can be estimated by thermoluminescent dosimeters placed in an anatomical phantom shielding.[4]

In one published study of women receiving radiotherapy during pregnancy,[44] 19 patients were irradiated during pregnancy and had normal births, although at least twice the rate of spontaneous abortion was observed as in a non-irradiated group.

It must be concluded that radiotherapy is best avoided in the adjuvant setting both following conservative surgery and as treatment to the chest wall in women with disease who are deemed to be at high risk for local recurrence. In both of these settings it is wise to delay radiotherapy until after delivery.

Chemotherapy

Chemotherapy use during pregnancy poses a theoretical risk to the fetus of both organ malformation and carcinogenesis,[45] although the limited data that exist, mainly from treatment of young women with Hodgkin's disease,[46] do not clearly support this. Certainly Sutton *et al.*[47] did not find any fetal abnormalities in 19 babies delivered following maternal chemotherapy for breast cancer. Doll *et al.* found an incidence of 19% for fetal malformations

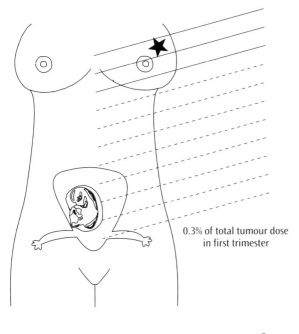

0.3% of total tumour dose
in first trimester

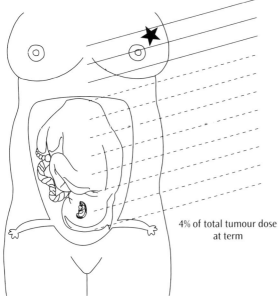

4% of total tumour dose
at term

Figure 28.3 *Radiation dose received by the fetus at various stages of gestation.*

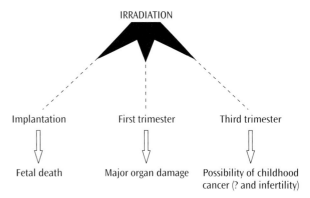

Figure 28.4 *Biological effects of radiation on the developing fetus.*

myelosuppression appear to be a problem in these infants.[38]

Some chemotherapeutic agents (e.g. the antimetabolite methotrexate) are inevitably teratogenic and should be avoided. Synergy between cytotoxic agents and radiotherapy may exist, and an increase in low-birth-weight babies following these treatments has been reported.[53]

Both adjuvant and up-front or 'neoadjuvant' chemotherapy can be used beyond the first trimester with reasonable safety. Despite this reassurance, many patients and indeed their physicians may feel reluctant to use these drugs during pregnancy, and so may wish to delay adjuvant treatment until after delivery. This would seem very reasonable if the delay will only be a matter of a few weeks. However, the length of permissable delay is in fact unknown, and delays of more than a few weeks could prove detrimental to the mother's outcome.

The long-term effects of sterility and neoplasm in the offspring are undocumented. Also awaiting clarification are the other long-term effects of these drugs on the child. For example, it is known that doxirubicin given to children with leukaemia may induce heart failure at a later date, and that the younger the child the higher the risk, but whether this occurs following maternal therapy is not known.

Hormone therapy

The use of hormonal agents in pregnancy is largely undocumented. Zeneca, the manufacturers of tamoxifen, have reported 50 pregnancies on tamoxifen, with 10 fetal abnormalities including two craniofacial defects. This potential for teratogenicity is supported by one case report in the literature of Goldenhar's syndrome (oculo-auriculo-vertebral dysplasia) occurring in an infant born to a woman taking tamoxifen.[54] Stilboestrol used in pregnant women can induce vaginal and testicular carcinomas in offspring, and it is feared that tamoxifen may exhibit this carcinogenic potential, although no abnormalities were reported in 85 women who became pregnant whilst on tamoxifen in the chemoprevention trial.[55]

if chemotherapy was given to the mother in the first trimester of pregnancy, falling to 2% if given after this.[48] Theriault *et al.* reported no fetal abnormalities in 12 pregnant women who were given FAC for breast carcinoma.[38] Berry *et al.* reported a series of 24 pregnant patients in their second or third trimester with primary or recurrent breast cancer who were safely given chemotherapy as part of their treatment.[49]

It is presumed that the placenta acts as a barrier to these drugs, although adriamycin can cross this barrier yet still does not appear to cause fetal abnormalities beyond the first trimester.[50–52] To date, no studies have been undertaken to measure the levels of these drugs in the amniotic fluid or cord blood, but neither hair loss nor

Jordan urges caution in the use of tamoxifen in women of child-bearing age.[56]

Treatment during lactation

Treatment should follow the same principles as in the non-pregnant patient.

Suppression of lactation prior to surgery is advisable to decrease breast size and vascularity. This can be achieved with 2.5 mg of bromocriptine for 2 weeks.

Cytotoxic agents are likely to be secreted in breast milk,[38] and thus again suppression of lactation is required before chemotherapy.

Many women find the postpartum months a physical and emotional strain even in normal circumstances. The additional burden of a life-threatening diagnosis and accompanying treatment means that the patient and her family are likely to need both psychological support and possibly social service input in terms of childcare. The patient's partner may also require support and time off work.

Treatment of advanced disease

Palliative treatment of the patient with advanced disease, with improvement in symptom control and quality of life, must be carefully balanced with management of the fate of the fetus.

In early pregnancy, termination of the pregnancy is usually recommended. Presentation with advanced disease in later pregnancy may present a challenge, often necessitating early planned delivery of the fetus by Caesarean section at 37 weeks. The nurse counsellor can play a pivotal role in co-ordination of treatment by the oncologist, surgeon, obstetrician and others involved.

PREGNANCY AFTER BREAST CANCER

The decision to have a child following a diagnosis of breast cancer must encompass the social, psychological and economic implications of a potentially limited lifespan.[57] The fact that only a very small proportion of women do so is probably a result of both the above considerations and the effect of treatment on fertility. There will also almost certainly be under-reporting of subsequent pregnancies if these are uneventful.[11] Siegal interviewed 50 women who had had breast cancer with regard to their reasons for not undertaking a further pregnancy.[58] The reasons given included fear of recurrence, fear of radiotherapy-induced birth defects, the belief that the child might be at increased risk of cancer, and the stress of childcare. The impact of the knowledge that they may have an inheritable defect from women with a genetic mutation such as BRCA1 is unknown.

Fertility

Tamoxifen frequently causes irregular periods in young women and increases serum oestradiol levels, but probably does not affect long-term fertility, nor does radiotherapy to the breast appear to affect fertility.

Chemotherapy is more likely to induce amenorrhoea and decrease fertility, although it does not increase spontaneous abortions or affect fetal health in subsequent pregnancies. Richards et al. found that whilst only 37% of women under the age of 40 years receiving CMF chemotherapy for breast cancer became amenorrhoeic, 97% of premenopausal women over the age of 40 years became so.[59] In a series of 21 women who had breast cancer diagnosed before the age of 35 years, 17 had received adjuvant chemotherapy, mainly six cycles of CMF. All of them subsequently achieved pregnancy.[60] It has been reported by Sutton et al.[47] that whilst 41% of women under 35 years of age receiving FAC chemotherapy developed amenorrhoea, one-third of these had cycles which returned after stopping the treatment. This study also found that 25 pregnancies occurred in 18 patients who had received this regimen (six of whom had had temporary amenorrhoea) a mean of 18 months after completing chemotherapy, and that there were no deleterious effects on the outcome for the patients.

In women who had become prematurely infertile as a result of treatment, it may be possible to conceive using pre-embryo donation techniques in which oestradiol and progesterone are given to the patient to stimulate her endometrium. Ova from another woman are then fertilized in vitro using the partner's sperm and implanted into the patient's receptive uterus.[61] Research is currently in progress which should ultimately allow cryopreservation of all or part of an ovary in women who are about to undergo treatment which will render them infertile. It is hoped that these ovaries may be reimplanted at a later date to allow ovarian function to be re-established (Schaterjee, personal communication). If in-vitro fertilization (IVF) is considered in women who have had breast cancer, it must be noted that there is a theoretical risk of increasing the rate of progression due to use of agents such as clomiphene and gonadotrophins. Arbour et al. found in an IVF clinic that 16 women developed breast cancer out of 950 women using these treatments. All of them were under the age of 48 years.[62]

For those women who remain infertile after breast cancer treatment, adoption may be an option, although historically adoption agencies may preclude individuals with a prior diagnosis of cancer.[63]

Prognosis

There is good evidence that breast cancer survivors who go on to become pregnant have a better outlook,[11,64] not just because they are in the self-selected cohort who live long enough to become pregnant, although there may be a 'healthy mother effect' in that those who are not well are unlikely to want to become pregnant.[65] Clark and Reid[11] found that over half of those who became pregnant following a diagnosis of breast cancer were alive at 15 years, compared to only 35% of 'control' 20- to 40-year-olds. Clark and Reid also found that the longer the interval between diagnosis and conception, the better the outlook, although those women who did best were those who had more than one child.

Other researchers have confirmed that there certainly seems to be no survival disadvantage in becoming pregnant for breast cancer survivors. Mignot *et al.* collected data on 68 women with a mean age of 32 years who conceived on average 21 months after diagnosis of breast carcinoma (1–87 months), and at 72 months of follow-up had seen 19% relapse, with an estimated 10-year survival of 71%.[66] This was not statistically significantly different from a 75% 10-year survival of age- and stage-matched controls. Ariel and Kempner[67] reported 47 patients who became pregnant subsequent to breast cancer, and found no increase in mortality. Recently, Kroman *et al.* identified 173 women from the Danish Cancer Registry who had become pregnant after a diagnosis of breast cancer, and found no evidence of a worse outcome.[68] A population-based case–control study of 53 women who became pregnant after a diagnosis of breast cancer showed no significant adverse effect on survival (relative risk = 0.80, 95% confidence intervals 0.3–2.3),[69] These studies do, however, highlight the fact that those who terminate a subsequent pregnancy demonstrate no survival advantage, and it has been suggested that they may fare worse. Nevertheless, several biases may be present, rendering the results less reliable and conclusive.[70]

Most authorities recommend a 2- to 3-year wait after the conclusion of treatment so that those with a poor prognosis, in whom disease is progressive or recurrent, can be identified. Contraception during this time should ideally be mechanical, as there may be some (albeit ill-defined) risk associated with using the combined oral contraceptive pill after breast cancer.

BREAST-FEEDING

Breast-feeding should be suppressed if a patient is receiving chemotherapy, because of the potential for milk contamination. However, breast-feeding in subsequent pregnancies is not contraindicated. Milk production in a breast which has undergone conservative surgery is theoretically possible, although poorly documented.[71,72] It is probably easier if the surgery has been to the periphery of the breast rather than centrally.

Radiotherapy does induce considerable changes in the normal breast epithelium which decrease the ability to lactate. In a study by Higgins and Haffty,[72] only one of 11 patients successfully breast-fed from the irradiated breast.

CONCLUSION

Breast cancer occurs with a similar frequency during pregnancy as it does in non-pregnant premenopausal women. It has a similar biology, and the survival rates in the two groups are comparable.

Treatment should therefore also be similar, and should not be delayed because of the pregnancy. Termination of the pregnancy is rarely indicated unless there is a risk to the fetus from chemotherapy or radiotherapy in the first trimester, or unless the patient has aggressive advanced disease.

The treatments for breast cancer can affect fertility, notably chemotherapy used in women over the age of 40 years. However, if a woman does become pregnant subsequent to a diagnosis of breast cancer her prognosis will not suffer and she may even paradoxically demonstrate an improved survival.

REFERENCES

1 White TT. Carcinoma of the breast in the pregnant and nursing patient. *Am J Obstet Gynecol* 1955; **69**: 1277–86.
2 Bunker ML, Peters MV. Breast cancer associated with pregnancy or lactation. *Am J Obstet Gynecol* 1963; **85**: 312–21.
3 Lethaby AE, O'Neill MA, Mason BH, Holdaway IM, Harvey VJ. Overall survival from breast cancer in women pregnant or lactating at or after diagnosis. Auckland Breast Cancer Study Group. *Int J Cancer* 1996; **67**: 751–5.
4 Petrek JA. Breast cancer during pregnancy. *Cancer* 1994; **74**: 518–27.
5 Gallenberg MM, Loprinzi CL. Breast cancer and pregnancy. *Semin Oncol* 1989; **16**: 369–76.
6 Ezzat A, Raja A, Berry J *et al.* Impact of pregnancy on non-metastatic breast cancer: a case–control study. *Clin Oncol* 1996; **8**: 367–70.
7 Saunders CM, Baum M. Breast cancer and pregnancy: a review. *J R Soc Med* 1993; **86**: 162–5.
8 Hermon C, Beral V. Breast cancer mortality rates are levelling off or beginning to decline in many western countries: analysis of time trends, age-cohort and age-period models of breast cancer mortality in 20 countries. *Br J Cancer* 1996; **73**: 955–60.
9 Kroman N, Wohlfahrt J, Andersen KW, Mouridsen HT, Westergaard T, Melbye M. Time since childbirth and prognosis in primary breast cancer: population-based study. *BMJ* 1997; **315**: 851–5.
10 Olson SH, Zauber AG, Tang J, Harlap S. Relation of time since last birth and parity to survival of young women with breast cancer. *Epidemiology* 1998; **9**: 669–71.
11 Clark RM, Reid J. Carcinoma of the breast in pregnancy and lactation. *Int J Radiat Oncol Biol Phys* 1978; **4**: 693–8.
12 Nugent P, O'Connell TX. Breast cancer and pregnancy. *Arch Surg* 1985; **120**: 1221–4.

13 Bonnier P, Romain S, Dilhuydy JM *et al.* Influence of pregnancy on the outcome of breast cancer: a case–control study. *Int J Cancer* 1997; **72**: 720–7.

14 McManus MJ, Welsch CW. The effect of oestrogen, progesterone, thyroxine and human placental lactogen on DNA synthesis of human breast ductal epithelium maintained in athymic nude mice. *Cancer* 1984; **54**: 1920–7.

15 Nagasawe H. Prolactin and estrogen in mammary tumorigenesis. *Cancer Growth Prog* 1989; **6**: 80–6.

16 Meduri G, Charnaux N, Loosfelt H *et al.* Luteinizing hormone/human chorionic gonadotrophin receptors in breast cancer. *Cancer Res* 1997; **57**: 857–64.

17 Bani D, Masini E, Bello MG, Bigazzi M, Sacchi TB. Relaxin activates the L-arginine-nitric oxide pathway in human breast cancer cells. *Cancer Res* 1995; **55**: 5272–5.

18 Purtillo DT, Hallgren HM, Yunis EJ. Depressed maternal lymphocyte response to phytohaemagglutinin in human pregnancy. *Lancet* 1972; **i**: 769.

19 Oliver RTD. Pregnancy and breast cancer. *Lancet* 1994; **344**: 471–2.

20 Potter JF, Schoeneman M. Metastasis of maternal cancer to the placenta and fetus. *Cancer* 1970; **25**: 380–8.

21 Wallack MK, Wolf JA, Bedwinck J *et al.* Gestational cancer of the female breast. *Curr Probl Cancer* 1983; **7**: 1–88.

22 Haagenson CD, Stout AP. Carcinoma of the breast: criteria for operability. *Ann Surg* 1943; **118**: 859–70.

23 Haagenson CD. The treatment and results of cancer of the breast at the Presbyterian Hospital, New York. *Am J Roentgenol* 1949; **62**: 328–34.

24 Ribeiro G, Jones DA, Jones M. Carcinoma of the breast associated with pregnancy. *Br J Surg* 1986; **73**: 607–9.

25 Petrek JA, Dukoff R, Rogatko A. Prognosis of pregnancy-associated breast cancer. *Cancer* 1991; **67**: 869–72.

26 De la Rochefordiere A, Asselain B, Campana F *et al.* Age as a prognostic factor in premenopausal breast carcinoma. *Lancet* 1993; **341**: 1039–43.

27 Peters MV. The effect of pregnancy in breast cancer. In: Forrest APM, Kunkler PB (eds) *Prognostic factors in breast cancer.* Baltimore, MD: Williams and Wilkins, 1968: 65–89.

28 Anderson BO, Petrek JA, Byrd DR, Senie RT, Borgen PI. Pregnancy influences breast cancer stage at diagnosis in women 30 years of age and younger. *Ann Surg Oncol* 1996; **3**: 204–11.

29 Guinee VF, Olsson H, Moller T *et al.* Effect of pregnancy on prognosis for young women with breast cancer. *Lancet* 1994; **343**: 1587–9.

30 Applewhite RR, Smith LR, DiVicenti F. Carcinoma of the breast with pregnancy and lactation. *Ann Surg* 1973; **39**: 101–4.

31 Byrd BF, Bayer DS, Robertson JC *et al.* Treatment of breast tumours associated with pregnancy and lactation. *Ann Surg* 1962; **155**: 940–7.

32 Samuels TH, Liu FF, Yaffe M, Haider M. Gestational breast cancer. *Can Assoc Radiol J* 1998; **49**: 172–80.

33 Montgomery TL. Detection and disposal of breast cancer in pregnancy. *Am J Obstet Gynecol* 1962; **85**: 312–19.

34 Max MH, Klamer TW. Breast cancer in 120 women under 35 years old. *Ann Surg* 1984; **50**: 23–5.

35 Finley JL, Silverman JF, Lannin DR. Fine-needle cytology of breast masses in pregnant and lactating women. *Diagn Cytopathol* 1989; **5**: 255–60.

36 Bottles K, Taylor RN. Diagnosis of breast masses in pregnant and lactating women by aspiration cytology. *Obstet Gynecol* 1985; **66**: 76–8.

37 Sainsbury JRC, Anderson TJ, Morgan DAL, Dixon JM. Breast cancer. *BMJ* 1994; **309**: 1150–3.

38 Theriault RL, Stallings CB, Buzdar AU. Pregnancy and breast cancer: clinical and legal issues. *Am J Clin Oncol* 1992; **15**: 535–9.

39 Kitchen PR, McLennan R. Breast cancer and pregnancy. *Med J Aust* 1987; **147**: 337–9.

40 Peterson H, Finster M. Anesthetic risk in the pregnant surgical patient. *Anesthesiology* 1979; **51**: 430–51.

41 Van der Vange N, Van Dongen JA. Breast cancer and pregnancy. *Eur J Surg Oncol* 1991; **17**: 1–8.

42 Stewart A, Kneale G. Radiation dose effects in relation to obstetric X-ray and childhood cancers. *Lancet* 1970; **1**: 1185.

43 Donegan WL. Mammary carcinoma and pregnancy. In: Donegan WL, Spratt JS (eds) *Cancer of the breast.* Philadelphia, PA: WB Saunders, 1985: 679–88.

44 Clark RM, Chua T. Breast cancer and pregnancy: the ultimate challenge. *Clin Oncol* 1989; **1**: 11–18.

45 Zemlickis D, Lishner M, Degendorfer P, Panzarella T, Sutcliffe SB, Koren G. Fetal outcome after *in utero* exposure to cancer chemotherapy. *Arch Intern Med* 1992; **152**: 573–6.

46 McKeen EA, Mulvihill JJ, Rosner F *et al.* Pregnancy outcome in Hodgkin's disease. *Lancet* 1979; **2**: 590.

47 Sutton R, Buzdar A, Fraschini G, Tashima C, Hortobagyi G. Pregnancy and offspring after adjuvant FAC chemotherapy in breast cancer patients. *Proc Annu Meet Am Cancer Res* 1988; **29**: A791.

48 Doll D, Ringenberg Q, Yarbro J. Management of cancer during pregnancy. *Arch Intern Med* 1988; **148**: 2058–64.

49 Berry DL, Theriault R, Holmes FA *et al.* Management of breast cancer during pregnancy using a standardized protocol. *J Clin Oncol* 1999; **17**: 855–61.

50 Williams PH, Van der Sijde R, Sleijfer DT. Combination chemotherapy and irradiation for stage IV breast cancer during pregnancy. *Gynecol Oncol* 1990; **36**: 281–4.

51 Denes A, Wallack M, Rigg L. *Adjuvant therapy of breast cancer during pregnancy.* In: Fourth International Conference on the Adjuvant Treatment of Breast Cancer.

52 Ebert U *et al.* Cytotoxic therapy and pregnancy. *Pharmacol Ther* 1997; **74**: 207–20.

53 Sweet DL, Kinzie J. Consequences of radiotherapy and antineoplastic therapy for the fetus. *J Reprod Med* 1976; **17**: 241–6.

54 Cullins SL, Pridjian G, Sutherland CM. Goldenhar's syndrome associated with tamoxifen given to the mother during gestation. *J Am Med Assoc* 1994; **271**: 1905–6.

55 Goodare H. Tamoxifen trial (letter). *Lancet* 1993; **342**: 444.

56 Jordan VC. The role of tamoxifen in the treatment and prevention of breast cancer. *Curr Probl Cancer* 1992; **16**: 129–76.

57 Collichio FA, Agnello R, Staltzer J. Pregnancy after breast cancer: from psychosocial issues through conception. *Oncology* 1998; **12**: 759–65, 769.

58 Siegal C. Pregnancy decision-making in breast cancer survivors. *J Psychol Oncol* 1997.

59 Richards MA, O'Reilly SM, Howell A *et al*. Adjuvant CMF in patients with axillary node-positive breast cancer. *J Clin Oncol* 1990; **8**: 2032–9.

60 Malamos NA, Stathopoulos GP, Keramopoulos A, Papadiamantis J, Vassilaros S. Pregnancy and offspring after the appearance of breast cancer. *Oncology* 1996; **53**: 471–5.

61 Saver MV, Paulson RJ, Lobo RA. Successful pre-embryo donation in ovarian failure after treatment for breast carcinoma. *Lancet* 1990; **335**: 723.

62 Arbour L, Narod S, Glendon G *et al*. *In-vitro* fertilisation and family history of breast cancer. *Lancet* 1994; **344**: 1235–6.

63 Ferrell BR, Hassey Dow K. Quality of life among long-term cancer survivors. *Oncology* 1997; **11**: 565–8.

64 Von Schoultz E, Johansson H, Wilking N, Rutqvist L-E. Influence of prior and subsequent pregnancy on breast cancer prognosis. *J Clin Oncol* 1995; **13**: 430–4.

65 Sankila R, Heinavaara S, Hakulinen T. Survival of breast cancer patients after subsequent term pregnancy: 'healthy mother effect'. *Am J Obstet Gynecol* 1994; **170**: 818–23.

66 Mignot L, Morran F, Sarrazin D, Varlaagne M, Gorins A, Morty M. Breast cancer and subsequent pregnancy. *Proc Annu Meet Am Soc Clin Oncol* 1986; **5**: 57.

67 Ariel IM, Kempner R. The prognosis of patients who become pregnant after mastectomy for breast cancer. *Int Surg* 1989; **74**: 185–7.

68 Kroman N, Jensen MB, Melbye M, Wohlfahrt J, Mouridsen HT. Should women be advised against pregnancy after breast cancer treatment? *Lancet* 1997; **350**: 319–22.

69 Velentgas P, Daling JR, Malone KE *et al*. Pregnancy after breast carcinoma: outcomes and influence on mortality. *Cancer* 1999; **85**: 2424–32.

70 Surbone A, Petrek JA. Childbearing issues in breast carcinoma survivors. *Cancer* 1997; **79**: 1271–8.

71 Varsos G, Yahalom J. Lactation following conservative surgery and radiotherapy for breast cancer. *J Surg Oncol* 1991; **46**: 141–4.

72 Higgins S, Haffty BG. Pregnancy and lactation after breast-conserving therapy for early-stage breast cancer. *Cancer* 1994; **73**: 2175–80.

73 Harrington SW. Carcinoma of the breast. *Ann Surg* 1937; **106**: 690–700.

74 Tretli S, Kvalheim G, Thoreson S *et al*. Survival of breast cancer patients diagnosed during pregnancy or lactation. *Br J Cancer* 1988; **58**: 382–4.

75 Greene FL, Leis HP. Management of breast cancer in pregnancy. *Proc Annu Meet Soc Clin Oncol* 1989; **8**: A94.

76 Ishida T, Yokoe T, Kasumi F *et al*. Clinicopathologic characteristics and prognosis of breast cancer patients associated with pregnancy and lactation: analysis of case–control study in Japan. *Jpn J Cancer Res* 1992; **83**: 1143–9.

29

An integrated policy for breast cancer management and research

I CRAIG HENDERSON

INTRODUCTION

To manage patients with breast cancer optimally, the health-care team must always utilize treatments that are known to prolong survival and/or palliate symptoms in a timely manner. The proper evaluation of a new treatment should be done at a time in the patient's course when the therapy is most likely to demonstrate a biological effect or, better yet, benefit the patient. These two imperatives must be coupled with other patient needs, most specifically the patient's need to know the truth and a need to be hopeful about her future – at least her immediate future. Not infrequently, these two needs of the patient conflict with one another and with the management and research imperatives. To serve their patients well and, at the same time, to contribute to better horizons for future breast cancer patients, the health-care team must clearly distinguish between the real benefits of established treatments and the patient's perceptions of these benefits. They must also know how to communicate this in a manner that allows the patient to participate in studies at appropriate times in her disease course, but does not compel her to enrol in a trial on the basis of false understanding of what benefits she might obtain.

BENEFITS FROM ESTABLISHED THERAPIES

None of the solid tumours are as treatable as breast cancer. There are not as many therapies either of proven

value or 'on the horizon' to treat lung, colon and ovarian cancers, and none of these other common tumour types benefit as much from the treatments that are available. None the less, the real benefits of treating breast cancer are still quite modest, and the public is demanding a sharp increase in the rate of progress towards preventing or improving the survival of patients with this disease. Only a small fraction of the findings that have appeared promising in laboratory experiments have eventually proved to be beneficial in the clinic. Clinical evaluation of new interventions is an obligate step. However, these evaluations must be performed without depriving the patient of the benefits of established treatments.

In 1997, the American Cancer Society estimated that approximately 180 200 patients with invasive and *in-situ* disease would be diagnosed with breast cancer and 43 900 patients would die. How many of the women diagnosed with breast cancer would die as a direct result of the disease if only symptomatic treatments were provided? What if no patients were treated with mastectomy, radiation therapy, endocrine therapy or chemotherapy? To my knowledge no one has attempted to estimate this number reliably in any formal fashion. In recent years, I have asked small groups of oncologists to provide 'guesstimates' based on their own understanding of and experience with the disease. The numbers have ranged from 51 000 to approximately 90 000 deaths. This implies that most cancer specialists believe that a substantial number of the women diagnosed with breast cancer each year have a benign disease (i.e. a disease incapable of causing the patient's death). For these patients, both conventional and experimental therapies are certain to do harm.

NATURE OF TREATMENT BENEFITS

Treatment may confer one of two benefits – an improvement in survival and/or palliation of symptoms. In most countries, medical societies appear to have accepted an ethical principle that no patient should unknowingly be deprived of treatment that will cure a disease such as breast cancer. In most cases, this principle is extended to state that no patient should be unknowingly deprived of a survival benefit. Controversy arises in the application of this principle when the evidence that the treatment prolongs survival is weak. Many therapies are employed because they *might* prolong survival, or because there is a public perception that the therapy will prolong survival.

It is equally difficult to determine the palliative value of a given treatment. By definition, palliation is subjective – only the patient can determine whether pain has been relieved. Double-blinded studies of placebo effect have demonstrated that the patient's perception of therapeutic value may be as important a component of palliation as the effect of the treatment on the disease. This creates two problems. First, the physician's recommendation to a patient regarding the potential palliative value of a treatment must be based on the subjective evaluation or perception of benefit by a different patient or group of patients. Because the placebo effect is as much a function of the patient as of the therapy, and because placebo effects vary enormously from one patient to another, it is uncertain how much the experience of previously treated patients applies to the patient at hand. Secondly, the placebo effect may be provided by an inactive therapy or an experimental therapy with uncertain benefit.

In general, therefore, an experimental intervention is unlikely to impart a survival benefit equal to or greater than that of an established treatment. This is because relatively few treatments impart a survival benefit. On the other hand, there are many clinical situations where a new and experimental treatment may provide palliation equal or even superior to conventional therapy if the patient perceives that this has an advantage.

SIZE OF TREATMENT BENEFITS

Formal studies of patient attitudes towards treatment have demonstrated that patients will tolerate considerable toxicity for very small gain. In one such study, cancer patients, physicians with varying levels of involvement in the treatment of cancer patients, nurses and the general public were asked to determine the minimum benefit they felt would be sufficient to make the toxicities of a treatment worthwhile.[1] A regimen was defined as 'intensive' if it caused severe nausea/vomiting, hair loss, tiredness or weakness, decreased sexual interest and required frequent injections and hospital admission for 3 or 4 days per month. A 'mild' regimen was defined as one that caused only slight nausea or vomiting, no alopecia, very little tiredness or weakness, and required only occasional injections and hospital admission for less than 1 day per month. Patients responded that they would consider a 1% chance of cure, a 12-month prolongation of life or a 10% chance that their symptoms would be relieved sufficient to justify the toxicities of intensive treatment (Table 29.1). A 1% chance of cure, a 3-month prolongation of life and only a 1% chance of symptom relief were considered sufficient to justify a mild treatment. In contrast, medical professionals and individuals without medical training and without a diagnosis of cancer all required much larger benefits to justify intensive treatment (Table 29.1). The patients in this study had a variety of different cancers, the most frequent being small-cell lung cancer.

A similar study was undertaken by Simes and his colleagues in Australia.[2] A total of 104 women who had completed adjuvant chemotherapy with cyclophosphamide, methotrexate and 5-fluorouracil (CMF) were asked if they considered the potential benefit sufficient to justify the toxicity. A prolongation of life by 1 year from 5 years without chemotherapy to 6 years with adjuvant CMF was sufficient for 77% of the patients (Table 29.2). However, a small percentage of the patients declared that their lives would have to be prolonged from 5 years to more than 20 years to justify the treatment![2] When the same patients were asked if an additional year of life from 15 years without treatment to 16 years with treatment justified the toxicities of adjuvant CMF, only 52%

Table 29.1 *Benefits sufficient to justify mild or severely toxic therapy in 100 UK patients with advanced breast cancer*

Respondent group	Minimum benefit sufficient to make toxicities of intensive treatment worthwhile		
	Chance of cure (%)	Prolongation of life (months)	Chance of relief (%)
Patients (n=100)	1	12	10
Controls (n=100)	50	24–60	75
Cancer doctors (n=148)	10	12	50
Cancer nurses (n=303)	50	24	50
General practitioners (n=790)	25	24	75

Source: Slevin *et al.*, 1990.[1] Reprinted with permission from the BMJ Publishing Group.

Table 29.2 *Benefits sufficient to justify the toxicities of chemotherapy in a group of 104 Australian women who had completed adjuvant CMF*

Hypothetical choice (without or with therapy) (survival period in years)	Percentage of patients opting for therapy
5 vs. 6	77
5 vs. 7	89
5 vs. 10	98
15 vs. 16	61
15 vs. 17	74
15 vs. 20	91
> 20	9

Source: Simes and Margrie, 1991.[2] Reproduced with permission from the NHMRC Clinical Trials Centre.

responded positively. This highlights the fact that when patients perceive their lower risk of dying of their disease, they may be less willing to accept the toxicity of treatment.

BASIC PRINCIPLES FOR INTEGRATING BREAST CANCER MANAGEMENT AND RESEARCH

There will be a limited number of times in each patient's course when the use of a new therapy is possible. To ensure that these opportunities are not missed, an innovative approach to treatment (or prevention) must be considered as one alternative at each and every decision point.

If, after considering all options, the physician concludes that:

- patient survival will not be compromised if a new treatment is employed; and
- the patient's symptoms may be palliated as well by a new treatment or a combination of conventional and innovative therapy

then a new treatment should be offered to the patient as one alternative.

This basic principle can only be employed if the clinician clearly understands which treatments prolong survival. In some cases the nature and magnitude of a survival benefit will also be important. For example, prolongation of life without a significant reduction in cause-specific mortality (i.e. without 'cure') will be insufficient to justify conventional therapies for some patients. In addition, it is often important to know whether a particular treatment will have the same impact when employed immediately or several months (or even years) later.

THERAPIES THAT AFFECT THE SURVIVAL OF BREAST CANCER PATIENTS

Prevention

No method of primary prevention has been reproducibly demonstrated to reduce the risk that a woman will develop breast cancer. The evidence that does exist is derived primarily from case–control and cohort studies. Possibly the most effective proactive measure to reduce breast cancer risk is regular exercise.[3] Oestrogen replacement therapy almost certainly decreases a woman's risk of dying of heart disease or osteoporosis, but may increase her risk of breast cancer.[4,5] Thus oestrogen use is certain to be a confounding factor in the evaluation of new approaches to primary prevention. There are at least two large randomized trials designed to determine whether the administration of tamoxifen will decrease a woman's chance of developing breast cancer. (However, neither of these trials is large enough to demonstrate reliably whether tamoxifen will decrease mortality from breast cancer.) In the American trial, women were precluded from using oestrogen while taking tamoxifen. In the European trial, women were allowed to take oestrogen, but this was used as a stratification category on enrolment. In the US Women's Health Initiative, the value of hormones, dietary fat, and nutritional supplements is being evaluated in a randomized trial. The effect of oestrogen use is a primary focus in this study. The varied approaches to the use of oestrogens in these studies highlight the uncertainty that exists about the effects of oestrogen on breast cancer incidence and mortality.

Note: To be credible, primary prevention studies must address the issue of oestrogen replacement, but there are insufficient data to permit conclusions that it should affect the design in any particular way.

Secondary prevention using mammography has been shown to reduce breast cancer mortality by approximately 30% in women aged 50 years or older. The benefits of screening mammography among younger women are smaller and less certain.[6] It is difficult to imagine a situation where the routine use of mammography at 1- to 3-year intervals in women aged 50 years or older would complicate the study of new methods of either prevention or treatment of breast cancer.

Note: It is clear that it would be unethical for any prevention or treatment study to proscribe mammography completely in this older age group.

Local treatment with surgery and/or radiotherapy for *in-situ* cancer

Retrospective studies in patients with ductal carcinoma *in situ* (DCIS) treated by biopsy only have observed long-term mortality rates in the range 0–23%.[7,8] These data were derived from studies performed before the widespread use of mammography, and they probably overestimate mortality from DCIS. Although it is widely perceived that DCIS is curable in 100% of patients treated by mastectomy, this is not necessarily true.[8] In historical series compiled by Haagensen, up to 4.5% of patients have been reported to die from breast cancer after an initial diagnosis of DCIS and treatment with mastectomy. At least 6 randomized trials comparing treatment with wide excision (lumpectomy, tylectomy) and the same surgery plus radiotherapy are currently in progress. The fact that no trial examines mastectomy in *in-situ* disease is evidence of a tacit agreement among breast cancer experts that the chances of a patient being 'cured' by mastectomy are probably no better than when breast-conserving therapy is used. A full report has been published for only one of the randomized trials comparing wide excision with the same surgery plus radiation therapy.[9] In this study, 818 women were randomized. There was a statistically significant reduction in the incidence of new cancers in the ipsilateral breast when radiotherapy was used, but after a mean follow-up of 43 months, only 3 patients had died, and all of them were in the lumpectomy plus radiotherapy arm. An update of these data was presented in March 1997 at a meeting of the Society of Surgical Oncology in Chicago; 35% of the patients had been followed for more than 8 years. Twelve deaths from metastatic breast cancer were observed, four among those randomized to lumpectomy alone and eight in the arm receiving lumpectomy plus radiotherapy.

On the basis of Haagensen's studies, lobular carcinoma *in situ* is increasingly being treated as a risk factor rather than as an obligate first step leading to invasive breast cancer.[9] There is no evidence that local treatment affects the survival of these patients.

Note: Treatment of lobular carcinoma *in situ* should not complicate the evaluation of new treatments for breast cancer. More extensive therapy will improve local control, but it has not been shown that more extensive therapy using radiation will reduce mortality from DCIS. Therefore, therapies other than full excision should neither complicate nor be a rationale for avoiding the evaluation of new treatments for ductal carcinoma *in situ*.

Local treatment of invasive cancer

Although the vast majority of medical professionals believe that a substantial percentage of breast cancer patients are cured by the use of surgery with or without radiotherapy, firm evidence to support this contention and to estimate the percentage of patients who might be cured is difficult to obtain. (For the purposes of this discussion, a cured patient is defined as one who would die of breast cancer without treatment but who, as a result of treatment, dies of some other cause after living out a normal lifespan.) The best evidence demonstrating that

the lives of some patients are prolonged as a result of local therapy comes from the randomized mammography trials. For example, mammography was relatively insensitive in the first of these trials conducted by the Health Insurance Plan (HIP) of New York in the early 1960s. As a result, the same number of cancers was diagnosed among the women randomized into the control group as in the mammography group – they were simply diagnosed later. None the less, a 25–30% reduction in mortality was observed.[10] Since no other therapies (e.g. adjuvant chemotherapy) were employed, this provides definitive evidence that survival is prolonged by the use of early compared to late mastectomy. The interval between screening examinations varied from 1 to 2.5 years in most of the randomized mammography trials. The optimal screening interval for any particular age group is not well defined.[11]

Shorter delays in the initiation of local therapy have recently been evaluated in several randomized trials. In each of these, patients were initially treated with either chemotherapy followed by surgery and radiation therapy, or with surgery followed by chemotherapy and radiation therapy. Several of the most important of these studies are described below. In one such study, radiotherapy was delayed for an average of 126 days after surgery, and there was a marginally significant increase in local failure rate[12] (see below).

Multiple randomized trials have compared more or less extensive surgery and surgery with or without radiotherapy. None of these trials have reproducibly shown that the extent of surgery, the type of surgery or the addition of radiation will affect survival. Possibly the most definitive trial among these is the National Surgical Adjuvant Breast and Bowel Project (NSABP)B-06, in which patients were randomized to receive either a lumpectomy alone, lumpectomy plus breast irradiation, or total mastectomy.[13]

Although patients treated with lumpectomy alone had a much higher frequency of ipsilateral breast recurrence, there was no significant difference in the incidence of distant recurrence or overall survival. The percentages remaining free of distant recurrence at 9 years were 59%, 60% and 63% for lumpectomy, lumpectomy plus radiation, and total mastectomy, respectively. In a randomized comparison of quadrantectomy and quadrantectomy plus radiotherapy, the rate of ipsilateral breast recurrence was only 3.8% at 3.5 years.[14] These authors concluded that quadrantectomy or very large excision involving approximately 25% of the breast may be sufficient to obtain optimal local control and survival for this older group of women.

Note: No experimental therapy should deprive a patient of all forms of local treatment; tumour excision is the minimum that should be given. A delay of several months might compromise the ability to control the disease locally, but the evidence from mammography trials indicates that delays of 6 months to 1 year (and possibly even longer) might not have a measurable effect on patient survival.

Adjuvant systemic therapy

Multiple trials have now demonstrated that the use of chemotherapy or hormone therapy soon after the diagnosis will prolong the survival of patients with operable breast cancer (stage I, II or IIIa, with or without lymphnode involvement).[15] However, it has not been shown that these adjuvant systemic therapies 'cure' early breast cancer. For many patients the prolongation of survival is plausibly measured in weeks or months.[16,17]

Although all patient *groups* appear to derive some benefit from adjuvant systemic therapy, the magnitude of the effect is proportional to the risk of developing recurrence. Patients at high risk of recurrence derive a greater benefit, but among low-risk patients the benefit may be very small indeed. It is almost certain that many patients, if not the majority of patients with early breast cancer, could not possibly benefit from adjuvant systemic therapy because micrometastases from the primary were not established prior to removal of the primary tumour or do not have the ability to grow at distant sites. For example, the latter might include tumours without the ability to secrete angiogenesis factors. However, these patients who would *not* benefit from adjuvant therapy cannot yet be reliably identified.

It is not clear whether the initiation of adjuvant therapy can be safely delayed for some time after the original diagnosis. Three recently completed randomized trials provide some insight into this question. In the oldest of these studies, one-third of 1229 patients were treated with peri-operative chemotherapy, another third with peri-operative chemotherapy followed by a 6-month course, and one-third treated with a 6-month course after an initial delay of 1 month.[18] The 1-month delay did not appear to compromise disease-free or overall survival of these patients. In a second study, 242 patients were treated with lumpectomy alone and then randomized to receive either chemotherapy followed by radiation therapy, or radiation therapy followed by chemotherapy.[12] In this study, chemotherapy was delayed by an average of 119 days if radiotherapy was given first, and radiotherapy was delayed by an average of 126 days if chemotherapy was given first. No overall survival differences were observed among these two groups of patients. However, there was a significant (P=0.05) difference in distant failure, with 24% of the patients treated with chemotherapy first experiencing a distant recurrence while, during this same time, 36% of those patients who were given radiation therapy first had a distant failure. Patients who had received chemotherapy first were more likely to have a local recurrence than patients who were initially treated with radiation therapy (14% vs. 5%, respectively; P=0.07). In the most recently reported of these trials, 1523 patients were randomized immediately after a fine-needle aspiration biopsy to receive either four cycles of adjuvant cyclophosphamide plus doxorubicin (CA) before surgery (often referred to as 'neoadjuvant therapy') followed by definitive surgery and radiotherapy, or to receive definitive surgery followed by adjuvant CA and radiotherapy.[19] Although it was thought that more patients were able to be safely treated with a breast-conserving treatment if neoadjuvant CA was given first, no difference in survival was observed between these two groups.

Note: It would be inappropriate to omit adjuvant systemic therapy for patients at some risk of breast cancer recurrence. However, each patient and physician must determine the level of risk below which they feel that the toxicities of therapy outweigh the benefit. The data shown in Table 29.2 suggest that *when* a woman is likely to die is a more important determinant in her decision to have adjuvant therapy than *whether* she is likely to die, or how great the benefit is likely to be. A delay of 1 or even several months is not likely to result in a measurable decrease in survival benefit from adjuvant therapy, but a delay much beyond that appears to compromise distant disease control, and will almost certainly eventually be shown to compromise survival as well.

Metastatic breast cancer

Most breast cancer experts assert that the primary goal of treatment for metastatic breast cancer is palliation rather than survival. However, A'Hern and his colleagues have provided elegant evidence that the treatment of metastases may prolong survival.[20] They correlated response rates and median survival in 50 randomized clinical trials in which the response to chemotherapy was significantly higher in one arm than in the other. They found that patients randomized to a regimen that produced a substantially higher response rate (e.g. 70%) might have a median survival nearly 6 months longer than that of a group of patients randomized to a regimen that induced only a 20% response rate (Table 29.3). In a subsequent analysis of a similar nature, A'Hern *et al.* demonstrated that the use of doxorubicin in combination with

Table 29.3 *Response rate and estimated median survival based on overview analysis of adjuvant chemotherapy trials*

Response rate in arm with higher response rate (%)		Estimated median survival (months)
Baseline	20	18.0
	30	21.4
	40	23.4
	50	24.4
	60	24.5
	70	23.6

Source: A'Hern *et al.*, 1988.[20] Reprinted with permission from Churchill Livingstone.

cyclophosphamide and 5-fluorouracil (CAF) significantly increased the odds of response by 44%, reduced the risk of treatment failure by 31%, and reduced the risk of dying by 22%.[21] These benefits are sufficient to justify the use of a 'mild' regimen for the patients in Slevin's study (see above). They may fall short of justifying an 'intensive regimen' (Table 29.3), but the patient should understand that a 6-month improvement in the median survival for all treated patients very probably reflects an increase in survival of 12 months or longer for some of the treated patients.

A second and equally important question is whether the timing of administration of effective systemic therapy is critical. Many patients are now diagnosed with metastases by routine physical examination, blood marker studies, serial bone scans or CT scans of various organs. No one has demonstrated that treating these asymptomatic patients will lead to a better overall survival than waiting until the first symptoms appear, nor has it been systematically evaluated whether there is any value in introducing endocrine treatments 'early or late' after recurrence. Multiple trials have demonstrated no difference in survival if patients are given chemotherapy immediately following the diagnosis of metastasis or only after a trial of endocrine treatment.[22]

Possibly the most relevant data on the introduction of new treatments for metastatic disease, as well as on the effect of delaying chemotherapy regimens that are known to be effective, have recently been reported by the Cancer and Leukemia Group B. A total of 342 patients were randomized to receive either CAF chemotherapy immediately after diagnosis of metastasis or 2–4 cycles of a phase II agent followed by CAF.[23,24] The phase II drugs that were evaluated in this trial included trimetrexate, intravenous melphalan, amonafide and carboplatin. When patients were randomized to a phase II agent first, they were evaluated for response after every two cycles. If there was evidence of progressive disease after the first two courses, the patient was crossed over to CAF therapy. If the patient's disease was stable or responding to the phase II agent, an additional two cycles were given before cross-over to CAF. The initial response rate to CAF was significantly higher than that to the phase II agents (Table 29.4). However, the cumulative response rate, the median duration of response and the median survival of patients treated initially with phase II agents were not significantly worse.

Note: Patients with metastatic breast cancer should not be deprived of treatment with an effective combination chemotherapy regimen at some point in their course. (Patients with receptor-positive disease or tumours characteristic of those that often respond to endocrine treatment should probably receive a course of endocrine therapy, too, despite the lack of definitive trials.) However, the precise time when a new therapy is introduced is probably not an important factor in determining outcome, and a delay of 3 to 4 months is not likely to affect survival.

THERAPIES KNOWN TO PALLIATE THE SYMPTOMS OF BREAST CANCER

By definition, palliation is subjective, and so, too, is the decision to employ a treatment which is predominantly or exclusively palliative.

There are a number of situations in which it is unlikely or quite certain that treatment will not improve the survival of patients with breast cancer. All of these might be subsumed under the heading 'Palliation.' They include the following.

More extensive surgery or radiotherapy to improve local control

Many patients find a local recurrence of their disease emotionally devastating. This argument may be the basis for more treatment decisions than any other in the overall management of breast cancer. In addition, it is often argued that many local recurrences that are unmanageable could have been prevented with more extensive primary treatment. This hypothesis has been tested in only one randomized trial.[25] This was the first randomized trial designed to evaluate any form of breast cancer treatment. Patients at the Christie Hospital in Manchester in the UK were treated with either a standard radical mastectomy of the Halsted type or the same surgery followed by orthovoltage radiotherapy to the chest

Table 29.4 *Response rate and survival of patients randomized in a Cancer and Leukemia Group B (CALGB) trial to either standard combination chemotherapy (cyclophosphamide, doxorubicin and 5-fluorouracil – CAF) or an initial trial of a new phase II agent for 2 to 4 courses followed by standard combination chemotherapy*

	Number of patients	Initial response (%)	Cumulative response (%)	Median duration (months)	Median survival (months)
CAF	164	55	55	9.6	18.1
Phase II → CAF	178	19	47	8.3	16.1
		$P \leqslant 0.05$	NS	NS	NS

Source: Costanza *et al.*, 1995.[24] Reproduced with permission from the American Society of Clinical Oncology.
NS, non-significant.

wall. Local recurrences among the patients randomized to surgery only were treated with radiotherapy at the time of recurrence. The local recurrence rate during the first 10 years of follow-up was 32% for patients treated with surgery only, and 19% for patients who received surgery and radiotherapy. However, the percentage of patients who had persistent local recurrence at the time of death was 16% for those randomized to surgery alone and 14% for those randomized to surgery and radiotherapy. This difference was not statistically significant. Although these data utilized treatment modalities that are not outmoded, the experiment has never been repeated using modern techniques.

Adjuvant systemic therapy to improve disease-free survival

A therapy that does not improve overall survival may increase the interval from diagnosis to first recurrence, while shortening the interval from first recurrence to death. This has been extensively studied by investigators in the International Breast Cancer Study Group (IBCSG),[26] who have defined a new endpoint – TWiST. This refers to time without symptoms (from the disease) or toxicity (from the therapy). TWiST is determined by summing all of the time during which the patient has no symptoms or toxicities, and subtracting from this the time during which the patient experiences any toxicity from adjuvant systemic therapy or therapy from metastatic disease. In general, the IBCSG has found a significant improvement in TWiST even for therapies that have no or only marginal survival benefits, such as adjuvant chemotherapy for post-menopausal women.

The same principle has recently been applied without formal calculation of TWiST by doctors at Duke University. They performed a randomized trial in which patients with metastatic breast cancer were first treated with conventional-dose chemotherapy.[27] Patients who went into complete clinical remission were randomized to receive high-dose chemotherapy and bone-marrow transplant immediately or after a second recurrence. A demonstration that early rather than delayed transplant would improve overall survival might have been taken as proof of principle and as justification for more routine use of high-dose chemotherapy and bone-marrow transplant for treatment of patients with metastatic breast cancer. However, the results of this trial demonstrated a statistically significant improvement in disease-free survival for the patients who received an early transplant, and a statistically significant improvement in overall survival for those who had a late transplant. The researchers at Duke University concluded that most patients would choose this improvement in disease-free survival in preference to an overall survival benefit. Neither the IBCSG nor practitioners at Duke University have formally surveyed patients regarding their opinions and the value of these benefits.

Treatment of asymptomatic disease

This patient group is steadily increasing in size, especially in the USA, because of the intensity with which breast cancer patients are followed up after completion of therapy. Frequently, patients know that they have had a recurrence of the disease but do not experience either pain or disability from this recurrence. This results from abnormalities in marker studies, such as CEA or CA-125, routine X-rays or scans. This cancer is often a relatively indolent disease, and patients may live for years with nodules in the lung, or even in the liver, without symptoms. Even the local recurrences, which frequently appear as painless nodules or thickening over the chest wall, may cause almost no symptoms other than patient anxiety. There are no randomized trials demonstrating that progressive and immediate treatment of these patients in the asymptomatic state will improve their survival. It is plausible that aggressive treatment in this setting will delay the onset of symptomatic metastases, and it has recently been shown in several randomized trials that the use of bisphosphonates may delay the onset of bone metastases. At the University Hospital in Heidelberg, 142 women with breast cancer and bone metastases were randomized to receive either bisphosphonate clodronate over 2 years or no treatment.[28] At a median follow-up of 3 years, significantly fewer women in the bisphosphonate group had developed distant metastases to either bone or other sites. However, no increased survival was evident in the treatment arm at that duration of follow-up.

Treatment of symptoms

This is the only category that represents true palliation. Radiation, endocrine and chemotherapies can all dramatically relieve pain, especially bone pain. Radiation therapy can reverse neurological symptoms and vomiting related to central nervous system metastases. A combination of surgery and radiation will usually control ulcerating, malodorous external lesions. There are no randomized trials comparing anti-cancer therapy with supportive treatments such as analgesics and tranquilizers. This has been done with other tumours where the effects of anti-cancer therapy are more marginal, and in those settings anti-cancer treatment has frequently been shown to be more effective (and even less costly) than supportive treatment. Randomized clinical trials include a quality-of-life component which has generally demonstrated that the more effective of two regimens will be associated with the best quality of life even when the more effective regimen is more toxic.[29–31] In one of these trials, patients were randomized to receive either 3 months of chemotherapy or continuous chemotherapy until progression of disease.[31] Continuous chemotherapy was associated with significantly more toxicity, but it also resulted in a higher response rate. Most quality-of-life measures were also significantly improved by the use of continuous chemotherapy. In this trial, there was a marginal survival advantage for the patients who were given continuous therapy as well. However, most randomized trials that have evaluated different durations of chemotherapy for the treatment of metastatic disease have failed to show a survival advantage for treatment durations longer than 6 months.[31–39]

The first three of the above palliation categories might be described as 'preventive palliation', since treatment is used in anticipation of symptoms that might never occur. Each of these represents situations in which a patient reasonably chooses an innovative therapy in preference or in addition to conventional therapy. As her survival would be unaffected, and true palliation can be provided when and if symptoms occur, she has very little to lose by choosing a new treatment at these decision points.

ALGORITHMS FOR INTRODUCING NEW TREATMENTS

Innovative therapies might be lumped into two broad classifications as follows. Category A includes treatments with uncertain and/or unknown benefit. Under conventional classifications, these would be phase I or II therapies. Category B includes effective therapies for which the benefit relative to more established treatments is still unknown. This could include some phase II and all phase III treatments.

As a fundamental principle, treatments in category A should be considered whenever a patient is at a decision point, or if there is no therapy that is known to prolong survival or palliate symptoms, or if the patient has no symptoms and there is no therapy known to prolong survival. Treatments in category B should be considered whenever the available therapies are known to have very

limited benefits in either improving survival or palliating symptoms. An innovative therapy in one of these two categories is appropriate at most clinical decision points.

An outline of key decision points in the course of the natural history of breast cancer is shown in Figure 29.1. The letter beside each of these decision points indicates which category of experimental treatment might be most appropriate.

Decision point 1

The number of women *who are aware* that they are at high risk of developing breast cancer is increasing. This has been exacerbated by the discovery of BRCA1 and BRCA2. These women are understandably anxious and desirous of some means of preventing breast cancer. No methods have been established, and all treatments therefore by definition belong to category A.

Decision point 2

Patients who present with locally advanced breast cancer, defined in this exercise as 'inoperable', include those with slowly growing disease that has spread to the skin or to deep structures. There is no evidence that treatment substantially prolongs the lives of these patients, or that there is an urgency to initiate therapy. These patients have often lived with their disease for many years. The use of a very innovative treatment in category A might be appropriate for many of these patients. This category also subsumes patients with inflammatory breast cancer. Although there are no randomized trials demonstrating an improvement in overall survival, the median duration of survival for patients diagnosed with this condition today is 3–4 years longer than it was a generation ago. Presumably this is due to the use of systemic therapy. Therefore a treatment in category B would be more appropriate.

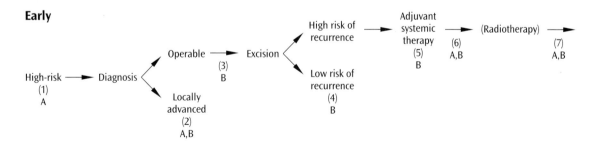

Figure 29.1 *An algorithm for deciding appropriate times for the introduction of innovative therapies.*

Decision point 3

Although patients with operable breast cancer should all undergo full excision of their tumour, there appears to be no harm in introducing treatments between the time of an incisional or fine-needle aspiration biopsy and definitive excision. As in the NSABP trial described above, new treatments, especially those in category B, might be introduced before complete excision.

Decision point 4

The benefits of adjuvant systemic therapy are questionable in many patients at low risk of recurrence. The introduction of any treatment, including innovative treatments, has at least as much potential for harming the patient as for benefiting them. Therefore it seems unwise to utilize treatments with no known anti-cancer potential in this group of patients, but trials comparing relatively non-toxic treatments with no therapy at all would still be appropriate.

Decision point 5

Patients at high risk of recurrence should receive systemic therapy, since it is known that this will prolong survival. However, the reduction in the annual odds of death and the absolute survival benefits are modest at best. For example, the difference in survival of treated compared to untreated patients will be in the range 5–10% in this population of patients. Therefore the introduction of therapies with a greater potential for prolonging survival is very appropriate.

Decision point 6

Maximum benefits from adjuvant systemic therapy can be obtained after a period of approximately 4 months. Patients at very high risk of recurrence are often very anxious because they recognize the limitations of conventional treatment. Many of these patients would be willing to participate in trials evaluating therapies that have not been demonstrated to be valuable in any setting. It is reasonable to speculate that some therapies might only be effective in the face of minimal tumour burden. This is the time when such treatments could be evaluated in randomized trials.

Decision point 7

Patients with operable breast cancer who undergo excision only (i.e. lumpectomy) will generally receive radiotherapy to improve local control. Long delays in the initiation of radiotherapy will compromise this outcome.

Innovative therapies, such as those described at decision point 6, should probably be administered after radiotherapy in this group of patients. This might apply equally well to patients who elect for adjuvant radiotherapy after mastectomy because of a high probability of recurrence, but timing in this setting has not been studied as carefully, and may not be as critical.[40]

Decision point 8

Patients with asymptomatic recurrences may be the ideal group in which to study new therapies with unproven efficacies. The presence of measurable or evaluable disease allows a quick assessment of the biological effects of treatment. Since these patients do not require palliation, and there is no evidence that survival is prolonged at this point in time, the use of an innovative therapy may be more than sufficient to palliate the patient's anxiety, which will be her major symptom at this time.

Decision point 9

Even after a symptomatic recurrence, a short course of treatment with a phase II therapy may be reasonable. Many of these patients are minimally symptomatic but recognize the limitations of conventional therapy. In the Cancer and Leukemia Group B trial described above, the use of an innovative therapy (with adequate monitoring of its ability to induce a response in sites of measurable disease) before the introduction of an established treatment that is more certain to palliate symptoms is unlikely to compromise the patient's survival. Many patients will feel that the additional hope engendered by the possibility that they are receiving something better will counterbalance the delay in the palliation of minimal symptoms and the inconvenience of a trial. In patients with symptomatic recurrences, the introduction of potentially more effective therapy is always justified. Conventional treatments that are currently available, especially the non-hormonal treatments, are limited in both their palliative potential and their impact on survival.

Decision point 10

The small survival benefits from the treatment of metastatic disease will most probably have been realized after the completion of 6–12 months of therapy. The patient and her physician should also be able to determine when maximum palliation has been achieved. Many physicians will discontinue treatment at this time. The introduction of an innovative therapy in either category A or B is appropriate for patients who are anxious to continue on some form of treatment at this point.

Decision point 11

This is the point at which new therapies have been conventionally introduced. Response rates are invariably low, as these patients have developed resistance to treatment over the months and years during which the disease has been slowly evolving. In many cases, prior treatment has induced resistance. These patients are often in greatest need of palliation. Thus in many ways this is the least desirable time to introduce new therapies. Almost no randomized trials have ever been conducted in this setting. However, one trial compared vinorelbine with intravenous alkeran.[41] Most of the patients in this trial had a life expectancy of less than 6 months, and all of them were considered resistant to doxorubicin. None the less, there was a statistically significant difference in median survival of approximately 1 month.

NEW TREATMENTS AS A SOURCE OF HOPE

In my experience, relatively few patients become resigned to death and continue to live without hope that some miracle will dramatically prolong their lives. When acceptance of death comes, it is usually quite late in the disease course.

The acceptance of the idea that all patients have a right to know the full truth about their disease and the limitations of any therapies that are available to treat it, the introduction of the randomized clinical trial which has demonstrated that most treatments once thought to have a great benefit have little or no value to the patient, and the increasingly widespread practice of evidence-based medicine by recently trained physicians make it very difficult for the medical care team to offer the cancer patient much hope. When physicians cannot or do not offer hope, patients tend to seek it elsewhere. This is reflected in the growing popularity of so-called 'alternative' medicine.

Experimental therapies can also offer the patient hope. However, this is a double-edged sword. On the one hand, if the physician or nurse offering the new treatment emphasizes the limitations of current knowledge about the treatment, and the fact that most new treatments do not ultimately prove to be beneficial, the medical team will not be able to compete successfully with the alternative medicine practitioner, who almost invariably believes passionately in his or her therapy and offers it without reservation. On the other hand, if the patient is allowed to believe that an experimental therapy has imparted benefits that it has not in fact done, it becomes increasingly difficult to evaluate the new treatment objectively in a properly controlled trial, especially a randomized trial. The experimental therapy may become an 'alternative medicine' of unproven value. High-dose chemotherapy and bone-marrow transplant for breast cancer are recent examples.

I believe this dilemma cannot be resolved entirely. The medical professional may allow the individual patient to feel that an experimental treatment in category A has been helpful, but he or she must never specifically confirm this or publicly state it until the phase III evaluation phase is complete. To do so would be inconsistent with the physician's commitment always to tell the patient the truth, and it would make it very difficult eventually to find the truth (i.e. to complete the phase III study).

A physician can ethically enrol a patient in a phase III trial only if he or she feels that the patient may be equally well served by any of the alternative treatments – in other words, when he or she is uncertain. I suspect that one reason why such a small percentage (3–6%) of all cancer patients enrol in phase III studies is because neither physician nor patient are comfortable with this state of 'uncertainty.' Often it is easier for patients to accept that they have a limited life expectancy than that they may live for many years anticipating a recurrence (i.e. 'waiting for the other shoe to drop'). I personally resolve this issue by dealing with the patient's need for hope in a variety of ways, including offering access to alternative approaches such as support groups, exercise programmes, etc., before discussing possible participation in a phase III study.

Thus treatments in category A (Figure 29.1) frequently offer patients hope. However, treatments in category B, especially those that are under evaluation in randomized clinical trials, rarely do so.

REFERENCES

1 Slevin ML, Stubbs L, Plant HJ *et al.* Attitudes to chemotherapy: comparing views of patients with cancer with those of doctors, nurses and general public. *BMJ* 1990; **300**: 1458–60.

2 Simes RJ, Margrie SJ. *Patient preferences for adjuvant chemotherapy in breast cancer.* NHMRC Clinical Trials Centre, 1991.

3 Bernstein L, Henderson BE, Hanisch R, Sullivan-Halley J, Ross RK. Physical exercise and reduced risk of breast cancer in young women. *J Natl Cancer Inst* 1994; **86**: 1371–2.

4 Dupont WD, Page DL. Menopausal estrogen replacement therapy and breast cancer. *Arch Intern Med* 1991; **151**: 67–72.

5 Steinberg KK, Thacker SB, Smith SJ *et al.* A meta-analysis of the effect of estrogen replacement therapy on the risk of breast cancer. *J Am Med Assoc* 1991; **265**: 1985–90.

6 Kerlikowske K, Grady D, Rubin SM, Sandrock C, Ernster V. Efficacy of screening mammography: a meta-analysis. *J Am Med Assoc* 1995; **273**: 149–54.

7 Haagensen C, Lane N, Lattes R, Bodian C. Lobular neoplasia (so-called lobular carcinoma *in situ*) of the breast. *Cancer* 1978; **42**: 737–69.

8 Henderson IC. What can a woman do about her risk of dying of breast cancer? *Curr Prob Cancer* 1990; **14**: 165–230.

9 Fisher B, Costantino J. Redmond C *et al.* Lumpectomy compared with lumpectomy and radiation therapy for the treatment of intraductal breast cancer. *N Engl J Med* 1993; **328**: 1581–6.

10 Shapiro S. Determining the efficacy of breast cancer screening. *Cancer* 1989; **63**: 1873–80.

11 Tabar L, Faberberg G, Day NE, Holmberg L. What is the optimum interval between mammographic screening examinations? An analysis based on the latest results of the Swedish Two-County Breast Cancer Screening Trial. *Br J Cancer* 1987; **55**: 547–51.

12 Recht A, Come S, Henderson I *et al.* Five-year results of a randomized trial testing the sequencing of chemotherapy and radiotherapy following conservative surgery for patients with early-stage breast cancer. *N Engl J Med* 1996.

13 Fisher B, Anderson S, Fisher ER *et al.* Significance of ipsilateral breast tumour recurrence after lumpectomy. *Lancet* 1991; **338**: 327–31.

14 Veronesi U, Luini A, Del Vecchio M *et al.* Radiotherapy after breast-preserving surgery in women with localized cancer of the breast. *N Engl J Med* 1993; **328**: 1587–91.

15 Early Breast Cancer Trialists' Collaborative Group. Systemic treatment of early breast cancer by hormonal, cytotoxic or immune therapy: 133 randomised trials involving 31 000 recurrences and 24 000 deaths among 75 000 women. *Lancet* 1992; **339**: 1–15, 71–85.

16 Henderson IC. Paradigmatic shifts in the management of breast cancer. *N Engl J Med* 1995; **332**: 951–3.

17 Henderson I. Adjuvant systemic therapy for early breast cancer. *Cancer* 1994; **74**: 401–9.

18 Goldhirsch A, Gelber RD. Randomized perioperative therapy in operable breast cancer: the Ludwig Trial V. In: Senn H-J, Goldhirsch A, Gelber RD, Osterwalder B (eds) *Recent results in cancer research – adjuvant therapy of primary breast cancer*. Berlin: Springer-Verlag, 1989: 43–53.

19 Fisher B. Effective therapy for primary breast cancer. *Proc Am Soc Clin Oncol* 1997; **16**: 127a.

20 A'Hern RP, Ebbs SR, Baum M. Does chemotherapy improve survival in advanced breast cancer? A statistical overview. *Br J Cancer* 1988; **57**: 615–18.

21 A'Hern RP, Smith IE, Ebbs SR. Chemotherapy and survival in advanced breast cancer: the inclusion of doxorubicin in Cooper type regimens. *Br J Cancer* 1993; **67**: 801–5.

22 Henderson IC. Endocrine therapy of metastatic breast cancer. In: Harris JR, Hellman S, Henderson IC, Kinne DW (eds) *Breast diseases*, 2nd edn. Philadelphia, PA: Lippincott Co., 1991: 559–603.

23 Costanza ME, Korzun AH, Henderson IC, Rice MA, Wood WC, Norton L. Amonafide: an active agent in metastatic breast cancer (CALGB 8642). *Proc Am Soc Clin Oncol* 1990; **9**: 31.

24 Costanza ME, Henderson IC, Berry D *et al.* A randomized comparison of single-agent induction chemotherapy vs. standard chemotherapy for stage IV breast cancer. *Proc Am Soc Clin Oncol* 1995; **14**: 116.

25 Easson EC. Post-operative radiotherapy in breast cancer. In: Forrest APM, Kunkler PB (eds) *Prognostic factors in breast cancer*. Edinburgh: E & S Livingstone Ltd, 1968: 119–27.

26 Gelber RD, Goldhirsch A, Cavalli F. Quality-of-life-adjusted evaluation of adjuvant therapies for operable breast cancer. *Ann Intern Med* 1991; **114**: 621–8.

27 Peters WP, Jones RB, Vredenburgh J *et al.* A large, prospective randomized trial of high-dose combination alkylating agents (CPB) with autologous cellular support (ABMS) as consolidation for patients with metastatic breast cancer achieving complete remission after intensive doxorubicin-based induction therapy (AFM). *Proc Am Soc Clin Oncol* 1996; **15**: 121.

28 Diel I, Solomayer EF, Goerner R, Gollan C, Wallwiener D, Bastea G. Adjuvant treatment of breast cancer patients with bisphosphonate clodronate reduces incidence and number of bone and non-bone metastases. *Proc Am Soc Clin Oncol* 1997; **16**: 130a.

29 Priestman TJ, Baum M. Evaluation of quality of life in patients receiving treatment for advanced breast cancer. *Lancet* 1976; **1**: 899–901.

30 Tannock IF, Boyd NF, DeBoer G *et al.* A randomized trial of two dose levels of cyclophosphamide, methotrexate and fluorouracil chemotherapy for patients with metastatic breast cancer. *J Clin Oncol* 1988; **6**: 1377–87.

31 Coates A, Gebski V, Bishop JF *et al.* Improving the quality of life during chemotherapy for advanced breast cancer. *N Engl J Med* 1987; **317**: 1490–5.

32 Smalley RV, Murphy S, Huguley CM, Bartolucci AA. Combination versus sequential five-drug chemotherapy in metastatic carcinoma of the breast. *Cancer Res* 1976; **36**: 3911–16.

33 Muss HB, Case LD, Richards III F *et al.* Interrupted versus continuous chemotherapy in patients with metastatic breast cancer. *N Engl J Med* 1991; **325**: 1342–8.

34 Harris AL, Cantwell BMJ, Carmichael J *et al.* Comparison of short-term and continuous chemotherapy (mitoxantrone) for advanced breast cancer. *Lancet* 1990; **335**: 186–90.

35 De Lena M, Zucali R, Viganotti G, Valagussa P, Bonadonna G. Combined chemotherapy–radiotherapy approach in locally advanced (T3b-T4) breast cancer. *Cancer Chemother Pharmacol* 1978; **1**: 53–9.

36 Ejlertsen B, Pfeiffer P, Pedersen D *et al.* Decreased efficacy of cyclophosphamide, epirubicin and 5-fluorouracil in metastatic breast cancer when reducing treatment duration from 18 to 6 months. *Eur J Cancer* 1993; **29A**: 527–31.

37 Cocconi G, Bisagni G, Bacchi M *et al.* A comparison of continuation versus late intensification followed by discontinuation of chemotherapy in advanced breast cancer. A prospective randomized trial of the Italian Oncology Group for Clinical Research (GOIRC). *Ann Oncol* 1990; **1**: 36–44.

38 Cocconi G, Bisagni G, Bacchi M *et al.* Prospective discontinuation of chemotherapy in advanced breast

carcinoma. Mature results of a randomized clinical trial. *Proc Am Soc Clin Oncol* 1989; **8**: 52.

39 Calabresi F, Di Lauro L, Marolla P *et al*. FAC +/– lonidamine (LND) in advanced breast cancer: results of a multicentric randomized clinical trial. *Proc Am Soc Clin Oncol* 1990; **9**: 20.

40 Griem KL, Henderson IC, Gelman R *et al*. The 5-year results of a randomized trial of adjuvant radiation therapy after chemotherapy in breast cancer treated with mastectomy. *J Clin Oncol* 1987; **5**: 1546–55.

41 Jones S, Winer E, Vogel C *et al*. Randomized comparison of vinorelbine and melphalan in anthracycline-refractory advanced breast cancer. *J Clin Oncol* 1995; **13**: 2567–74.

Index

Note: *Italicised page references* refer to figures. **Bold page references** refer to tables.